Cancer Immunotherapy: Research and Practice

Cancer Immunotherapy: Research and Practice

Edited by Molly Finch

hayle
medical

New York

Hayle Medical,
750 Third Avenue, 9th Floor,
New York, NY 10017, USA

Visit us on the World Wide Web at:
www.haylemedical.com

ISBN: 978-1-63241-840-1

Cataloging-in-Publication Data

Cancer immunotherapy : research and practice / edited by Molly Finch.
p. cm.
Includes bibliographical references and index.
ISBN 978-1-63241-840-1
1. Cancer--Immunotherapy. 2. Cancer--Immunotherapy--Research. 3. Cancer--Immunological aspects.
4. Cancer--Treatment. I. Finch, Molly.
RC271.I45 C36 2020
616.994 061--dc23

Table of Contents

Permissions

List of Contributors

Index

Preface

The main aim of this book is to educate learners and enhance their research focus by presenting diverse topics covering this vast field. This is an advanced book which compiles significant studies by distinguished experts in the area of analysis. This book addresses successive solutions to the challenges arising in the area of application, along with it; the book provides scope for future developments.

Cancer immunotherapy is a growing field of oncology that is concerned with the artificial stimulation of the immune system for the treatment of cancer. This is achieved by enhancing the body's natural ability to fight cancer. In cancer immunotherapy, antibody proteins of the immune system detect cancer cells by binding to them. The chief difference between normal and modified immunotherapy antibodies lies in the fact that while the former binds to external pathogens, the latter binds to tumor antigens thereby identifying and marking the cancer cells for the immune system to kill or inhibit their growth. Cancer immunotherapy can be passive, hybrid or active. Hybrid therapy is a combination of active and passive therapies. In active immunotherapy, the immune system is directed to attack tumor cells by targeting tumor antigens. Passive immunotherapies improve existing anti-tumor responses by using lymphocytes, cytokines and monoclonal antibodies. Some of the approved immunotherapy antibodies are nivolumab, alemtuzumab, ofatumumab, ipilimumab and rituximab. This book elucidates new techniques and applications of cancer immunotherapy in a multidisciplinary manner. It explores all the important aspects of cancer immunotherapy research and practice in the present day scenario. It will prove to be immensely beneficial to students and researchers in this field.

It was a great honour to edit this book, though there were challenges, as it involved a lot of communication and networking between me and the editorial team. However, the end result was this all-inclusive book covering diverse themes in the field.

Finally, it is important to acknowledge the efforts of the contributors for their excellent chapters, through which a wide variety of issues have been addressed. I would also like to thank my colleagues for their valuable feedback during the making of this book.

Editor

Tumor Mouse Model Confirms MAGE-A3 Cancer Immunotherapeutic as an Efficient Inducer of Long-Lasting Anti-Tumoral Responses

Catherine Gérard*, Nathalie Baudson, Thierry Ory, Jamila Louahed

GlaxoSmithKline Vaccines, Rixensart, Belgium

Abstract

Purpose: MAGE-A3 is a potential target for immunotherapy due to its tumor-specific nature and expression in several tumor types. Clinical data on MAGE-A3 immunotherapy have raised many questions that can only be addressed by using animal models. In the present study, different aspects of the murine anti-tumor immune responses induced by a recombinant MAGE-A3 protein (recMAGE-A3) in combination with different immunostimulants (AS01, AS02, CpG7909 or AS15) were investigated.

Experimental Design and Results: Based on cytokine profile analyses and protection against challenge with MAGE-A3-expressing tumor, the combination recMAGE-A3+AS15 was selected for further experimental work, in particular to study the mechanisms of anti-tumor responses. By using MHC class I-, MHC class II-, perforin-, B-cell- and IFN-γ- knock-out mice and CD4+ T cell-, CD8+ T cell- and NK cell- depleted mice, we demonstrated that CD4+ T cells and NK cells are the main anti-tumor effectors, and that IFN-γ is a major effector molecule. This mouse tumor model also established the need to repeat recMAGE-A3+AS15 injections to sustain efficient anti-tumor responses. Furthermore, our results indicated that the efficacy of tumor rejection by the elicited anti-MAGE-A3 responses depends on the proportion of tumor cells expressing MAGE-A3.

Conclusions: The recMAGE-A3+AS15 cancer immunotherapy efficiently induced an antigen-specific, functional and long-lasting immune response able to recognize and eliminate MAGE-A3-expressing tumor cells up to several months after the last immunization in mice. The data highlighted the importance of the immunostimulant to induce a Th1-type immune response, as well as the key role played by IFN-γ, CD4+ T cells and NK cells in the anti-tumoral effect.

Editor: Ramon Arens, Leiden University Medical Center, Netherlands

Funding: The funders had role in study design, data collection and analysis, decision to publish, or preparation of the manuscript. GlaxoSmithKline Biologicals SA was the funding source and was involved in all stages of the study conduct and analysis. GlaxoSmithKline Biologicals SA also funded all costs associated with the development and publishing of the present manuscript. JL was involved in study supervision at all stages. All authors were involved in study design, review of study reports, data analysis and interpretation. NB and TO conducted the study and were involved in data generation. All authors were involved in drafting and approval of the manuscript.

Competing Interests: I have read the journal's policy and have the following conflicts: CG, NB, TO, JL are employees of GlaxoSmithKline Vaccines. CG and JL declare stock ownership in the GlaxoSmithKline group of companies. CG and JL are also inventor on patents owned by GlaxoSmithKline group of companies (WO/2013/096430).

* E-mail: catherine.gerard@gsk.com

Introduction

Ever since William Coley's observations in the 19th century that cancer may be treated by mobilizing the patient's own immune system, the ultimate goal for cancer immunologists has been to reproducibly achieve this in patients. The mutated aberrant proteins, re-activated or over-expressed in tumor cells, represent potential "tumor antigens" that can be targeted by the immune system [1–3].

Aberrant gene promoter demethylation is an important mechanism by which the expression of normally silent genes is re-activated in tumor cells. This is the case for the *MAGEA* family of genes that are normally expressed during embryonic life [4] and in the placenta [5,6], but are silent in normal adult tissues, except in the germline cells of the testis [5].

MAGE-A3, a member of this MAGE-A family, is an attractive tumor antigen, as i) it is almost exclusively expressed in tumors,

eliminating the risk of mounting an active immune response against normal tissues (germ cells of the testis are the only normal cells expressing MAGE-A3, but they are devoid of classical HLA class I–II molecules and hence have no antigen presentation capabilities, which exclude the development of immune-related toxicity upon MAGE-A3 immunotherapy), ii) it is expressed in many different cancer types, and iii) it is naturally immunogenic, as CD8+ T lymphocytes specific for MAGE-A3 were found to infiltrate tumor sites in melanoma patients [7].

Clinical data generated over the last decade using different immunotherapeutic approaches showed that delivering MAGE-A3 as a purified recombinant protein formulated with an immunostimulant may be a promising approach [8–11]. Nevertheless, despite encouraging results, many issues remain to be solved to further improve MAGE-A3-specific immunotherapy. In particular, improving the MAGE-A3-immunostimulant combination to induce long lasting anti-tumor immune responses remains essential. In addition, the precise mechanisms and key immune effectors leading to tumor rejection are not known, and no clear immune correlate for clinical efficacy has yet been determined. Nor is it known to which extent the focal pattern of MAGE-A3 expression within a tumor can limit clinical efficacy. Such questions and hypotheses cannot reasonably be addressed in clinical trials, due to the long duration and limited number of patients. Therefore, pre-clinical studies remain essential to guide the clinical development of MAGE-A3-specific immunotherapy.

We addressed some of these questions in the present study. In a first series of experiments, mice were immunized with recombinant MAGE-A3 (recMAGE-A3) formulated with different immunostimulants: AS01, AS02, AS15 or CpG7909. AS15 was selected from this panel for further investigation, due to its capacity to drive the immune system towards a Th1-type immune response and the resulting anti-tumor activity against MAGE-A3-expressing tumor cells. Mice were therefore immunized with the selected recMAGE-A3+AS15 formulation in another series of experiments to evaluate i) the key effectors involved in the anti-tumor activity, ii) the influence of booster injections and iii) the impact of tumor heterogeneity -i.e. the proportion of tumor cells expressing MAGE-A3- on this anti-tumor activity.

Materials and Methods

Ethics Statement

Experiments were carried out in GlaxoSmithKline Vaccines laboratories or by GlaxoSmithKline staff at Armand Frappier Institute (IAF - Canada). Animal studies disclosed in this manuscript were ethically reviewed and approved by the GlaxoSmithKline Vaccines' Belgian ethical Committee for Animal Experimentation or by the Ethics Committee of the IAF. They were conducted in accordance with European Directive 2010/63/EU, the CCAC standards (Canadian council for Animal Care), and the GlaxoSmithKline Vaccines Policy on the Care, Welfare and Treatment of Animals. Both GlaxoSmithKline Vaccine facility and IAF are AAALAC (Association for Assessment and Accreditation of Laboratory Animal Care) accredited. All efforts were made to minimize suffering: tumors exceeding a maximum allowable size of 17 mm×17 mm, ulceration, tumor necrosis, convulsion, morbidity and circling behavior were conditions requiring euthanasia by intra-peritoneal injection with barbituric acid derivative (overdose).

Antigen Description, Production and Purification

The fusion protein ProtD–MAGE-A3-His, also abbreviated recMAGE-A3, contains the first 127 residues of protein D derived from *Haemophilus influenzae* at its N-terminus to improve the protein expression in a bacterial system, and a sequence of histidine residues at its C-terminus to facilitate the fusion protein purification.

The production of recMAGE-A3 was performed in the *Escherichia coli* strain AR58, as described previously [11]. Another recombinant MAGE-A3 protein, consisting of the first 314 amino acids of MAGE-A3 followed by 6 histidine residues, was produced in baculovirus [11]. This protein, referred to as bacMAGE-A3, was used in the monitoring of the immune responses.

Description of the Immunostimulants

AS02 consists of an oil-in-water emulsion containing 3-*O*-desacyl-4′-monophosphoryl lipid A (MPL, GlaxoSmithKline Vaccines, Rixensart, Belgium), a Toll-like receptor (TLR)-4 agonist, and QS-21 (*Quillaja saponaria* Molina fraction 21, Antigenics Inc, a wholly owned subsidiary of Agenus Inc,

Lexington, MA, USA), which is a molecule of the saponin family [12]. AS01 is an Adjuvant System containing MPL, QS-21 and liposome. AS15 contains MPL, QS-21, liposome, and the TLR-9 ligand CpG7909 (synthetic oligodeoxyribonucleotides [ODNs] containing unmethylated CpG motifs; herein referred to as CpG).

Mouse Strains and Immunizations

C57BL/6 or CB6F1 (hybrid between C57BL/6 and BALB/c) female mice (6–8 week-old) were purchased from Harlan (Horst, The Netherlands) and kept in specific pathogen-free conditions.

Mice were usually injected 2 or 4 times intra-muscularly at 2-week intervals with 1 or 10 μg of recMAGE-A3 in 50 μl of immunostimulant.

To study long-term protection, mice received 2 injections of either recMAGE-A3+AS15 or phosphate-buffered solution (PBS) at 2-week intervals. Eight weeks after the second immunization, the animals were challenged with a TC1-MAGE-A3 tumor (see description of the tumor cells below; *Tumor models and challenges*). On Day 150, 80 days after tumor challenge, tumor-free animals from the recMAGE-A3+AS15 group were randomized and allocated to two groups. One group received four booster injections of recMAGE-A3+AS15 at a 4-week interval and the other group received injections of PBS following the same schedule. Thirty days after the last injection, mice underwent a tumor challenge in the same flank, and tumor growth was monitored during 46 days (up to Day 319). Additionally, tumor cells were injected into a group of ten PBS-immunized mice, as a positive control for tumor growth.

To assess the role of IFN-γ, perforin and MHC class I or II molecules in tumor protection following MAGE-A3 immunotherapy, immunodeficient mice were used with the same immunization schedules as described above. The following strains were purchased from the Jackson Institute: IFNγ-knocked out (KO) mice (B6.129S7-Ifngtm1Ts/J), MHC class I-KO (B6.129P2-b2mtm1Unc), MHC class II-KO (B6.129S2-H2-dIAb1-Ea00451), B cell-KO (B6.129S2.IgHmTm1Cgn) and perforin-KO mice (C57BL/6-Prf1 tm1Sdz/J).

To assess the potential role of T cells, recMAGE-A3-immunized C57BL/6 mice were depleted of CD4$^+$ or CD8$^+$ T cells by injecting 0.5 mg rat anti-mouse antibodies (GK1.5 [TIB-207 from ATCC] and 2.43 [TIB-210 from ATCC], respectively) one week before the tumor challenge and then weekly during the course of the experiment. NK cell depletion was achieved by injecting the anti-Asialo GM1 antibody (Cedarlane) twice a week starting at day 49 (i.e. 7 days before tumor challenge) and until the end of the experiment (0.1 ml per injection). Depletions were verified by flow cytometry (data not shown). Control antibodies with similar isotypes to the depleting antibodies were used as negative controls.

Tumor Models and Challenges

TC1-MAGE-A3 cells are murine tumor cells genetically modified to express human MAGE-A3. TC1 tumor cells (obtained from Dr T. Wu, John Hopkins University) are interesting as they recapitulate the different steps leading to a tumorigenic cell line. Originally, the TC1 tumor cell line was generated from C57BL/6 primary lung epithelial cells immortalized by transfection of the *Hpv-16 e6* and *e7* genes, and transformed with an activated *Ras* oncogene [13]. These cells were transfected with a pcDNA3 plasmid containing *MAGEA3* cDNA and the *zeocin* selection gene. Clones resistant to zeocin treatment were tested for *MAGEA3* expression by RT-PCR and for MHC class I expression by flow cytometry (data not shown). The best clone showing reproducible tumorigenicity in mice was chosen.

For each challenge, the animals received a subcutaneous injection of 2×10^6 TC1-MAGE-A3 cells (200 µl in the flank). Individual tumor growth was recorded twice a week, by measuring the product of the 2 main diameters of the tumor during the monitoring phase, starting 7 days after the day of challenge. Mice were sacrificed during the study when the tumor size reached 289 mm^2. In such case, the value of the last measurement obtained prior to sacrifice was carried forward to the next time point(s).

To determine whether a threshold percentage of MAGE-A3-expressing tumor cells is needed to elicit tumor rejection by the immune system, PBS-sham-immunized mice and mice immunized with recMAGE-A3+AS15 were challenged with TC1 parental cells (100% MAGE-A3-negative cells), TC1-MAGE-A3 cells (100% MAGE-A3 expressing cells), or different ratios of TC1/TC1-MAGE-A3: i.e. 10/90, 50/50 or 90/10%, respectively.

Cytokine Production

Isolated mouse splenocytes were cultured in the presence of 1 µg/ml bacMAGE-A3. After 72 h, the concentrations of IL-2, IL-4, IL-5, IFN-γ and TNF-α in the supernatants were measured by cytometric bead array (CBA, Pharmingen cat n° 551287), according to the manufacturer's instructions.

Intracellular Cytokine Staining and Flow Cytometry

Peripheral blood mononuclear cells isolated from immunized animals were stimulated in vitro in 96-round bottom well plates with either medium (no stimulation) or a pool of fifty-seven 15 mer peptides overlapping by 10 amino acids, covering the entire sequence of MAGE-A3 (1 µg/ml for each peptide), in a final volume of 200 µl of RPMI, 5% fetal calf serum (FCS) containing rabbit anti-mouse anti-CD49d and anti-CD28 antibodies (Becton Dickinson, BD n° 553154 and n° 553295 respectively; final concentration: 1 µg/ml each). After 2 h of incubation at 37°C, the secretion of cytokines was blocked by the addition of 50 µl brefeldin (Golgi Plug, BD n° 555029: 1/1000 in RPMI 5% FCS). Cells were transferred to a 96-conical bottom well plate, centrifuged and washed with 250 µl PBS containing 1% FCS (FACS buffer). The cell pellets were incubated for 10 min at 4°C in the presence of rat anti-mouse CD16/CD32 (2.4G2, BD n° 553142; 0.5 mg/ml) to block Fcγ receptors. CD4$^+$ and CD8$^+$ T cells were stained for 30 min at 4°C by adding 50 µl phycoery-thrin-labeled rat anti-mouse CD4 monoclonal antibody (BD n° 556616) or peridinin chlorophyll protein-labeled rat anti-mouse CD8 monoclonal antibody (BD n° 553036). After a washing step, the cells were fixed in 200 µl of cytoFix-cytoPerm solution (BD n° 554722) for 20 min at 4°C and permeabilized by adding permWASH solution (BD n° 554723). After centrifugation, cells were incubated 2 h at 4°C with 50 µl of a mix of allophycocyanin-labeled anti-IFN-γ (BD n° 554413). Cells were washed, centri-fuged and resuspended in FACS buffer before flow cytometry analysis (LSR2 from BD). Gating was done on T cells, and a total of approximately 20,000 CD4$^+$ T cells were acquired. The data were expressed as percentages of MAGE-A3-specific IFN-γ-producing CD4$^+$ or CD8$^+$ T cells amongst the total population of CD4$^+$ or CD8$^+$ T cells, respectively, after subtraction of control medium value.

Statistical Analyses

Cytokine analyses were performed using an ANOVA with group as factor after log-transformation of the data. For other analyses, the statistical model was a repeated ANOVA with group, time and group-by-time interaction as factors; the correlation between two measurements from the same mice is assumed to be autoregressive, i.e. correlations decline exponentially with time. Variances were assumed to be different across groups but identical across time points. Comparisons of the mean tumor sizes were made at the last time point.

Results

Immune and Anti-tumor Responses in Mice Immunized with recMAGE-A3 Combined with Different Immunostimulants

After four immunizations of C57BL/6 mice with recMAGE-A3, alone or formulated with an immunostimulant (AS01, AS02, CpG or AS15), both humoral and cellular immune responses were assessed. The antibody response was low after immunization with recMAGE-A3 alone, compared with immunization with rec-MAGE-A3 formulated with an immunostimulant (Figure S1). The humoral responses induced by recMAGE-A3 formulated with different immunostimulants were considered equivalent, irrespec-tive of the immunostimulant. Similarly, no major differences were observed between the immunostimulants in their ability to induce T-cell responses as evaluated by lympho-proliferation experiments (Figure S2).

In contrast, relevant differences between the immunostimulants were observed when the in vitro cytokine production by splenocytes isolated from immunized animals was measured by CBA in the culture supernatants (Figure 1). Despite the low number of mice (n = 2 or 3) in each group, our results showed that AS15 induces a clear bias towards a Th1 profile, characterized by higher IFN-γ/IL-5 and TNF-α/IL-5 ratios, comparatively to AS01, AS02 and CpG. This observation was associated with a higher production of IL-2 induced by AS15 comparatively to the other immunostim-ulants.

After 4 immunizations with PBS or recMAGE-A3 formulated with different immunostimulants, the mice were challenged subcutaneously with TC1-MAGE-A3 tumor cells and in vivo tumor growth was followed during 4 weeks. In mice treated with PBS, a progressive growth of the tumors was seen (Figure 2). Different outcomes were observed for the mice immunized with recMAGE-A3, depending on the associated immunostimulant. Mice were not protected against tumor growth when AS02 was used and were poorly protected with AS01 or CpG. However, tumor growth was controlled in the mice immunized with recMAGE-A3+AS15. Not only was tumor size reduced in this group, but 3/5 mice were tumor-free when tumors were assessed four weeks after the tumor challenge.

The specificity of this anti-tumor response was established by showing that mice immunized with recMAGE+AS15 were not able to eradicate TC1 cells transfected with an irrelevant antigen (TC1-Her2/neu) injected in the same conditions as the TC1-MAGE-A3 cells (data not shown). We also observed that AS15 had to be present in every injection to efficiently stimulate anti-MAGE-A3 immunity (data not shown).

Based on the entire set of data comparing the different immunostimulants, we selected AS15 for all subsequent experi-ments with recMAGE-A3, as it induced a Th1-biased immune response and was the most efficient against the growth of MAGE-A3-expressing tumor cells.

Immunization with recMAGE-A3+AS15 Elicits Long-term Protection

An important aspect in the generation of an anti-tumor immune response is the induction of long-term immune memory that is capable of providing long-term protection against tumor recur-rences. In preliminary experiments in mice, we observed that

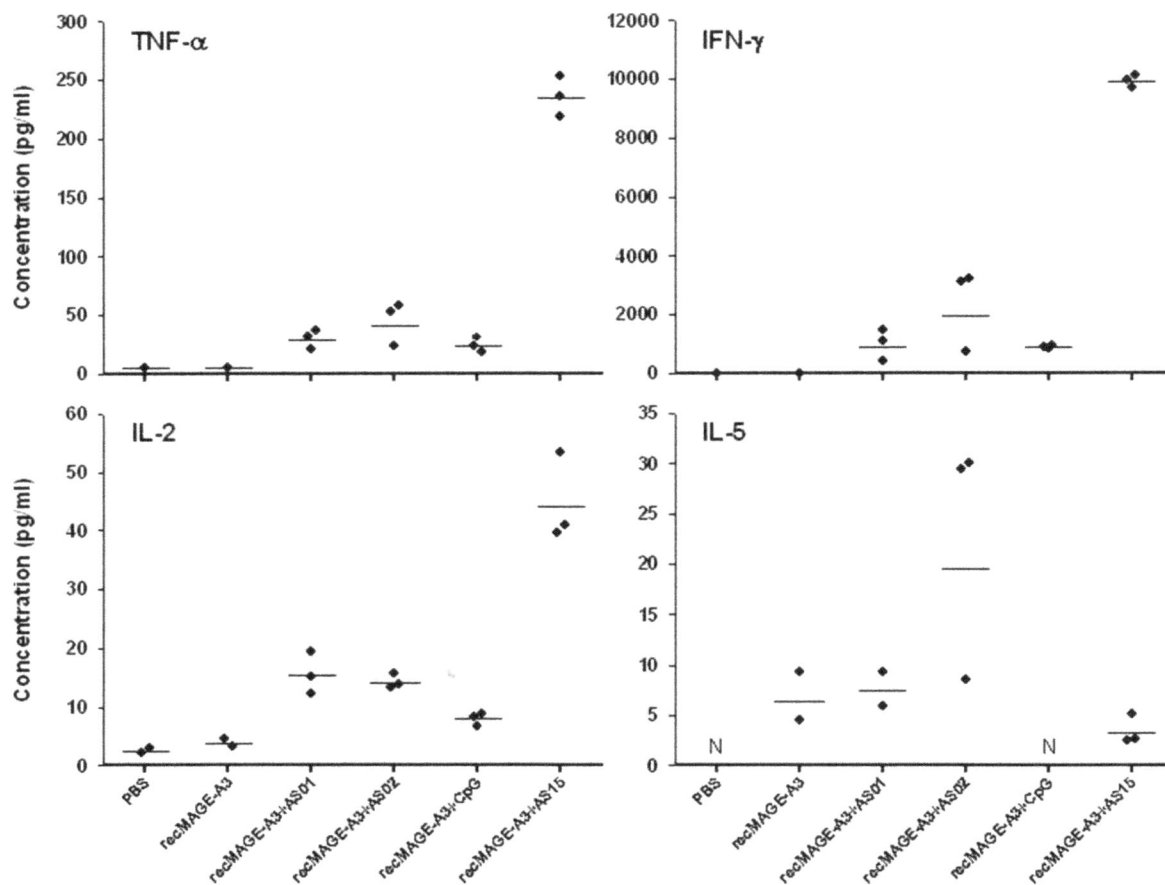

Figure 1. Cytokine production by isolated splenocytes from C57BL/6 mice immunized with recMAGE-A3 alone or formulated with different immunostimulants. The mice were immunized on Days 0, 14, 28 and 42 with recMAGE-A3 (10 µg of antigen) alone or recMAGE-A3 formulated with different immunostimulants, and re-stimulated *in vitro* by bacMAGE-A3. Cytokine production was measured by cytometric bead array (CBA) after 72 h of culture. Each dot represents a mouse, and bars are geomeans. N, not done.

increasing the number of recMAGE-A3+AS15 injections was necessary to better protect mice against the tumor challenge, suggesting that sustaining the immune response by repeated injections may be needed for improved efficacy (data not shown).

We set up an experiment to evaluate whether immunization with recMAGE-A3+AS15 was able to induce such long-term immune memory and whether boosters were necessary (Figure 3A). To this end, mice were immunized on Days 0 and 14 with either PBS or recMAGE-A3+AS15. Immunization with recMAGE-A3+AS15 induced IFN-γ-producing antigen-specific CD4$^+$ and CD8$^+$ T cells (Figure 4). After the challenge with TC1-MAGE-A3 tumor cells, all PBS-immunized mice developed a tumor and were sacrificed, whereas 52 of 60 recMAGE-A3+AS15-immunized mice rejected the tumor and remained tumor-free for at least two months (Figure 3A).

At this stage, 50 of the 52 tumor-free mice were randomly allocated to two groups. One group received PBS and the other group recMAGE-A3+AS15. Immune responses were evaluated at Day 166, 7 days after the first booster. In the group having received a PBS booster, the CD4$^+$ and CD8$^+$ T-cell responses at Day 166 (5 months after the first two immunizations with recMAGE-A3+AS15) were lower than the responses at Day 21 (one week after the first two immunizations with recMAGE-A3+AS15) (Figure 4). This illustrates the decrease in immune responses over time. In contrast, a single recMAGE-A3+AS15 booster

injection was sufficient to raise the levels of cytokine-producing CD4$^+$ T cells up to at least the levels measured at Day 21. In addition, the levels of CD8$^+$ T cells were increased up to 5-fold compared with the levels measured one week after the first two immunizations (Figure 4) and the MAGE-A3–specific CD8$^+$ T cells producing IFN-γ represented up to 20% of the CD8$^+$ T cell pool.

After four monthly boosters, the 50 mice were tumor-challenged. At this stage, a third group of 10 mice receiving only PBS was introduced as a control for tumor growth. No IFN-γ-producing antigen-specific CD4$^+$ and CD8$^+$ T cells were detected in this control group.

In the group that received boosters of PBS, only low levels of IFN-γ-producing antigen-specific CD4$^+$ T cells were observed (residual from the first two MAGE-A3+AS15 injections given 9 months earlier). However, 19 of these 25 mice remained tumor-free after the challenge, indicating that a long-term immune memory had been raised, and that mice were still protected almost one year after the last immunization. In the group of mice boosted monthly with recMAGE-A3+AS15 all 25 mice remained tumor-free (Figure 3B). These data suggest that there was a benefit of giving booster injections with recMAGE-A3+AS15, even if a long-lasting and efficient immune response was induced by the first immunization.

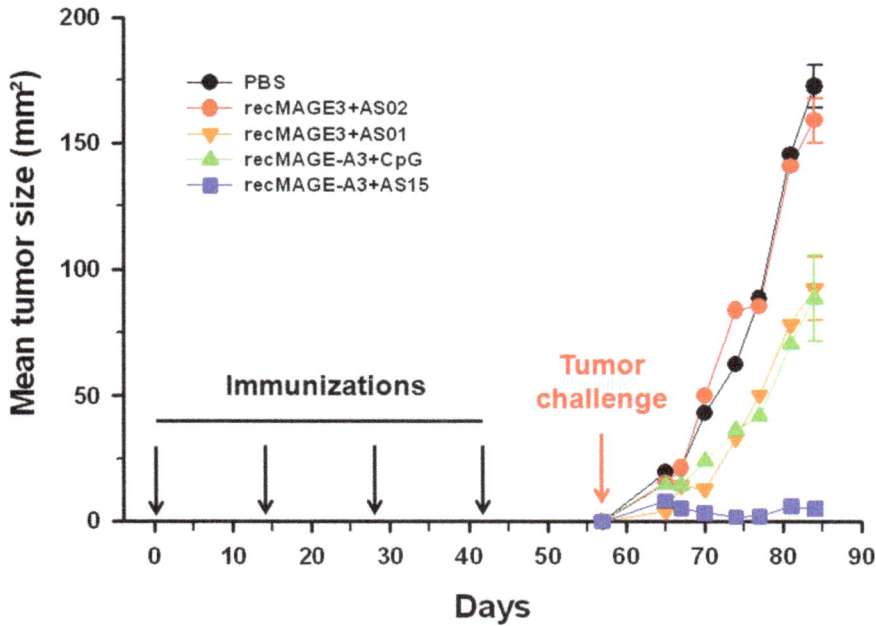

Figure 2. Tumor growth after tumor challenge in C57BL/6 mice immunized with recMAGE-A3 formulated with different immunostimulants. The mice (n = 5) were immunized with recMAGE-A3 (10 μg of antigen) formulated with different immunostimulants and challenged with TC1-MAGE-A3 cells. On day 84, standard errors of the mean are shown and the number of mice remaining tumor-free is indicated for each group. On Day 84, the recMAGE-A3+AS15 group was found different from any other group (p<0.01). Also, tumor growth rate was decreased in the recMAGE-A3+AS15 group, compared with the other groups (p<0.01).

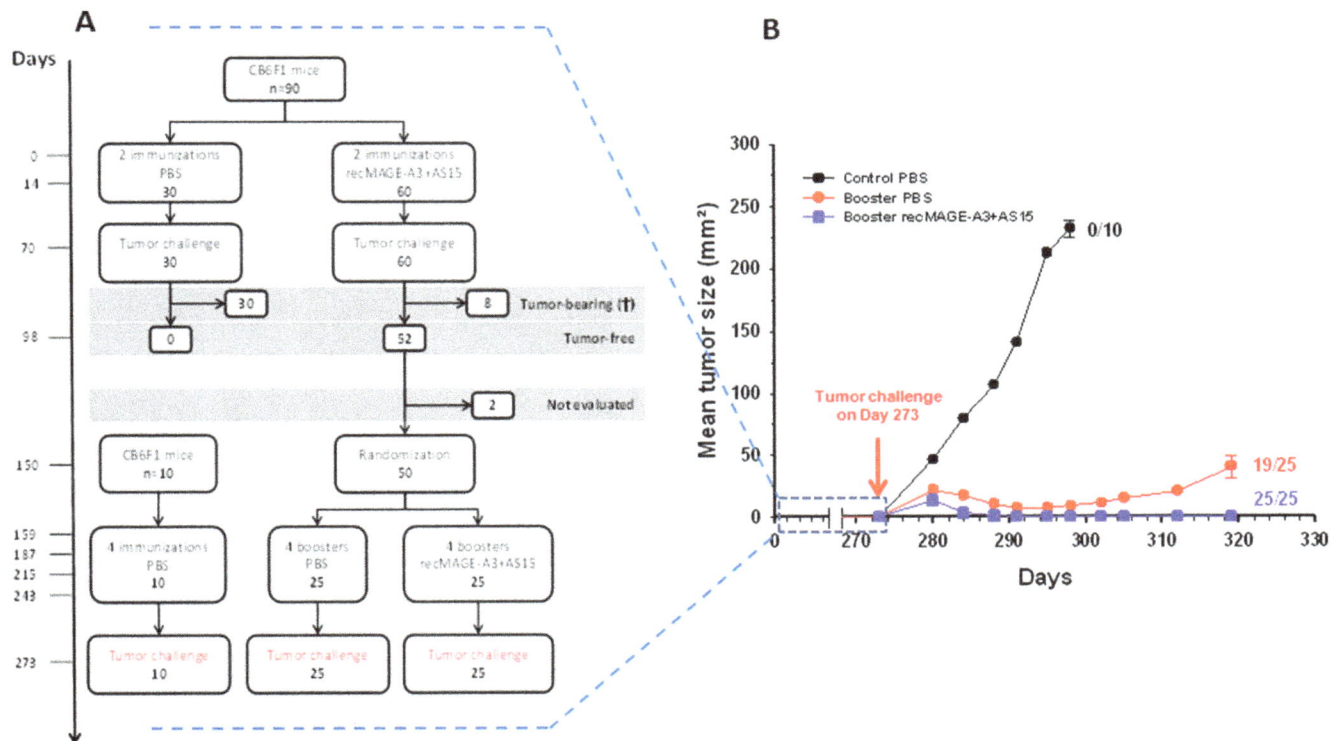

Figure 3. Persistence of protection after immunization with recMAGE-A3+AS15. A. Study design and sample size (CB6F1 mice) at the different steps are shown. Immunizations were made with 1 μg of antigen. B. After the second tumor challenge, tumor growth was followed for 46 days. At the end of the experiment (Day 319), standard errors of the mean are shown and the number of tumor-free mice is indicated for each group.

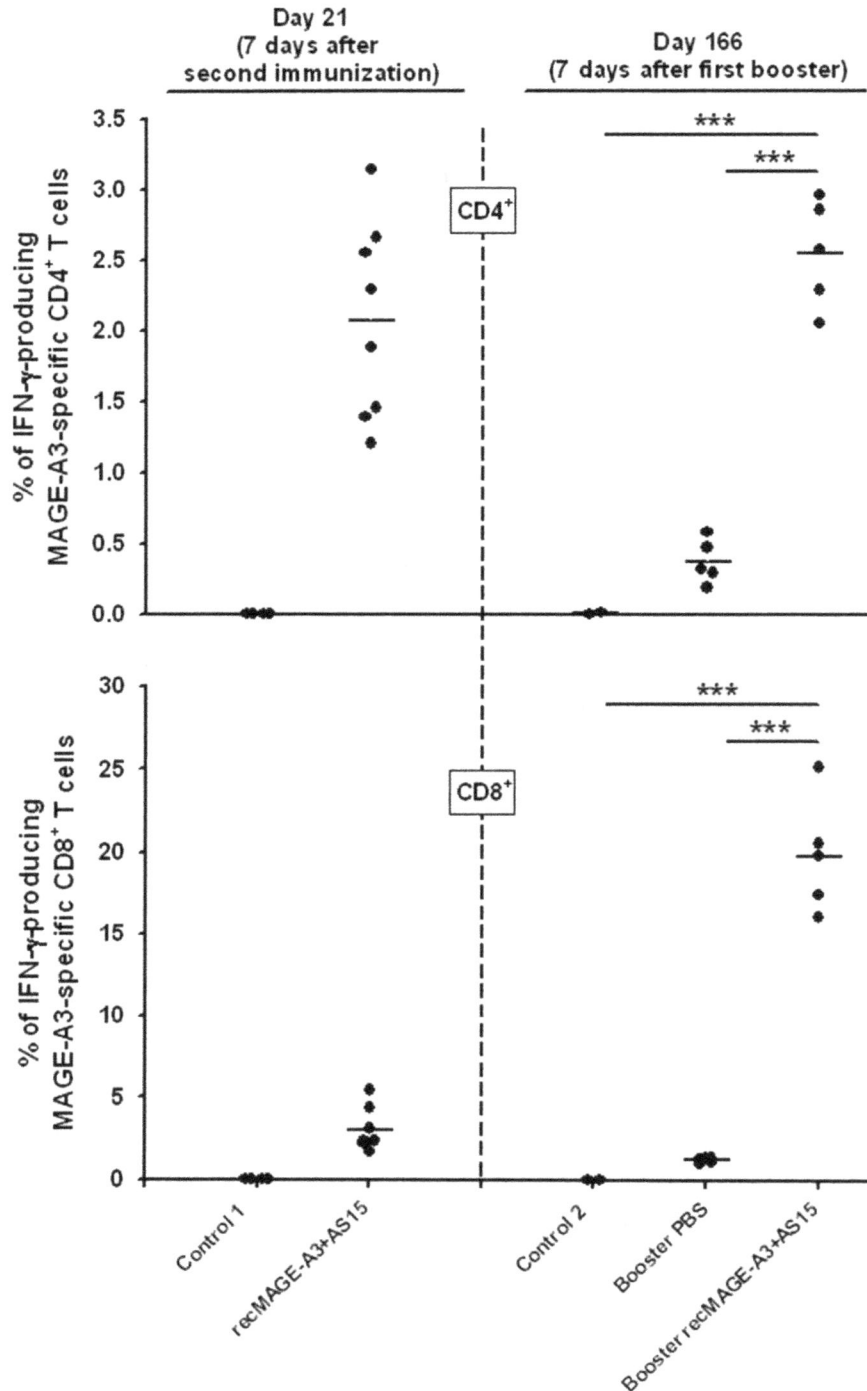

Figure 4. Percentage of IFN-γ-producing MAGE-A3-specific CD4⁺ and CD8⁺ T cells. CB6F1 mice were treated as shown in Figure 3A. Briefly, mice were tumor-challenged after two immunizations with recMAGE-A3+AS15 or PBS (Control 1). Mice of the MAGE-A3+AS15 group remaining tumor-free received either PBS boosters or recMAGE-A3+AS15 boosters. A new control group received PBS (Control 2). Blood samples were taken on Day 21 (7 days after the second immunization) and on day 166 (7 days after the first booster injection). Blood samples were pooled and the amounts of MAGE-A3-specific IFN-γ-producing CD4⁺ and CD8⁺ T cells were determined by intra-cellular staining and flow cytometry. Data are expressed as the percentage of total CD4⁺ and total CD8⁺ T cells after subtraction of the control medium values, which represented around 0.02% when measuring CD4⁺ T cells and 0.1% when measuring CD8⁺ T cells, respectively; each dot is a pool of 3 samples at Day 21 and each dot is a pool of 5 samples on Day 166. *** = p<0.001.

In a subsequent long-term experiment, we determined that AS15 was necessary in each booster to optimally protect the animals against tumor growth (data not shown).

CD4+ T Cells, NK Cells, IFN-γ and MHC Class II are the Cell Subpopulations and Molecular Effectors Involved in recMAGE-A3+AS15-induced Tumor Protection

In an attempt to identify the cells or the effector mechanisms that might be responsible for the protection against the tumor, a series of experiments was conducted in mice either KO or depleted of specific cell types. The different groups of deficient mice received two or four immunizations of recMAGE-A3+AS15 at a two-week interval before they were challenged with TC1-MAGE-A3 cells. As shown in Figure 5, B cell-KO, MHC Class I-KO and perforin-KO mice remained protected by recMAGE-A3+AS15 immunizations. In contrast, tumor protection was impacted in NK and CD4+ T cell-depleted mice, and in IFN-γ-KO and MHC class II-KO mice. These results identified the CD4+ T cells and NK cells as key cell populations in the tumor rejection mechanism. IFN-γ was also identified as a critical molecular effector. Although the exact source of IFN-γ is not known, it further emphasizes the importance of inducing a Th1-biased anti-tumor immune response.

Tumor Growth Inhibition Depends on the Proportion of MAGE-A3-expressing Cells in the Tumor

Expression of MAGE antigens is not necessarily homogeneous in a tumor, showing focal staining in immunohistochemistry [14], probably because not all cells express MAGE-A3 at the same time and at the same level. As this phenomenon is expected to have an impact on the efficacy of recMAGE-A3+AS15 immunization, we evaluated whether recMAGE-A3+AS15 was able to protect mice against a tumor that is not composed of 100% MAGE-A3-expressing cells.

After immunization with PBS or recMAGE-A3+AS15, mice were challenged with different ratios of TC1 parental tumors and TC1-MAGE-A3-expressing cells (0–10–50–90 and 100%) (Figure 6). Results showed that all tumor mixtures grew evenly in mice sham-immunized with PBS. Likewise, the growth of a MAGE-A3-negative tumor was not impacted by recMAGE-A3+AS15 immunization. In contrast, recMAGE-A3+AS15 immunization protected against tumor growth during the 25 days following tumor challenge even when only 10% of the TC1 cells expressed MAGE-A3. The same applied when 50% of the cells, and beyond, expressed MAGE-A3. However, while all mice challenged with 100% MAGE-A3-expressing cells remained tumor-free up to 57 days after the challenge, relapses were observed in the mice challenged with tumors that contained MAGE-A3-negative cells. The intensity of the phenomenon was dependent on the percentage of MAGE-A3-negative cells in the challenging tumor. In the group challenged with 90% MAGE-A3-expressing cells, 2/9 mice showed a relapse. The mean tumor size in this group was not statistically different from that of the group receiving 100% MAGE-A3-expressing TC1 cells. In contrast, in the group challenged with 50% of MAGE-A3-expressing cells, 6/9 mice had relapsed on Day 112, and in the group challenged with 10% of MAGE-A3-expressing cells, relapses were observed in 7/9 mice on Day 112. The mean tumor size in these groups was statistically different from that of the group receiving 100% of MAGE-A3-expressing TC1 cells, with the highest mean tumor size among all relapsed animals observed in mice challenged with 10% MAGE-A3-expressing cells.

Discussion

In the present study, we evaluated the potential of recMAGE-A3 formulated with different immunostimulants. Both the induced immune responses and their capacity to inhibit tumor growth were analyzed. For the functional experiments, the anti-tumor potential of MAGE-A3 immunizations was evaluated in a prophylactic setting with non-tumor-bearing mice rather than a therapeutic setting in order to more closely mimic the clinical situation of adjuvant treatment for cancer patients. Indeed, in the adjuvant setting, the patients first undergo surgery, and are considered free of tumor when they receive the immunization schedule. Although mouse models may not entirely reflect the human situation, partly due to intrinsic differences between the two immune systems [15] and because mice have not been primed by a primary tumor, injection of TC1-MAGE-A3 cells was selected as a tumor model to characterize the impact of the immune responses that have been induced by recMAGE-A3–based immunization. With this model, the different immunostimulants could be evaluated and at least part of the mechanisms of tumor rejection could be unraveled.

Our first and reproducible observation was that the injection of recMAGE-A3 alone did not induce protective immune responses, recMAGE-A3 being weakly immunogenic by itself. High antibody titers and detectable T-cell priming were only achieved when recMAGE-A3 was formulated with an immunostimulant. The need for recombinant proteins or peptide antigens to be mixed with immunostimulants to overcome their poor intrinsic immunogenicity is a common observation. The role of immunostimulants is essential in stimulating innate immunity and to shape the subsequent adaptive immune response [16]. This parallels other observations in clinical trials in which recMAGE-A3 was injected either alone or formulated with the immunostimulant AS02 [17].

In our study, after 4 immunizations, all immunostimulants were efficient at stimulating B cells to produce MAGE-A3-specific antibodies, as measured by enzyme-linked immunosorbent assay, and to stimulate cellular immune responses, as measured by lymphoproliferation. However, not all of the formulations performed equally in protecting the animals against a tumor challenge. Among the panel of immunostimulants tested, AS15 was the most efficient at controlling tumor size, with also a majority of animals remaining tumor-free. AS15 is the complex combination of multiple immunostimulatory molecules, targeting different immune cells. This liposome-based immunostimulant contains MPL, a detoxified derivative of LPS with TLR4 agonistic properties, QS-21, a saponin, and CpG, which is an oligodeoxy-nucleotide with a phosphorothioate backbone and unmethylated CpG motifs (CpG ODN 7909) that binds to TLR9. These components are potent activators of innate immunity, known to induce cellular immunity and anti-tumor immune responses [18–20]. MPL and QS-21 have been shown to act synergistically to induce cell-mediated immune responses [21]. Our data show that the addition of CpG to MPL and QS-21 further strengthen anti-tumor cellular immunity. Analysis of the cytokine profiles of the MAGE-A3-specific T cells revealed a peculiarity of the AS15-induced response, compared with the responses induced by the other immunostimulants. AS15 was indeed shown to induce a strong Th1-type cytokine profile, with particularly high TNF-α and IFN-γ production, two archetypal Th1 cytokines. Earlier reports on MAGE-A3- [22] or MAGE-A6-expressing tumors.

[23] highlighted the association between disease progression and Th2-polarized immune response. It was then shown that patients with active disease of any stage were skewed towards Th2-type responses against MAGE-A6 epitopes. In contrast, Th1-polarized responses were associated with no disease progression

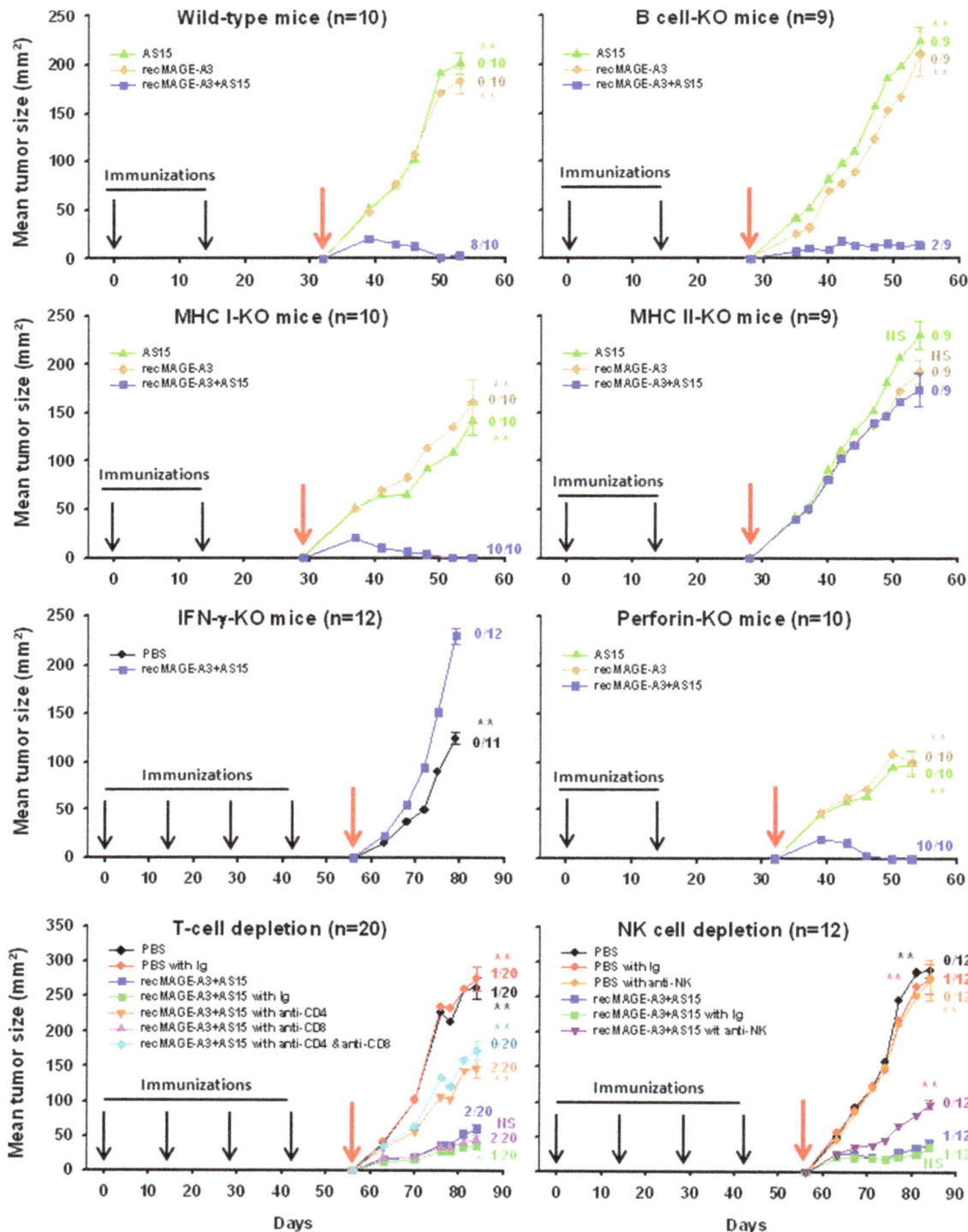

Figure 5. Tumour growth after tumor challenge in wild-type C57BL/6 mice, different knocked-out (KO) or cell-depleted C57BL/6 mice, immunized with either PBS, MAGE-A3 alone, AS15 alone or recMAGE-A3+AS15 (as indicated). In cell depletion experiments, control isoptypes (Ig) similar to the antibody used to deplete T cell or NK cells were used. The number of animals per group is indicated in each graph title. The red arrow indicates the time of tumor challenge. At the last time point, standard errors of the mean are shown and the number of tumor-free mice is indicated for each group. The mean tumor size of each group was statistically compared with that of the recMAGE-A3+AS15 group at the last time point (* = p<0.01; ** = p<0.001; NS = not significant).

[23]. Taken together, these observations highlight the importance of a Th1-type immune response in anti-tumoral immunity, and may explain the strong protection afforded by AS15, an inducer of

Th1 responses, against tumor challenge in our study. Such activity may be linked to the combined effect of CpG that stimulates plasmacytoid dendritic cells through TLR-9 activation [24],

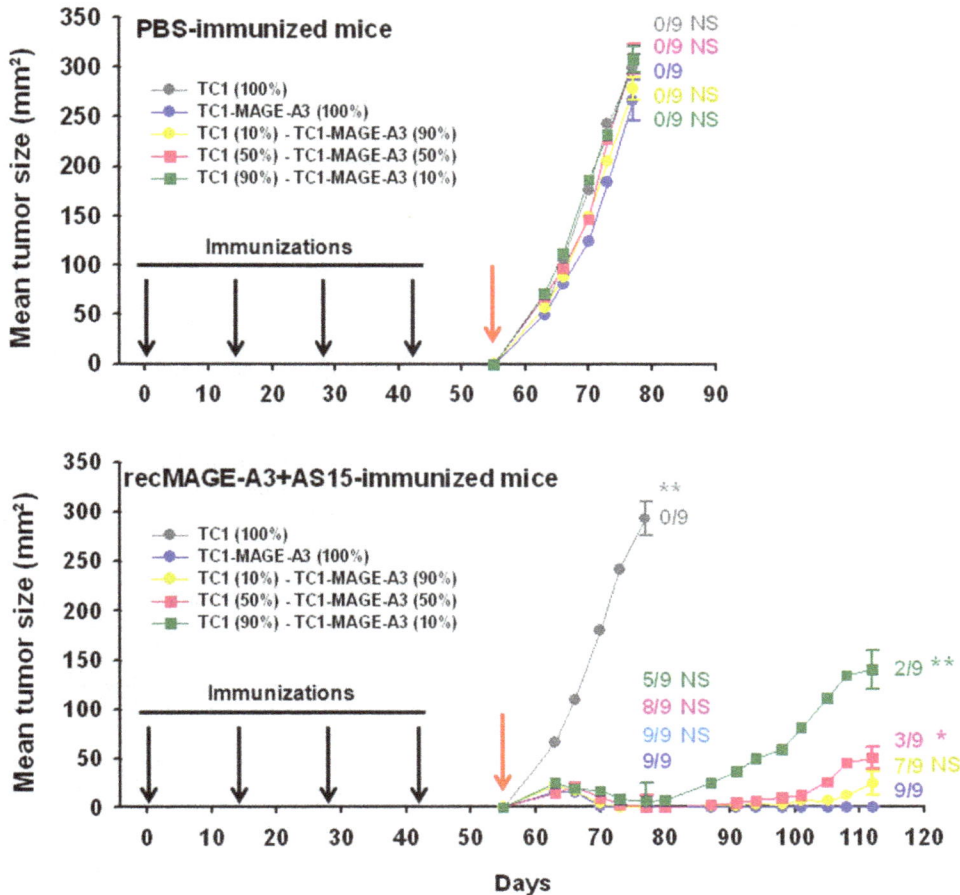

Figure 6. Tumor growth in C57BL/6 mice immunized with PBS (n = 9) or recMAGE-A3+AS15 (n = 9) and challenged with tumor cells containing various percentages (from 0 to 100%) of MAGE-A3-expressing cells. The mice immunized with recMAGE-A3+AS15 (1 μg of antigen) were followed up to Day 112. On Days 77 and 112, standard errors of the mean are shown and the number of tumor-free mice is indicated for each group. Statistical comparisons of the mean tumor size of each group with that the TC1-MAGE-A3 (100%) group on Days 77 and 112 are shown (* = p<0.01; ** = p<0.001; NS = not significant). Red arrow: day of challenge.

leading to enhanced T cell responses, and of the TLR-4 ligand MPL, which potentiates Th1 pathway.

By using a panel of immunodeficient mice, we tried to determine the main actors in tumor growth abrogation. Our data suggested that B cells, and thus antibody responses, were not needed to inhibit tumor growth. This might be expected as MAGE-A3 is an intracellular protein not directly accessible to antibodies for cell killing by antibody-dependent cell-mediated cytotoxicity. More surprising was the observation that CD8[+] T cells do not seem to be essential in this *MAGEA3*-transfected tumor model, as demonstrated in CD8[+] T cell-depleted mice or perforin-KO mice. Cytotoxic CD8[+] T cells are often considered as the most important cell type responsible for the elimination of tumor cells. Indeed, tumor cells, being MHC class I-positive but in most of the cases MHC class II-negative, can logically only be directly targeted by the MHC class I-restricted CD8[+] T cells. This statement has been supported by experimental results, such as the capacity of CD8[+] T cells isolated from tumor infiltrates and passively transferred to patients after *in vitro* expansion to eliminate advanced bulky tumors [25]. In contrast, our results suggest the CD4[+] T cells to be critical effectors in this *MAGEA3*-transfected tumor model. This is not an isolated finding, as it is in line with earlier reports showing the importance of this T-cell subset in

tumor eradication in mouse models [26–28]. There are also findings in humans suggesting that this T-cell population plays a relevant role in tumor regression, as clinical efficacy has been reported after passive transfer of CD4[+] T cells specific for NY-ESO-1 isolated from a melanoma tumor site [29]. The involvement of CD4[+] T cells is not illogical, given their known central role in orchestrating the different phases of the adaptive immune response and the cross-talk they establish with other immune cells, especially the antigen-presenting cells. These actions are driven through MHC class II antigen presentation, and we observed here that MHC class II-deficient, but not MHC class I-deficient mice, cannot eradicate the tumor, which is further indication of the involvement of the CD4[+] rather than the CD8[+] T-cell subset. The mechanisms by which the CD4[+] T cells may act are not clear, and different hypotheses can be put forward. Help provided by CD4[+] T cells stimulates the expansion of a heterogeneous immune population of effector cells that are able to target different facets of tumorigenesis, acting together against tumor growth. One hypothesis relies on a CD4[+] T cell-driven delayed type hypersensitivity (DTH)-like reaction. Antigen-presenting cells are thus attracted to the site of the tumor, capture tumor cell debris and present tumor antigens to CD4[+] T cells through MHC class II [30]. Upon activation, T cells produce various cytokines and chemokines, attracting inflammatory cells like macrophages, granulocytes, eosinophils, and NK cells in the vicinity of the tumor [26,31,32]. Also particularly relevant was the observation that both CD4[+] T cells and NK cells are necessary for an anti-tumor response [33]. Our results are in line with these observations, as there was a reduced impact on tumor growth in recMAGE-A3+AS15-immunized NK cell-deficient mice.

Among the various cytokines that can be produced by CD4[+] cells and NK cells, IFN-γ was shown to play an essential role in tumor eradication. Indeed, IFN-γ-KO mice were unable to kill the tumor cells in our experiments. IFN-γ is produced at different stages of the immune response. It is found as early as during the initial innate response, as the result of the activation of antigen-presenting cells by certain Toll-like receptor ligands. In this regard, we have demonstrated here the capacity of AS15 to stimulate IFN-γ production. We observed measurable levels of IFN-γ in the serum of mice as early as 24 h after recMAGE-A3+AS15 injection (data not shown). IFN-γ is also produced during the development and amplification of the adaptive response. MAGE-A3-specific CD4[+] T cells were shown to produce cytokines upon in vitro re-stimulation with MAGE-A3 protein or peptides. It is not the first time that a critical role is attributed to IFN-γ in controlling tumor growth (for review see [34]). Several groups have demonstrated that IFN-γ pathway-deficient mice are more prone to developing tumors [35–37], although the exact role played by this cytokine in tumor immuno-surveillance is not fully unraveled. IFN-γ regulates many different biological processes, and some of them may modify the tumor microenvironment, ultimately abrogating tumor growth. IFN-γ can inhibit cell proliferation [38,39], promote apoptosis [40,41], exert cytotoxic activity on tumor cells through the production of oxygen derivatives and nitric oxide [42,43], and promotes the induction of inhibitors of angiogenesis by tumor cells [44,45]. IFN-γ also has the capacity to stimulate the expression of MHC markers at the surface of malignant cells, which facilitate targeting and eradication by the host immune system (for review, see [46]). It is likely that these combined actions of IFN-γ facilitated the anti-tumor effect in our tumor challenge model. Of note, immunization with AS01 or CpG, which induced fewer IFN-γ-producing cells than immunization with AS15, did not afford full protection against a tumor challenge, highlighting a potential association between the level of IFN-γ and the level of protection.

Our work in mice demonstrated that recMAGE-A3+AS15 immunization induces a long-term immune memory, able to recognize and eliminate MAGE-A3-expressing tumor cells up to several months after the last immunization. The present study focused on the anti-tumor effect against TC1-MAGE-A3 tumors, but tumor protection was also obtained against other MAGEA3 -transfected murine cell lines (B16-MAGE-A3 melanoma or CT26-MAGE-A3 colon carcinoma) (data not shown). Although protection was still afforded several months after the last immunization, a higher level of protection was observed if recMAGE-A3+AS15 boosters were given to sustain and even increase the levels of MAGE-A3-specific T cells. In a separate series of experiments, we showed that AS15 was necessary not only in priming, but also in booster injections. Indeed, less IFN-γ and/or IL-2-producing CD4[+] T cells were detected, and concomitantly, less efficiency against tumor challenge was found when the booster injections were carried out without AS15 (data not shown). Similarly, an earlier MAGE-A3 study in human demonstrated the need to use an immunostimulant for priming, even if the immunostimulant is used in boosters [47]. This implies that additional spaced booster injections would be needed to sustain long-term anti-tumoral immunity, and each booster injection must be formulated with the immunostimulant in the clinical situation.

In clinical trials, patients are often enrolled based on the levels of MAGEA3 gene expression, but the pattern of MAGE-A3 protein expression, which is not necessarily homogeneous in tumors, as demonstrated previously by immunohistochemistry [14], is not taken into account. MAGE antigens show focal expression, meaning that in an early metastasis, at the time when patients receive treatment, not all cells necessarily express MAGE-A3.

Consequently, it is reasonable to assume that tumors with a low percentage of MAGE-A3-expressing cells would be more difficult to control by anti-MAGE-A3 immune responses. We attempted to mimic this situation in mice, trying to determine the percentage of MAGE-A3-expressing tumor cells below which the elicited immune responses cannot be effective. Surprisingly, our results showed that tumor growth can still be controlled in the short term even if only 10% of cells in the tumor mass express MAGE-A3. How MAGE-A3-negative cells can be targeted after MAGE-A3 immunization is not clear. One hypothesis is that this phenomenon results from immune responses to other antigens expressed by the TC1 tumor cells, through the mechanism of antigen/epitope spreading [48,49]. However, after several weeks, we observed a number of relapses in mice that harbored tumors with MAGE-A3-negative cells. Furthermore, the lower the percentage of MAGE-A3-expressing cells in the tumor, the higher the number of relapses and the larger the tumor size, suggesting that the phenomenon is probably due to the outgrowth of MAGE-A3-negative tumor cells. If the hypothesis is true, this also implies that the potential immune responses raised by antigen/epitope spreading would not remain efficient on the long-term, in contrast to those induced by recMAGE-A3+ AS15 immunization.

The potential of MAGE-A3 as target for cancer immunother-apy was used early in clinical trials [9,11]. The immunostimulant in these trials was AS02, and some clinical activity was observed, especially in less advanced melanoma patients (no visceral metastasis) expressing either HLA – A1– A2 or B44. These results prompted the evaluation of recMAGE-A3+AS02 in a double-blind, randomized, placebo-controlled phase II study involving patients with completely resected MAGE-A3-expressing stage IB or II Non-Small Cell Lung Cancer (NSCLC) [10]. Another proof-of-concept phase II study was conducted in metastatic melanoma patients [8]. In this clinical study, the two immunostimulants AS02 and AS15 were compared and the results highlighted the superiority of AS15 over AS02 to elicit efficient anti-tumoral responses, with higher specific antibody titers and more robust T-cell induction. In particular, CD4[+] T cells were shown to be major players in the observed clinical activity. This is in line with the results described in mice in the present study.

Altogether, the clinical results parallel those obtained with our tumor challenge model in mice. Our data support the use of AS15 as immunostimulant in combination with the recMAGE-A3 protein. This study highlights that pre-clinical studies are complementary to clinical development, as they can provide further information regarding the potential key effector mecha-nisms involved in tumor rejection and thus potentially helping in the design of recMAGE-A3-based immunotherapy in the clinical setting. Such a translational approach between preclinical and clinical data will continue to support the development of the MAGE-A3 immunotherapy, which is now under evaluation in two large, double blind, randomized phase III trials for the treatment of NSCLC (MAGRIT, NCT00480025) and melanoma (DERMA, NCT00796445).

Supporting Information

Figure S1　Antibody titers determined in C57BL/6 mice (n = 10 per group) immunized at 4 occasions with control saline, recMAGE-A3 alone, recMAGE-A3+AS01, rec-MAGE-A3+AS02, recMAGE-A3+CpG or recMAGE-A3+AS15. Results are expressed as mid-point titers (dilution at the inflexion point of the optical density (OD)/sample dilution curve). Each dot represents a mouse and horizontal bars are geomeans. Statistical analysis: The recMAGE-A3 alone group is different from all other groups. The humoral responses induced by recMAGE-A3 formulated with an immunostimulant were considered equivalent, irrespective of the immunostimulant, as the ratio of the geometric mean titers between groups were close to 1 and all 95% CI comprised between 0.5 and 2.

Figure S2　Lymphoproliferation performed on splenocytes isolated from C57BL/6 mice (n = 3) immunized at 4 occasions with control saline, recMAGE-A3 alone, recMAGE-A3/AS01, recMAGE-A3/AS02, recMAGE-A3/CpG or recMAGE-A3/AS15. Briefly, 2×10^5 spleen cells were plated in quadruplicate in a 96-well microplate, in RPMI medium containing 1% normal mouse serum. After 72 h of stimulation with bacMAGE-A3 (1 μg/ml), 1 μCi ^{3}H thymidine was added. Sixteen hours later, cells were harvested onto filter plates.

Incorporated radioactivity was counted in a β-counter and the stimulation indices were calculated. Stimulation with ConA (2 μg/ml) was included as positive control. Each dot represents a mouse and horizontal bars are geomeans.

Table S1　The ARRIVE Guidelines Checklist.

Acknowledgments

The authors thank the "Preclinical Cancer Immunology" group (GlaxoSmithKline Vaccines, Laval, Canada), the "R&D Formulation Development" group (GlaxoSmithKline Vaccines, Rixensart, Belgium), Yves Renaux, André De Groote, Aurélie Delplanque, Carole François and Romain Piccininno for technical assistance, Marie-Pierre Malice for the statistical analyses, Pascal Cadot and Virginie Durbecq (XPE Pharma & Science, on behalf of GlaxoSmithKline Vaccines) and Ulrike Krause for providing medical writing services and editorial support in preparing this manuscript.

Author Contributions

Conceived and designed the experiments: CG NB TO JL. Performed the experiments: NB TO. Analyzed the data: CG NB TO JL. Contributed reagents/materials/analysis tools: NB TO. Wrote the paper: CG NB TO JL.

References

1. van der Bruggen P, Traversari C, Chomez P, Lurquin C, De Plaen E, et al. (1991) A gene encoding an antigen recognized by cytolytic T lymphocytes on a human melanoma. Science 254(5038): 1643–1647.
2. Van Pel A, Boon T (1982) Protection against a nonimmunogenic mouse leukemia by an immunogenic variant obtained by mutagenesis. Proc Natl Acad Sci USA 79(15): 4718–4722.
3. Van Pel A, van der Bruggen P, Coulie PG, Brichard VG, Lethé B, et al. (1995) Genes coding for tumor antigens recognized by cytolytic T lymphocytes. Immunol Rev 145: 229–250.
4. Hudolin T, Kastelan Z, Derezić D, Basić-Jukić N, Cesare Spagnoli G, et al. (2009) Expression of MAGE-A1, MAGE-A3/4 and NY-ESO-1 cancer-testis antigens in fetal testis. Acta Dermatovenerol Croat 17(2): 103–107.
5. De Plaen E, Arden K, Traversari C, Gaforio JJ, Szikora JP, et al. (1994) Structure, chromosomal localization, and expression of 12 genes of the MAGE family. Immunogenetics 40(5): 360–369.
6. Jungbluth AA, Silva WA Jr, Frosina D, Zaidi B, et al. (2007) Expression of cancer-testis (CT) antigens in placenta. Cancer Immun 7: 15.
7. Gaugler B, Van den Eynde B, van der Bruggen P, Romero P, Gaforio JJ, et al. (1994) Human gene MAGE-3 codes for an antigen recognized on a melanoma by autologous cytolytic T lymphocytes. J Exp Med 179(3): 921–930.
8. Kruit WH, Suciu S, Dreno B, Mortier L, Robert C, et al. (2013) Selection of immunostimulant AS15 for active immunization with MAGE-A3 protein: results of a randomized phase II study of the European Organisation for Research and Treatment of Cancer Melanoma Group in Metastatic Melanoma. J Clin Oncol 31(19): 2413–2420.
9. Marchand M, Punt CJ, Aamdal S, Escudier B, Kruit WH, et al. (2003) Immunisation of metastatic cancer patients with MAGE-3 protein combined with adjuvant SBAS-2: a clinical report. Eur J Cancer 39(1): 70–77.
10. Vansteenkiste J, Zielinski M, Linder A, Dahabreh J, Gonzalez EE, et al. (2013) Adjuvant MAGE-A3 immunotherapy in resected non-small-cell lung cancer: phase II randomized study results. J Clin Oncol 31(19): 2396–2403.
11. Vantomme V, Dantinne C, Amrani N, Permanne P, Gheysen D, et al. (2004) Immunologic Analysis of a Phase I/II Study of Vaccination with MAGE-3 Protein Combined with the AS02B Adjuvant in Patients with MAGE-3-Positive Tumors. J Immunother 27(2): 124–135.
12. Garçon N, Chomez P, Van Mechelen M (2007) GlaxoSmithKline Adjuvant Systems in vaccines: concepts, achievements and perspectives. Expert Rev Vaccines 6(5): 723–739.
13. Lin KY, Guarnieri FG, Staveley-O'Carroll KF, Levitsky HI, August JT, et al. (1996) Treatment of established tumors with a novel vaccine that enhances major histocompatibility class II presentation of tumor antigen. Cancer Res 56(1): 21–26.
14. Jungbluth AA, Busam KJ, Kolb D, Iversen K, Coplan K, et al. (2000) Expression of MAGE-antigens in normal tissues and cancer. Int J Cancer 85(4): 460–465.
15. Mestas J, Hughes CC (2004) Of mice and not men: differences between mouse and human immunology. J Immunol 172(5): 2731–2738.
16. Garcon N, Van Mechelen M (2011) Recent clinical experience with vaccines using MPL-and QS-21-containing Adjuvant Systems. Expert Rev Vaccines 10(4): 471–486.
17. Atanackovic D, Altorki NK, Stockert E, Williamson B, Jungbluth AA, et al. (2004) Vaccine-induced CD4$^+$ T cell responses to MAGE-3 protein in lung cancer patients. J Immunol 172(5): 3289–3296.
18. Chu RS, Targoni OS, Krieg AM, Lehmann PV, Harding CV (1997) CpG oligodeoxynucleotides act as adjuvants that switch on T helper 1 (Th1) immunity. J Exp Med 186(10): 1623–1631.
19. den Brok MH, Sutmuller RP, Nierkens S, Bennink EJ, Toonen LW, et al. (2006) Synergy between in situ cryoablation and TLR9 stimulation results in a highly effective in vivo dendritic cell vaccine. Cancer Res 66(14): 7285–7292.
20. Krieg AM, Yi AK, Matson S, Waldschmidt TJ, Bishop GA, et al. (1995) CpG motifs in bacterial DNA trigger direct B-cell activation. Nature 374(6522): 546–549.
21. Garçon N, Heppner DG, Cohen J (2003) Development of RTS,S/AS02: a purified subunit-based malaria vaccine candidate formulated with a novel adjuvant. Expert Rev Vaccines 2(2): 231–238.
22. Marturano J, Longhi R, Russo V, Protti MP (2008) Endosomal proteases influence the repertoire of MAGE-A3 epitopes recognized in vivo by CD4+ T cells. Cancer Res 68(5): 1555–1562.
23. Tatsumi T, Kierstead LS, Ranieri E, Gesualdo L, Schena FP, et al. (2002) Disease-associated bias in T helper type 1 (Th1)/Th2 CD4(+) T cell responses against MAGE-6 in HLA-DRB10401(+) patients with renal cell carcinoma or melanoma. J Exp Med 196(5): 619–628.
24. Nierkens S, den Brok MH, Garcia Z, Togher S, Wagenaars J, et al. (2011) Immune adjuvant efficacy of CpG oligonucleotide in cancer treatment is founded specifically upon TLR9 function in plasmacytoid dendritic cells. Cancer Res 71(20): 6428–6437.
25. Rosenberg SA, Restifo NP, Yang JC, Morgan RA, Dudley ME (2008) Adoptive cell transfer: a clinical path to effective cancer immunotherapy. Nat Rev Cancer 8(4): 299–308.
26. Hock H, Dorsch M, Diamantstein T, Blankenstein T (1991) Interleukin 7 induces CD4+ T cell-dependent tumor rejection. J Exp Med 174(6): 1291–1298.
27. Lauritzsen GF, Weiss S, Dembic Z, Bogen B (1994) Naive idiotype-specific CD4+ T cells and immunosurveillance of B-cell tumors. Proc Natl Acad Sci USA 91(12): 5700–5704.
28. Rakhra K, Bachireddy P, Zabuawala T, Zeiser R, Xu L, et al. (2010) CD4(+) T cells contribute to the remodeling of the microenvironment required for sustained tumor regression upon oncogene inactivation. Cancer Cell 18(5): 485–498.
29. Hunder NN, Wallen H, Cao J, Hendricks DW, Reilly JZ, et al. (2008) Treatment of metastatic melanoma with autologous CD4+ T cells against NY-ESO-1. N Engl J Med 358(25): 2698–2703.
30. Corthay A, Skovseth DK, Lundin KU, Røsjø E, Omholt H, et al. (2005) Primary antitumor immune response mediated by CD4+ T cells. Immunity 22(3): 371–383.

31. Greenberg PD (1991) Adoptive T cell therapy of tumors: mechanisms operative in the recognition and elimination of tumor cells. Adv Immunol 49: 281–355.

32. Hung K, Hayashi R, Lafond-Walker A, Lowenstein C, Pardoll D, et al. (1998) The central role of CD4(+) T cells in the antitumor immune response. J Exp Med 188(12): 2357–2368.

33. Perez-Diez A, Joncker NT, Choi K, Chan WF, Anderson CC, et al. (2007) CD4 cells can be more efficient at tumor rejection than CD8 cells. Blood 109(12): 5346–5354.

34. Dunn GP, Koebel CM, Schreiber RD (2006) Interferons, immunity and cancer immunoediting. Nat Rev Immunol 6(11): 836–848.

35. Kaplan DH, Shankaran V, Dighe AS, Stockert E, Aguet M, et al. (1998) Demonstration of an interferon gamma-dependent tumor surveillance system in immunocompetent mice. Proc Natl Acad Sci USA 95(13): 7556–7561.

36. Street SE, Cretney E, Smyth MJ (2001) Perforin and interferon-gamma activities independently control tumor initiation, growth, and metastasis. Blood 97(1): 192–197.

37. Street SE, Trapani JA, MacGregor D, Smyth MJ (2002) Suppression of lymphoma and epithelial malignancies effected by interferon gamma. J Exp Med 196(1): 129–134.

38. Bromberg JF, Horvath CM, Wen Z, Schreiber RD, Darnell JE Jr (1996) Transcriptionally active Stat1 is required for the antiproliferative effects of both interferon alpha and interferon gamma. Proc Natl Acad Sci USA 93(15): 7673–7678.

39. Chin YE, Kitagawa M, Su WC, You ZH, Iwamoto Y, et al. (1996) Cell growth arrest and induction of cyclin-dependent kinase inhibitor p21 WAF1/CIP1 mediated by STAT1. Science 272(5262): 719–722.

40. Chin YE, Kitagawa M, Kuida K, Flavell RA, Fu XY (1997) Activation of the STAT signaling pathway can cause expression of caspase 1 and apoptosis. Mol Cell Biol 17(9): 5328–5337.

41. Xu X, Fu XY, Plate J, Chong AS (1998) IFN-gamma induces cell growth inhibition by Fas-mediated apoptosis: requirement of STAT1 protein for up-regulation of Fas and FasL expression. Cancer Res 58(13): 2832–2837.

42. Williamson BD, Carswell EA, Rubin BY, Prendergast JS, Old LJ (1983) Human tumor necrosis factor produced by human B-cell lines: synergistic cytotoxic interaction with human interferon. Proc Natl Acad Sci USA 80(17): 5397–5401.

43. Fransen L, Van der Heyden J, Ruysschaert R, Fiers W (1986) Recombinant tumor necrosis factor: its effect and its synergism with interferon-gamma on a variety of normal and transformed human cell lines. Eur J Cancer Clin Oncol 22(4): 419–426.

44. Coughlin CM, Salhany KE, Gee MS, LaTemple DC, Kotenko S, et al. (1998) Tumor cell responses to IFNgamma affect tumorigenicity and response to IL-12 therapy and antiangiogenesis. Immunity 9(1): 25–34.

45. Qin Z, Blankenstein T (2000) CD4+ T cell–mediated tumor rejection involves inhibition of angiogenesis that is dependent on IFN gamma receptor expression by nonhematopoietic cells. Immunity 12(6): 677–686.

46. Seliger B, Ruiz-Cabello F, Garrido F (2008) IFN inducibility of major histocompatibility antigens in tumors. Adv Cancer Res 101: 249–276.

47. Atanackovic D, Altorki NK, Cao Y, Ritter E, Ferrara CA, et al. (2008) Booster vaccination of cancer patients with MAGE-A3 protein reveals long-term immunological memory or tolerance depending on priming. Proc Natl Acad Sci USA 105(5): 1650–1655.

48. Corbière V, Chapiro J, Stroobant V, Ma W, Lurquin C, et al. (2011) Antigen spreading contributes to MAGE vaccination-induced regression of melanoma metastases. Cancer Res 71(4): 1253–1262.

49. Lally KM, Mocellin S, Ohnmacht GA, Nielsen MB, Bettinotti M, et al. (2001) Unmasking cryptic epitopes after loss of immunodominant tumor antigen expression through epitope spreading. Int J Cancer 93(6): 841–847.

2

EGFRvIII-Specific Chimeric Antigen Receptor T Cells Migrate to and Kill Tumor Deposits Infiltrating the Brain Parenchyma in an Invasive Xenograft Model of Glioblastoma

Hongsheng Miao[1], Bryan D. Choi[1,2], Carter M. Suryadevara[1], Luis Sanchez-Perez[1], Shicheng Yang[1], Gabriel De Leon[1,3], Elias J. Sayour[1,2], Roger McLendon[2,4], James E. Herndon II[5], Patrick Healy[5], Gary E. Archer[1,2,4], Darell D. Bigner[1,2,4], Laura A. Johnson[1,4¤], John H. Sampson[1,2,4*]

1 Duke Brain Tumor Immunotherapy Program, Division of Neurosurgery, Department of Surgery, Duke University Medical Center, Durham, North Carolina, United States of America, 2 Department of Pathology, Duke University Medical Center, Durham, North Carolina, United States of America, 3 Department of Molecular Cancer Biology, Duke University Medical Center, Durham, North Carolina, United States of America, 4 The Preston Robert Tisch Brain Tumor Center, Duke University Medical Center, Durham, North Carolina, United States of America, 5 Department of Biostatistics and Bioinformatics, Duke University Medical Center, Durham, North Carolina, United States of America

Abstract

Glioblastoma (GBM) is the most common primary malignant brain tumor in adults and is uniformly lethal. T-cell-based immunotherapy offers a promising platform for treatment given its potential to specifically target tumor tissue while sparing the normal brain. However, the diffuse and infiltrative nature of these tumors in the brain parenchyma may pose an exceptional hurdle to successful immunotherapy in patients. Areas of invasive tumor are thought to reside behind an intact blood brain barrier, isolating them from effective immunosurveillance and thereby predisposing the development of "immunologically silent" tumor peninsulas. Therefore, it remains unclear if adoptively transferred T cells can migrate to and mediate regression in areas of invasive GBM. One barrier has been the lack of a preclinical mouse model that accurately recapitulates the growth patterns of human GBM in vivo. Here, we demonstrate that D-270 MG xenografts exhibit the classical features of GBM and produce the diffuse and invasive tumors seen in patients. Using this model, we designed experiments to assess whether T cells expressing third-generation chimeric antigen receptors (CARs) targeting the tumor-specific mutation of the epidermal growth factor receptor, EGFRvIII, would localize to and treat invasive intracerebral GBM. EGFRvIII-targeted CAR (EGFRvIII+ CAR) T cells demonstrated in vitro EGFRvIII antigen-specific recognition and reactivity to the D-270 MG cell line, which naturally expresses EGFRvIII. Moreover, when administered systemically, EGFRvIII+ CAR T cells localized to areas of invasive tumor, suppressed tumor growth, and enhanced survival of mice with established intracranial D-270 MG tumors. Together, these data demonstrate that systemically administered T cells are capable of migrating to the invasive edges of GBM to mediate antitumor efficacy and tumor regression.

Editor: Maria G. Castro, University of Michigan School of Medicine, United States of America

Funding: This work was supported by grants from the National Institutes of Health: 1R01CA177476-01 (J.H. Sampson), 5R01-CA135272-05 (J.H. Sampson), 5P50-NS020023- 30 (D.D. Bigner and J.H. Sampson), 3R25-NS065731-03S1 (J.H. Sampson), 1F30CA177152-01 (B.D. Choi). Additional support was provided by the Pediatric Brain Tumor Foundation (D.D. Bigner and J.H. Sampson), Ben and Catherine Ivy Foundation (J.H. Sampson), Voices Against Brain Cancer (L.A. Johnson), American Brain Tumor Association (L.A. Johnson), and Duke Cancer Institute (J.H. Sampson and B.D. Choi). The funders had no role in study design, data collection and analysis, decision to publish, or preparation of the manuscript.

Competing Interests: The authors have declared that no competing interests exist.

* E-mail: john.sampson@duke.edu

¤ Current address: Translational Research Program, Abramson Family Cancer Research Institute, Perelman School of Medicine, University of Pennsylvania, Philadelphia, Pennsylvania, United States of America

Introduction

Glioblastoma (GBM) is the most common form of primary malignant brain tumor in adults and remains one of the most deadly neoplasms. Despite multimodal therapy including maximal surgical resection, radiation, and temozolomide (TMZ), the median overall survival is less than 15 months [1]. Moreover, these therapies are non-specific and are ultimately limited by toxicity to normal tissues [2]. In contrast, immunotherapy promises an exquisitely precise approach, and substantial evidence suggests that T cells can eradicate large, well-established tumors in mice and humans [3–7].

Chimeric antigen receptors (CARs) represent an emerging technology that combines the variable region of an antibody with T-cell signaling moieties, and can be genetically expressed in T cells to mediate potent, antigen-specific activation. CAR T cells carry the potential to eradicate neoplasms by recognizing tumor cells regardless of major histocompatibility complex (MHC) presentation of target antigen or MHC downregulation in tumors, factors which allow tumor-escape from treatment with ex vivo expanded tumor-infiltrating lymphocytes (TILs) [8] and T-cell receptor (TCR) gene therapy [9,10]. Clinical trials utilizing CARs in other tumor systems including renal cell carcinoma [11], indolent B-cell and mantle cell lymphoma [12], neuroblastoma [13], acute lymphoblastic leukemia [14], and chronic lymphoid leukemia [15] have verified their remarkable potential. However, severe adverse events, including patient deaths, have occurred from administration of CAR T cells when directed against tumor antigens simultaneously expressed on normal tissues [16,17].

The tumor-specific variant of the epidermal growth factor receptor, EGFRvIII, is a type III in-frame deletion mutant of the wild-type receptor that is exclusively expressed on the cell surface of GBMs and other neoplasms but is absent on normal tissues [18–20]. Unlike previous CARs, an EGFRvIII-specific construct carries the potential to eliminate tumor cells without damaging normal tissue due to the tumor specificity of its target antigen. Thus, as a tumor-specific CAR, EGFRvIII-targeted CARs (EGFRvIII⁺ CARs) should be able to employ the previously demonstrated potency of CAR T cells both precisely and safely against tumor when implemented into the clinic.

Despite their promise, the utility of CAR therapy against brain tumors has been questioned due to the concept of central nervous system (CNS) immune privilege. This dogma has since been challenged, as T cells are now known to infiltrate CNS parenchyma in the context of neuropathology and neuroinflammation where the blood brain barrier (BBB) is known to be disrupted [21,22]. GBM in particular has been implicated in BBB dysfunction through its modulation of the local brain microenvironment, owing in part to both the inevitable disruption of natural brain architecture by bulky tumor masses and their inherent pathologic characteristics that increase the permeability of microvessels, thereby compromising BBB integrity [23]. While it is reasonable to suspect that T cells and chemotherapeutic agents may gain entry to tumor cores through these regions of increased permeability, the long-term therapeutic benefits of this rationale have been marred by the fact that GBM is predisposed to the development of highly invasive neoplastic peninsulas that are removed from main tumor masses, residing within normal brain areas that are protected by regions of intact BBB [24–26]. This may explain the failure of therapeutic regimens that depend on BBB permeability for targeted treatment delivery, where main tumor cores are discriminately subjected to therapy while invasive tumor cells are able to evade clinical intervention and tumor recurrence becomes inevitable [27].

It recent years, preclinical evaluations of GBM therapy have correlated only poorly with their clinical counterpart [28], and it has been increasingly difficult to reconcile this apparent discrepancy in efficacy. One explanation may be the lack of a suitable preclinical GBM model in which tumor engraftment adequately mimics the invasive features and physiological growth patterns found in the clinical scenario. Human tumor xenografts are often criticized due to their production of large, well-circumscribed, non-invasive intracranial masses (e.g. U87MG [29–31]), characteristics that impede their use as an adequate platform for evaluating novel therapies against GBM. Thus, identifying a preclinical model that accurately recapitulates human GBM is a critical first step to evaluating the efficacy of novel therapies designed to target highly invasive gliomas arising *de novo* in the brain.

To address these issues in the current study, we developed a model system to examine the efficacy of CAR T-cell therapy using a brain tumor explant that more precisely reflects clinically relevant growth patterns of GBM. D-270 MG is a tumor line derived directly from a patient's primary GBM by direct orthotopic transplant and is known to naturally express EGFRvIII [32]. In order to monitor the *in vivo* efficacy of EGFRvIII⁺ CAR T cells against D-270 MG intracranial xenografts, we produced a cell line that co-expresses firefly luciferase (FLuc) and GFP, D-270MG^FLuc/GFP, which retains the pathological features of human GBM and displays homogeneous levels of EGFRvIII expression. Here, we present data to demonstrate that D-270MG^FLuc/GFP xenografts display the invasive nature and hallmark characteristics of human GBM, making it an ideal preclinical model for the evaluation of this CAR-based strategy. We show that EGFRvIII⁺ CAR T cells are capable of recognizing D-270MG^FLuc/GFP cells in an antigen-specific manner *in vitro* and are capable of migrating into the invasive edges of intracerebral D-270MG^FLuc/GFP tumors in NOD.Cg-*Prkdc^scid Il2rg^tm1Wjl*/SzJ (NSG) mice. Importantly, our results indicate that treatment of D-270MG^FLuc/GFP tumors with EGFRvIII⁺ CAR T cells significantly inhibited tumor growth and prolonged survival in NSG mice. Taken together, these observations in our novel model system demonstrate that adoptively transferred EGFRvIII⁺ CAR T cells can readily traffic *in vivo* to the invasive edges of GBM to mediate antigen-specific tumor regression.

Results

D-270MG^FLuc/GFP xenograft is highly invasive in NSG mice

In order to evaluate the antitumor efficacy of systemically delivered EGFRvIII⁺ CAR T cells against invasive intracerebral GBM tumors, we utilized the D-270MG^FLuc/GFP xenograft, which was isolated directly from a patient's primary GBM tumor and has been previously validated to naturally express EGFRvIII [20,32]. We first sought to histologically evaluate and compare the characteristic growth patterns of D-270MG^FLuc/GFP tumor with U87MG.ΔEGFR, a xenograft derived from a previously described human glioma cell subline [33,34] that is among the most frequently used models in preclinical studies of GBM. U87MG.ΔEGFR is an EGFRvIII⁺ stably transfected subline of the parental human malignant astrocytoma cell line U87MG, which does not naturally express EGFRvIII. NSG mice received intracerebral tumor implants and were sacrificed after seven days. Brains were formalin-fixed, paraffin-embedded, and 5 μm sections were stained with hematoxylin and eosin (H&E). NSG mice with no tumors were used as a control (**Fig. 1a**). Here, we show that U87MG.ΔEGFR xenografts produce tumors with well-defined boundaries that can be clearly delineated from normal brain (**Fig. 1b, c**). In stark contrast, D-270MG^FLuc/GFP tumors exhibit expanding borders with small perivascular streams of cells radiating from central tumor masses, and even subarachnoid infiltration of tumor cells (**Fig. 1d, e, f**). We found that D-270MG^FLuc/GFP xenografts reveal an invasive nodular proliferation of malignant cells with reduced eosinophilic cytoplasm and large nuclei with prominent nucleoli. We also observed focal areas of necrosis and frequent mitotic activity in tumors. Altogether, these data demonstrate that the *in vivo* phenotype of D-270MG^FLuc/GFP xenografts is consistent with the classic features of human GBM. Moreover, the *in vivo* growth patterns of this model recapitulate the diffuse and infiltrative nature of tumors found in patients, making D-270MG^FLuc/GFP an exemplary model for evaluating this CAR-based platform.

T cells expressing EGFRvIII⁺ CARs recognize D-270MG^FLuc/GFP tumors that naturally express EGFRvIII

Effective T-cell recognition and antitumor activity requires antigen-specific receptor expression and engagement of tumorigenic antigens. Therefore, we sought to determine if EGFRvIII⁺

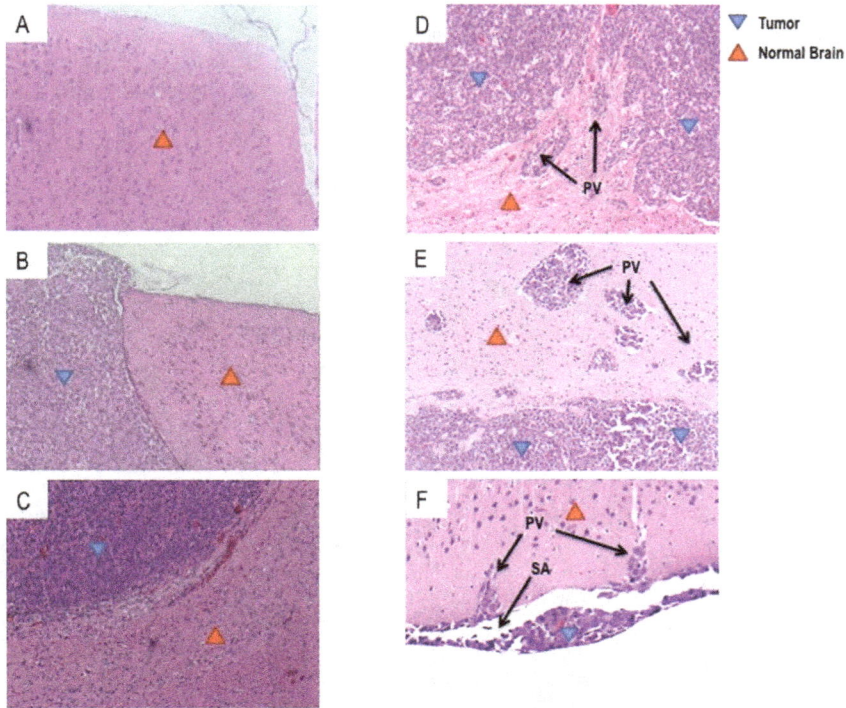

Figure 1. D-270MG$^{FLuc/GFP}$ xenograft is highly invasive in NSG mice. NSG mice received intracerebral tumor implants (D-270MG$^{FLuc/GFP}$/ 1×10^4 cells or U87MG.ΔEGFR/1×10^4 cells) and were sacrificed after seven days. Histological analysis by H&E staining of (**a**) non-tumor bearing brain, (**b, c**) established U87MG.ΔEGFR and (**d, e, f**) D-270MG$^{FLuc/GFP}$ intracerebral malignant gliomas in NSG mice is shown. Figures delineate tumor vs. normal brain and demonstrate perivascular (PV) and subarachnoid (SA) infiltration. Images are representative of tumors obtained and analyzed from six mice (n = 6). x20 magnification.

CAR T cells would recognize D-270MG$^{FLuc/GFP}$ tumor cells, given their natural expression of EGFRvIII. Towards this end, we obtained human peripheral blood lymphocytes (PBLs) from patients and transduced them with a previously-described retrovirus encoding a third-generation EGFRvIII$^+$ CAR containing the humanized 139 anti-human EGFRvIII single-chain variable fragment in tandem with the hCD28-41BB-CD3æ chain signaling domain [35]. Following transduction, we determined surface expression by flow cytometry, and T cells were found to efficiently express the EGFRvIII$^+$ CAR construct on their cell surface (**Fig. 2a**). In order to assess antigen-specificity of EGFRvIII$^+$ CAR T cells, we first quantitatively assessed levels of EGFRvIII expression in D-270MG$^{FLuc/GFP}$, U87MG.ΔEGFR (EGFRvIII$^+$), and U87MG (EGFRvIII$^-$) control tumor cells. We found similar levels of EGFRvIII expression between D-270MG$^{FLuc/GFP}$ and U87MG.ΔEGFR tumor cells (**Fig. 2b**). Next, antigen-specific reactivity against EGFRvIII was determined in co-culture assays; while EGFRvIII$^+$ CAR T cells did not secrete observable levels of the type 1 cytokine interferon-gamma (IFN-γ) in response to the U87MG (EGFRvIII$^-$) tumor cell line, they did produce IFN-γ in the presence of the U87MG.ΔEGFR (EGFR-vIII$^+$) cell line as measured by intracellular staining (ICS) (**Fig. 2c; P = 0.0004;** two-way ANOVA). Untransduced T cells alone showed no IFN-γ production versus either target. Importantly, recognition of the D-270MG$^{FLuc/GFP}$ cell line was observed only by EGFRvIII$^+$ CAR T cells and not by untransduced T cells (**Fig. 2d;** P = 0.002; one-way ANOVA). These data corroborate the specificity of EGFRvIII$^+$ CAR T cells and demonstrate their ability to elicit antitumor activity upon interaction with D-270MG$^{FLuc/GFP}$ tumors.

EGFRvIII$^+$ CAR T cells effectively migrate to invasive GBM tumors

Effective therapy in a clinical setting requires that systemically administered T cells effectively migrate to and encounter tumor cells *in vivo*. Unlike cancers of the periphery, GBM tumors rarely metastasize outside of the brain, instead shedding neoplastic cells that migrate away from main tumor cores and develop into highly invasive peninsulas residing within the normal brain, hiding within regions of intact BBB [24–26]. Although T cells are able to access bulky GBM lesions through dysfunction of the local BBB, it is unknown if they can effectively migrate into the invading tumor deposits that may reside behind an intact BBB. Therefore, we sought to evaluate the capacity of EGFRvIII$^+$ CAR T cells to localize to D-270MG$^{FLuc/GFP}$ intracerebral tumors, which closely mirror the invasive architecture of human GBM (**Fig. 1d–f**). To examine this, human donor PBLs were transduced with the external *Gaussian* luciferase (extGLuc) retrovirus or underwent a dual transduction with both the extGLuc and EGFRvIII$^+$ CAR retroviruses for use in bioluminescence imaging (BLI) analysis [36]. Following transduction, T cells were cultured *in vitro* prior to systemic infusion into NSG mice bearing established orthotopic D-270MG$^{FLuc/GFP}$ tumors. Imaging analysis two (**Fig. 3a**) and nine (**Fig. 3b**) days after T-cell injection revealed extGLuc signals in the brain area, demonstrating localization of EGFRvIII$^+$ CAR T cells to the tumor site. We also sought to evaluate whether EGFRvIII-specificity was necessary for efficient T-cell localization to tumor, and to do this, we compared the trafficking patterns of extGluc$^+$ EGFRvIII$^+$ T cells (**Fig. 3a,b**) with extGluc$^+$ T cells (**Fig. 3c,d**) in NSG mice bearing D-270MG$^{FLuc/GFP}$ tumors. We found that extGluc-only T cells (EGFRvIII$^-$) failed to efficiently

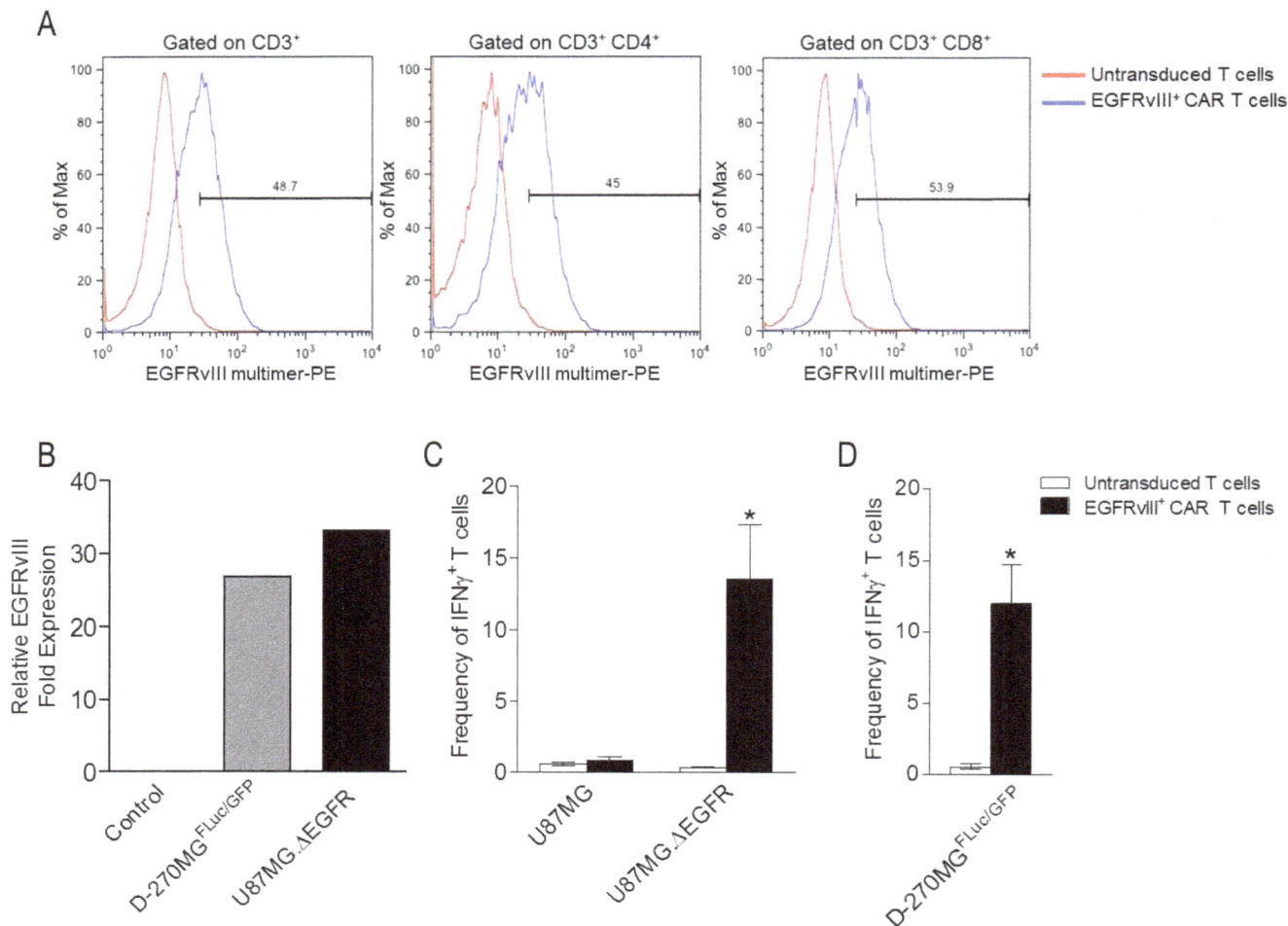

Figure 2. T cells expressing EGFRvIII⁺ CARs recognize D-270MG^{FLuc/GFP} tumors that naturally express EGFRvIII. (a) Cells were stained for EGFRvIII⁺ CARs to detect cell-surface expression using EGFRvIII multimer-PE. Negative staining controls were conducted by staining untransduced T cells from the same donor. EGFRvIII CAR⁺ T cells were gated on CD3⁺ (left), CD3⁺ CD4⁺ (middle), and CD3⁺ CD8⁺ (right). (**b**) Expression levels of EGFRvIII were quantified in D-270MG^{FLuc/GFP} and U87MG.ΔEGFR tumor cells using qRT PCR. U87MG (EGFRvIII⁻) tumor cells were used as a control. (**c**) In order to assess EGFRvIII specificity, untransduced T cells or EGFRvIII⁺ CAR T cells were co-cultured with U87MG or U87MG.ΔEGFR tumor cells. Quantification of cells positive for ICS of IFN-γ⁺ is shown. The effect of T-cell transduction on frequency of IFN-γ⁺ cells significantly differs between U87MG and U87MG.ΔEGFR tumor cells ($P = 0.0004$; two-way ANOVA). (**c**) To evaluate D-270MG^{FLuc/GFP} tumor cell recognition, untransduced T cells or EGFRvIII⁺ CAR T cells were co-cultured with D-270MG^{FLuc/GFP}. Quantification of cells positive for ICS of IFN-γ⁺ is shown. The effect of T-cell transduction on frequency of IFN-γ⁺ cells significantly differs between untransduced T cells and EGFRvIII⁺ CAR T cells ($P = 0.002$; one-way ANOVA). EGFRvIII⁺ CAR T cells were also cultured alone (no target) as a control, and quantification of cells positive for ICS of IFN-γ⁺ was negligible (data not shown). Data represent one of two ($n = 2$) experiments with similar results.

migrate across the BBB, whereas extGluc⁺ EGFRvIII⁺ CAR T cells rapidly localized in the brain. This suggests a necessity of EGFRvIII⁺ CAR expression for brain-trafficking or accumulation in NSG mice bearing D-270MG^{FLuc/GFP} tumors. A separate group of mice were also sacrificed nine days after T-cell injection and tumor tissue was submitted for immunohistochemical analysis. **Figure 3E** shows that systemically administered EGFRvIII⁺ CAR T cells successfully migrated to the invasive edges of intracerebral tumor, particularly in areas of peninsula formation at the leading edge of tumor invasion. NSG mice receiving saline were used as a control (**Fig. 3F**). These results demonstrate that, in our model of invasive GBM, adoptively transferred EGFRvIII⁺ CAR T cells have the capacity to traffic to invasive areas of tumor thought to reside beyond the BBB.

In vivo systemic delivery of EGFRvIII⁺ CAR T cells delays tumor growth and prolongs survival

We sought to determine the therapeutic effect of systemically administered EGFRvIII⁺ CAR T cells against invasive intracerebral gliomas *in vivo*. Utilizing the NSG mouse model, D-270MG^{FLuc/GFP} xenografts were implanted intracerebrally and allowed to engraft for three days prior to intravenous infusion with EGFRvIII⁺ CAR T cells. D-270MG^{FLuc/GFP} cells were monitored using BLI every three days. No significant difference was observed between groups of mice that were either left untreated or infused with non-specific control CAR T cells. However, there was a significant delay in tumor growth in EGFRvIII⁺ CAR T-cell treatment groups compared to untreated and control CAR T cells, as detected by serial BLI recordings of tumor-cell photon emissions (**Fig. 4a**; $P < 0.0001$; mixed model). Tumors were not visible in any group until day 11, at which point tumors began growing in

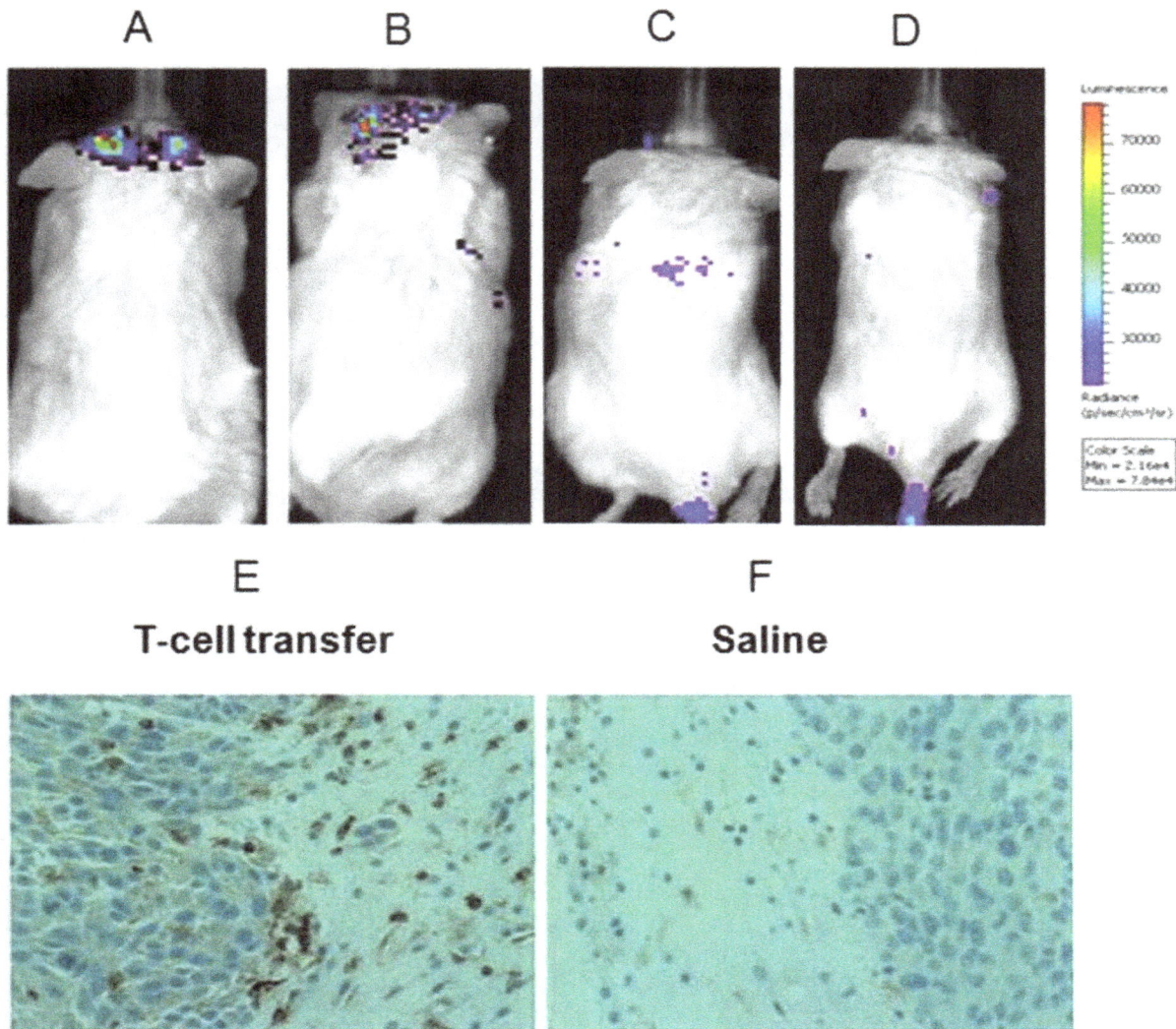

Figure 3. EGFRvIII⁺ CAR T cells effectively migrate to invasive GBM tumors. 1×10^7 extGLuc⁺ EGFRvIII⁺ CAR T cells were administered systemically to D-270MG$^{FLuc/GFP}$ tumor-bearing mice, and T-cell trafficking and/or accumulation near tumor was monitored using BLI on days 2 (**a**) and 9 (**b**). To assess the role of antigen-specificity on T-cell localization at the site of tumor, 1×10^7 extGLuc-only T cells were systemically administered to a separate group of tumor-bearing mice and monitored for trafficking and/or accumulation near tumor using BLI on day 7 (**c, d**). NSG mice treated with extGLuc⁺ EGFRvIII⁺ CAR T cells (**e**) or saline (**f**) were sacrificed on day 9, and brains were harvested, formalin-fixed, and paraffin-embedded. 5 μm coronal sections were immunostained with rabbit anti-human CD3 antibody and counterstained with hematoxylin. Images are representative of tumors obtained and analyzed from four mice (n = 4). Data represent one of two (n = 2) experiments with similar results.

control and untreated mice. Complete suppression of tumor growth was evident in mice treated with EGFRvIII⁺ CAR T cells until day 17, but grew to achieve BLI values similar to untreated mice by day 26 (**Fig. 4a**). These growth kinetics translated into an 8–9 day survival advantage in mice treated with EGFRvIII⁺ CAR T cells when compared to both untreated mice and those receiving control CAR T cells (**Fig. 4b**; P<0.0001; generalized Wilcoxon test). Together, these preclinical results suggest that systemically administered third-generation EGFRvIII⁺ CAR T cells can inhibit invasive brain tumor growth and prolong survival.

Discussion

The therapeutic benefits of CAR-based adoptive cell therapy have been widely demonstrated in patients suffering with cancer [7,13–15]. Since its introduction, CAR design has evolved

significantly to mediate a potent and robust T-cell immune response when directed against tumors in the periphery [6,37]. Importantly, we demonstrate here that similar immune responses can be achieved against established tumors in the immunologically privileged brain, even when directed against highly invasive cancers that are considered prone to immune evasion. The molecular properties and phenotype of GBM make it an extraordinarily difficult malignancy to treat from an immunologic perspective. Its invasive nature behind the BBB could confer a relatively high degree of isolation from immune activity, allowing tumors to grow silently with limited immune surveillance. Unlike previous studies, we have sought to examine the efficacy of adoptive T-cell therapy using the D-270MG$^{FLuc/GFP}$ xenograft, which we demonstrate possesses diffuse intraparenchymal and perivascular invasion, consistent with the histopathological hallmarks of human GBM. Furthermore, unlike cell lines engineered

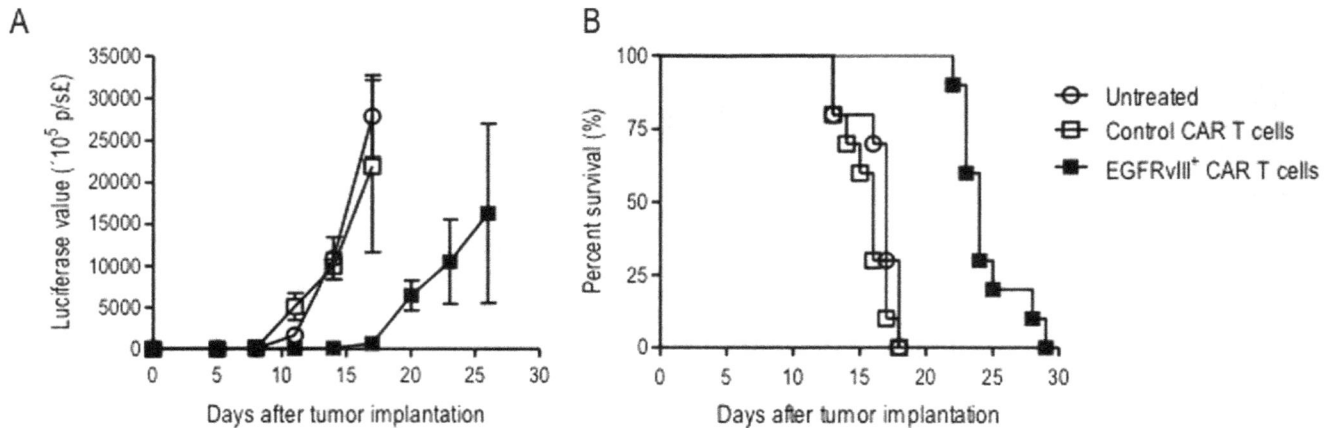

Figure 4. *In vivo* **systemic delivery of EGFRvIII⁺ CAR T cells delays tumor growth and prolongs survival.** NSG mice were implanted with 1×10^4 D-270MG$^{FLuc/GFP}$ tumor cells intracranially, randomized into three groups (n = 6-8), and monitored for tumor growth and survival. $5.0 - 10 \times 10^6$ T cells were administered intravenously 3 days after tumor implantation. (**a**) Normalized BLI values associated with longitudinal monitoring of tumor growth for untreated, control CAR T-cell, and EGFRvIII⁺ CAR T-cell groups are shown (value = mean ± SD). The pattern of change in log BLI values significantly differs between the three treatment groups (P<0.0001; mixed model). (**b**) The survival of animals treated with EGFRvIII⁺ CAR T cells was significantly prolonged (P<0.0001; generalized Wilcoxon test) when compared to other treatment groups. Data represent one of two (n = 2) experiments with similar results.

to express EGFRvIII, such as U87MG.ΔEGFR, D-270 MG was isolated from a primary tumor that naturally expressed EGFRvIII and has maintained expression *ex vivo* and *in vivo*. This lends greater credence to its more accurate recapitulation of the clinical scenario.

We demonstrate here that EGFRvIII⁺ CAR T cells recognize tumors naturally expressing EGFRvIII, such as D-270MG$^{FLuc/GFP}$. We show that these EGFRvIII⁺ CAR T cells recognize tumor cells in an antigen-specific manner *in vitro* as measured by ICS (**Fig. 2c, d**). It is important to note that we measured a 10–15% frequency of IFN-γ⁺ cells in our *in vitro* ICS assays, which is less than our recorded frequency of CD3⁺ CAR⁺ T cells. This has been a consistent and expected result under the culture, transduction, and assay protocols described here. One explanation may be the varied differentiation states of CD3⁺ CAR⁺ T cells, since different stages of activation can alter the incubation time required for T-cell secretion of IFN-γ. We have found that longer incubation times (greater than the 18 h described here) and altered tumor : T cell ratios yield frequencies> 50%, and we suspect that this is due to the inclusion of more cells occupying a greater spectrum of activation. However, we chose the assay conditions described here since incubation times>18 h decrease cell viability, and 18 h incubations have yielded consistent results to date [38].

Our data show that systemically delivered EGFRvIII⁺ CAR T cells have the capacity to migrate to invasive tumor deposits within the CNS. T-cell migration across endothelium requires molecular cues provided by chemokine-chemokine receptor interaction and engagement of adhesion molecules, which are thought to be independent of TCR engagement [39,40]. The cross-reactivity of murine adhesion molecules and chemokines with human T cells and their chemokine receptors is known to be limited [41], and although this could have negatively impacted T-cell localization, we instead observed a substantial influx of T cells into the invasive tumor. We are currently evaluating the contribution of tumor-derived human chemokines and EGFRvIII-specificity on CAR T cells to further elucidate the steps required for effective T-cell migration across the BBB in the invasive areas of GBM.

Importantly, we show here that systemically administered EGFRvIII⁺ CAR T cells have the capacity to inhibit tumor

growth and prolong survival of mice with established D-270MG$^{FLuc/GFP}$ tumors (**Fig. 4a, b**). Despite the evidence of an effective, antigen-specific immune response, it is important to note that brain tumors ultimately continued to grow and caused death even in mice receiving EGFRvIII⁺ CAR T cells (**Fig. 4b**). Normalized BLI values from these treated mice eventually reached comparable values to untreated and CAR control groups, indicating tumor growth after a period of dormancy likely mediated by antitumor T-cell activity (**Fig. 4a**). One possible explanation is the loss or functional loss of EGFRvIII⁺ CAR T cells in this model. To test the antitumor efficacy of EGFRvIII⁺ CAR T cells *in vivo*, we chose an NSG mouse model, which has the advantage of evaluating promising preclinical therapies in an animal system using human tumor tissue. However, one major drawback of this approach is the fact that human T cells often have a limited lifespan and functional half-life in the murine background. For this reason, we sought to monitor T-cell persistence over time *in vivo* by BLI analysis. However, we unexpectedly found the administration of coelenterazine to be toxic at the manufacturer's recommended dosage, and as such, terminated BLI measurements after day 9 (**Fig. 3a, b**). Our studies demonstrate that, despite this potential for CAR T cell loss, EGFRvIII⁺ CAR T cells were able to persist long enough to migrate to and mediate antitumor activity against invasive intracranial tumors. We are currently evaluating host conditioning regimens to support enhanced and long-term human T-cell survival and function in NSG mice, since these factors could, in theory, potentiate antitumor efficacy.

A second possible explanation for the eventual recurrence of tumor in our model is the concept of antigen-loss, wherein therapeutic pressure selects for tumor cells that do not express the target antigen. This explanation would be consistent with two recent clinical studies where recurrence in patients treated with CARs [42] or a vaccine targeting a single antigen [43] was characterized by outgrowth of antigen-loss variants. As such, given the theoretical limitations of targeting single tumor antigens, future efforts will likely focus on the identification of additional GBM-specific targets and multimodal therapies designed to target several antigens simultaneously through CAR-mediated or alternative

T-cell-based approaches. Additional areas of further investigation may include determining factors involved in eliciting broader endogenous immune responses through mechanisms such as epitope spreading, which has emerged as a critical factor during clinical trials of immunotherapy for melanoma [44].

In the current study, we have demonstrated that systemically administered and tumor-specific EGFRvIII$^+$ CAR T cells effectively migrate to areas of tumor invasion and mediate efficacy in a murine model of invasive human glioma. This work contributes to the rapidly growing literature supporting the utility of adoptively transferred CAR T cells targeting tumor-specific antigens as a potent treatment modality for invasive brain tumors.

Materials and Methods

Human GBM cell lines and xenografts

We utilized the previously described human glioma cell line, U87MG [29–31], which does not express EGFRvIII, and subline U87MG.ΔEGFR [33,34], which was stably transfected to express EGFRvIII. We also utilized the D-270 MG cell line, which was propagated directly as a xenograft from a primary human GBM harvested from a patient and has previously been shown to naturally express EGFRvIII [20,32]. Briefly, mechanically minced tumor tissue was enzymatically dissociated into single cells using the Papain Dissociation System. After wash, tissue was homogenized and passed through a 75 μm cell strainer, re-suspended with freezing medium containing 90% fetal bovine serum (FBS) and 10% dimethyl sulfoxide and frozen in individual vials using standard procedures. For further experimentation, cells were thawed at 37°C, washed, and counted with trypan blue per standard practice.

Animals

NSG mice were obtained (Charles River Laboratories, Wilmington, MA) and bred under standard conditions at Duke University Medical Center (DUMC). Mice were kept and utilized under the accordance of protocols approved by the Duke University Institutional Animal Care and Use Committee (IACUC). All mice used in this study were healthy females between 6–8 weeks of age weighing 0.020–0.025 kg and were randomized to experimental or control groups. Mice were routinely monitored for health (every 2 days) and qualified for euthanasia if they demonstrated an inability to ambulate to food and water (i.e. in lateral recumbency and unable to right itself), or if they were unable to move forward two steps when prompted gently by touching a finger to the hind area. Moribund mice were humanely euthanized when they met these endpoints using CO_2 asphyxiation followed by decapitation as approved by our Duke University IACUC protocol. In accordance with this protocol, mice did not receive any analgesics or anesthetics.

Human PBLs

Human PBLs used in this study were obtained from normal volunteers at Duke University Medical Center. The use of PBLs was approved under protocol 0009043 by the Duke University School of Medicine Institutional Review Board (irb.mc.duke.edu). Approved protocols conform to the Declaration of Helsinki protocols. All patients signed a written informed consent. PBLs were cultured in AIM-V medium (Life Technologies, Grand Island, NY) supplemented with 10% human AB serum (Valley Biomedical Inc., Winchester, VA), 50 units/mL penicillin, 50 μg/mL streptomycin (Life Technologies, Grand Island, CA) and 300 IU/mL interleukin-2 (IL-2) and maintained at 37°C with 5% CO_2.

EGFRvIII$^+$ CARs and extGLuc retroviral vector transduction

The extGLuc retroviral vectors were supplied by Renier Brentjens of Memorial Sloan-Kettering Cancer Center, New York, NY. The EGFRvIII$^+$ CAR and extGLuc retroviral vectors were utilized to generate EGFRvIII$^+$ CAR T cells and exGluc$^+$ EGFRvIII$^+$ CAR T cells. The transduction procedures have previously been described [36,45,46]. Briefly, peripheral blood mononuclear cells (PBMCs) from healthy donors and GBM patients (post-resection, prior to treatment) were thawed and cultured in AIM-V medium supplemented with 5% human AB serum, plus antibiotics, 300 IU/mL IL-2, and 50 ng/mL OKT-3. After 48 hours, T cells (0.25×10^6/mL) were transduced with a retroviral supernatant containing either the extGLuc, EGFRvIII$^+$ CAR, or both vectors spun onto RetroNectin (Takara Bio Inc, Japan) coated non-tissue culture treated 6-well plates twice on two consecutive days as described by the manufacturer. Transduced cells were allowed to expand in AIM-V medium as above, without OKT-3.

Rapid Expansion Protocol

Transduced PBLs (or untransduced control PBLs from same donor) were expanded *in vitro* using rapid expansion protocol (REP) [47]. Briefly, T cells were cultured in complete AIM-V medium plus 10% human AB serum, 300 IU/mL IL-2, and 50 ng/mL OKT-3 in the presence of 100x excess 5000 rads irradiated allogeneic PBMC feeder cells, and allowed to expand 10–14 days.

Lentiviral transduction of D-270 MG with firefly-luciferase-GFP gene

The D-270 MG tumor cell line was transduced with a lentiviral vector encoding the firefly luciferase (FLuc) and EGFP genes linked by 2A peptide driven by an internal murine stem cell virus (MSCV) promoter. Briefly, lentiviral vectors were generated by transient transfection of HEK 293T cells with a four-plasmid system [48]. Six hours post-transfection, plates were washed twice with phosphate-buffered saline (PBS) and 20 mL fresh medium was added. The supernatant was collected 30–48 hours post-transfection and cell debris was removed by centrifugation at 6000 g for 10 minutes, followed by filtration on 0.45 μm polyvinylidene fluoride filters. The lentiviral supernatant was kept at −80°C. D-270 MG cells were then quickly thawed at 37°C, washed, counted with trypan blue, and re-suspended in the lentiviral supernatant and zinc medium with 10% FBS and incubated at 37°C with 5% CO_2 overnight. D-270MG$^{FLuc/GFP}$ tumor cells were cell sorted based on GFP expression. Expression of FLuc was confirmed by data acquisition using the IVIS 100 *in vivo* BLI system (Caliper Life Sciences, Hopkinton, MA) coupled with Living Image software (PerkinElmer, Waltham, MA). EGFRvIII expression levels by D-270MG$^{FLuc/GFP}$ and U87MG.ΔEGFR tumor cells were measured by qRT PCR as previously described [49].

Cell surface CAR expression and ICS of transduced T cells

Cells were stained for EGFRvIII$^+$ CARs to detect cell-surface expression using an EGFRvIII multimer-PE as previously described [50]. Negative staining controls were conducted by staining untransduced cells from the same donor. ICS was performed by co-culturing T cells with tumors 1:1 over 18 hours with the BD GolgiPlug protein transport inhibitor containing brefeldin A (BD Sciences, San Jose, CA) in RPMI-1640 medium plus 10% FBS. Following co-culture, cells were submitted to surface staining for CD3, CD8 and intracellular IFN-γ stain using the BD Cytofix/Cytoperm method (BD Biosciences, San Jose, CA).

Monitoring tumor growth and T-cell trafficking using BLI

To monitor tumor growth, 24 NSG mice underwent intracranial implantation of 1×10^4 D-270MG$^{FLuc/GFP}$ tumor cells in 5 μl PBS and methocell mixer using stereotactic coordinates 2 mm lateral and 4 mm intraparenchymal from the bregma on experimental day 0. Tumor growth was analyzed every three to five days for 26 days by BLI as previously described [51] until the study was terminated. Briefly, BLI was performed by injecting mice intraperitoneally with 150 mg D-luciferin/kg (Xenogen, Hopkinton, MA) 10 minutes prior to imaging and photon emission (photons s^{-1} cm^{-2} sr^{-1}) was recorded. To monitor T-cell trafficking, T cells were transduced with the extGLuc or co-transduced with the EGFRvIII$^+$ CAR and extGLuc retroviral vectors as described above (see *EGFRvIII$^+$ CARs and extGLuc retroviral vector transduction*). Mice receiving T cells were injected with $5.0 - 10\times10^6$ cells intravenously via the tail vein and imaged on days 2 and 9 after infusion. Briefly, 250 μg coelenterazine (NanoLight Technology, Pinetop, AZ) was injected IV in mice receiving either saline or EGFRvIII$^+$ extGLuc$^+$ CAR T cells and imaged within 90 seconds by measuring BLI. We obtained image data sets and measurement of signal intensity by using the IVIS 100 *in vivo* BLI system and through region of interest analysis using Living Image Software with normalized images displayed on each data set according to color intensity. Mean BLI values for control and treatment groups were calculated and plotted according to the corresponding day of imaging.

H&E Staining and Immunohistochemistry

In order to evaluate tumor architecture and growth patterns, NSG mice received intracerebral tumor implants (D-270MG$^{FLuc/GFP}$/1×10^4 cells or U87MG.ΔEGFR/1×10^4 cells) and were sacrificed after seven days. Brains were harvested, formalin-fixed and paraffin-embedded. 5 μm sections were stained with H&E. To evaluate

T-cell migration to the invasive edge of tumor, we utilized two experimental groups, which included four tumor-bearing mice treated with saline or extGLuc$^+$ EGFRvIII$^+$ CAR 1×10^7 T cells. Mice were euthanized on day 9. Brains were harvested, formalin-fixed and paraffin-embedded. 5 μm coronal sections were immunostained with rabbit anti-human CD3 antibody (Thermo Lab Vision, Clone RM9107S) as recommended by the manufacturer at a 1:100 dilution and counterstained with hematoxylin.

Statistical methods

Statistical differences in group percentage cytotoxicity and bioluminescence were evaluated by either a one-way analysis of variance (ANOVA) model or a two-way ANOVA model with interaction. The Kaplan Meier estimator was used to generate survival curves, and differences between survival curves were calculated using a generalized Wilcoxon test. Patterns of change in normalized BLI values on the log scale over time were evaluated using a mixed model that included main effects for time and treatment group along with a time interaction with treatment group. This model accounted for within animal correlation of measurements by using a 1st degree autoregressive covariance structure.

Acknowledgments

We extend our gratitude to Steven A. Rosenberg and Richard A. Morgan of the Surgery Branch at the National Cancer Institute for providing us with the EGFRvIII$^+$ CAR construct and Renier J. Brentjens of Memorial Sloan-Kettering Cancer Center for providing us with the extGluc retrovirus used in this study. We also thank Alina Boesteanu for providing histology images of U87MG.ΔEGFR xenograft implants and David Snyder for his contribution to animal care.

Author Contributions

Conceived and designed the experiments: HM BDC CMS LSP GA DB LAJ JHS. Performed the experiments: HM LSP SY GD EJS. Analyzed the data: RM JEH PH. Contributed reagents/materials/analysis tools: LSP LAJ JHS. Wrote the paper: HM BDC LSP CMS LAJ.

References

1. Stupp R, Mason WP, van den Bent MJ, Weller M, Fisher B, et al. (2005) Radiotherapy plus concomitant and adjuvant temozolomide for glioblastoma. N Engl J Med 352: 987–996.
2. Imperato JP, Paleologos NA, Vick NA (1990) Effects of treatment on long-term survivors with malignant astrocytomas. Ann Neurol 28: 818–822.
3. Johnson LA, Morgan RA, Dudley ME, Cassard L, Yang JC, et al. (2009) Gene therapy with human and mouse T-cell receptors mediates cancer regression and targets normal tissues expressing cognate antigen. Blood 114: 535–546.
4. Hong JJ, Rosenberg SA, Dudley ME, Yang JC, White DE, et al. (2010) Successful treatment of melanoma brain metastases with adoptive cell therapy. Clin Cancer Res 16: 4892–4898.
5. Robbins PF, Morgan RA, Feldman SA, Yang JC, Sherry RM, et al. (2011) Tumor regression in patients with metastatic synovial cell sarcoma and melanoma using genetically engineered lymphocytes reactive with NY-ESO-1. J Clin Oncol 29: 917–924.
6. Rosenberg SA (2011) Cell transfer immunotherapy for metastatic solid cancer—what clinicians need to know. Nat Rev Clin Oncol 8: 577–585.
7. Kochenderfer JN, Dudley ME, Feldman SA, Wilson WH, Spaner DE, et al. (2012) B-cell depletion and remissions of malignancy along with cytokine-associated toxicity in a clinical trial of anti-CD19 chimeric-antigen-receptor-transduced T cells. Blood 119: 2709–2720.
8. Rosenberg SA, Yang JC, Robbins PF, Wunderlich JR, Hwu P, et al. (2003) Cell transfer therapy for cancer: lessons from sequential treatments of a patient with metastatic melanoma. J Immunother 26: 385–393.
9. Zitvogel L, Tesniere A, Kroemer G (2006) Cancer despite immunosurveillance: immunoselection and immunosubversion. Nat Rev Immunol 6: 715–727.
10. Kalos M, June CH (2013) Adoptive T cell transfer for cancer immunotherapy in the era of synthetic biology. Immunity 39: 49–60.
11. Lamers CH, Sleijfer S, Vulto AG, Kruit WH, Kliffen M, et al. (2006) Treatment of metastatic renal cell carcinoma with autologous T-lymphocytes genetically retargeted against carbonic anhydrase IX: first clinical experience. J Clin Oncol 24: e20–22.
12. Till BG, Jensen MC, Wang J, Qian X, Gopal AK, et al. (2012) CD20-specific adoptive immunotherapy for lymphoma using a chimeric antigen receptor with both CD28 and 4-1BB domains: pilot clinical trial results. Blood 119: 3940–3950.
13. Pule MA, Savoldo B, Myers GD, Rossig C, Russell HV, et al. (2008) Virus-specific T cells engineered to coexpress tumor-specific receptors: persistence and antitumor activity in individuals with neuroblastoma. Nat Med 14: 1264–1270.
14. Brentjens RJ, Davila ML, Riviere I, Park J, Wang X, et al. (2013) CD19-targeted T cells rapidly induce molecular remissions in adults with chemotherapy-refractory acute lymphoblastic leukemia. Sci Transl Med 5: 177ra138.
15. Porter DL, Levine BL, Kalos M, Bagg A, June CH (2011) Chimeric antigen receptor-modified T cells in chronic lymphoid leukemia. N Engl J Med 365: 725–733.
16. Brentjens R, Yeh R, Bernal Y, Riviere I, Sadelain M (2010) Treatment of chronic lymphocytic leukemia with genetically targeted autologous T cells: case report of an unforeseen adverse event in a phase I clinical trial. Mol Ther 18: 666–668.
17. Morgan RA, Yang JC, Kitano M, Dudley ME, Laurencot CM, et al. (2010) Case report of a serious adverse event following the administration of T cells transduced with a chimeric antigen receptor recognizing ERBB2. Mol Ther 18: 843–851.
18. Wikstrand CJ, Hale LP, Batra SK, Hill ML, Humphrey PA, et al. (1995) Monoclonal antibodies against EGFRvIII are tumor specific and react with breast and lung carcinomas and malignant gliomas. Cancer Res 55: 3140–3148.
19. Heimberger AB, Hlatky R, Suki D, Yang D, Weinberg J, et al. (2005) Prognostic effect of epidermal growth factor receptor and EGFRvIII in glioblastoma multiforme patients. Clin Cancer Res 11: 1462–1466.
20. Wong AJ, Ruppert JM, Bigner SH, Grzeschik CH, Humphrey PA, et al. (1992) Structural alterations of the epidermal growth factor receptor gene in human gliomas. Proc Natl Acad Sci U S A 89: 2965–2969.
21. Engelhardt B (2006) Molecular mechanisms involved in T cell migration across the blood-brain barrier. Journal of Neural Transmission 113: 477–485.

22. Banks WA, Erickson MA (2010) The blood-brain barrier and immune function and dysfunction. Neurobiology of Disease 37: 26–32.

23. Rascher G, Fischmann A, Kroger S, Duffner F, Grote EH, et al. (2002) Extracellular matrix and the blood-brain barrier in glioblastoma multiforme: spatial segregation of tenascin and agrin. Acta Neuropathol 104: 85–91.

24. Ajay D, Sanchez-Perez L, Choi BD, De Leon G, Sampson JH (2012) Immunotherapy with tumor vaccines for the treatment of malignant gliomas. Curr Drug Discov Technol 9: 237–255.

25. Claes A, Idema AJ, Wesseling P (2007) Diffuse glioma growth: a guerilla war. Acta Neuropathol 114: 443–458.

26. Giese A, Westphal M (1996) Glioma invasion in the central nervous system. Neurosurgery 39: 235–250; discussion 250–232.

27. Agarwal S, Manchanda P, Vogelbaum MA, Ohlfest JR, Elmquist WF (2013) Function of the blood-brain barrier and restriction of drug delivery to invasive glioma cells: findings in an orthotopic rat xenograft model of glioma. Drug Metab Dispos 41: 33–39.

28. Vauleon E, Avril T, Collet B, Mosser J, Quillien V, et al. (2010) Overview of Cellular Immunotherapy for Patients with Glioblastoma. Clinical and Developmental Immunology 2010.

29. Hashizume R, Ozawa T, Dinca EB, Banerjee A, Prados MD, et al. (2010) A human brainstem glioma xenograft model enabled for bioluminescence imaging. J Neurooncol 96: 151–159.

30. Miura FK, Alves MJ, Rocha MC, da Silva R, Oba-Shinjo SM, et al. (2010) Xenograft transplantation of human malignant astrocytoma cells into immuno-deficient rats: an experimental model of glioblastoma. Clinics (Sao Paulo) 65: 305–309.

31. Candolfi M, Curtin JF, Nichols WS, Muhammad AG, King GD, et al. (2007) Intracranial glioblastoma models in preclinical neuro-oncology: neuropatholog-ical characterization and tumor progression. J Neurooncol 85: 133–148.

32. Bigner SH, Humphrey PA, Wong AJ, Vogelstein B, Mark J, et al. (1990) Characterization of the epidermal growth factor receptor in human glioma cell lines and xenografts. Cancer Res 50: 8017–8022.

33. Nishikawa R, Ji XD, Harmon RC, Lazar CS, Gill GN, et al. (1994) A mutant epidermal growth factor receptor common in human glioma confers enhanced tumorigenicity. Proc Natl Acad Sci U S A 91: 7727–7731.

34. Lal A, Glazer CA, Martinson HM, Friedman HS, Archer GE, et al. (2002) Mutant epidermal growth factor receptor up-regulates molecular effectors of tumor invasion. Cancer Res 62: 3335–3339.

35. Morgan RA, Johnson LA, Davis JL, Zheng Z, Woolard KD, et al. (2012) Recognition of glioma stem cells by genetically modified T cells targeting EGFRvIII and development of adoptive cell therapy for glioma. Hum Gene Ther 23: 1043–1053.

36. Santos EB, Yeh R, Lee J, Nikhamin Y, Punzalan B, et al. (2009) Sensitive in vivo imaging of T cells using a membrane-bound Gaussia princeps luciferase. Nat Med 15: 338–344.

37. Sadelain M, Brentjens R, Riviere I (2013) The basic principles of chimeric antigen receptor design. Cancer Discov 3: 388–398.

38. Choi BD, Suryadevara CM, Gedeon PC, Herndon Ii JE, Sanchez-Perez L, et al. (2014) Intracerebral delivery of a third generation EGFRvIII-specific chimeric antigen receptor is efficacious against human glioma. J Clin Neurosci 21: 189–190.

39. Engelhardt B, Ransohoff RM (2012) Capture, crawl, cross: the T cell code to breach the blood-brain barriers. Trends Immunol 33: 579–589.

40. Ransohoff RM (2009) Chemokines and chemokine receptors: standing at the crossroads of immunobiology and neurobiology. Immunity 31: 711–721.

41. Mestas J, Hughes CC (2004) Of mice and not men: differences between mouse and human immunology. J Immunol 172: 2731–2738.

42. Grupp SA, Kalos M, Barrett D, Aplenc R, Porter DL, et al. (2013) Chimeric antigen receptor-modified T cells for acute lymphoid leukemia. N Engl J Med 368: 1509–1518.

43. Sampson JH, Heimberger AB, Archer GE, Aldape KD, Friedman AH, et al. (2010) Immunologic escape after prolonged progression-free survival with epidermal growth factor receptor variant III peptide vaccination in patients with newly diagnosed glioblastoma. J Clin Oncol 28: 4722–4729.

44. Butterfield LH, Ribas A, Dissette VB, Amarnani SN, Vu HT, et al. (2003) Determinant spreading associated with clinical response in dendritic cell-based immunotherapy for malignant melanoma. Clin Cancer Res 9: 998–1008.

45. Hughes MS, Yu YY, Dudley ME, Zheng Z, Robbins PF, et al. (2005) Transfer of a TCR gene derived from a patient with a marked antitumor response conveys highly active T-cell effector functions. Hum Gene Ther 16: 457–472.

46. Morgan RA, Dudley ME, Yu YY, Zheng Z, Robbins PF, et al. (2003) High efficiency TCR gene transfer into primary human lymphocytes affords avid recognition of melanoma tumor antigen glycoprotein 100 and does not alter the recognition of autologous melanoma antigens. J Immunol 171: 3287–3295.

47. Riddell SR, Greenberg PD (1990) The use of anti-CD3 and anti-CD28 monoclonal antibodies to clone and expand human antigen-specific T cells. J Immunol Methods 128: 189–201.

48. Yang S, Cohen CJ, Peng PD, Zhao Y, Cassard L, et al. (2008) Development of optimal bicistronic lentiviral vectors facilitates high-level TCR gene expression and robust tumor cell recognition. Gene Ther 15: 1411–1423.

49. Yoshimoto K, Dang J, Zhu S, Nathanson D, Huang T, et al. (2008) Development of a real-time RT-PCR assay for detecting EGFRvIII in glioblastoma samples. Clin Cancer Res 14: 488–493.

50. Sampson JH, Choi BD, Sanchez-Perez L, Suryadevara CM, Snyder DJ, et al. (2013) EGFRvIII mCAR-modified T cell therapy cures mice with established intracerebral glioma and generates host immunity against tumor-antigen loss. Clin Cancer Res.

51. Szentirmai O, Baker CH, Lin N, Szucs S, Takahashi M, et al. (2006) Noninvasive bioluminescence imaging of luciferase expressing intracranial U87 xenografts: correlation with magnetic resonance imaging determined tumor volume and longitudinal use in assessing tumor growth and antiangiogenic treatment effect. Neurosurgery 58: 365–372; discussion 365–372.

3

Identification of Special AT-Rich Sequence Binding Protein 1 as a Novel Tumor Antigen Recognized by CD8+ T Cells: Implication for Cancer Immunotherapy

Mingjun Wang[1,2✎], Bingnan Yin[1✎], Satoko Matsueda[2✎], Lijuan Deng[1], Ying Li[2], Wei Zhao[1], Jia Zou[1], Qingtian Li[1], Christopher Loo[1], Rong-Fu Wang[1,2], Helen Y. Wang[1,2*]

1 Center for Inflammation and Epigenetics, The Methodist Hospital Research Institute, Houston, Texas, United States of America, 2 Center for Cell and Gene Therapy, Baylor College of Medicine, Houston, Texas, United States of America

Abstract

Background: A large number of human tumor-associated antigens that are recognized by CD8+ T cells in a human leukocyte antigen class I (HLA-I)-restricted fashion have been identified. Special AT-rich sequence binding protein 1 (SATB1) is highly expressed in many types of human cancers as part of their neoplastic phenotype, and up-regulation of SATB1 expression is essential for tumor survival and metastasis, thus this protein may serve as a rational target for cancer vaccines.

Methodology/Principal Findings: Twelve SATB1-derived peptides were predicted by an immuno-informatics approach based on the HLA-A*02 binding motif. These peptides were examined for their ability to induce peptide-specific T cell responses in peripheral blood mononuclear cells (PBMCs) obtained from HLA-A*02+ healthy donors and/or HLA-A*02+ cancer patients. The recognition of HLA-A*02+ SATB1-expressing cancer cells was also tested. Among the twelve SATB1-derived peptides, SATB1$_{565-574}$ frequently induced peptide-specific T cell responses in PBMCs from both healthy donors and cancer patients. Importantly, SATB1$_{565-574}$-specific T cells recognized and killed HLA-A*02+ SATB1+ cancer cells in an HLA-I-restricted manner.

Conclusions/Significance: We have identified a novel HLA-A*02-restricted SATB1-derived peptide epitope recognized by CD8+ T cells, which, in turn, recognizes and kills HLA-A*02+ SATB1+ tumor cells. The SATB1-derived epitope identified may be used as a diagnostic marker as well as an immune target for development of cancer vaccines.

Editor: Silke Appel, University of Bergen, Norway

Funding: This work was in part supported by grants from National Cancer Institute, National Institutes of Health and Cancer Research Institute, and The Methodist Hospital Research Institute. The funders had no role in study design, data collection and analysis, decision to publish, or preparation of the manuscript.

Competing Interests: The authors have declared that no competing interests exist.

* E-mail: ywang4@tmhs.org

✎ These authors contributed equally to this work.

Introduction

One of the most promising approaches in cancer therapy relies on harnessing the immune system to eradicate malignant cells [1], the success of which relies largely on the identification of suitable tumor-associated antigens (TAA) for generating effective cancer vaccines. It has been well-established that tumor cells express TAAs that can be recognized by CD8+ T cells in the context of human leukocyte antigen class I (HLA-I) molecules. A large number of TAAs and TAA-derived epitopes have been identified [2,3], with some of these proteins and peptide derivatives already in clinical vaccine trials. Recent approvals of the immunotherapy-based vaccine/drug sipuleucel-T (Provenge) and ipilimumab (Yervoy) by the Food and Drug Administration (FDA) represent milestones in the field of cancer immunotherapy [4,5]. And a phase III clinical trial of the gp100 peptide for melanoma also yielded highly encouraging results [6]. In addition, work from two independent groups underlined the importance of tumor-specific antigens in eliciting immune responses against a developing tumor [7,8], undoubtedly further intensifying the efforts to search for novel tumor antigens for cancer immunotherapy.

Despite such promising results, success in cancer vaccine trials on the whole has been sporadic [9–11]. During the last couple of years, several TAAs that are expressed in different types of neoplasia have been identified [2,3]. However, the majority of the antigens described thus far are dispensable for the survival and growth of the tumor cells, with the exception of a few TAAs such as telomerase [12], survivin [13] and anti-apoptotic members of the Bcl-2 family (Bcl-2, Bcl-X(L) and Mcl-2) [14]. Tumor cells may therefore have escaped surveillance by the immune system through loss and/or down-regulation of tumor antigens [15]. Consequently, targeting TAAs that are essential for survival and growth of tumor cells may better prevent immunoselection of antigen-loss variants as a result of vaccination and improve the efficacy of cancer immunotherapy [15,16]. Such immunogenic tumor antigens that elicit minimal immune escape therefore represent the most optimal vaccine candidates for immunotherapy of cancer.

Special AT-rich sequence binding protein 1 (SATB1) is a nuclear factor that functions as a global chromatin organizer. It regulates gene expression by folding chromatin into loop domains, and tethering DNA domains to the SATB1 network structure [17]. SATB1 appeared to be over-expressed in aggressive breast cancer cell lines but absent or undetectable in normal and immortalized human mammary epithelial cells, suggesting a role of SATB1 in reprogramming chromatin organization and ultimately transcriptional profiles of breast tumors to promote growth and metastasis [18]. In addition, higher levels of SATB1 expression were associated with many other types of cancer, including laryngeal squamous cell carcinoma [19], endometrioid endometrial cancer [20], hepatocellular carcinoma [21], rectal cancer [22], cutaneous malignant melanoma [23], gastric cancer [24,25], ovarian cancer [26], prostate cancer [27], lung cancer [28] and glioma [29]. Up-regulation of SATB1 in these types of cancers can promote tumor growth and metastasis. Since SATB1 is essential for tumor growth/survival and metastasis, immune escape by loss or down-regulation of SATB1 expression may impair sustained tumor cell growth and/or metastasis, thus making SATB1 an attractive target for anticancer vaccines against various types of cancers that express SATB1.

In this report, we describe the identification of SATB1-derived T cell epitopes for T cell recognition using an immuno-bioinformatics approach. We selected twelve peptides that were predicted to bind to the HLA-A*02 molecule. They were synthesized and evaluated in vitro for their ability to stimulate T cells in PBMCs from healthy subjects and/or cancer patients based on interferon-γ (IFN-γ) release. One of these peptides, SATB1$_{565-574}$, was found to induce IFN-γ release in peripheral T cells from both healthy subjects and cancer patients. Importantly, SATB1$_{565-574}$ -specific T cells were able to recognize and kill HLA-A*02$^+$, SATB1-expressing tumor cells in an HLA-I-dependent manner. These results demonstrate the validity of the immuno-bioinformatics approach and suggest SATB1$_{565-574}$ may represent a new tumor-specific epitope for cancer immunotherapy.

Materials and Methods

Healthy Donors and Cancer Patients

HLA-A*02$^+$ prostate or ovarian cancer patients and ten HLA-A*02$^+$ healthy subjects were enrolled in this study after written informed consent was obtained. All protocols were approved by the Institutional Review Board (IRB) at the Baylor College of Medicine prior to commencing studies. 20 mL of peripheral blood was obtained from each person, and peripheral blood mononuclear cells (PBMCs) were isolated by density gradient centrifugation using Lymphoprep (Nycomed Pharma AS; Oslo, Norway). Freshly isolated PBMCs were cryopreserved for later use in 1 mL freezing medium containing 90% FCS and 10% dimethyl sulfoxide (DMSO) at -140°C. HLA-A*02 expression in PBMCs obtained from cancer patients and healthy subjects was verified by flow cytometry with FITC-labeled HLA-A*02 mAb BB7.2 (BD Pharmingen; San Diego, CA, USA).

Cell Lines

All breast cancer cell lines (MCF-7, CAMA-1, MDA-MB-134VI, MDA-MB-175VII, MDA-MB-361, DU4475, MDA-MB-231, MDA-MB-436, MDA-MB-453, MDA-MB-468), T2 cells (an HLA-A*02$^+$ TAP-deficient cell line), prostate cancer cell lines (PC3, LNCaP and DU145), ovarian cancer cell line Ovcar-3 and lymphoma cell line Jeko-1 were purchased from American Type Culture Collection (ATCC; Manassas, VA, USA). An ovarian cancer cell line Skov-1 [30,31] was a gift from Dr. Kunle Odunsi

(Roswell Park Cancer Institute, NY, USA); a lymphoma cell line L1236 [32,33] was a gift from Dr. Catherine M. Bollard (Baylor College of Medicine, Houston, USA). All cell lines were maintained in RPMI-1640 medium (Mediatech; Manassas, VA, USA), supplemented with 10% FBS, 1% L-glutamine, and 1% penicillin and streptomycin.

Peptides

Twelve SATB1-derived peptides (Table 1) were predicted using BIMAS (http://www-bimas.cit.nih.gov/molbio/hla_bind/), SYF-PEITHI (http://www.syfpeithi.de/), and Rankpep (http://bio.dfci.harvard.edu/Tools/rankpep.html) based on the HLA-A*02 binding motif. Epitopes that were predicted by at least two of these algorithms were selected for further testing. The peptides were synthesized by a solid-phase method using a peptide synthesizer (AApptec, Inc.; Louisville, KY, USA), purified by reverse-phase high-performance liquid chromatography and validated by mass spectrometry. The synthesized peptides were dissolved in DMSO at a concentration of 10 mg/mL and stored at -80°C until further use. One peptide (SATB1$_{544-552}$) was excluded from the study due to the difficulty of peptide synthesis.

In vitro Stimulation of Peptide-specific T Cells in PBMCs

PBMCs (1×10^5 cells/well) from either healthy subjects or cancer patients were incubated with standard peptide concentrations of 20 µg/mL per peptide [34–37] in 96-well U-bottom microplates (BD; Franklin Lakes, NJ, USA) in 200 µL of T-cell medium (TCM), consisting of RPMI 1640 (Mediatech; Manassas, VA, USA), 10% human AB serum (Valley Biomedical, Winchester, USA), 50 µM of 2-mercaptoethanol, 100 IU/mL of interleukin-2 (IL-2), and 0.1 mM MEM nonessential amino acid solution (Invitrogen; grand island, NY, USA). Half of the TCM was removed and replaced with fresh TCM containing peptides (20 µg/mL) every 5 days. After 14 days of culture, the cells were harvested and tested for their ability to produce IFN-γ in response to T2 cells (1×10^4 cells/well), which were pre-loaded with either SATB1 peptide (5 µg/mL) or a control peptide (an irrelevant HLA-A*02 binding EBV peptide: GLCTLVAML) as a negative control. After 18 hours of incubation, supernatants were collected, and IFN- γ release was determined by ELISA assay.

Rapid Expansion Protocol (REP) for SATB1 Peptide-specific T Cells

SATB1 peptide-specific T cells were expanded by a rapid expansion protocol (REP) as previously described [38] with a slight modification. Briefly, on day 0, 0.1–0.5$\times 10^6$ SATB1 peptide-specific T cells were cultured in a T25 flask with 20 mL RPMI-1640 supplemented with 10% human AB serum, 50 µM of 2-mercaptoethanol, 30 ng/mL OKT3 antibody (Ortho Biotech; Bridgewater, NJ, USA) and 30 ng/mL anti-CD28 antibody (R&D Systems; Minneapolis, MN, USA), together with 20×10^6 irradiated allogeneic PBMCs and 5×10^6 irradiated Epstein Barr Virus (EBV) transformed B cells as feeder cells. Flasks were incubated upright at 37°C in 5% CO_2. IL-2 (300 IU/mL) was added on day 1, and on day 5, half of the cell culture supernatant was removed and replenished with fresh medium containing 300 IU/mL IL-2. 14 days after initiation of the REP, cells were harvested and cryopreserved for future experiments.

Depletion of CD4$^+$ or CD8$^+$ T Cells from PBMCs

CD4$^+$ T cells or CD8$^+$ T cells were positively depleted from PBMCs according to the manufacturer's instruction using monoclonal anti-CD4-coated or monoclonal anti-CD8-coated Dyna-

       Cancer Immunotherapy: Research and Practice

Table 1. A list of predicted HLA-A*02 binding peptides derived from SATB1.

SATB1 peptides	HLA restriction	Position	Sequence	Binding score BIMAS[a]	SYFPEITHI[b]	Rankpep[c]
SATB1$_{105-113}$	HLA-A2	105113	MLFNQLIEM	71.872	21	87
SATB1$_{658-666}$	HLA-A2	658–666	ILQSFIQDV	1033.404	27	86
SATB1$_{544-552}$	HLA-A2	544–552	TLWENLSMI	816.565	25	95
SATB1$_{156-164}$	HLA-A2	156–164	MLQDVYHVV	298.138	22	88
SATB1$_{514-522}$	HLA-A2	514–522	ALFAKVAAT	63.417	25	80
SATB1$_{325-333}$	HLA-A2	325–333	QLLNQQYAV	257.342	24	81
SATB1$_{315-323}$	HLA-A2	315–323	QLVNQQLVM	2.037	15	73
SATB1$_{72-80}$	HLA-A2	72–80	TMLPVFCVV	144.784	22	69
SATB1$_{623-631}$	HLA-A2	623–631	RLPPRQPTV	69.552	25	54
SATB1$_{565-574}$	HLA-A2	565–574	AIYEQESNAV	125.472	25	11.261
SATB1$_{196-205}$	HLA-A2	196–205	LLKDMNQSSL	5.211	24	10.011
SATB1$_{214-223}$	HLA-A2	214–223	SMISSIVNST	12.379	23	7.812

Note: [a] Predicted T(1/2) of disassociation in minutes;
[b]and [c] Higher values represent better binders.

beads (Dynal Biotech ASA; Oslo, Norway). PBMCs depleted of CD4$^+$ T or CD8$^+$ T cells were verified by flow cytometry.

ELISA Assay

Cytokine release was measured by coating 96-well ELISA plates (Thermo Fisher Scientific; Rochester, NY, USA) with 1 μg/mL anti-human IFN-γ (Pierce Biotechnology; Rockford, IL, USA) overnight at 4°C. The plate was washed six times with PBS containing 0.05% Tween-20 (wash solution) to remove unbound coating antibody, and blocked with 1% BSA/PBS at room temperature for 2 hrs. Afterwards, 50 μL supernatant was added to each well and incubated at room temperature for 1 hr, then 50 μL of 0.5 μg/mL biotinylated anti-human IFN-γ (Pierce Biotechnology; Rockford, IL, USA) was added and plates were incubated for an additional 1 hr at room temperature. After incubation, plates were washed and incubated for 30 min with Poly-HRP-Streptavidin (Thermo Fisher Scientific; Rochester, NY, USA) diluted 1:5000 in PBS/1% BSA. Plates were washed and 100 μL of TMB substrate solution (Sigma-Aldrich Co.; St. Louis, MO, USA) was added per well. The colorimetric reaction was stopped using 2N H$_2$SO$_4$ and plates were read at 450 nm using an ELISA plate reader.

RNA Extraction and RT-PCR

RNA extraction and RT-PCR was carried out as reported previously [39]. In brief, total RNA was extracted from cancer cells with 1 mL Trizol reagent (Invitrogen; Carlsbad, CA, USA). Three micrograms of RNA was reverse-transcribed to cDNA in 30 μl volume and 1 μl of each cDNA was used in subsequent PCR reaction with a pair of SATB1 specific primers: Primer 1:5′-TGCAAAGGTTGCAGCAACCAAAAGC-3′; 5′-AACATGGA-TAATGTGGGGCGGCCT-3′. GAPDH was used as loading control: primer 1:5′-TGATGACATCAAGAAGGTGGTGAAG-3′; Primer 2:5′-TCCTTGGAGGCCATGTGGGCCAT-3′. The PCR reaction was carried out under the following conditions: 95°C for 1 min, 95°C for 40 s, 60°C for 30 s, 72°C for 40 s, total 40 cycles, 72°C for 5 min, and GAPDH was run for 25 cycles. Equal amounts of PCR products were then loaded and detected by gel electrophoresis.

Western Blot

Whole cell extracts were prepared and resolved in SDS-PAGE gels. The proteins were transferred to PVDF membrane (Bio-Rad Laboratories, Inc., Hercules, CA, USA) and further incubated with the SATB1 antibody (BD Biosciences, San Jose, CA, USA). LumiGlo Chemiluminescent Substrate System from KPL (Gaithersburg, MD, USA) was used for protein detection.

FACS Analysis

Cells (0.5×10^6) were stained with either FITC-anti-CD8, PE-Cy5-anti-CD4 (Both from eBioscience, San Diego, CA, USA) or FITC-anti-HLA-A*02 (BD Pharmingen; San Diego, CA, USA) in PBS containing 2% FBS on ice for 30 min, and then washed twice in PBS. Afterwards, cells were re-suspended in 500 μl PBS and analyzed using a FACScalibur machine. For DimerX HLA-A*02:Ig staining, SATB1 reactive CD8$^+$ T cells were incubated with purified HLA-A*02:Ig dimer (BD Biosciences, San Jose, CA, USA) loaded with a given peptide, and then stained with FITC anti-mouse IgG1 (BD Biosciences, San Jose, CA, USA). Flow cytometry was performed on a FACScalibur machine.

Cytotoxicity Assay

SATB1-derived peptide-specific T cells were tested for cytotoxicity against peptide-loaded T2 cells, two HLA-A*02$^+$ SATB1$^+$ cancer cell lines (Skov-1 and Jeko-1) and an HLA-A*02 negative SATB1$^+$ PC3 cell line as a negative control by a lactate dehydrogenase (LDH) assay (Promega; Madison, WI, USA). The assay was performed in accordance with the manufacturer's instructions. LDH release was calculated based on the following formula:

Cytotoxicity (%) = (Experimental − Effector Spontaneous − Target Spontaneous LDH release)/(Target Maximum − Target Spontaneous LDH release)×100.

Spontaneous release was determined by using the supernatant of the target cells alone or effector cells alone, and the maximum release was determined by using the supernatant of target cells incubated with a lysis solution included in LDH kit.

Statistics

Student's t-test was used to analyze quantitative differences between the experimental wells and controls in ELISA assays. $P<0.05$ was considered significant.

Results

SATB1 mRNA is Expressed in a Variety of Cancers

To examine whether SATB1 is expressed in cancer cells, mRNA expression for SATB1 in various types of tumor cells was performed by RT-PCR. As shown in Figure 1, SATB1 mRNA was highly expressed in a variety of cancers including breast cancer, ovarian cancer, prostate cancer as well as lymphoma. While the normal prostate epithelial cell line, PNT1A did not express SATB1 mRNA.

Induction of SATB1-derived Peptide-specific CTLs in Healthy Donors

First, we obtained PBMCs from 10 HLA-A*02$^+$ healthy donors to determine whether SATB1-reactive T cell precursors were present in these healthy subjects. The cells were stimulated *in vitro* for two weeks with each of the SATB1-derived peptides containing HLA-A*02-binding motif (Table 1). At the end of peptide stimulation, supernatants from the cultures were analyzed by ELISA to detect IFN-γ release in response to T2 cells pulsed with or without corresponding peptides. As shown in Table 2, nearly all of the 11 SATB1-derived peptides (10/11) were capable of inducing peptide-specific T cell responses in at least one of the healthy subjects. In particular, the peptide SATB1$_{565-574}$ induced higher level of IFN-γ release (>900 pg/mL) in 4 out of 10 healthy subjects, indicating its high immunogenicity and potential in expanding antigen-specific T cells in healthy subjects.

Presence of SATB1-derived Peptide Specific CTLs in Cancer Patients

Our analysis indicated that peptide-specific T cells against SATB1$_{565-574}$ were found in ~60% of healthy subjects, we therefore reasoned that CTL precursors that could recognize this peptide might also be abundant in PBMCs from cancer patients. To test our hypothesis, we examined whether peptide SATB1$_{565-574}$ could induce peptide-specific CTLs from PBMCs of HLA-A*02$^+$ ovarian cancer patients. PBMCs from three HLA-A*02$^+$ ovarian cancer patients were collected and stimulated *in vitro* with peptide SATB1$_{565-574}$. As shown in Table 3, peptide SATB1$_{565-574}$ was able to induce peptide-specific CTLs from PBMCs of ovarian cancer patients, indicating that the peptide is highly immunogenic not only in healthy subjects but also in cancer patients. We also determined whether this peptide candidate could induce peptide-specific CTLs from PBMCs of HLA-A*02$^+$ prostate cancer patients. As was the case with ovarian cancer patients, peptide SATB1$_{565-574}$ similarly induced peptide-specific CTLs from PBMCs of 5 prostate cancer patients as well (Table 3), indicating CTL precursors that recognize this peptide are abundant in PBMCs from cancer patients.

SATB1-derived Peptide Induced CD8$^+$ T Cell-dependent Responses

To further analyze SATB1$_{565-574}$ peptide-specific T cells, we next expanded SATB1$_{565-574}$ peptide-specific T cells identified in Tables 2 and 3 in order to obtain a sufficient number of these cells. To this end, we performed peptide titration experiments to determine the optimal peptide concentration for loading T2 cells for T cell recognition. As shown in Figure 2A, T2 cells could be sensitized by peptide SATB1$_{565-574}$ but not a control EBV peptide for T cell recognition at a concentration of 0.08 μg/mL, and the binding sites of HLA-A*02 molecules on T2 cells became saturated at 5 μg/mL. Further increasing the concentrations of SATB1$_{565-574}$ failed to enhance production of IFN-γ. Therefore, we consistently used the peptide concentration of 5 μg/mL for pre-loading T2 cells in our ELISA assays. The expanded T cells maintained antigen-specificity and secreted significant amounts of IFN-γ after stimulation with T2 cells pulsed with the corresponding peptides, but not with a control EBV peptide (Figures 2A and B). To obtain direct evidence on the subsets of the responding T cells depicted in Figure 2B, the expanded SATB1 peptide-reactive PBMCs were depleted for either CD4$^+$ T cells (Figure 2C) or CD8$^+$ T cells (Figure 2D) prior to incubation with peptides for ELISA assays. As shown in Figure 2E, CD8$^+$ T cells, not CD4$^+$ T cells (Figure 2F), obtained from expanded PBMCs responded to SATB1$_{565-574}$ pulsed T2 cells, indicating that the T cell response induced by SATB1$_{565-574}$ was dependent on CD8$^+$ T cells. Furthermore, dimerX HLA-A*02:Ig staining (Figure 2G and H) and IFN-γ intracellular staining (Figure S1) also demonstrated that SATB1$_{565-574}$ induced peptide specific, HLA-A*02 restricted CD8$^+$ T cell-dependent responses.

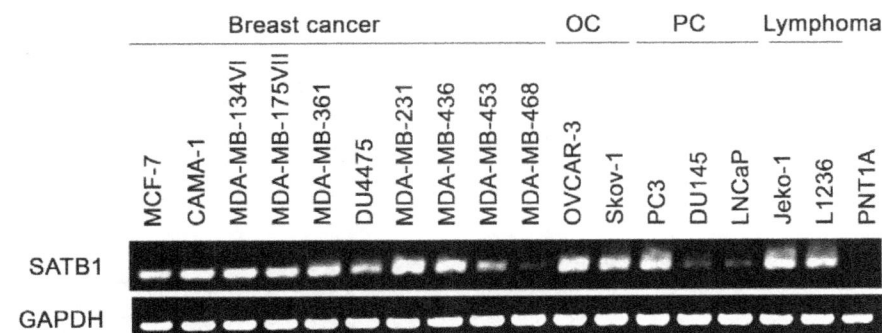

Figure 1. SATB1 mRNA was highly expressed in various types of cancers. The mRNA expression for SATB1 in different cell lines was determined by RT-PCR. The breast cancer cell lines (MCF-7, CAMA-1, MDA-MB-134VI, MDA-MB-175VII, MDA-MB-361, DU4475, MDA-MB-231, MDA-MB-436, MDA-MB-453 and MDA-MB-468), prostate cancer (PC) cell lines (PC3, LNCaP and DU145), ovarian cancer (OC) cell lines (Ovcar-3 and Skov-1), lymphoma cell lines (Jeko-1 and L1236) and a normal prostate epithelial cell line PNT1A were included as a control. Results are representative of three independent experiments.

Table 2. Recognition of the peptides by in vitro-stimulated T cells from the PBMCs of ten HLA-A*02$^+$ healthy subjects.

	# 1	# 2	# 3	# 4	# 5	# 6	# 7	# 8	# 9	# 10
SATB1$_{105-113}$	0	0	467	0	138	0	0	677	0	0
SATB1$_{658-666}$	0	0	0	0	127	0	0	0	106	0
SATB1$_{156-164}$	582	152	109	109	0	0	0	0	465	168
SATB1$_{514-522}$	172	0	259	0	0	0	0	0	203	0
SATB1$_{325-333}$	366	0	823	147	112	0	0	729	111	0
SATB1$_{315-323}$	0	0	0	0	0	0	0	0	0	0
SATB1$_{72-80}$	208	0	0	171	0	0	0	742	132	214
SATB1$_{623-631}$	0	0	0	93	316	116	0	0	0	301
SATB1$_{565-574}$	**1106**	**0**	**0**	**906**	**954**	**90**	**0**	**1032**	**0**	**99**
SATB1$_{196-205}$	352	0	0	0	0	0	0	0	0	0
SATB1$_{214-223}$	0	0	0	0	0	0	0	1061	0	0

Note: Values denote concentrations of IFN-γ (pg/ml) in the supernatants of T cells stimulated with SATB1 peptide-loaded T2 cells minus that of T cells stimulated with unloaded T2 cells.

Recognition and Killing of Cancer Cells by the SATB1-derived Peptide-specific CD8$^+$ T Cells in an HLA-I Restricted Manner

Based on our results thus far, SATB1$_{565-574}$ specific CD8$^+$ T cells were used in subsequent experiments. To determine whether SATB1-derived peptide-specific T cells were able to recognize and kill HLA-A*02$^+$, SATB1-expressing cancer cells, we used an HLA-A*02$^-$ SATB1 mRNA positive prostate cancer cell line PC3 (as a negative control) and five HLA-A*02$^+$ SATB1 mRNA positive cancer cell lines. The expression of SATB1 mRNA in these 6 cell lines was previously examined by RT-PCR (Figure 1) and HLA-A*02 expression was verified by flow cytometry (Figure 3A). In addition, we also checked the expression of SATB1 protein among these cell lines (Figure 3B), and found that all cancer cell lines expressed SATB1 protein except PC3 and Ovcar-3. Therefore, Ovcar-3 was also regarded as a negative control. As shown in Figure 4A, SATB1$_{565-574}$ -specific T cells could recognize HLA-A*02$^+$ SATB1 expressing Skov-1 and Jeko-1 cells, but not PC3 or Ovcar-3 cells. The other two HLA-A*02$^+$ SATB1 expressing cancer cell lines (CAMA-1, MDA-MB-231) could only be recognized when they were pre-treated with IFN-γ (Figure 4B), suggesting that either enhanced HLA-A*02 expression on the cell surfaces (Figure S2) or induction of immunoproteasomes by IFN-γ, may facilitate the presentation of the correct epitope to cell surfaces for T cell scrutiny. In contrast, normal cells, including PNT1A and autologous PBMCs, could not be recognized by SATB1$_{565-574}$ -specific T cells (Figure 4A). In addition, SATB1$_{565-574}$-specific T cells did not recognize in vitro-differentiated Th subsets, including Th1, Th2 and Th17 cells (Figure S3).

To determine whether the recognition of cancer cells by SATB1$_{565-574}$-specific CD8$^+$ T cells was HLA-I restricted, we co-cultured SATB1$_{565-574}$ -specific T cells with either Skov-1 or Jeko-1 cells in the presence of either anti-HLA-I mAb (W6/32) or anti-HLA-II mAb. As shown in Figure 4C and D, T cell responses were completely inhibited by the addition of anti-HLA-I mAb, but not anti-HLA-II (HLA-DP mAb), which suggests that the recognition of tumor cells by SATB1$_{565-574}$-specific CD8$^+$ T cells is HLA-I restricted.

To further examine whether SATB1$_{565-574}$-specific CD8$^+$ T cells were able to kill HLA-A*02$^+$, SATB1-expressing cancer cells, we performed cytotoxicity assays. As shown in Figure 4E, SATB1$_{565-574}$-specific T cells killed T2 cells pulsed with SATB1$_{565-574}$, but not T2 cells alone or those pulsed with a control EBV peptide. Importantly, SATB1$_{565-574}$-specific T cells were able to kill HLA-A*02$^+$, SATB1 expressing Skov-1 and Jeko-1 cells, but not HLA-A*02$^-$ PC3 cells (Figure 4F and G). These results suggest that SATB1$_{565-574}$ -specific T cells recognize a T cell epitope that is endogenously processed and presented by tumor cells.

Discussion

It is well-established that CD8$^+$ T cells play a critical role in controlling tumor development and progression. Peptide epitopes derived from TAAs can be recognized as antigens by T cells in the context of MHC-I molecules [40,41]. Identification of ideal TAAs and their peptides that are recognized by T cells are essential for the development of effective cancer vaccines. Ideal TAAs such as anti-apoptotic proteins [14], telomerase [12] and survivin [13], being mandatory for tumor growth/survival, may represent

Table 3. Recognition of the peptide by in vitro-stimulated T cells from the PBMCs of HLA-A*02$^+$ cancer patients.

	Ovarian cancer patients			Prostate cancer patients				
	MD	CH	EL13	#1	#2	#3	#4	#5
SATB1$_{565-574}$	1000	16	231	1813	1946	873	1194	242

Note: Values denote concentrations of IFN-γ (pg/ml) in the supernatants of T cells stimulated with SATB1 peptide-loaded T2 cells minus that of T cells stimulated with unloaded T2 cells.

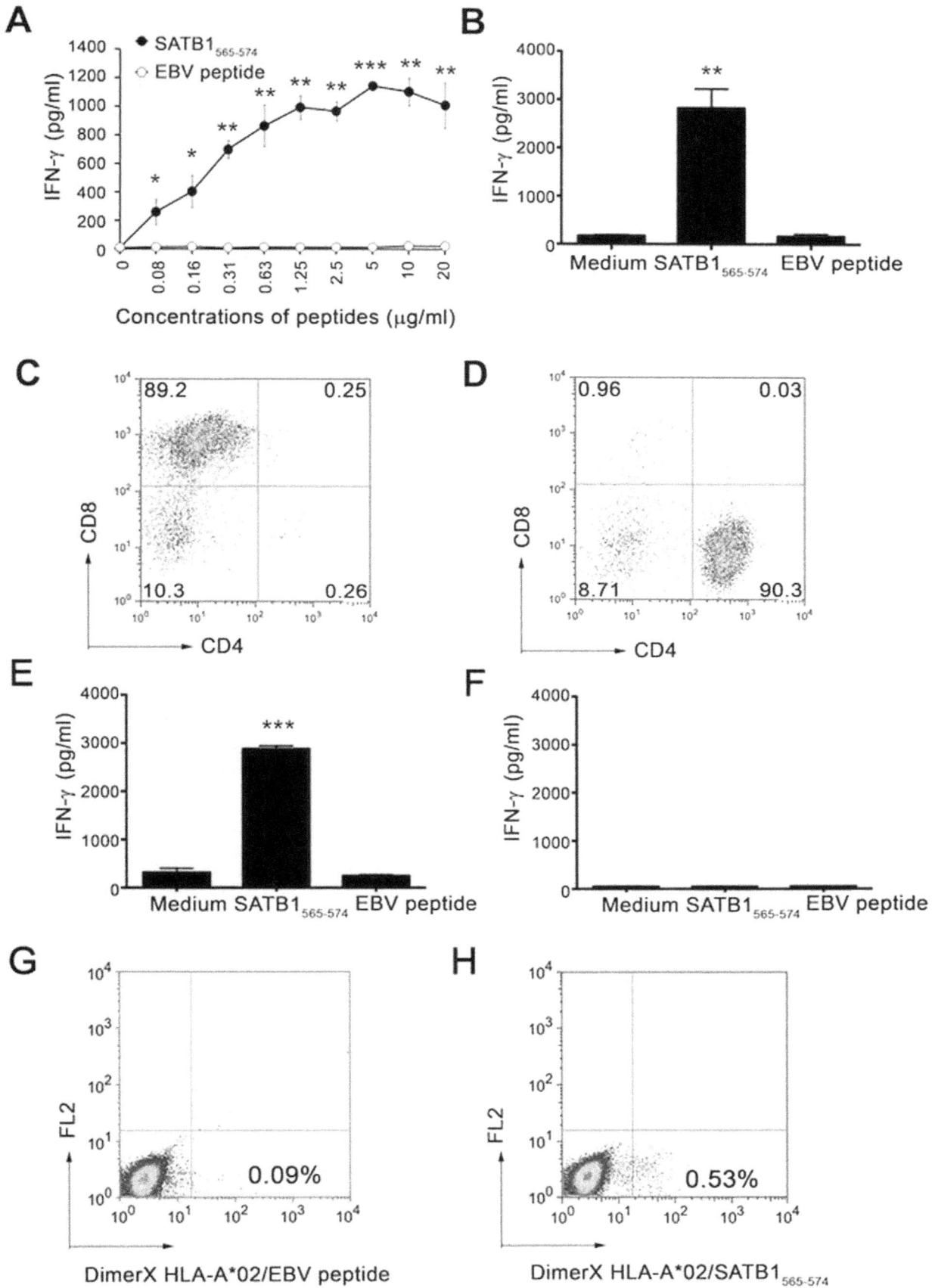

Figure 2. SATB1-derived peptide SATB1$_{565-574}$ induced CD8$^+$ T cell-dependent responses. The recognition of T2 cells pre-loaded with titrated concentrations of peptides (0–20 µg/ml) by expanded SATB1$_{565-574}$-specific T cells from healthy donor #1 was tested by ELISA assay (A). The expanded SATB1-reactive PBMCs (B) were co-incubated with T2 cells (1×10^4 cells/well) alone in complete medium (CM), or with T2 cells pre-loaded with either SATB1$_{565-574}$ (5 µg/mL) or a control EBV peptide as a negative control. Cells were incubated for 18–24 hours, the IFN-γ secretion in the supernatant was determined by ELISA assay. SATB1-reactive PBMCs depleted of CD4$^+$ T cells (C) and SATB1-reactive PBMCs depleted of CD8$^+$ T cells (D) were verified by flow cytometry. The recognitions of T2 cells pulsed with SATB1$_{565-574}$ by SATB1-reactive PBMCs depleted of either CD4$^+$ T cells (E) or CD8$^+$ T cells (F) were determined by ELISA. SATB1 reactive CD8$^+$ T cells were incubated with purified HLA-A2:Ig dimer loaded with a control EBV peptide (G) or with peptide SATB1$_{565-574}$ (H), and then stained with FITC anti-mouse IgG1. Cells were analyzed using a FACScalibur machine. Data (from A, B, E and F) are plotted as means ± SD. Results are representative of at least three independent experiments. *$P<0.05$, **$P<0.01$, ***$P<0.001$ versus controls (T2 cells alone or T2 cells pulsed with a control EBV peptide).

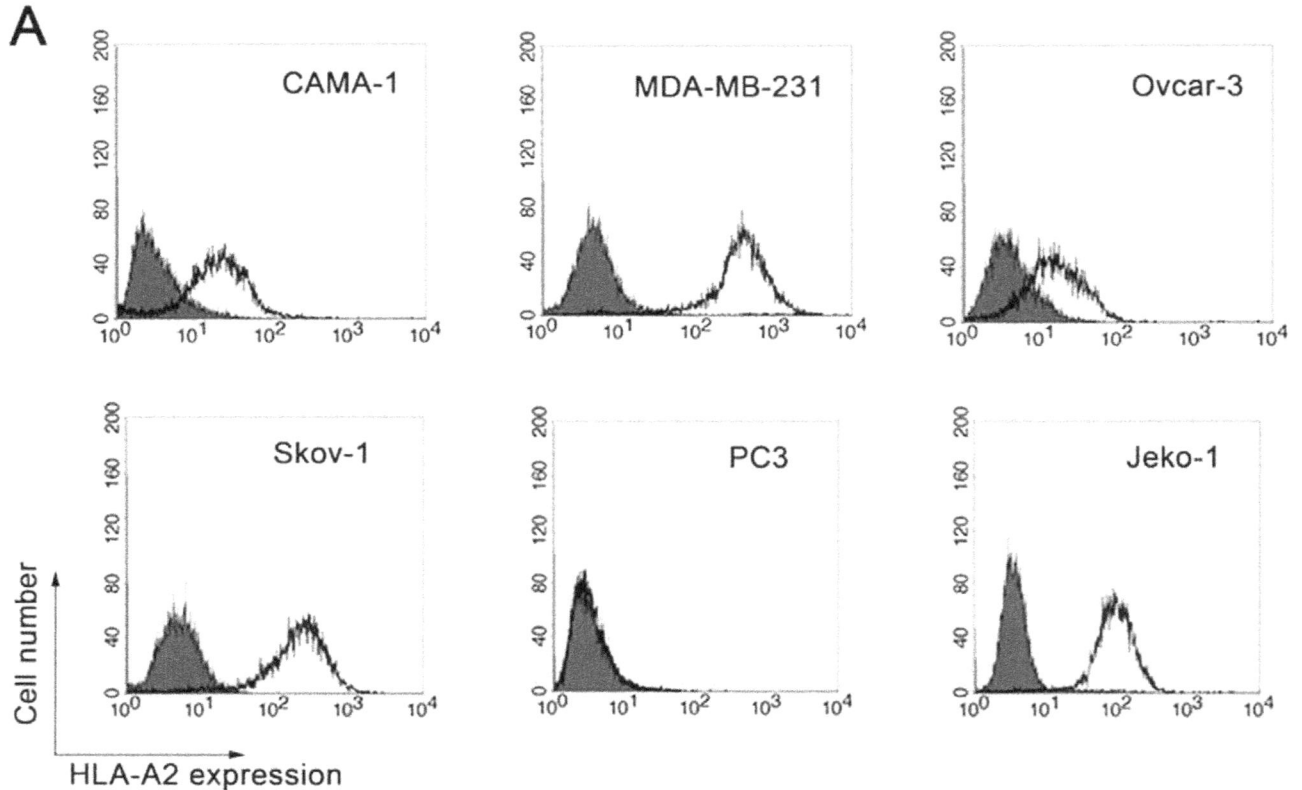

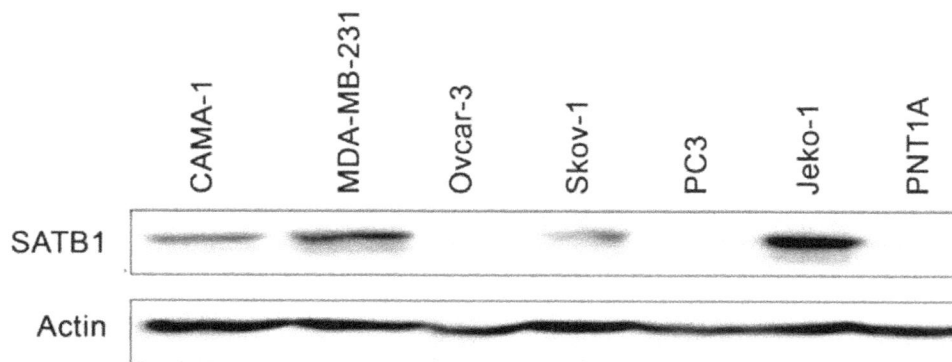

Figure 3. HLA-A*02 and SATB1 protein expression in tumor cell lines. (A) Cells were stained with FITC-anti-HLA-A*02 in PBS containing 2% FBS. Then, cells were washed and re-suspended in PBS and analyzed using a FACScalibur machine. (B) The expression of SATB1 protein in various tumor cells was determined by western blot. Actin was used as a loading control.

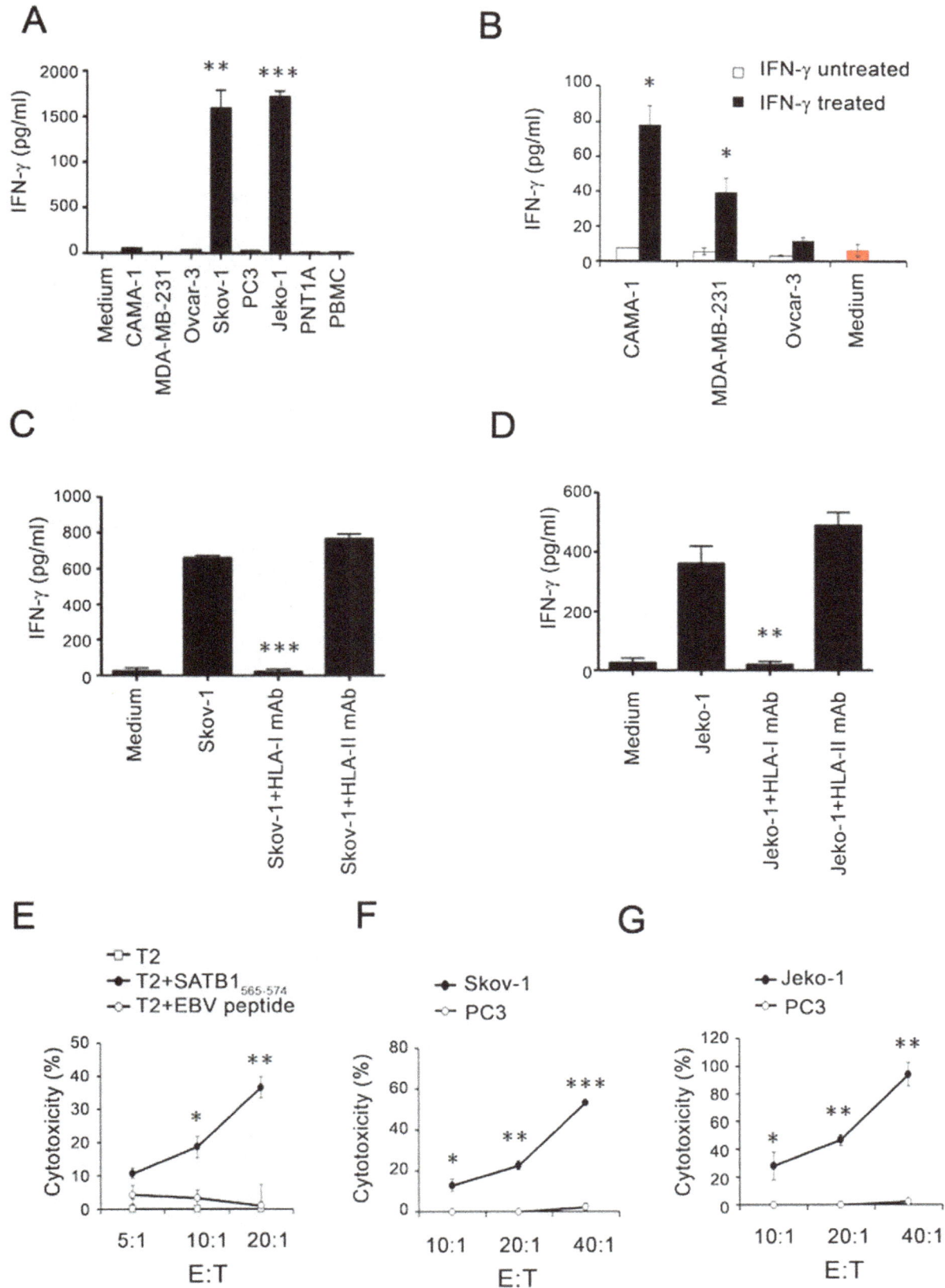

Figure 4. SATB1$_{565-574}$-specific CD8$^+$ T cells recognized and killed HLA-A*02$^+$ SATB1-expressing cancer cells in a HLA-I dependent manner. (A) SATB1$_{565-574}$-specific T cells from healthy donor #1 were cultured alone in medium or co-incubated with various types of tumor cells as well as normal cells (PNT1A and PBMC); (B) Tumor cells were pretreated without or with IFN-γ (10 ng/mL) for 48 hours before incubation with

SATB1$_{565-574}$-specific T cells. SATB1$_{565-574}$-specific T cells were cultured in medium alone as a negative control (red column); To block HLA-dependent responses, either anti-HLA-I mAb (W6/32) or HLA-II mAb was added into cell cultures during incubation of SATB1$_{565-574}$-specific T cells with Skov-1 (C) or Jeko-1 cells (D). Cells were incubated for 18–24 hours, the IFN-γ secretion in the supernatant was determined by ELISA assay. SATB1$_{565-574}$-specific CD8$^+$ T cells were tested for cytotoxicity against T2 cells pulsed with or without peptides (E), Skov-1 (F) and Jeko-1 (G) by the LDH assay. HLA-A*02 negative PC3 cells were used as a negative control in the LDH assay. Data from A–G are plotted as means ± SD. Results are representative of three independent experiments. *P<0.05, **P<0.01, ***P<0.001 versus controls.

optimal targets for vaccine mediated immunotherapy of cancer. SATB1 is highly expressed in many types of human cancers and up-regulation of SATB1 expression is essential for tumor survival and metastasis, thus SATB1 represents one of such ideal TAAs.

The aim of the current study was to identify HLA-A*02 binding SATB1-derived epitopes recognized by CD8$^+$ T cells in PBMCs of healthy subjects and cancer patients. Twelve SATB1-derived peptides were predicted using BIMAS, SYFPEITHI, and Rankpep based on the HLA-A*02 binding motif. Peptides that were predicted by at least 2 of 3 programs were selected for further testing for their ability to stimulate PBMCs from healthy subjects and/or cancer patients. Further studies showed that 10 out of 11 synthesized SATB1-derived peptides were capable of inducing peptide-specific T cell responses in at least one out of 10 healthy subjects. Specifically, SATB1$_{565-574}$ was found to induce higher level of IFN-γ release (>900 pg/mL) in 4 out of 10 healthy subjects, indicating that this peptide may be immunogenic and potentially capable of expanding antigen-specific T cells in healthy subjects. Furthermore, SATB1$_{565-574}$ induced frequently specific T cell responses in PBMCs of ovarian cancer patients as well as in PBMCs from prostate cancer patients. Importantly, SATB1$_{565-574}$ peptide-specific T cells recognized and killed HLA-A*02$^+$ SATB1-expressing Jeko-1, Skov-1 cells as well as IFN-γ-treated breast cancer cell lines (CAMA-1 and MDA-MB-231), suggesting this peptide is naturally processed by cancer cells.

SATB1 is a global chromatin organizer and transcription factor and has emerged as a key factor integrating higher-order chromatin architecture with gene regulation [42]. SATB1 promotes tumor growth and metastasis by reprogramming chromatin organization and transcription profiles, and is highly expressed in a variety of cancers including breast cancer [18], laryngeal squamous cell carcinoma [19], endometrioid endometrial cancer [20], hepatocellular carcinoma [21], rectal cancer [22], cutaneous malignant melanoma [23], gastric cancer [24,25], ovarian cancer [26], prostate cancer [27], lung cancer [28] and glioma [29]. In tumor cells with high levels of SATB1, genes that promote tumor progression and metastasis were up-regulated, whereas genes that inhibit tumor metastasis were repressed [17]; while silencing of SATB1 greatly reduced the invasive and metastatic capacity of cancer cells [43]. Thus SATB1 is required and essential for tumor growth/survival and metastasis, and down-regulation or loss of SATB1 expression may impair sustained tumor growth and metastasis. These characteristics make SATB1 an attractive target for development of effective cancer vaccines against various types of cancer. Here, we have described an HLA-A*02 binding SATB1-derived epitope, SATB1$_{565-574}$. This is, to our knowledge, the first report to identify and characterize a SATB1-derived epitope that is recognized by CD8$^+$ T cells.

Although SATB1$_{565-574}$ peptide-specific T cells recognized and killed HLA-A*02$^+$ SATB1-expressing Jeko-1 and Skov-1 cells, however, they did not directly recognize the other two HLA-A*02$^+$ SATB1$^+$ breast cancer cells tested in this study including CAMA-1 and MDA-MB-231. These differences may arise from the different cell types harboring different sets of proteasomes [44], thus leading to different repertoire of peptides associated with MHC-I in different cell types. Indeed, when CAMA-1 and MDA-

MB-231 were pretreated with an inducer of immunoproteasomes-IFN-γ, they could then be recognized by SATB1$_{565-574}$ peptide-specific T cells (Figure 4B), suggesting that IFN-γ may enhance induction of immunoproteasomes, thus leading to the correct presentation of SATB1$_{565-574}$ to the tumor cell surface for T cell scrutiny. The enhanced expression of HLA-A*02 on cell surface by IFN-γ (Figure S2) is another possibility that make treated tumor cells recognized by SATB1$_{565-574}$ peptide-specific T cells.

It should be noted that SATB1 is not only highly expressed in various types of malignant tumor, its expression was also detectable in thymocytes and progenitor cells including osteoblasts, the basal layer of the epidermis, amyloblasts, and embryonic stem cells [45–47]. These cells may be targeted by vaccine-induced SATB1-peptide specific CD8$^+$ T cells. However, the fact that SATB1$_{565-574}$-specific T cell responses are easily induced in healthy donors as well as cancer patients, suggests that a high frequency of SATB1-specific CD8$^+$ T cell precursors is present in the circulation, which indicates that anti-cancer vaccines targeting SATB1 may be safe and may not induce autoimmunity. Indeed, SATB1$_{565-574}$ peptide-specific T cells did not recognize autologous PBMC in vitro (Figure 4A). Furthermore, although SATB1 plays an important role during T cell differentiation, SATB1$_{565-574}$ -specific T cells did not recognize in vitro-differentiated Th cell subsets, including Th1, Th2 and Th17 cells (Figure S3). Besides, the peptide SATB1$_{565-574}$ -HLA-I complexes on the surface of normal cells may be too low to reach the threshold for T cell scrutiny; while in cancer cells, over-expression of SATB1 results in increased presentation of the peptide on the cell surface for T cell recognition. Thus, the difference in SATB1 expression on normal and malignant cells may explain the reason that SATB1-specific T cells in healthy donors do not cause autoimmunity, SATB1-targeted immunotherapy is expected to be safe to treat cancer patients. Nevertheless, the risk of autoimmunity induced by SATB1-targeted immunotherapy should be still considered in future clinic trials and impact of SATB1-specific T cells on developing T cells in vivo needs further exploration.

The FDA has recently approved a cancer vaccine, Sipuleucel-T, for the treatment of patients with advanced prostate cancer based on a phase III study [4]. Sipuleucel-T is prepared from autologous PBMCs containing antigen presenting cells that are incubated with a recombinant protein composed of a PAP linked to granulocyte-macrophage colony-stimulating factor (GM-CSF). Sipuleucel-T presumably works in part by augmenting PAP-specific CD8$^+$ T cell responses, further demonstrating the importance of tumor antigen-specific CD8$^+$ T cells induced by cancer vaccines. So far, Sipuleucel-T is the first cellular immunotherapeutic agent approved by the FDA to be used for the treatment of cancer patients. The FDA approval of Sipuleucel-T as a therapeutic cancer vaccine not only validates the efficacy of cancer immunotherapy, but also provides a strong impetus in the field of cancer immunology [1]. Therefore, identification and development of more novel TAAs including SATB1 and peptide derivatives recognized by CTLs is definitely essential to facilitate the development of effective cancer vaccines. Although, a large number of human TAAs have been identified in melanoma and other types of cancer [2], much less is known about ovarian and lymphoma tumor antigens, thus impeding the development of cancer immunotherapy for patients with ovarian cancer and lymphoma. In this study, we find that SATB1 is also highly expressed in ovarian cancer cells and lymphoma cells, and importantly SATB1-specific T cells can recognize and kill these cancer cells, suggesting that identification of SATB1 as a tumor antigen has important implications for the development of potentially therapeutic vaccines against ovarian cancer, lymphoma and other types of cancer as well.

In summary, we have identified a novel SATB1-derived CD8$^+$ T cell epitope SATB1$_{565-574}$. Since SATB1 expression is strongly up-regulated in various types of cancer, SATB1$_{565-574}$ may serve as a diagnostic tool or an immunotherapeutic target of cancer vaccines for ovarian cancer, lymphoma and other types of cancer.

Supporting Information

Figure S1 SATB1$_{565-574}$ induced peptide-specific CD8$^+$ T cell-dependent responses. SATB1$_{565-574}$- reactive T cells were co-cultured with T2 cells loaded with EBV peptide as a negative control (A) or peptide SATB1$_{565-574}$ (B) in the presence of GolgiStop in a 48-well plate for 4 hrs at 37°C. Cells were then stained with FITC conjugated anti-CD8 and PE conjugated anti-IFN-γ, and analyzed on a FACScalibur machine.

Figure S2 IFN-γ enhanced expression of HLA-A*02 molecules on surfaces of tumor cells. Cells were pre-treated without (Green line) or with (red line) IFN-γ at 10 ng/mL for 48 hours, and then were stained with FITC-anti-HLA-A*02. Afterwards, cells were re-suspended in 500 μl PBS and analyzed using a FACScalibur machine. The grey histograms represent isotype controls.

Figure S3 SATB1$_{565-574}$ -specific T cells were not able to recognize in vitro-differentiated Th cell subsets. Different T cell subsets (Th1, Th2, Th17 and PBMC) were co-incubated without or with SATB1$_{565-574}$ -specific CD8$^+$ T cells (0.1×10^6) in 96-well plate, respectively. Cells were incubated for 18–24 hours, the IFN-γ secretion in the supernatant was determined by ELISA assay. T2 cells loaded with SATB1$_{565-574}$ were used as positive control. ***$P < 0.001$ versus control (SATB1$_{565-574}$–specific T cells stimulated with unloaded T2 cells).

File S1 Supplemental Materials and Methods.

Acknowledgments

We would like to thank Drs. Dan Liu and Adebusola Alagbala Ajibade for the critical reading of this manuscript.

Author Contributions

Conceived and designed the experiments: MW BY SM RFW HYW. Performed the experiments: MW BY SM LD YL WZ JZ QL CL. Analyzed the data: MW SM RFW HYW. Wrote the paper: MW RFW HYW.

References

1. Mellman I, Coukos G, Dranoff G (2011) Cancer immunotherapy comes of age. Nature 480: 480–489.
2. Novellino L, Castelli C, Parmiani G (2005) A listing of human tumor antigens recognized by T cells: March 2004 update. Cancer immunology, immunotherapy : CII 54: 187–207.
3. Cheever MA, Allison JP, Ferris AS, Finn OJ, Hastings BM, et al. (2009) The prioritization of cancer antigens: a national cancer institute pilot project for the acceleration of translational research. Clinical cancer research : an official journal of the American Association for Cancer Research 15: 5323–5337.
4. Kantoff PW, Higano CS, Shore ND, Berger ER, Small EJ, et al. (2010) Sipuleucel-T immunotherapy for castration-resistant prostate cancer. The New England journal of medicine 363: 411–422.
5. Hodi FS, O'Day SJ, McDermott DF, Weber RW, Sosman JA, et al. (2010) Improved survival with ipilimumab in patients with metastatic melanoma. The New England journal of medicine 363: 711–723.
6. Schwartzentruber DJ, Lawson DH, Richards JM, Conry RM, Miller DM, et al. (2011) gp100 peptide vaccine and interleukin-2 in patients with advanced melanoma. The New England journal of medicine 364: 2119–2127.
7. DuPage M, Mazumdar C, Schmidt LM, Cheung AF, Jacks T (2012) Expression of tumour-specific antigens underlies cancer immunoediting. Nature 482: 405–409.
8. Matsushita H, Vesely MD, Koboldt DC, Rickert CG, Uppaluri R, et al. (2012) Cancer exome analysis reveals a T-cell-dependent mechanism of cancer immunoediting. Nature 482: 400–404.
9. Rosenberg SA (2011) Cell transfer immunotherapy for metastatic solid cancer—what clinicians need to know. Nature reviews Clinical oncology 8: 577–585.
10. Lesterhuis WJ, Haanen JB, Punt CJ (2011) Cancer immunotherapy–revisited. Nature reviews Drug discovery 10: 591–600.
11. Di Lorenzo G, Buonerba C, Kantoff PW (2011) Immunotherapy for the treatment of prostate cancer. Nature reviews Clinical oncology 8: 551–561.
12. Beatty GL, Vonderheide RH (2008) Telomerase as a universal tumor antigen for cancer vaccines. Expert review of vaccines 7: 881–887.
13. Andersen MH, Svane IM, Becker JC, Straten PT (2007) The universal character of the tumor-associated antigen survivin. Clinical cancer research : an official journal of the American Association for Cancer Research 13: 5991–5994.
14. Straten P, Andersen MH (2010) The anti-apoptotic members of the Bcl-2 family are attractive tumor-associated antigens. Oncotarget 1: 239–245.
15. Riker A, Cormier J, Panelli M, Kammula U, Wang E, et al. (1999) Immune selection after antigen-specific immunotherapy of melanoma. Surgery 126: 112–120.
16. Campoli M, Chang CC, Ferrone S (2002) HLA class I antigen loss, tumor immune escape and immune selection. Vaccine 20 Suppl 4: A40–45.
17. Kohwi-Shigematsu T, Poterlowicz K, Ordinario E, Han HJ, Botchkarev VA, et al. (2012) Genome organizing function of SATB1 in tumor progression. Seminars in cancer biology.
18. Han HJ, Russo J, Kohwi Y, Kohwi-Shigematsu T (2008) SATB1 reprogrammes gene expression to promote breast tumour growth and metastasis. Nature 452: 187–193.
19. Zhao XD, Ji WY, Zhang W, He LX, Yang J, et al. (2010) Overexpression of SATB1 in laryngeal squamous cell carcinoma. ORL; journal for oto-rhino-laryngology and its related specialties 72: 1–5.
20. Mokhtar NM, Ramzi NH, Yin-Ling W, Rose IM, Hatta Mohd Dali AZ, et al. (2012) Laser capture microdissection with genome-wide expression profiling displayed gene expression signatures in endometrioid endometrial cancer. Cancer investigation 30: 156–164.
21. Tu W, Luo M, Wang Z, Yan W, Xia Y, et al. (2012) Upregulation of SATB1 promotes tumor growth and metastasis in liver cancer. Liver international : official journal of the International Association for the Study of the Liver 32: 1064–1078.
22. Meng WJ, Yan H, Zhou B, Zhang W, Kong XH, et al. (2012) Correlation of SATB1 overexpression with the progression of human rectal cancer. International journal of colorectal disease 27: 143–150.
23. Chen H, Takahara M, Oba J, Xie L, Chiba T, et al. (2011) Clinicopathologic and prognostic significance of SATB1 in cutaneous malignant melanoma. Journal of dermatological science 64: 39–44.
24. Cheng C, Lu X, Wang G, Zheng L, Shu X, et al. (2010) Expression of SATB1 and heparanase in gastric cancer and its relationship to clinicopathologic features. APMIS : acta pathologica, microbiologica, et immunologica Scandinavica 118: 855–863.
25. Lu X, Cheng C, Zhu S, Yang Y, Zheng L, et al. (2010) SATB1 is an independent prognostic marker for gastric cancer in a Chinese population. Oncology reports 24: 981–987.
26. Xiang J, Zhou L, Li S, Xi X, Zhang J, et al. (2012) AT-rich sequence binding protein 1: Contribution to tumor progression and metastasis of human ovarian carcinoma. Oncology letters 3: 865–870.
27. Mir R, Pradhan SJ, Galande S (2012) Chromatin organizer SATB1 as a novel molecular target for cancer therapy. Current drug targets.
28. Zhou LY, Liu F, Tong J, Chen QQ, Zhang FW (2009) [Expression of special AT-rich sequence-binding protein mRNA and its clinicopathological significance in non-small cell lung cancer]. Nan fang yi ke da xue xue bao = Journal of Southern Medical University 29: 534–537.
29. Chu SH, Ma YB, Feng DF, Zhang H, Zhu ZA, et al. (2012) Upregulation of SATB1 is associated with the development and progression of glioma. Journal of translational medicine 10: 149.

30. Fogh J, Wright WC, Loveless JD (1977) Absence of HeLa cell contamination in 169 cell lines derived from human tumors. Journal of the National Cancer Institute 58: 209–214.

31. Fogh J, Trempe G (1975) New human tumor cell lines; Fogh J, editor. New York: Plenum Publishing Corp.

32. Kanzler H, Hansmann ML, Kapp U, Wolf J, Diehl V, et al. (1996) Molecular single cell analysis demonstrates the derivation of a peripheral blood-derived cell line (L1236) from the Hodgkin/Reed-Sternberg cells of a Hodgkin's lymphoma patient. Blood 87: 3429–3436.

33. Wolf J, Kapp U, Bohlen H, Kornacker M, Schoch C, et al. (1996) Peripheral blood mononuclear cells of a patient with advanced Hodgkin's lymphoma give rise to permanently growing Hodgkin-Reed Sternberg cells. Blood 87: 3418–3428.

34. Zeng G, Wang X, Robbins PF, Rosenberg SA, Wang RF (2001) CD4(+) T cell recognition of MHC class II-restricted epitopes from NY-ESO-1 presented by a prevalent HLA DP4 allele: association with NY-ESO-1 antibody production. Proceedings of the National Academy of Sciences of the United States of America 98: 3964–3969.

35. Wang M, Lamberth K, Harndahl M, Roder G, Stryhn A, et al. (2007) CTL epitopes for influenza A including the H5N1 bird flu; genome-, pathogen-, and HLA-wide screening. Vaccine 25: 2823–2831.

36. Hammond AS, Klein MR, Corrah T, Fox A, Jaye A, et al. (2005) Mycobacterium tuberculosis genome-wide screen exposes multiple CD8 T cell epitopes. Clinical and experimental immunology 140: 109–116.

37. Matsueda S, Wang M, Weng J, Li Y, Yin B, et al. (2012) Identification of prostate-specific g-protein coupled receptor as a tumor antigen recognized by CD8(+) T cells for cancer immunotherapy. PloS one 7: e45756.

38. Dudley ME, Wunderlich JR, Shelton TE, Even J, Rosenberg SA (2003) Generation of tumor-infiltrating lymphocyte cultures for use in adoptive transfer therapy for melanoma patients. Journal of immunotherapy 26: 332–342.

39. Weng J, Ma W, Mitchell D, Zhang J, Liu M (2005) Regulation of human prostate-specific G-protein coupled receptor, PSGR, by two distinct promoters and growth factors. Journal of cellular biochemistry 96: 1034–1048.

40. Van den Eynde BJ, Boon T (1997) Tumor antigens recognized by T lymphocytes. International journal of clinical & laboratory research 27: 81–86.

41. Boon T, Coulie PG, Van den Eynde B (1997) Tumor antigens recognized by T cells. Immunology today 18: 267–268.

42. Pavan Kumar P, Purbey PK, Sinha CK, Notani D, Limaye A, et al. (2006) Phosphorylation of SATB1, a global gene regulator, acts as a molecular switch regulating its transcriptional activity in vivo. Molecular cell 22: 231–243.

43. Yamayoshi A, Yasuhara M, Galande S, Kobori A, Murakami A (2011) Decoy-DNA against special AT-rich sequence binding protein 1 inhibits the growth and invasive ability of human breast cancer. Oligonucleotides 21: 115–121.

44. Toes RE, Nussbaum AK, Degermann S, Schirle M, Emmerich NP, et al. (2001) Discrete cleavage motifs of constitutive and immunoproteasomes revealed by quantitative analysis of cleavage products. The Journal of experimental medicine 194: 1–12.

45. Alvarez JD, Yasui DH, Niida H, Joh T, Loh DY, et al. (2000) The MAR-binding protein SATB1 orchestrates temporal and spatial expression of multiple genes during T-cell development. Genes & development 14: 521–535.

46. Fessing MY, Mardaryev AN, Gdula MR, Sharov AA, Sharova TY, et al. (2011) p63 regulates Satb1 to control tissue-specific chromatin remodeling during development of the epidermis. The Journal of cell biology 194: 825–839.

47. Savarese F, Davila A, Nechanitzky R, De La Rosa-Velazquez I, Pereira CF, et al. (2009) Satb1 and Satb2 regulate embryonic stem cell differentiation and Nanog expression. Genes & development 23: 2625–2638.

4

Phase I Clinical Trial of Fibronectin CH296-Stimulated T Cell Therapy in Patients with Advanced Cancer

Takeshi Ishikawa[1,2], Satoshi Kokura[1,2]*, Tatsuji Enoki[3], Naoyuki Sakamoto[1], Tetsuya Okayama[1,2], Mitsuko Ideno[3], Junichi Mineno[3], Kazuko Uno[4], Naohisa Yoshida[1], Kazuhiro Kamada[1], Kazuhiro Katada[1], Kazuhiko Uchiyama[1], Osamu Handa[1], Tomohisa Takagi[1], Hideyuki Konishi[1], Nobuaki Yagi[1], Yuji Naito[1], Yoshito Itoh[1], Toshikazu Yoshikawa[2]

1 Department of Molecular Gastroenterology and Hepatology, Graduate School of Medical Science, Kyoto Prefectural University of Medicine, Kyoto, Japan, 2 Department of Cancer ImmunoCell Regulation, Kyoto Prefectural University of Medicine, Kyoto, Japan, 3 Center for Cell and Gene Therapy, Takara Bio Inc, Otsu, Japan, 4 Division of Basic Research, Louis Pasteur Center for Medical Research, Kyoto, Japan

Abstract

Background: Previous studies have demonstrated that less-differentiated T cells are ideal for adoptive T cell transfer therapy (ACT) and that fibronectin CH296 (FN-CH296) together with anti-CD3 resulted in cultured cells that contain higher amounts of less-differentiated T cells. In this phase I clinical trial, we build on these prior results by assessing the safety and efficacy of FN-CH296 stimulated T cell therapy in patients with advanced cancer.

Methods: Patients underwent fibronectin CH296-stimulated T cell therapy up to six times every two weeks and the safety and antitumor activity of the ACT were assessed. In order to determine immune function, whole blood cytokine levels and the number of peripheral regulatory T cells were analyzed prior to ACT and during the follow up.

Results: Transferred cells contained numerous less-differentiated T cells greatly represented by CD27+CD45RA+ or CD28+CD45RA+ cell, which accounted for approximately 65% and 70% of the total, respectively. No ACT related severe or unexpected toxicities were observed. The response rate among patients was 22.2% and the disease control rate was 66.7%.

Conclusions: The results obtained in this phase I trial, indicate that FN-CH296 stimulated T cell therapy was very well tolerated with a level of efficacy that is quite promising. We also surmise that expanding T cell using CH296 is a method that can be applied to other T- cell-based therapies.

Editor: William C. S. Cho, Queen Elizabeth Hospital, Hong Kong

Funding: This study was partially supported by JSPS KAKENHI Grant Number 23590891. The funders had no role in study design, data collection and analysis, decision to publish, or preparation of the manuscript. No additional external funding received for this study.

Competing Interests: Takeshi Ishikawa, Satoshi Kokura, Tetsuya Okayama, and Toshikazu Yoshikawa have an affiliation with a donation-funded department from TAKARA BIO Inc.

* E-mail: s-kokura@koto.kpu-m.ac.jp

Introduction

Adoptive T cell transfer (ACT) is currently one of the few immunotherapies that can induce objective clinical responses in a significant number of patients with metastatic solid tumors [1]. The intrinsic properties of the ACT population, particularly its state of differentiation, are said to be crucial to the success of ACT-based approaches [2–5]. Less differentiated T cells have a higher proliferative potential and are less prone to apoptosis than more differentiated cells. Less differentiated T cells express receptors such as the IL-7 receptor α-chain (IL-7Rα), therefore these cells have the potential to proliferate and become fully activated in response to homeostatic cytokines such as IL-7 [6]. Results from prior clinical studies demonstrated a significant correlation between tumor regression and the percentage of persistent ACT transferred cells in the peripheral blood [3,7]. These findings

suggest that the persistence and proliferative potential of transferred T cells play a role in clinical response and that less-differentiated T cells are ideal for ACT transfer therapy. Using a standard rapid expansion protocol, T cells for ACT are usually expanded with a high dose of IL-2 and CD3-specific antibody for about 2 weeks. T cells using this protocol induce progressive T cell differentiation towards a late effector state. However, although IL-2 is essential for the persistence and growth of T cell it also has undesirable qualities, such as its ability to promote the terminal differentiation of T cells [8]. As a result, the currently used procedure results in phenotypic and functional changes of T cells that make them less optimal for mediating antitumor responses in vivo. In light of this, developing new methods to obtain less differentiated T cells is crucial for improving current T-cell-based therapies so that patients can develop a long-lasting positive immune response.

It has been reported that fibronectin (FN), a major extracellular matrix protein, functions not only as an adhesion molecule but also as a signal inducer via binding to integrins expressed on T cells [9,10]. FN acts together with anti-CD3 to induce T cell proliferation, which is thought to depend on integrin very late activation antigen-4 (VLA-4)/CS1 interactions [11,12]. Recombinant human fibronectin fragment (FN-CH296, RetroNectin) has been widely used for retroviral gene therapy to enhance gene transfer efficiency. FN-CH296 was also reported to be able to stimulate peripheral blood T cell growth in vitro when used together with anti-CD3 and IL-2. Anti-CD3/IL-2/FN-CH296-stimulated T cells contained a higher quantity of less-differentiated T cells and in vivo persistence of these cells was significantly higher than cells stimulated by other methods [13]. These observations led us to apply FN-CH296-mediated stimulation to less differentiated phenotype T cells to generate 'fit T cells' [2,14] which are ideal for ACT. In this way, we proceeded to evaluate the safety and efficacy of FN-CH296-stimulated T cell therapy in patients with advanced cancer.

Methods

The protocol for this trial and supporting TREND checklist are available as supporting information; see Checklist S1 and Protocol S1.

Study Design

The clinical protocol was approved by the ethics committee of Kyoto Prefectural University of Medicine and was conducted in accordance with the Declaration of Helsinki and Ethical Guidelines for Clinical Research (the Ministry of Health, Labor and Welfare, Japan). The primary objective of this phase I clinical trial was to assess the safety and adverse-event profiles of FN-CH296-stimulated T cell therapy in patients with advanced cancer. Our secondary objective was to assess the antitumor activity of ACT therapy. This study was conducted as a standard 3+3 phase I design that investigated the dose limiting toxicities (DLTs) occurring over a 28-day period after the second infusion of cultured lymphocytes. DLT was defined as grade ≥ 3 for any adverse event related to the infusion of cultured cells. We used an accelerated titration design to assess the safety of the number of adoptive lymphocytes at 1×10^9 (cohort 1), 3×10^9 (cohort 2), and 9×10^9 (cohort 3) per person. If no DLTs were observed in the first cohort of patients, a second cohort of 3 patients were treated at the next higher dose. If DLT was observed in at least one patient, the cohort was expanded to 6 patients. If ≥ 2 DLTs were noted in the initial or expanded cohort, no further dose escalations were performed and the maximally tolerated dose (MTD) was considered to have been exceeded. There was no intra-patient dose escalation in this study.

Written informed consent was obtained from all patients. This study is registered in the UMIN Clinical Trials Registry with the identifier UMIN000001835.

Patients

Patients enrolled in this trial fulfilled the following eligibility criteria: histologically or cytologically confirmed esophageal cancer, gastric cancer, colorectal cancer, pancreatic cancer, biliary tract cancer or non-small lung cancer; residual disease after standard treatment with no other curative treatment options available; no plans to receive chemotherapy other than oral fluorouracil prodrugs, radiation therapy or biological response modifiers; between 20 to 80 years of age; an Eastern Cooperative Oncology Group (ECOG) performance status of 2 or less; a life

expectancy of at least three months; at least four weeks since their last chemotherapy or radiation therapy; and adequate hematologic, hepatic, renal and cardiac function.

The exclusion criteria were as follows: presence of uncontrolled infection; a history of autoimmune disease or severe hypersensitivity; presence of serious complications such as unstable angina, or myocardial infarction within six months of cancer onset, interstitial pneumonia or pulmonary fibrosis with radiological findings, presence of marked ascites or pleural effusion, ileus, active other malignancy, severe mental impairment, pregnancy or lactation, and a medical history of severe hypersensitivity.

Preparation of the FN-CH296-stimulated T cells

Peripheral blood (50–70 mL) was taken from cancer patients. Peripheral blood mononuclear cells (PBMCs) were separated using Ficoll-Paque PREMIUM (GE Healthcare, Tokyo, Japan). Subsequently, $3–8 \times 10^7$ cells were re-suspended in culture medium in a CultiLife215 bag (Takara Bio, Otsu, Japan) that was pre-coated with both anti-CD3 and FN-CH296 (RetroNectin®, Takara Bio), which is a recombinant fragment of human fibronectin. Cells were cultured in a serum-free medium, GT-T551 (Takara Bio), which was supplemented with 0.6–1.2% heat-inactivated autologous plasma and 200 U/mL of recombinant IL-2 (Proleukin; Novartis Pharma, Nürnberg, Germany). On day 4, the cells were transferred to a CultiLife Eva bag (Takara Bio), and GT-T551 medium that was supplemented with 0.6–1.2% heat-inactivated autologous plasma and 200 U/mL of IL-2 was added. On day 7, GT-T551 medium containing 200 U/mL of IL-2 was added. On day 10, the cells were harvested and re-suspended in 50–90 mL of cryopreserved solution consisting of CP-1 (Kyokutou Seiyaku, Tokyo, Japan), RPMI1640 (KOHJIN BIO, Sakado, Japan) and human serum albumin (Albuminar; CSL Behring, PA, USA) to create the final cell product. In order to obtain the determined number of adoptive lymphocytes, the patients in cohorts 1 and 2 needed a one-time lymphocyte culture, and the patients in cohort 3 needed three lymphocyte cultures. Cultured lymphocytes were frozen and stored at $-80°C$ until the time of transfusion.

Before infusing patients, cell products were assessed for ① viability by trypan blue exclusion assay ② for sterility by the BacT/ALERT (bioMérieux, Durham, NC, USA) microbiological detection system, and ③ endotoxin by a kinetic turbidimetric LAL assay. Both sterility and endotoxin tests were contracted to FALCO Biosystems (Kyoto, Japan). Further, phenotypic markers of a small aliquot of final products were examined after the freeze-thawing. Thus, these markers are considered to be almost similar to those of the infused cells.

Whole Blood Cytokine Assays

Immune function was tested using venous blood obtained from patients prior to administering them with cultured cells (baseline) and during the follow up which occurred 4 weeks after the 2nd and 6th cultured cell infusion (Fig. 1). Methods for quantifying IFN-α production in whole human blood have been described previously [15]. Briefly, heparinized peripheral blood was cultured with Sendai virus (500 HA/mL) within 8 h after the blood sample was taken. The blood–virus mixture was incubated at 37°C for 20 h, and IFN-α activity in the supernatants was quantified by a bioassay. Other cytokines were quantified according to procedures described previously [16,17]. Heparinized whole blood was diluted 4-fold with Eagle's minimal essential medium (Nissui Pharmaceutical Co. Ltd., Tokyo, Japan) and stimulated with phytohemagglutinin-P (PHA-P, 25 µg/mL, Wako Pure Chemical Ind., Osaka, Japan). Samples were incubated at 37°C for 48 h, after which the supernatants were harvested by centrifugation at $800 \times g$ for

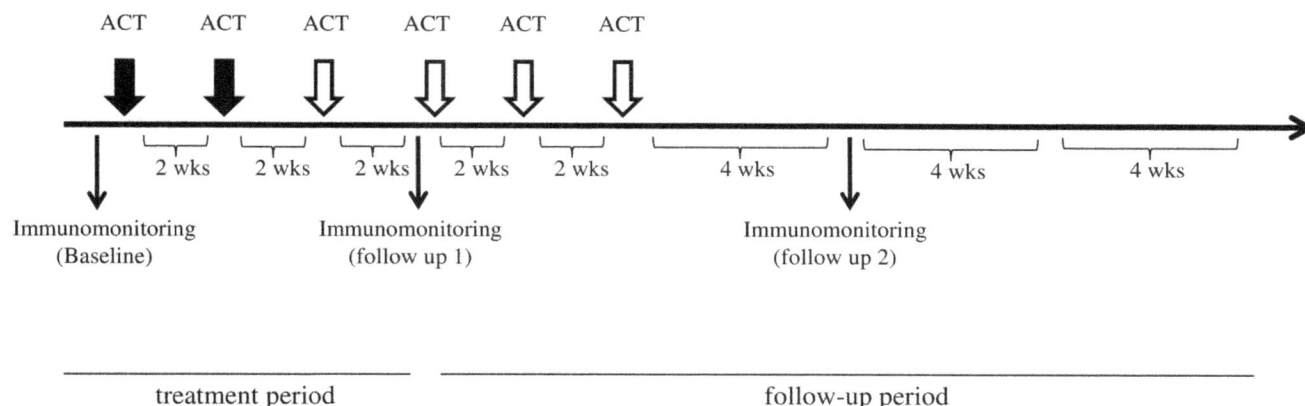

Figure 1. Treatment protocol. Subjects received CH296-stimulated T-cell therapy on days 1 and 15. We conducted safety evaluations for the first 6 weeks of treatment. Patients who wished to continue the treatment received up to 4 further treatments every 2 weeks. To test immune function, venous blood was obtained from subjects before the start of therapy (baseline) and during follow-up one which occurred at 4 weeks (2 treatments) and after 6 cultured cell administrations.

10 min, and then stored at $-80°C$ until they were required for analysis. Cytokine levels in the samples were measured with a Bio-Plex multiplex cytokine array system (; Bio-Rad Laboratories, CA, USA) according to the manufacturer's instructions. The Multiplex Th1/Th2 bead kit (Bio-Rad Laboratories) measured the following cytokines: IL-2, IL-4, IL-5, IL-10, IL-12(p70), IL-13, Tumor Necrosis Factor (TNF)-α, IFN-γ, and granulocyte–monocyte colony-stimulating factor (GM-CSF). Data acquisition and analysis were conducted with the Bio-Plex Manager Software, version 5.0. Since the levels of cytokines without PHA-P-stimulation were extremely low (data not shown), we only assessed those with PHA-P-stimulation in this study.

Flow Cytometric Analysis

The cells were stained with FITC-, phycoerythrin (PE)-, Phycoerythrin-TexasRed (ECD)-, or Phycoerythrin-Cyanin (PC5)-conjugated mAb specific for CD3, CD4, CD8, CD27, CD45RA, CD56, HLA-DR (Beckman Coulter, Marseille, France), CD28, NKG2D (eBioscience, CA, USA) and CCR7 (R&D systems, MN, USA). To determine the regulatory T cell (Treg), we used the following antibodies: PE-Cy^{TM}5 mouse anti-human CD4, PE mouse anti-human CD25, and Alexa Fluor® 488 mouse anti-human Foxp3 (BD Biosciences Pharmingen, CA, USA). Cells were incubated at 5°C for 30 min, then washed with phosphate-buffered saline and analyzed by Cytomics FC500 (Beckman Coulter). For Foxp3 detection, cells were permeabilized overnight in Fix/Perm buffer (eBioscience) and then stained with anti-Foxp3. Data acquisition and analysis were conducted with the CXP Software, version 2.2 (Beckman Coulter). The flow data was analyzed by the following method: lymphocyte gates were determined visually in FSC/SSC dot plot after which gates with a positive region of CD3, HLA-DR were determined by staining cells with isotype control antibodies. The others (CD4, CD8, CD28, CD45RA, CD56, CD28, NKG2D and CCR7) were determined visually at a valley point of histogram or dot plot. Tregs phenotype was defined as CD4+ CD25+Foxp3+ cell.

Study Treatment

Frozen cells were rapidly thawed at 37°C in a water bath with gentle agitation. Patients were infused intravenously for 30 min on an outpatient basis at Kyoto Prefectural University Hospital. Patients were monitored for acute toxic effects for at least one hour

after infusion before they were discharged. Cultured lymphocytes were administered on days 1 and 15, and we conducted immune-monitoring to evaluate the safety of the treatment 4 weeks after the 2nd adoptive cell transfer was done. Two transfers are usually sufficient to assess the safety of novel ACT however since further treatments can be beneficial, patients could receive up to four more transfers every two weeks unless they had unacceptable toxic effects, disease progression, or withdrew consent (Fig. 1).

Toxicity and Efficacy Assessment

Safety and toxicity was determined based on regular patient interviews, laboratory tests and physical examinations. Toxic effects were monitored according to the National Cancer Institute Common Toxicity Criteria (NCI-CTC VERSION 3.0). The relationship between adoptive cell transfer and toxicity was evaluated based on the characteristics of ACT side effects compared with those of oral fluorouracil prodrugs.

Antitumor activity was evaluated based on actual tumor response. For efficacy assessment, computed tomography (CT) was performed before the start of ACT treatment, four weeks after the 2nd infusion of cultured lymphocytes and thereafter, every 4 weeks for three months. Responses were defined according to the Response Evaluation Criteria in Solid Tumors (RECIST VERSION 1.0) criteria.

Statistical Analysis

A Wilcoxon signed ranks test was used to compare the results before and after treatment. Spearman correlation coefficient method was used to assess a possible linear association between two continuous variables. P values less than 0.05 were considered significant. All statistical analyses were performed with SPSS software (version 20) for Windows (IBM Corporation, Illinois, U.S.A.).

Results

Patient Characteristics

From May 2009 to December 2009, ten cancer patients were enrolled in this study. One patient discontinued due to a rapid worsening of his general condition before starting treatment. Thus nine patients were eligible for the study and assigned to three treatment cohorts. The patients' clinical features are listed in

Table 1. Patient characteristics.

No.	Cohort	Age (years)	Gender	Disease	ECOG/PS	Prior treatment	Combined treatment (chemotherapy)
1	Cohort 1	52	M	colonic cancer	0	1st line, mFOLFOX62nd line, S-1	S-1
2	Cohort 1	62	M	pancreatic cancer	1	1st line, GEM2nd line, S-1	S-1
3	Cohort 1	60	M	gastric cancer	0	1st line, S-1	S-1
4	Cohort 2	72	F	rectal cancer	0	1st line, mFOLFOX62nd line, Capectabine	S-1
5	Cohort 2	61	F	bile duct cancer	1	1st line, GEM2nd line, S-1	S-1
6	Cohort 2	75	M	lung cancer	1	1st line, GEM/CDDP2nd line, DTX	none
7	Cohort 3	48	M	hepatocellular carcinoma	1	1st line, 5-FU/CDDP	none
8	Cohort 3	43	M	bile duct cancer	1	1st line, GEM2nd line, GEM/S-1	S-1
9	Cohort 3	53	M	rectal cancer	1	1st line, mFOLFOX6+bevacizumab2nd line, FOLFIRI 3rd line, CPT-11+cetuximab	S-1

ECOG = Eastern Cooperative Oncology Group.
PS = performance status.

Table 1. The median age was 60 years (range 43–75), and all patients had an ECOG performance score of 0 or 1. Three patients had colorectal cancer, two had bile duct cancer, and one patient each had pancreatic cancer, gastric cancer, hepatocellular carcinoma, and lung cancer. Of the nine patients, seven had received S-1 (an oral fluoropyrimidine) monotherapy that was combined with ACT therapy. All patients underwent two infusions of cultured cells, and eight patients who wished to continue treatment completed a further 4 T-cell infusions. Of nine patients, one (Patient no. 9) did not wish to continue the treatment, so he received two infusions of cultured cells in total.

Phenotype of Transferred Cells

Cells expanded a mean of 394.0-fold (range, 292.5-554.5-folds) during the 10-day culture period. The mean cultured cell viability was 97.4% (range 95.7-98.5%). Changes in cell-surface phenotype after culture are shown in Figure 2. Before stimulation, PBMCs contained approximately 45% CD4+ cells and 25% CD8+ cells. The ratio of CD8 cells significantly increased to almost 60% after culture, whereas CD4+ cell ratio showed a decrease. The ratio of CD27+CD45RA+ and CD28+CD45RA+ cells which was expressed in less-differentiated T cells, significantly increased to almost 60% after culture, whereas there was no significant change in the ratio of CCR7+CD45RA+ cells. Both CD3+HLA-DR+ and CD8+NKG2D+ cell population which are activation markers for lymphocytes, significantly increased after culture. On the other hand, CD3-CD56+ (NK cell) and CD3+CD56+ cell population (NKT cell) were insignificant after culture (mean of 0.73% and 2.16% respectively). The transferred cell phenotype of each case is shown in Table 2. The large majority of transferred cells were CD3 positive (98.1% as mean), and there were very few CD3-CD56+ cells (0.73% as mean). The ratios of CD4+, CD8+, and CD8+NKG2D+ cells in transferred cells were 36.2%, 60.3%, and 53.7%, respectively. As for less-differentiated T cell phenotype, CD27+CD45RA+, CD28+CD45RA+, and CCR7+CD45RA+ cells were 59.5%, 60.0%, and 22.4%, respectively. The proportion of these less-differentiated T cell phenotype was markedly different among patients, particularly, the proportion in patient 2 was considerably low (Table 2). Ratios of CD27+CD45RA+, CD28+CD45RA+, and CCR7+CD45RA+ transferred cells (after culture) strongly correlated with those of PBMCs (before culture) (Fig. 3).

Toxicity

The adverse events reported in this study are shown in Table 3. One patient, who was administered S-1, experienced grade 3 neutropenia however, this episode was considered to be related to S-1 and not to ACT. Grade two or lower level hematologic toxicities were observed mainly in patients administered with S-1, and these hematological toxicities were mostly transient. Non-hematological events including fatigue and anorexia were observed, but these were all mild. No ACT-related severe or unexpected toxicities were observed. Thus, no DLT was observed in this phase I study.

Clinical Outcome

One patient (no.4) achieved complete response (CR). The CR patient suffered from lymph node recurrence after a rectal cancer operation and she was treated with mFOLFOX6 as first line chemotherapy. Subsequently, she was treated with Capecitabine as second line chemotherapy, but intrapelvic lymph node metastasis was detected by FDG-PET. The patient then received ACT therapy combined with S-1. Three months after 6 infusions of cultured T cells, the lesion completely disappeared. Patient no.8

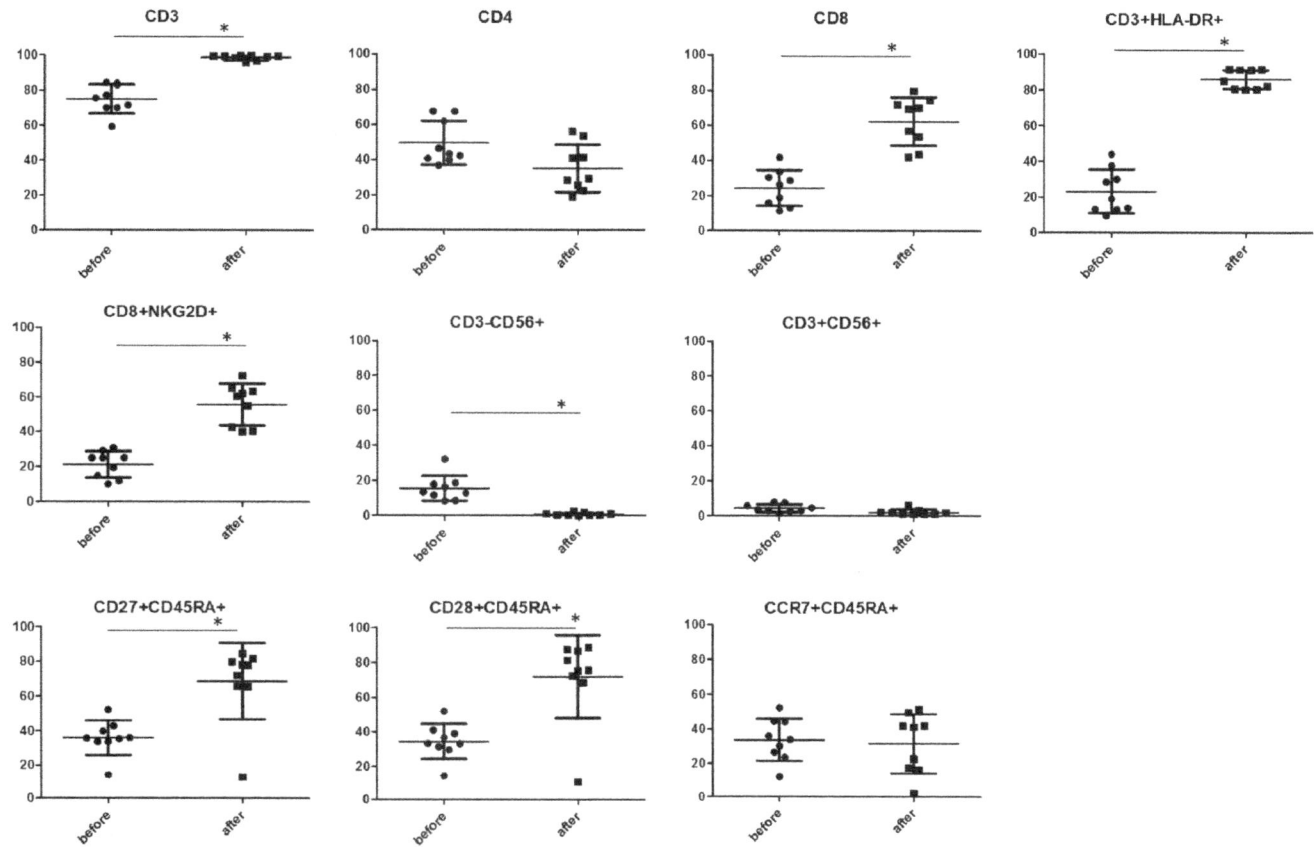

Figure 2. Changes in cell-surface phenotype after culture. PBMCs were stimulated with anti-CD3/CH-296. On day 10, cultured cells were harvested for transfusion. Cell-surface phenotypes of PBMCs or cultured cells were analyzed by flow cytometry. The average results from nine subjects are shown. In all panels, the lines represent the mean or standard deviation. *P<0.05.

experienced partial response (PR). He had refractory bile duct cancer, and was treated with GEM as first line chemotherapy followed by GEM/S-1 as 2nd line chemotherapy. However, 17 months after starting chemotherapy, the size of the primary tumor increased and metastases in the cervical vertebra were detected. He then underwent ACT therapy combined with S-1. Two

months after 6 infusions of ACT, the size of the primary tumor in his liver decreased by 35% and metastatic lesions in the cervical vertebra completely disappeared by FDG-PET.

Of the 9 patients, one (11.1%) exhibited CR, one (11.1%) had PR, 4 (44.4%) had stable disease (SD), and 3 (33.3%) had progressive disease (PD) (Table 4). The response rate was 22.2%

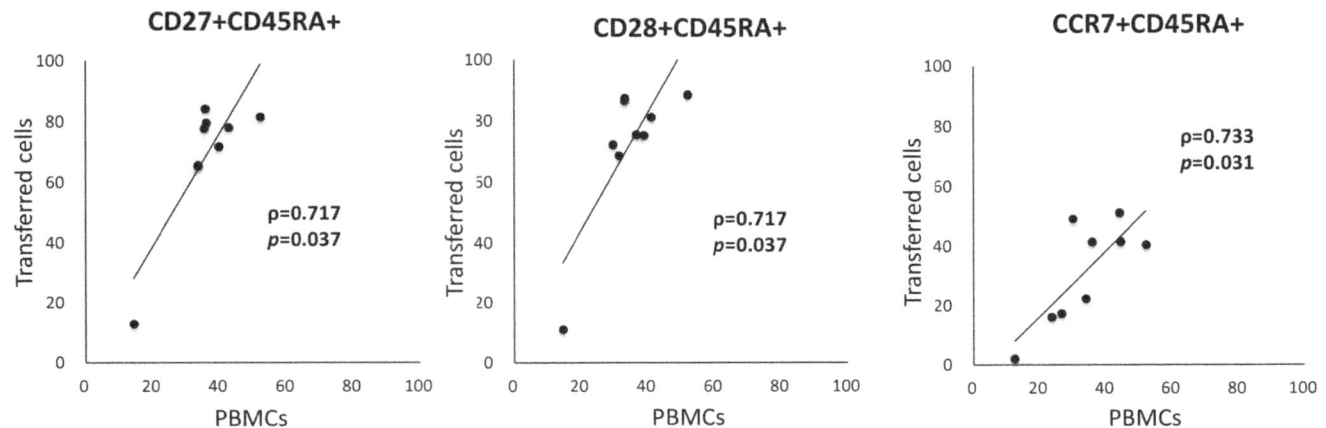

Figure 3. Correlation between the number of less-differentiated T-cell surface markers of transferred cells (after culture) and those of PBMCs (before culture). The comparison was done in terms of cell-surface markers (i.e. CD27+CD45RA+, CD28+CD45RA+, CCR7+CD45RA+).

Table 2. Characteristics of infused cells.

Patinet No.	CD3$^+$	CD4$^+$	CD8$^+$	CD3$^+$HLA-DR$^+$	CD8$^+$NKG2D$^+$	CD3-CD56$^+$	CD3$^+$CD56$^+$	CD27$^+$CD45RA$^+$	CD28$^+$CD45RA$^+$	CCR7$^+$CD45RA$^+$
1	99.45	28.41	70.09	81.87	63.27	0.38	1.99	77.83	75.57	41.67
2	96.52	41.37	53.51	80.10	42.52	2.33	6.32	12.91	11.03	2.03
3	98.35	44.16	52.14	87.18	45.02	1.15	1.19	35.37	33.64	9.87
4	99.41	26.83	68.72	91.74	59.93	0.39	1.65	68.25	54.41	28.33
5	99.68	41.21	53.48	93.18	50.06	0.36	1.62	56.06	63.96	16.67
6	99.50	44.85	48.92	85.80	45.19	0.41	2.65	57.03	60.33	16.47
7	99.30±0.47	27.59±2.53	70.875±1.62	91.16±0.06	62.97±3.17	0.55±0.33	1.37±0.37	65.66±0.06	70.45±2.59	16.84±0.87
8	99.74±0.06	21.37±3.56	77.27±3.58	86.22±7.26	68.98±4.86	0.08±0.04	1.00±0.19	85.25±1.36	88.46±2.47	25.44±4.16
9	95.88±4.82	50.21±8.12	47.50±8.26	82.04±2.48	44.92±8.52	0.96±0.69	1.66±1.26	77.22±4.96	81.74±6.64	44.56±5.91

Patient no. 1 to 6 needed a one-time culture and patients 7 to 9 underewent three lymphocyte cultures.
Values are expressed as mean±SD.

(95% confidence interval (CI) 2.8 ? 60.0%) and the disease control rate (DCR; CR+PR+SD) was 66.7% (95% CI 29.9 – 92.5%).

Immune Monitoring

To determine the immune responses in patients receiving novel ACT, whole blood cytokine assays and peripheral Treg analysis, which could be useful in immune monitoring[18–20], were done using venous blood obtained from patients. There was no marked change in whole blood cytokine levels (Fig. 4A) in patients after they were infused with cultured cells; however, there was a decrease in IL-4, IL-5 and IL-13 after the treatment. The levels of IFN-γ, TNF-α, IL-2, IL-12 and GM-CSF in cohort 3 increased after the treatment; in particular, the levels of IFN-γ, IL-12 and GM-CSF increased a multiple of 10 or more times. Next, we evaluated whole blood cytokine levels according to objective tumor response. The levels of IFN-γ, IL-2, IL-12 and GM-CSF in patients with PR/CR increased more than twice after the treatment, while those levels in patients with SD or PD decreased or did not change significantly post treatment (Fig. 4B).

As for Tregs, both the number and proportion of these cells in the peripheral blood showed no significant change after treatment when they were evaluated according to cohort or tumor response (Fig. 4A, B).

Discussion

The results presented in this study indicate that FN-CH296-stimulated T cell therapy was very well tolerated in our patient sample. No significant ACT-related grade 3 or 4 adverse events occurred in any patient and the ACT produced tumor regression in 2 patients: CR in one patient with rectal cancer and PR in another with bile duct cancer. The response rate was 22.2% and the DCR was 66.7%. Despite the size of the sample, these results are promising.

The findings of previous mouse studies and clinical trials demonstrated that less-differentiated T cells may be the optimal

Table 3. Maximum toxicity per patient.

	Any Grade (with S-1)	Grade 3–4 (with S-1)
Hematological		
Neutropenia	3 (3)	1 (1)
Lymphopenia	2 (1)	0
Anemia	5 (5)	0
Thrombocytopenia	8 (6)	0
Increased aspartate aminotransferase	1 (1)	0
Increased alanine aminotransferase	1 (1)	0
Increased alkaline phosphatase	3 (3)	0
Increased total bilirubin	6 (5)	0
Non-hematological		
Fatigue	3 (3)	0
Anorexia	3 (3)	0
Nausea	1 (1)	0
Diarrhea	2 (2)	0
Mucositis	2 (2)	0

Table 4. Tumor response.

No. of patients	Response				Response rate (%) (95% CI)
	CR	PR	SD	PD	
9	1	1	4	3	22.2 (2.8–60.0)

CR = complete response; PR = partial response; SD = stable disease; PD = progressive disease; 95% CI = 95% confidence interval.

population for ACT-based immunotherapies because of their in vivo persistence, high proliferative potential, receptiveness to homeostatic and costimulatory signals, their homing to secondary lymphoid tissues and their ability to secrete IL-2 [2–5]. Added to this, Yu et al. have reported that FN-CH296 acting with anti-CD3 induce T cell proliferation. These evidence suggests thats FN-CH296/anti-CD3 stimulation can be an efficient way to generate a large number of less-differentiated T cells suitable for ACT resulting in higher and longer persistence in vivo [13].

CD45RA, CD27, CD28, and CCR7 are known to be highly expressed in less-differentiated T cells. Based on human viral infection studies, a linear model of T cell differentiation has been proposed wherein CD27+CD28+CD45RA+ naïve cells progress through a CD27+CD28+CD45RA- early antigen-experienced phenotype and then proceeds to a CD27+CD28-CD45RA−/+ intermediate phenotype and finally to CD27-CD28-CD45RA+/− late antigen-experienced phenotype. This linear movement leads to an increase in cytotoxic potential and a reduction in cell proliferation [21]. CD27 and CD28 are costimulatory molecules that act in concert with T cell receptor (TCR) to support T cell expansion [22]. It has been suggested that CD28-expressing T cells secrete IL-2 and induce antiapoptotic molecules [23]. In recent times, the role of CD28 expression in ACT-based clinical trials has been getting closer attention and more detailed investigations are being done. Analysis of persisting and non-persisting TIL clones indicate preferential survival of the clonotypes expressing high levels of CD28, implicating a survival advantage for transferred T cells with CD28+ less-differentiated phenotype [4,5]. CD27 can also augment TCR-induced T cell

proliferation and is required for the generation and maintenance of memory T cells in vivo [24]. There is evidence that the frequency of T cells expressing CD27 increases gradually after ACT and may be associated with the long-term maintenance of a stable number of tumor-specific T cells in responding patients [25]. In this phase I clinical trial, the frequencies of both CD27+CD45RA+ and CD28+CD45RA+ cells increased significantly after culture and their population in transferred cells were about 60%. On the other hand, the frequency of CCR7+CD45RA+ cells, which were also expressed in less-differentiated T cells, did not change after culture for unknown reasons. The ratios of the less-differentiated phenotype T cells (i.e. CD27+CD45+, CD28+CD45RA+, and CCR7+CD45RA+ cells) in transferred cells differed greatly for each patient. A strong positive correlation was found between the ratios of CD27+CD45RA+ ($\rho = 0.717$, $p = 0.037$), CD28+CD45RA+ ($\rho = 0.717$, $p = 0.037$), CCR7+CD45RA+ ($\rho = 0.733$, $p = 0.031$) cells in transferred cells and those in PBMCs (before culture). It is necessary to improve upon or find new methods that can efficiently generate large numbers of less-differentiated T cells even in cases where there are few less-differentiated T cells. Consistent with previous reports [13], we found that stimulation with FN-CH296/anti-CD3 preferentially expanded CD8+ cells in this study. It is generally believed that the predominant tumoricidal effector mechanism is the cytotoxic killing effect of CD8+ T cells, however, despite the research done to date, the impact of the preferential proliferation of CD8 T cells on cancer immunotherapy still needs much further investigation.

Previous studies have demonstrated that IFN-γ plays an important role in cancer immunotherapy and IFN-γ expression of T cells is considered to be highly correlated with therapeutic success. We have also demonstrated that the assay of whole blood IFN-γ levels was an efficient method for evaluating clinical response to cancer immunotherapies [19] [20]. In this study, whole blood IFN-γ levels in cohort 3 increased up to 10 or more times after 6 infusions of cultured cells. Whole blood IFN-γ levels in PR or CR cases increased more than twice, whereas those in PD or SD cases saw no significant increase after the treatment. The finding in our prior study [20] that the increase in whole blood IFN-γ levels after ACT was independently related to overall

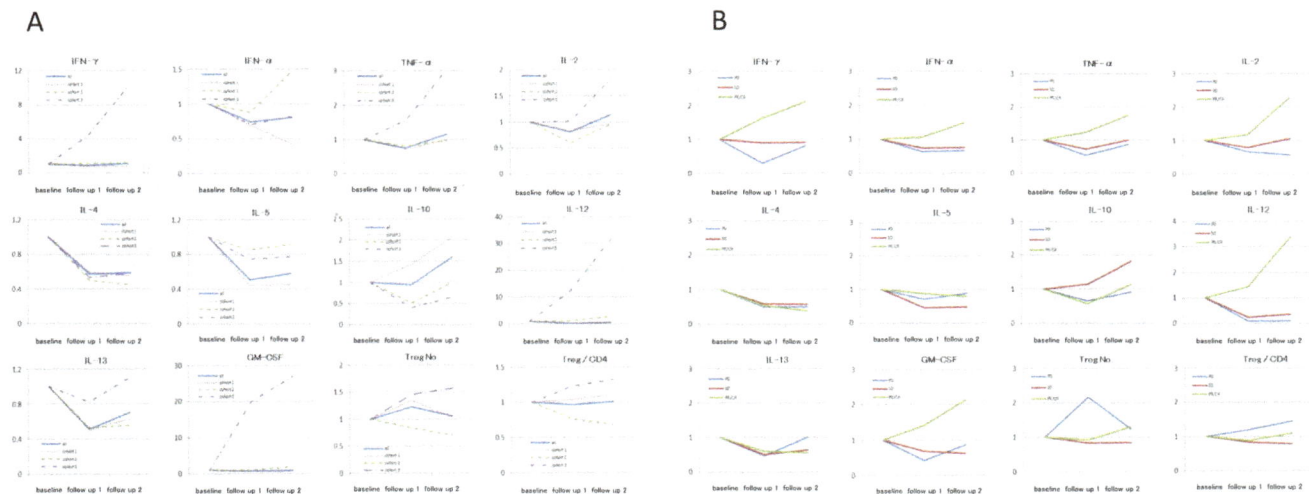

Figure 4. Longitudinal plots of whole blood cytokine levels plotted according to the deviation of cytokine levels from the baseline. Mean cytokine levels in subjects in each cohort (A) and levels for the various tumor responses (B) are shown.

survival in cancer patients emphasizes the relevance of the results gained in this study.

While no significant correlation between the number of infused less-differentiated T cells and whole blood IFN-γ levels was not confirmed probably due to small sample sizes, we surmise that less-differentiated T cells may contribute to the elevation of IFN-γ levels. Future studies are needed to explore the effect of the number of CD27+CD45RA+, CD28+CD45+ and CCR7+CD45RA+ cells on the whole blood IFN-γ levels.

In addition to IFN-γ other Th1 cytokine levels such as IL-2, IL-12 and TNF-α also increased in patients in cohort 3, and in patients with PR/CR, whereas Th2 cytokine levels such as IL-4, IL-5 and IL-13 decreased after the treatment. Besides, whole blood GM-CSF level increased in patients in cohort 3 and in patients who experienced PR/CR. It was previously reported that cell-mediated immunity is preferentially activated by Th1 cytokines, whereas Th2 cytokines suppresses cell-mediated immunity [26]. GM-CSF is a pleiotropic cytokine that stimulates dendritic cells (DCs) and promotes uptake of tumor antigens by DCs leading to T-cell cross-priming and activating the immune system against specific antigens [27,28]. Consequently, based on the results from the immune-monitoring done in this present study, we are inclined to believe that the fibronectin CH296-stimulated T cell therapy may exert anti-tumor effects by activating cell-mediated immunity. Although we recently demonstrated that ACT has the potential to reduce the number of Tregs [29], in the analysis done in this study, the number of peripheral Tregs did not change significantly post treatment.

Responsiveness to immune-based therapies varies among tumor types. While melanoma and renal-cell cancer are classically considered to be immunogenic, most epithelial malignancies are not immunogenic and respond poorly to immunotherapy. In our sample, all nine patients had epithelial malignancies such as gastrointestinal cancers and lung cancer which are traditionally considered as refractory to immunotherapy. It should be noted that objective response was observed in patients with rectal cancer and bile duct cancer. It remains unclear if this novel ACT has therapeutic potential for multiple tumor types. Additional studies are needed to determine the breadth of activity of this novel ACT in human malignancies.

In this phase I clinical trial, we demonstrated the safety of FN-CH296-stimulated T cell therapy in patients with advanced cancer. The results were promising with a response rate of 22.2% and DCR of 66.7%. ACT technology is a platform with high potential that can be further improved. Modification of T cells with transgenes encoding T cell receptors (TCRs) or chimeric antigen receptors (CARs) allows tumor specificity to be conferred on functionally distinct T cell subsets [30,31]. FN-CH296 stimulation could be efficient at generating large numbers of engineered T cells with less-differentiated phenotype. We surmise that T cell expansion using FN-CH296 could be applicable to various T cell based therapies such as engineered T cell therapy.

Author Contributions

Conceived and designed the experiments: TI SK TE JM. Performed the experiments: TI SK TE MI TO NS. Analyzed the data: TI SK TE MI. Contributed reagents/materials/analysis tools: TI TE MI KU. Wrote the paper: TI TE. Intellectual input and data analysis support: NY K. Kamada K. Katada KU OH TT HK NY YN YI TY.

References

1. Childs RW, Barrett J (2004) Nonmyeloablative allogeneic immunotherapy for solid tumors. Annu Rev Med 55: 459–475.
2. Gattinoni L, Klebanoff CA, Palmer DC, Wrzesinski C, Kerstann K, et al. (2005) Acquisition of full effector function in vitro paradoxically impairs the in vivo antitumor efficacy of adoptively transferred CD8+ T cells. J Clin Invest 115: 1616–1626.
3. Robbins PF, Dudley ME, Wunderlich J, El-Gamil M, Li YF, et al. (2004) Cutting edge: persistence of transferred lymphocyte clonotypes correlates with cancer regression in patients receiving cell transfer therapy. J Immunol 173: 7125–7130.
4. Zhou J, Shen X, Huang J, Hodes RJ, Rosenberg SA, et al. (2005) Telomere length of transferred lymphocytes correlates with in vivo persistence and tumor regression in melanoma patients receiving cell transfer therapy. J Immunol 175: 7046–7052.
5. Huang J, Khong HT, Dudley ME, El-Gamil M, Li YF, et al. (2005) Survival, persistence, and progressive differentiation of adoptively transferred tumor-reactive T cells associated with tumor regression. J Immunother 28: 258–267.
6. Weng NP, Levine BL, June CH, Hodes RJ (1995) Human naive and memory T lymphocytes differ in telomeric length and replicative potential. Proc Natl Acad Sci U S A 92: 11091–11094.
7. Dudley ME, Wunderlich JR, Robbins PF, Yang JC, Hwu P, et al. (2002) Cancer regression and autoimmunity in patients after clonal repopulation with antitumor lymphocytes. Science 298: 850–854.
8. Refaeli Y, Van Parijs L, London CA, Tschopp J, Abbas AK (1998) Biochemical mechanisms of IL-2-regulated Fas-mediated T cell apoptosis. Immunity 8: 615–623.
9. Ruoslahti E (1988) Fibronectin and its receptors. Annu Rev Biochem 57: 375–413.
10. Hynes RO (1992) Integrins: versatility, modulation, and signaling in cell adhesion. Cell 69: 11–25.
11. Nojima Y, Rothstein DM, Sugita K, Schlossman SF, Morimoto C (1992) Ligation of VLA-4 on T cells stimulates tyrosine phosphorylation of a 105-kD protein. J Exp Med 175: 1045–1053.
12. Sato T, Tachibana K, Nojima Y, D'Avirro N, Morimoto C (1995) Role of the VLA-4 molecule in T cell costimulation. Identification of the tyrosine

phosphorylation pattern induced by the ligation of VLA-4. J Immunol 155: 2938–2947.
13. Yu SS, Nukaya I, Enoki T, Chatani E, Kato A, et al. (2008) In vivo persistence of genetically modified T cells generated ex vivo using the fibronectin CH296 stimulation method. Cancer Gene Ther 15: 508–516.
14. Gattinoni L, Powell DJ, Jr., Rosenberg SA, Restifo NP (2006) Adoptive immunotherapy for cancer: building on success. Nat Rev Immunol 6: 383–393.
15. Uno K, Nakano K, Maruo N, Onodera H, Mata H, et al. (1996) Determination of interferon-alpha-producing capacity in whole blood cultures from patients with various diseases and from healthy persons. J Interferon Cytokine Res 16: 911–918.
16. Takeshi Ishikawa SK, Naoyuki Sakamoto, Tsuguhiro Matsumoto, Jun Funaki, Satoko Adachi, et al. (2011) Adoptive cellular therapy enhances the helper T cell response and reduces the number of regulatory T cells. Experimental and Therapeutic Medicine 2: 737–743.
17. Ishikawa T, Kokura S, Sakamoto N, Okajima M, Matsuyama T, et al. (2012) Relationship between circulating cytokine levels and physical or psychological functioning in patients with advanced cancer. Clin Biochem 45: 207–211.
18. Liyanage UK, Moore TT, Joo HG, Tanaka Y, Herrmann V, et al. (2002) Prevalence of regulatory T cells is increased in peripheral blood and tumor microenvironment of patients with pancreas or breast adenocarcinoma. J Immunol 169: 2756–2761.
19. Ishikawa T, Kokura S, Sakamoto N, Matsumoto T, Funaki J, et al. (2011) Adoptive cellular therapy enhances the helper T cell response and reduces the number of regulatory T cells. Exp Ther Med 2: 737–743.
20. Ishikawa T, Kokura S, Sakamoto N, Okayama T, Endo M, et al. (2013) Whole blood interferon-gamma levels predict the therapeutic effects of adoptive T-cell therapy in patients with advanced pancreatic cancer. Int J Cancer.
21. Appay V, Dunbar PR, Callan M, Klenerman P, Gillespie GM, et al. (2002) Memory CD8+ T cells vary in differentiation phenotype in different persistent virus infections. Nat Med 8: 379–385.
22. Hamann D, Baars PA, Rep MH, Hooibrink B, Kerkhof-Garde SR, et al. (1997) Phenotypic and functional separation of memory and effector human CD8+ T cells. J Exp Med 186: 1407–1418.

23. Acuto O, Michel F (2003) CD28-mediated co-stimulation: a quantitative support for TCR signalling. Nat Rev Immunol 3: 939–951.

24. Hendriks J, Gravestein LA, Tesselaar K, van Lier RA, Schumacher TN, et al. (2000) CD27 is required for generation and long-term maintenance of T cell immunity. Nat Immunol 1: 433–440.

25. Powell DJ, Jr., Dudley ME, Robbins PF, Rosenberg SA (2005) Transition of late-stage effector T cells to CD27+ CD28+ tumor-reactive effector memory T cells in humans after adoptive cell transfer therapy. Blood 105: 241–250.

26. Romagnani S (1991) Human TH1 and TH2 subsets: doubt no more. Immunol Today 12: 256–257.

27. Metcalf D, Begley CG, Johnson GR, Nicola NA, Vadas MA, et al. (1986) Biologic properties in vitro of a recombinant human granulocyte-macrophage colony-stimulating factor. Blood 67: 37–45.

28. Dranoff G (2004) Cytokines in cancer pathogenesis and cancer therapy. Nat Rev Cancer 4: 11–22.

29. Matsumoto T, Kokura S, Ishikawa T, Funaki J, Adachi S, et al. (2011) Decrease of the regulatory T-cell population by adoptive T-cell transfer in a mouse colorectal cancer transplant model. Oncol Res 19: 543–554.

30. Stroncek DF, Berger C, Cheever MA, Childs RW, Dudley ME, et al. (2012) New directions in cellular therapy of cancer: a summary of the summit on cellular therapy for cancer. J Transl Med 10: 48.

31. Turtle CJ, Hudecek M, Jensen MC, Riddell SR (2012) Engineered T cells for anti-cancer therapy. Curr Opin Immunol 24: 633–639.

5

A Novel and Effective Cancer Immunotherapy Mouse Model using Antigen-Specific B Cells Selected In Vitro

Tatsuya Moutai, Hideyuki Yamana, Takuya Nojima¤, Daisuke Kitamura*

Division of Molecular Biology, Research Institute for Biomedical Sciences (RIBS), Tokyo University of Science, Noda, Chiba, Japan

Abstract

Immunotherapies such as adoptive transfer of T cells or natural killer cells, or monoclonal antibody (MoAb) treatment have recently been recognized as effective means to treat cancer patients. However, adoptive transfer of B cells or plasma cells producing tumor-specific antibodies has not been applied as a therapy because long-term culture and selective expansion of antigen-specific B cells has been technically very difficult. Here, we describe a novel cancer immunotherapy that uses B-cell adoptive transfer. We demonstrate that germinal-center-like B cells (iGB cells) induced in vitro from mouse naïve B cells become plasma cells and produce IgG antibodies for more than a month in the bone marrow of non-irradiated recipient mice. When transferred into mice, iGB cells producing antibody against a surrogate tumor antigen suppressed lung metastasis and growth of mouse melanoma cells expressing the same antigen and prolonged survival of the recipients. In addition, we have developed a novel culture system called FAIS to selectively expand antigen-specific iGB cells utilizing the fact that iGB cells are sensitive to Fas-induced cell death unless their antigen receptors are ligated by membrane-bound antigens. The selected iGB cells efficiently suppressed lung metastasis of melanoma cells in the adoptive immunotherapy model. As human blood B cells can be propagated as iGB cells using culture conditions similar to the mouse iGB cell cultures, our data suggest that it will be possible to treat cancer-bearing patients by the adoptive transfer of cancer-antigen-specific iGB cells selected in vitro. This new adoptive immunotherapy should be an alternative to the laborious development of MoAb drugs against cancers for which no effective treatments currently exist.

Editor: Yoshiki Akatsuka, Fujita Health University, School of Medicine, Japan

Funding: This work was supported by Takeda Science Foundation, Grants-in-Aid for Scientific Research (B) (22390097) from Japan Society for the Promotion of Science (JSPS) and Grants-in-Aid for Scientific Research on Priority Areas (22021042) from The Ministry of Education, Culture, Sports, Science and Technology of Japan (MEXT) (to DK), and by Grants-in-Aid for JSPS Fellows (to TM). The funders had no role in study design, data collection and analysis, decision to publish, or preparation of the manuscript.

Competing Interests: The authors have declared that no competing interests exist.

* E-mail: kitamura@rs.noda.tus.ac.jp

¤ Current address: Department of Immunology, Duke University Medical Center, Durham, North Carolina, United States of America

Introduction

Immunotherapy has recently become more widely accepted as an effective means to treat cancer patients. The main player in cell-mediated cancer immunotherapy has been cytotoxic T lymphocytes (CTLs) directed against tumor cells, which recognize via their T-cell receptor (TCR) a particular peptide derived from a tumor antigen (Ag) presented by MHC I on the tumor cells. Such T cells from excised tumor tissues or patients' blood are selectively expanded in vitro on syngeneic Ag presenting cells (APCs) expressing the tumor Ag with cytokines like IL-2 and then transferred back into the patients [1,2]. Relatively non-specific versions of cellular immunotherapy have also been clinically tested, including those using T cells and NK cells expanded through stimulation with IL-2 and anti-CD3 antibodies (Abs), with/without additional cytokines [3,4]. Recently, in-vitro expanded dendritic cells (DCs), which are very efficient APC, have also been used to stimulate tumor-Ag-specific CTLs as well as CD4+ T cells in vivo [5–7]. These therapies based on adoptive cell transfer have thus far not been commonly adopted as an option for cancer therapy since their clinical success has been limited while they require time-consuming laboratory work, including individual cell culture for several weeks in a quality-controlled clean room.

On the other hand, Ab-based immunotherapy has been growing rapidly as a promising cancer immunotherapy. Indeed, more than a dozen monoclonal Abs (MoAbs) are currently approved for the treatment of cancer in humans [8–10]. As an anti-cancer drug, MoAbs have tremendous merits as compared to chemotherapy since they target only the cells expressing specific Ags. The biochemical nature and biological features of each isotype of Abs are well known, and so are the mechanisms by which they mediate target cell lysis, namely, Ab-dependent cellular cytotoxicity (ADCC) and complement-dependent cytotoxicity (CDC) [11,12]. As naturally existing proteins in all individuals, Abs are expected to have fewer side effects and, as such, it is easier to predict their performance as a drug. As compared to the cell-mediated immunotherapies described above, Ab-mediated immunotherapy is simpler to perform if the supply of the MoAb is adequate. However, the MoAb drugs also have drawbacks: they are expensive and their development is still challenging, requiring considerable time and cost, from animal immunization, through screening of hybridomas, to gene cloning and recombination methods for their humanization, which is necessary to avoid an immune response by the recipient [10,13]. Tumor Ags that MoAb drugs target are typically transmembrane proteins, which are often difficult to prepare as a soluble immunogen. Moreover, even with humanized MoAbs, residual mouse-derived segments of the V-region can be antigenic in humans and induce human anti-mouse Abs [14]. Because of these issues, pharmaceutical companies tend to limit MoAb targets to those expressed by relatively common cancers.

Given the aforementioned merits of MoAb drugs and the merits of adoptive cell transfer therapies as being primarily custom-made and costing less to develop, it seems plausible to develop a therapy to transfer patient-derived plasma cells that produce tumor-Ag-specific, completely human Ab. However, we are unaware of any case where such a therapy has been successful. Plasma cells are terminally differentiated cells and thus are unable to grow in culture. Instead, B cells, a direct precursor of plasma cells, could be used for the transfer. However, even B cells have proven difficult to expand in a sufficient number for adoptive transfer therapy. In addition, it has not been established whether and to what extent the transferred B cells can survive and differentiate into plasma cells in vivo.

Usually, MoAbs are derived from Ag-specific hybridomas, hybrid cells between splenic B cells from repeatedly immunized animals and a fusion partner plasmacytoma cell line. In the animal immunized with a given Ag, Ag-bound B cells are activated and proliferate to form germinal centers (GCs) in the spleens or lymph nodes. In the GCs, the B cells undergo isotype switching and somatic hypermutation of immunoglobulin genes to increase affinity of their Ag receptors (B-cell receptor, BCR). Among them, the B cells expressing BCR specific to the immunized Ag are selectively expanded and differentiated into memory B cells or long-lived plasma cells (LLPCs) [15,16]. Upon a final booster immunization, the Ag-specific memory B cells are activated and proliferate to become plasmablasts, which usually form the Ag-specific hybridomas. Thus, although Ag-specific memory B cells can be found in a considerable number in immunized individuals, antigen-specific B cells are usually rare in non-immunized individuals. Therefore, any B-cell adoptive transfer therapy would require a method to selectively expand the rare tumor-Ag-specific B cells from the extremely polyclonal peripheral B cells of the patients.

To develop a system to selectively expand tumor-Ag-specific B cells for adoptive transfer therapy, we utilized the induced GC B (iGB) cell culture system that we recently reported [17]. In this system, mouse naïve B cells are cultured successively with IL-4 and IL-21 on a feeder cell line expressing CD40L and BAFF (40 LB), resulting in the extensive proliferation (up to 10,000 fold in 8 days) of class-switched B cells with a GC phenotype, termed iGB cells. After culture with IL-21 and transfer into irradiated mice, the iGB cells differentiate into plasma cells and tend to colonize the bone marrow (BM) and secrete Abs [17]. By adapting this system to human B cells, it would be possible to prepare large numbers of human B cells that would produce completely human Abs when transferred into patients. Toward our goal of establishing B-cell-mediated adoptive transfer therapy for cancer, we have evaluated in a mouse model how much and for how long the transferred iGB cells produce Ab in non-irradiated mice, and whether they inhibit growth of cancer cells that express an Ag recognized by the same Ab in vivo. In addition, by applying the iGB culture technique, we have developed a system to select relatively rare B cells that bind to a membrane-bound Ag, and showed that the selected B cells are effective in the adoptive transfer cancer immunotherapy model.

Results

iGB Cells Colonize the Bone Marrow and Produce Ab after Transfer into Non-irradiated Mice

As we reported previously, most iGB cells after the secondary culture with IL-21 have undergone class switching and express either IgG1 or IgE by day 8. Very few of them express IgM, IgG2b or IgA, and almost none express IgG2c or IgG3 (Figure 1A). We showed previously that the iGB cells differentiate to plasma cells in the bone marrow (BM) when they were transferred into irradiated mice. Here we evaluated the Ab production from the iGB-derived plasma cells in non-irradiated mice. The iGB cells were generated from Hy10 mice, which carry a hen egg lysozyme (HEL)-specific heavy chain (VDJ9) and light chain (κ5) genes in knock-in and transgenic configurations, respectively [18]. Among the iGB cells, IgE$^-$ CD138$^-$ HEL-binding (HEL$^+$) cells were FACS-purified and transferred into non-irradiated C57BL/6 (B6) mice, which were bled weekly to measure the concentration of anti-HEL IgG1. As shown in Figure 1B, a high level of HEL-specific IgG1 was detected in the sera a week after the transfer, and then it gradually declined to a low but still detectable level (>1 μg/ml) by 10 weeks. Anti-HEL IgG1 was undetectable in the sera of the control mice that received iGB cells derived from WT B6 mice. Significant numbers of anti-HEL IgG1 Ab-producing cells (APCs) were detected in the BM, but very few in the spleen, of mice that received the Hy10-derived iGB cells 4 weeks previously (Figure 1C). Anti-HEL Ab of IgG2b class, but not of IgG2c or IgG3 (data not shown), was also detectable a week after transfer with Hy10-derived iGB cells but not with WT iGB cells (Figure 1D). Although the exact concentration of the IgG2b anti-HEL could not be estimated because of the lack of a standard isotype-matched anti-HEL Ab, the IgG2b titer was far lower than that of anti-HEL IgG1 (data not shown). Taken together, these data indicate that in-vitro generated iGB cells are able to differentiate into plasma cells that colonize the BM of non-irradiated mice and can continue to produce Ab there for at least 4 weeks.

iGB Cells Inhibit Lung Metastasis of Mouse Melanoma Cells in vivo

These results suggest a possible application of the iGB cell culture system to clinical use, namely in Ab-mediated cancer therapy. We tested this possibility with a well-studied mouse model of tumor metastasis using the B16 mouse melanoma cell line. We used B16 cells with a membrane-anchored form of HEL (mHEL) [19] as a surrogate tumor Ag, and generated a transfectant clone with homogeneous HEL expression on the cell surface, termed B16-mHEL (Figure 2A). We tested whether HEL-specific iGB cells could inhibit metastasis and growth of the B16-mHEL cells in vivo by producing anti-HEL Abs. Since the HEL-binding affinity of the Hy10 spleen B cells is known to be heterogeneous [18], we sorted those strongly binding HEL from Hy10 spleen B cells and cultured them on 40 LB feeder cells for 3 days with IL-4 and subsequently for 3 days with IL-21 to make iGB cells. Spleen B cells from WT B6 mice were also cultured in parallel. IgE$^-$ CD138$^-$ B cells sorted from the Hy10 iGB (Hy10-iGB) or WT iGB (WT-iGB) cells, or PBS only as a control, were then injected i.v. into non-irradiated B6 mice that had received B16-mHEL 24 h before (Figure 2B). Lungs of the recipient mice were inspected 3 weeks later. The lungs of the mice that received WT iGB cells or PBS only, had numerous clumps of widely disseminated tumor cells, mostly fusing with each other to form indistinguishable masses. By contrast, only a few small clumps of tumor cells were found in mice that had received Hy10 iGB cells (Figure 2C). As a control, mice

A.

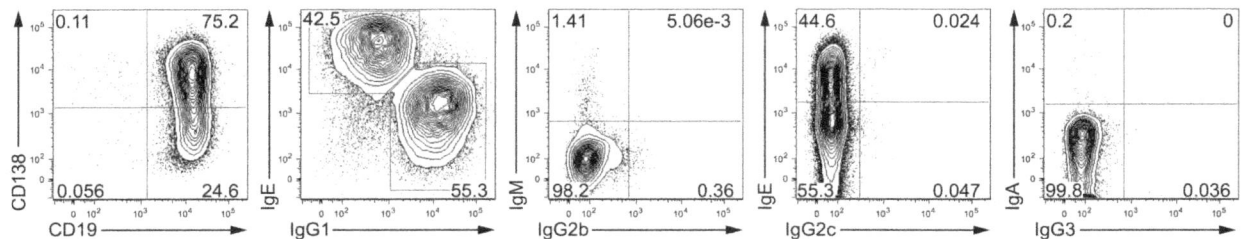

B.

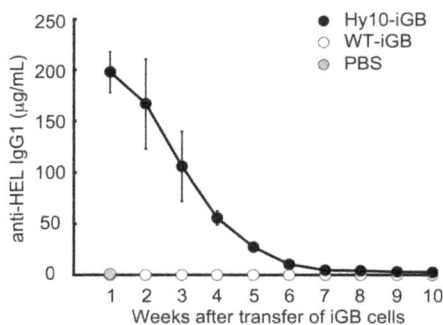

C.

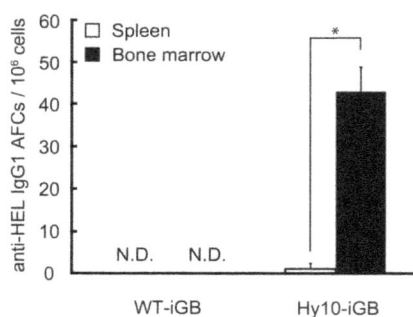

D.

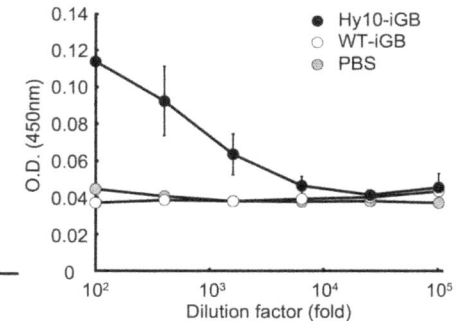

Figure 1. Evaluation of the capacity of iGB cells to differentiate and produce Ab in non-irradiated mice. (A) Splenic B cells from C57BL/6 mice were cultured for 4 days with IL-4, then for 4 days with IL-21 on 40 LB cells. The expression of Ig isotypes, CD19 and CD138 on the expanded iGB cells was analyzed by flow cytometry. Data represent the cells within the lymphocyte gate defined by side- and forward scatter. Numbers indicate the percentages of the iGB cells in the quadrants or windows. Data shown are representative of three independent experiments. (B) Naïve, HEL-binding or total B cells from the spleens of Hy10 or WT C57BL/6 mice, respectively, were cultured as in (A). After the culture, iGB cells were harvested and CD138$^-$ IgE$^-$ iGB cells (2×10^7 cells/mouse) were purified and transferred i.v. into non-irradiated C57BL/6 mice. PBS was also injected as a control. These mice were bled at the indicated weeks after transfer and the serum anti-HEL IgG1 concentration was determined by ELISA. The data are expressed as the mean $\pm$ S.D. of individual serum of mice (n = 5 for each group). Data is representative of two independent experiments. (C) HEL-binding or total B cells were cultured and transferred into non-irradiated mice as in (B). Four weeks after the transfer, the numbers of AFCs secreting HEL-binding IgG1 among spleen or bone-marrow cells were determined by ELISPOT assay. The mean number $\pm$ S.D. of the AFCs in 10^6 spleen or BM cells is indicated by each bar. Shown are collective data from three independent experiments, each using 3 recipient mice per group. *p<0.001. N.D.: not detected. (D) Anti-HEL IgG2b titers in the serum samples (10-fold dilutions) obtained at 1 week in (B) were determined by ELISA. Each value is the mean $\pm$ S.D. of the samples (n = 5 per each group). Data are representative of two independent experiments.

inoculated with parental B16 cells developed numerous lung tumors even when treated with Hy10 iGB cells (data not shown).

Long-term observation of the same set of mice revealed that the mice transferred with Hy10 iGB cells survived significantly longer than those transferred with WT iGB cells or only PBS (Figure 2D). Among these mice, serum anti-HEL IgG1 was detected at relatively high concentration in the early period of the time course only in the mice transferred with Hy10 iGB cells, although the Ab concentration gradually declined (Figure 2E). We could show by flow cytometry that the anti-HEL IgG1 was bound to the B16-mHEL cells taken from lung tumors ex vivo 3 weeks after the transfer of Hy10 iGB cells (Figure 2F and 2G). Collectively, these data indicate that HEL-specific Abs produced by iGB-cell-derived plasma cells directly inhibited colonization and/or growth of B16-mHEL cells in the lung and prolonged survival of the recipient mice. Possible mechanisms for the Ab-mediated tumor suppression and possible causes for the eventual death of the treated mice are discussed below.

Development of a Culture System to Selectively Expand Ag-specific iGB Cells

The results of these in vivo studies suggested that it could be possible to use iGB-cell-mediated tumor therapy in humans. Toward this end, it would be necessary to select presumably rare B

cells with specificity for a given tumor Ag. Therefore, we first attempted to develop a model system to enrich and expand Ag-specific mouse B cells present at low levels in the polyclonal B cell pool. We designed a system based on Fas/FasL-mediated apoptosis, since essentially all iGB cells express Fas [17] and are sensitive to Fas-mediated apoptosis (data not shown). In addition, iGB cells become resistant to Fas-mediated apoptosis when their IgG1 BCR is ligated with membrane-bound Ag (data not shown), as previously reported for activated IgM$^+$ B cells [20]. Therefore, only Ag-binding iGB cells should survive under conditions where Fas is engaged (Figure 3A). To test this hypothesis, we prepared a model system and generated two new feeder cell lines, 40 LB cells stably expressing a surrogate Ag mHEL (40 LB-mHEL) and those stably expressing mHEL and FasL (40 LB-mHEL-FasL). We initiated the iGB cell cultures on conventional 40 LB feeder cells with a mixture of spleen B cells from CD45.1$^+$ Hy10 mice and CD45.2$^+$ WT mice at a ratio of 1:99. After the successive culture with IL-4 and IL-21 on 40 LB cells (expansion), the expanded iGB cells were plated onto 40 LB-mHEL feeder cells and cultured for 6 hours (Ag-stimulation), and then replated on 40 LB-mHEL-FasL for 8 hours (selection), and finally on 40 LB for 5 days (recovery), with IL-21 present throughout after the expansion phase. These specific conditions were determined after many trials with various settings (Figure 3B). After the expansion phase, we confirmed that

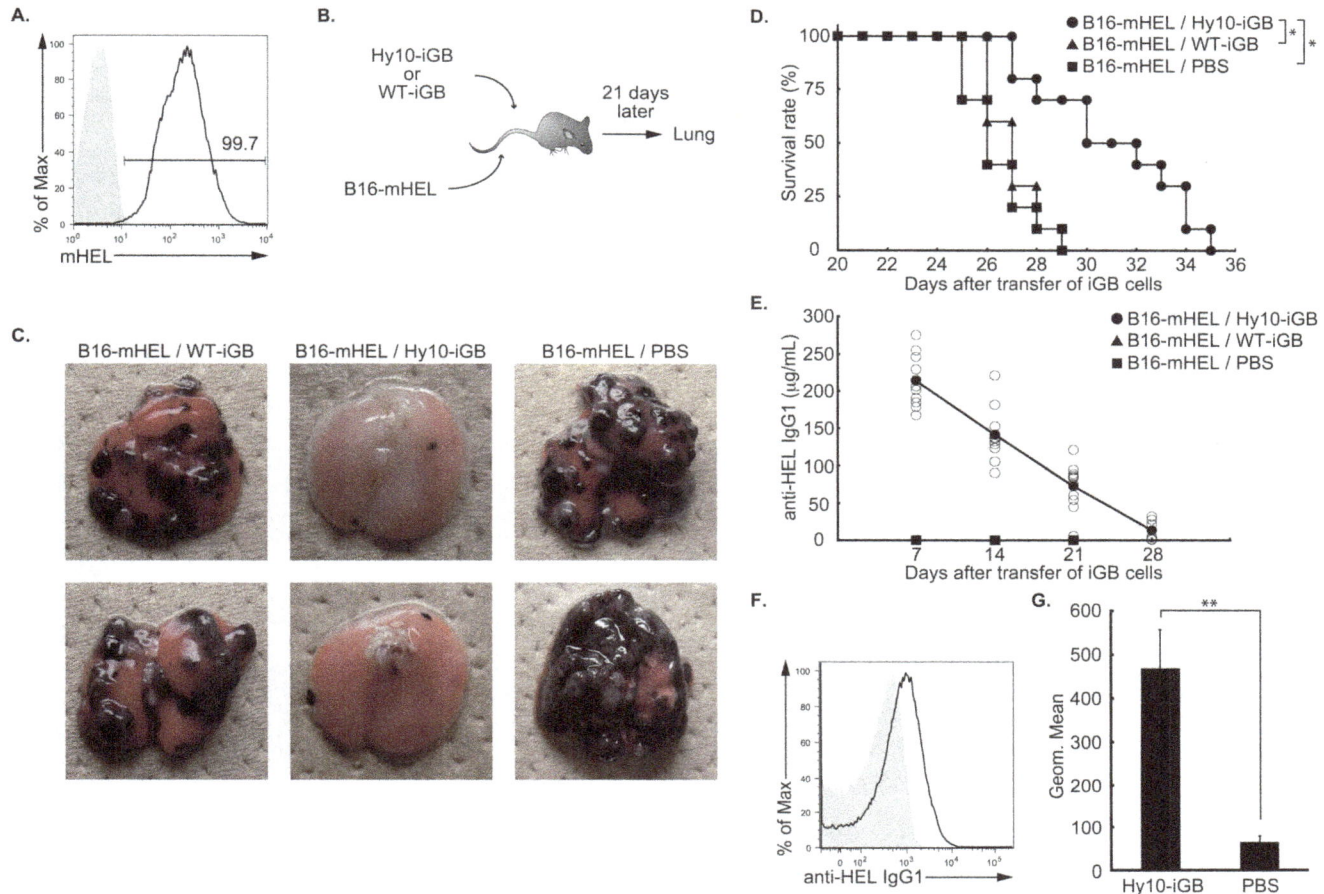

Figure 2. HEL-specific iGB cells inhibit lung metastasis of B16 melanoma cells expressing HEL in mice. (A) Expression of HEL Ag on the B16 melanoma cells transfected with an mHEL expression vector (B16-mHEL). B16-mHEL cells were stained with anti-HEL IgG1 MoAb (black line) or isotype-matched control MoAb (shaded), followed by APC-conjugated anti-mouse IgG1 Ab, and analyzed by flow cytometry. The number indicates the percentage of mHEL-expressing cells. Data is a representative of two independent experiments. (B) Experimental strategy. IgE$^-$ CD138$^-$ iGB cells (2×10^7 cells/mouse) derived from HEL-binding splenic B cells of Hy10 mice (Hy10-iGB) or total splenic B cells of WT C57BL/6 mice (WT-iGB), or PBS alone were transferred i.v. into non-irradiated C57BL/6 mice, which had been transferred i.v. with B16-mHEL (C, D, E) or B16-mHEL-GFP (F, G) cells (2×10^5 cells/mouse) 24 hours before. (C) Photographs of the lungs of the recipient mice described in (B) 3 weeks after the transfer. Images of two mice randomly selected from ten per group are shown. When possible, lungs of the rest of the mice were visually inspected on the day of death. In the non-treated groups, there was fusion of individual metastases into very large tumor masses, making it meaningless to count the number of tumors. (D) Survival rate of the same set of mouse groups (n = 10 per group) as in (B) was compared using LogRank test. *p<0.001. (E) Concentration of serum anti-HEL IgG1 in the same mice used in (D) was determined by ELISA at the indicated time points. Open and closed symbols indicate the values of individual samples and averages of each group, respectively. Data in (D) and (E) are representative of four similar experiments. (F) Binding of anti-HEL IgG1 to B16-mHEL cells in the lung of tumor bearing mice. Lungs of mice that had received Hy10 iGB cells (black line) or PBS (shaded) and B16-mHEL-GFP cells (2×10^5 cells/mouse) as in (B) were excised 3 weeks after the transfer. Single cell suspensions from the lungs were stained with anti-mouse IgG1-APC and analyzed by FACSCantoII. Representative histograms of the samples gated on GFP$^+$ cells are shown. (G) Summary of the experiments shown in (F). Bars represent averages ± S.D. of geometric means (Geom. Mean) of APC fluorescence intensity of the GFP$^+$ cells from mice of each group (n = 3). Data are representative of two independent experiments. **p<0.05.

the proportion of CD45.1$^+$ HEL-binding cells remained at 1% (Figure 3C). The proportion remained the same after the Ag-stimulation culture, and did so in the control culture on 40 LB feeder cells as well, although the intensity of HEL staining became lower in the former probably because the BCR was internalized (Figure 3D, "selected"). After the subsequent selection and recovery phases, however, the proportion of CD45.1$^+$ HEL-binding cells increased up to ~80% on average, whereas no enrichment was seen after the parallel control culture on 40 LB cells ("non-selected"). The selected iGB cells mostly expressed BCR of IgG1 isotype (data not shown). Using the "selected" protocol, on average 3×10^5 HEL-binding B cells were recovered from the culture that began with 10^4 such cells among 10^6 B cells

in total (Figure 3E and 3F). Thus, we have established a selection culture protocol that enables efficient enrichment and expansion of Ag specific B cells that are present as a small population among a vast majority of non-specific polyclonal B cells. We call this selection system the "Fas-mediated antigen-specific iGB cell selection (FAIS) system". We have also succeeded in enriching iGB cells specific for the hapten 4-hydroxy-3-nitrophenyl acetyl (NP), initially present at ~5%, up to ~80% by essentially the same system using the FasL-expressing 40 LB cells displaying NP-conjugated protein on their surface (data not shown).

Next we examined whether fewer Ag-specific B cells in a non-specific pool could be enriched, anticipating the possibility of using this system for clinical application. This time, we started the

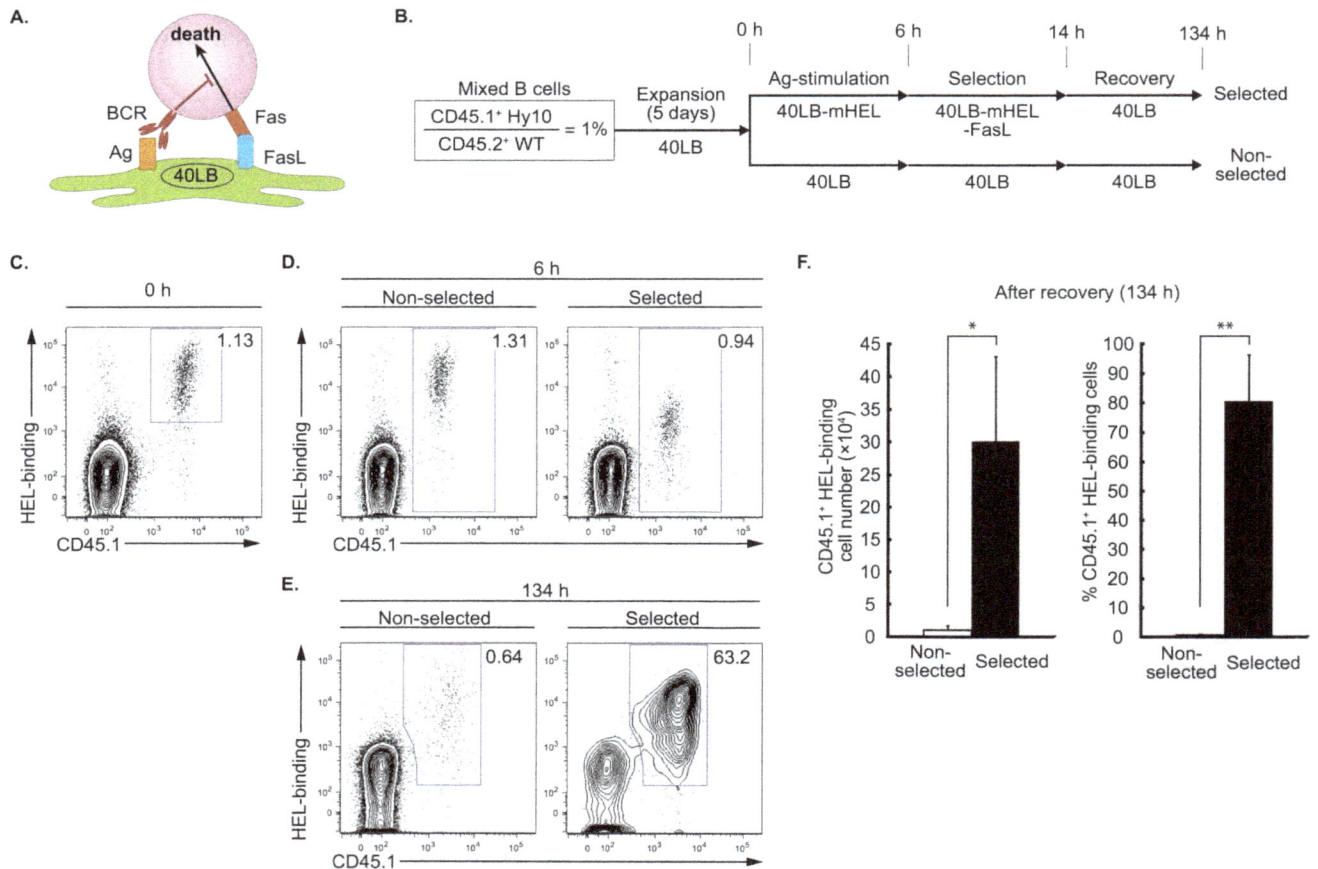

Figure 3. Culture system to selectively expand Ag-specific iGB cells. (A) Schematic representation of the principle of Fas-mediated Ag-specific iGB cell selection (FAIS) system. Only iGB cells whose BCR are ligated with Ag presented on feeder cells become resistant to death via Fas ligation by FasL on the same feeder cells. (B) Protocol for the FAIS system. Splenic B cells from CD45.1[+] Hy10 mice and CD45.2[+] WT mice were mixed at a ratio of 1:99 (1%), and cultured on a 40 LB feeder layer with IL-4 for 3 days and subsequently with IL-21 for 2 days. The resultant iGB cells were step-wise cultured on feeder layers of 40 LB-mHEL for 6 h (Ag-stimulation), 40 LB-mHEL-FasL for 8 h (selection), and 40 LB for 120 h (recovery) in the "selected" protocol. In the "non-selected" protocol, the appropriate number of iGB cells was replated on a feeder layer of 40 LB cells with the same timing as the "selected" protocol. At each time of replating, iGB cells were isolated from the feeder, IgE[+] and CD138[+] cells in both protocols. (C–E) Representative flow cytometric profiles (HEL-binding vs. CD45.1; gated on CD19[+] cells) of the mixed iGB cells before the Ag-stimulation phase (0 h; C), after the Ag-stimulation phase (6 h; D), and after the recovery phase (134 h; E). At each time point, purified iGB cells were stained with biotinylated HEL and streptavidin-APC, anti-CD19 and anti-CD45.1 Abs and analyzed by flow cytometry. The profiles of iGB cells cultured by "selected" (left) or "non-selected" (right) protocol are shown. The numbers in each window represents the percentage of Hy10 iGB cells (CD45.1[+], HEL-binding) among total CD19[+] iGB cells. Data are representative of three independent experiments. (F) The absolute number (left) and percentage (right) of the Hy10 iGB cells after the recovery culture with either the non-selected or selected protocol as determined by the analysis shown in (E) are shown as averages ± S.D. of three independent experiments. *$p<0.05$. **$p<0.01$.

cultures with CD45.1[+] Hy10 splenic B cells mixed at a frequency of 0.1 or 0.01% in 1×10^6 WT B6 splenic B cells (CD45.2[+]), a frequency that was confirmed just before the Ag-stimulation culture of the iGB cells (Figure 4A). Each B-cell mixture was cultured according to the FAIS system ("selected") or merely on 40 LB cells as a control ("non-selected"). After the recovery culture, the HEL-binding iGB cells were enriched to ~40% and ~10% when they were initially present at 0.1% and 0.01%, respectively (Figure 4B and 4C). These data suggest that very rare Ag-specific B cells, as few as 1 in 10^4, could be enriched and expanded by repeating the FAIS culture protocol.

In-vitro Selected Ag-specific iGB Cells Suppress Tumor Growth in vivo

Finally, we tested whether the in-vitro selected iGB cells are an effective anti-tumor therapy in the melanoma metastasis model in mice. CD45.1[+] HEL-binding B cells from Hy10 mice were mixed with CD45.2[+] polyclonal B cells from WT B6 mice at a ratio of 1:99 and cultured in the FAIS system or on 40 LB cells as a non-selected control, as described in Figure 3 (Figure 5A). After the recovery culture, the frequency of the HEL-binding iGB cells reached 85%, a more than 400-fold enrichment, after the FAIS culture compared to in the control culture (Figure 5B). We transferred these iGB cells (2×10^7) either selected or non-selected, or only PBS, into non-irradiated B6 mice that had been transferred with 2×10^5 B16-mHEL cells. Three weeks later, B16-mHEL cells were disseminated throughout the lungs and formed numerous clumps of various sizes in the mice that had received non-selected iGB cells or PBS. By contrast, only a small number of tumors, mostly small in size, were observed in lungs of the mice that had received the selected iGB cells (Figure 5C). These data indicate that iGB cells selected in vitro based on their Ag binding specificity are still capable of differentiating into

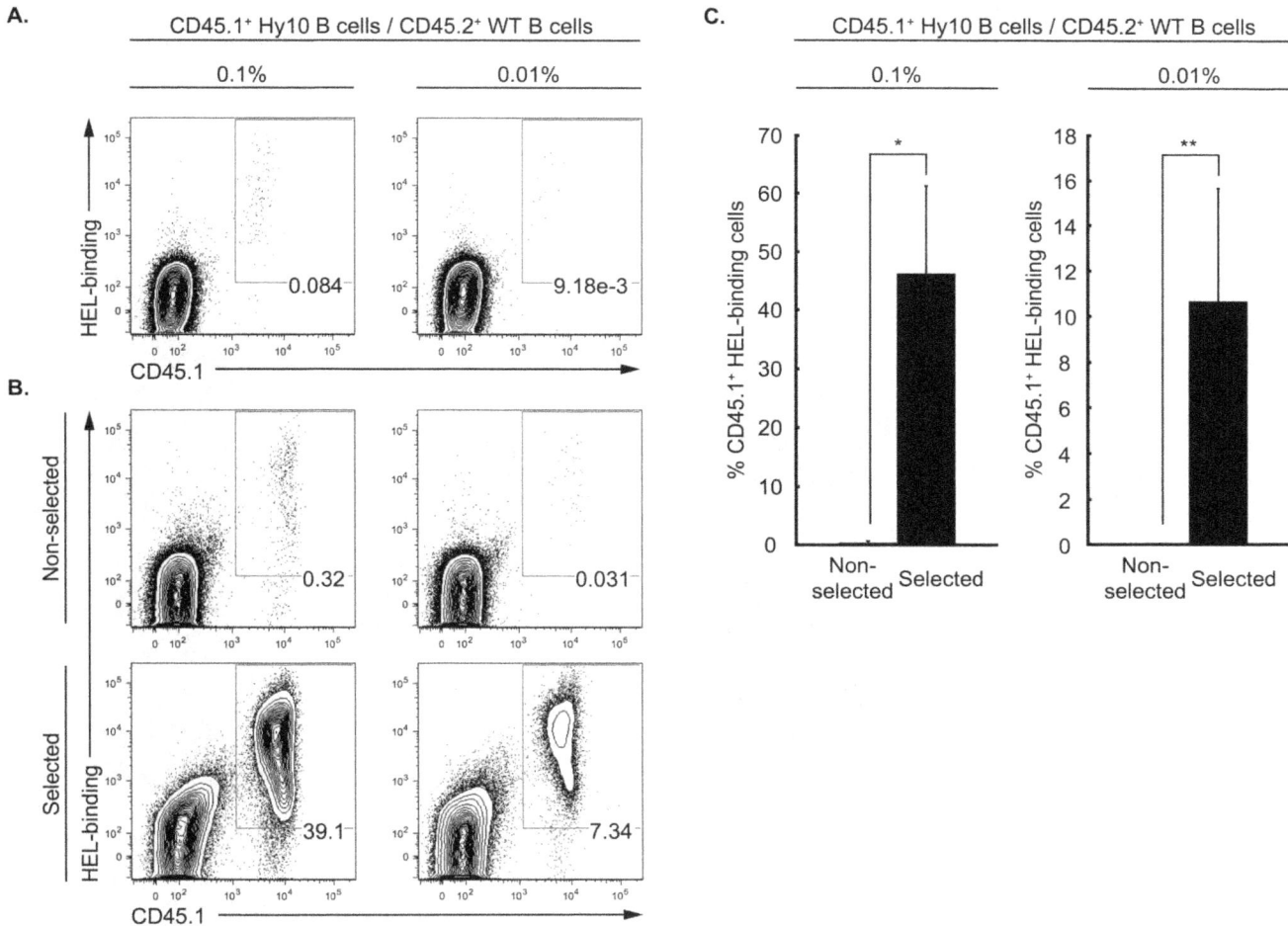

Figure 4. FAIS system can enrich very rare Ag-specific iGB cells. (A and B) Splenic B cells from CD45.1⁺ Hy10 mice were mixed at a frequency of 0.1% or 0.01% with 1×10^6 CD45.2⁺ WT splenic B cells. The mixed cells (1×10^6) were cultured as described in Figure 3B. Shown are flow cytometric profiles (HEL-binding vs. CD45.1; gated on CD19⁺ cells) of the mixed cells before the Ag-stimulation phase (0 h; A) and after the recovery phase (134 h; B) in a representative experiment. The number indicated in each window indicates the percentage of Hy10 iGB cells (CD45.1⁺, HEL-binding) among total CD19⁺ iGB cells. (C) The percentage of Hy10 iGB cells after recovery culture in either non-selected or selected protocol initiated from the mixing ratio of 0.1% (left panel, n = 3) or 0.01% (right panel, n = 2), as determined by the analysis shown in (B), are indicated as averages ±S.D. of independent experiments. *p<0.01. **p<0.05.

plasma cells in vivo and inhibiting growth of tumor cells that express the same Ag.

Discussion

Based on results using our mouse model, here we propose a new system of adoptive transfer cancer immunotherapy using B cells. With this system, one can expand naïve B cells to produce a large number of GC-like B (iGB) cells and from them, infrequent Ag-specific B cells can be selected and further expanded by the FAIS system for use in adoptive transfer therapy. We showed that the transferred iGB cells colonized the bone marrow and produced Ab, mainly of the IgG1 class, for several weeks. Using this system, we showed an example of an effective cancer treatment. The transfer of iGB cells specific for a surrogate tumor Ag (HEL) suppressed metastasis and growth in the lungs of melanoma cells expressing the same Ag and prolonged the survival of the recipient mice. If this system can be adapted to work with human B cells, the B-cell adoptive transfer should be a very attractive alternative to MoAb in cancer immunotherapy: it will require a shorter period of time from the identification of a tumor Ag to launch the

treatment of patients than producing a humanized MoAb, therefore will serve as a custom-made therapy that could target diseases of low incidence. In addition, human-derived iGB cells should produce complete human Ab in the recipient.

In the present study, it remains to be formally demonstrated how the transfer of iGB cells resulted in the suppression of melanoma growth in the lungs. Considering the high serum titer of the HEL-specific IgG1 sustained at least 4 weeks after the transfer (Figures 1B and 2E) and the binding of such IgG1 to the HEL-expressing melanoma cells ex vivo (Figure 2F and 2G), the tumor suppression is likely to be mediated by the anti-HEL IgG1 produced by the iGB-cell-derived plasma cells. Thus, the mechanisms responsible for the tumor suppression may be ADCC and/or CDC, the same mechanisms ascribed to MoAb drugs in vivo [9,10]. In this regard, previous studies comparing various isotypes of mouse MoAbs for their anti-tumor effects in vivo as well as in vitro demonstrated that IgG1 showed moderate effects in vivo and in ADCC, but not in CDC, whereas IgG2a was the most effective in most cases, with IgG2b and IgG3 being variable among the reports using different sets of MoAbs and target cells

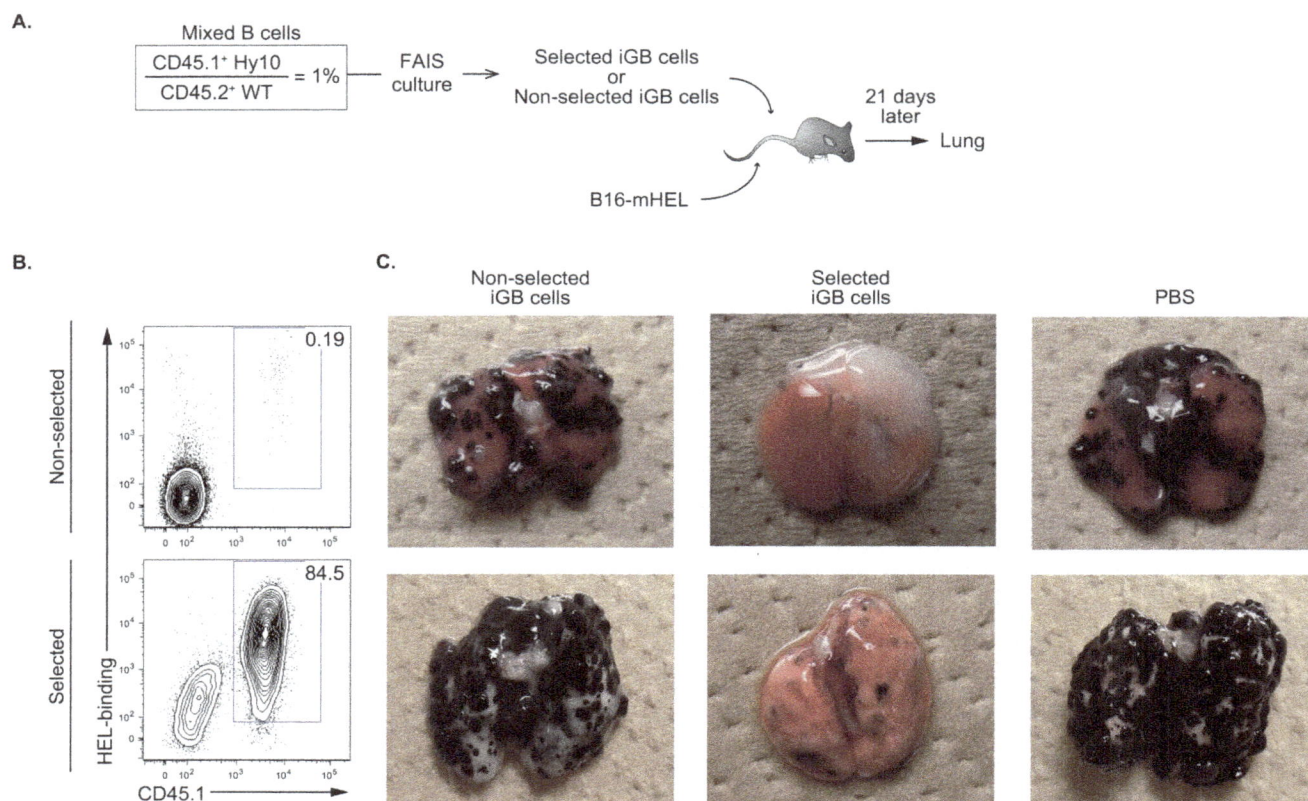

Figure 5. In-vitro selected antigen-specific iGB cells suppress tumor growth in vivo. (A) Experimental strategy. A 1:99 mixture of splenic B cells from CD45.1+ Hy10 mice and CD45.2+ WT mice was subjected to the FAIS system as described in Figure 3B. The selected or non-selected iGB cells after the recovery phase, or PBS alone, were injected into non-irradiated C57BL/6 mice that had been transferred i.v. with B16-mHEL cells, as described in Figure 2B. (B) Representative flow cytometric profiles (HEL-binding vs. CD45.1) of iGB cells after the recovery phase of the "selected" and "non-selected" protocols. The numbers in each window indicate the percentage of the Hy10 iGB cells (CD45.1+, HEL-binding; gated on CD19+ cells) among total CD19+ iGB cells. (C) Photographs of the lungs of the mice treated as in (A) 3 weeks after the transfer. Representative images of two mice out of three are shown.

[21–24]. Thus, the propensity of the B cells derived from our mouse iGB cell culture system to switch almost exclusively to either IgG1 or IgE isotypes may have limited the efficacy of the therapy in our mouse model; all the mice, even those treated with the Ag-specific iGB cells, eventually died. It should be noted that such mice died with huge clumps of melanoma tumors in the peritoneal cavity, but only a few small tumors were found in their lungs even at death (data not shown), indicating that the anti-tumor activity of Ab isotypes may differ depending on the tissues being infiltrated. Considering a future application for humans, feasibility of iGB cells would depend on the IgG subtype to which human iGB cells would switch in the iGB cell culture.

The success of adoptive B-cell transfer immunotherapy for cancer will depend on how efficiently the tumor-Ag-specific iGB cells can be selected and propagated. For this, we developed a new system to select and expand rare Ag-specific B cells in vitro, termed the FAIS system. This system is based on the characteristics of the iGB cells: first, iGB cells grow enormously and robustly on a 40 LB feeder layer; second, essentially all of them express Fas receptor and die when plated on 40 LB feeder cells expressing FasL; third, they become resistant to the Fas-signal when their BCR is pre-stimulated by a cognate Ag bound on the feeder cells. This system is so simple that, once cancer-specific Ag is identified that can be expressed on the feeder cells, it would be easily testable if B cells binding the Ag can be obtained. Our preliminary data

show that human blood B cells can grow and express Fas in a similar culture condition, suggesting that the FAIS system may be applied to human B cells. It remains to be determined how high the affinity of BCR is required for the B cells to be selected out by this system. If the B cells with moderate affinity would be selected, the FAIS system would have to be improved to enable a controllable V gene mutagenesis by AID and repeatable selection-expansion cycles, in order to obtain B cells with a BCR whose affinity to Ag is high enough for clinical applications.

The Ag-specific B cells selected by the FAIS system could also serve as a source of complete human MoAbs, which would be more desirable than "humanized" murine MoAbs, which have mouse/human hybrid V regions, possibly lessening their original affinity to Ags, and making them more immunogenic to humans than the fully human MoAbs [13]. In addition, our system requires less time, cost, and technical skills compared to the conventional methods such as the "humanized" MoAbs, phage display technologies [25,26] or the lymphocyte microwell-array system [27–29]. Phage display technology depends on the quality of the Ab cDNA libraries, which consist of a huge number of random combinations of H and L chains. The lymphocyte microwell-array system requires special devices to detect single cells that emit faint fluorescence. Recently, Spits, Beaumont and colleagues have reported a system to efficiently expand human B cells in vitro and generate human MoAbs from them. They immortalized blood memory B cells by expressing conditionally active STAT5 or Bcl-6/Bcl-xL and cultured the cells with IL-21 on feeder cells expressing CD40 L. From the expanded cells, those binding to viral or bacterial Ags were selected by fluorescence activated cell sorting or limiting dilution methods [30–32]. They used B cells from humans or "humanized" mice previously infected or immunized with such pathogens, in which the frequency of Ag-specific memory B cells may be relatively high. It is unknown whether the same system can be applied for selecting presumably rare B cells specific for tumor Ags from unimmunized individuals. Based on the results shown here, our FAIS system may be able to enrich Ag-specific B cells that are as rare as 0.01% in a non-specific B-cell pool, and possibly even less if repeated selection procedures are possible. In addition, our system does not require purified Ags; it is only necessary to express Ags on the feeder cell line by gene transduction. This is advantageous over the other methods described above since most of the target Ags for MoAb immunotherapies are transmembrane proteins that are often difficult to prepare as soluble Ags. Another advantage over the methods requiring in-vivo immunization would be that the in-vitro system is free of T-cell-mediated self-tolerance and therefore may allow the expansion of B cell clones that react with self tumor Ags.

Materials and Methods

Ethics Statement

All mouse procedures were performed in accordance with the regulations of the Tokyo University of Science on animal care and use, under the protocols approved by the Animal Care and Use Committee of the Tokyo University of Science (approved protocol #S13009). In the survival study, the tumor-recipient mice were checked daily in the mornings and evenings, and we euthanized the mice when mice could not move owing to the tumor before sacrificing them.

Mice

C57BL/6 mice were purchased from Japan SLC. Hy10 (formerly called HyHEL10) mice carrying a HEL-specific V_H knock-in (VDJ9 ki) allele and an Ig-κ transgene (κ5 tg) [18,33] were backcrossed to the congenic C57BL/6-CD45.1 strains. Mice 8–10 weeks of age were used for experiments unless indicated otherwise. All mice were maintained in our mouse facility under specific pathogen-free conditions. When we dissected the mice, mice were killed by cervical dislocation under anesthesia with Isoflurane in all mouse experiments.

Plasmid Construction and Retroviral Transduction

A cDNA encoding a membrane-bound form of HEL (mHEL) excised from pcDNA3-mHEL (a gift of Dr. R. Brink [19]) was inserted into pMX-IRES-GFP [34] to make pMX-mHEL-IRES-GFP. An shRNA sequence targeting the Fas 3′UT sequence, 5′ gtgttctctttgccagcaaat-3′, was inserted into pSIREN-RetroQ vector (Clontech), to make a retroviral vector pSIREN-RetroQ-shFas. An eGFP sequence in the pMX-IRES-GFP vector was replaced with a cDNA consisting of extracellular and transmembrane domains of human CD8 (hCD8) to make pMX-IRES-hCD8. A FasL cDNA was inserted into the pMX-IRES-hCD8 to make pMX-FasL-IRES-hCD8. The retroviral vectors were transfected into packaging cells, PLAT-E [34], using FuGENE (Roche). On the next day, the supernatants were added to target cells in the presence of 10 μg/mL DOTAP Liposomal Transfection Reagent (Roche).

Cell Lines

B16 mouse melanoma cells [35] were transfected with the pcDNA3-mHEL plasmid by lipofection using Trans IT-LT1 (Takara), and cultured with G418 (2 mg/ml, Wako). Drug-resistant stable clones (B16-mHEL) were subsequently selected. B16 cells were retrovirally transduced with the pMX-mHEL-IRES-GFP, and then cloned by limiting dilution method to establish B16-mHEL-GFP cells. 40 LB, Balb/c 3T3 fibroblasts expressing exogenous CD40-ligand and BAFF, have been described previously [17]. 40 LB cells were transduced with the pMX-mHEL-IRES-GFP vector, and a single clone expressing mHEL and eGFP, termed 40 LB-mHEL, was selected by limiting dilution. To express FasL, 40 LB cells were first transduced with the pSIREN-RetroQ-shFas vector. The resultant Fas-knocked-down cells (40 LB-Fas⁻) were then transduced with the pMX-FasL-IRES-hCD8 vector and a single clone expressing FasL and hCD8 (40 LB-FasL cells) was selected by limiting dilution. Finally, the 40 LB-FasL cells were transduced with the pMX-mHEL-IRES-GFP vector to obtain a single clone expressing mHEL and eGFP (40 LB-mHEL-FasL). B16 and 40 LB cells, and their derivatives, were maintained in D-MEM medium (high glucose; Wako) supplemented with 10% FBS, 100 units/ml penicillin, and 100 μg/ml streptomycin (GIBCO) in a humidified atmosphere at 37°C with 5% CO_2.

Isolation of Cells

Naïve B cells were purified from the spleens of the mice mentioned above ("Mice") by 2-step negative sorting, first by an iMag system (BD Biosciences) using biotinylated MoAbs against CD43 (S7: BD Pharmingen), CD4, CD8α, CD11b, CD49b (DX5), Ter-119 (BioLegend), and streptavidin-particle-DM (BD Biosciences) and then by passing of the unbound cells through a MACS LS column (Miltenyi Biotec), yielding B cells of >97% purity. B cells strongly binding HEL were purified from naïve B cells of Hy10 mice prepared as above by sorting the cells brightly stained with biotinylated-HEL plus streptavidin-APC and with CD19-PE/Cy7 (BioLegend) with FACSAria II (BD Biosciences). HEL (Sigma) was conjugated with biotin using EZ-Link Biotinylation kit (Pierce). iGB cells were purified by removing the feeder cells, IgE⁺ cells and plasmablasts/plasma cells with an iMag system as described previously [17] using primary MoAbs against H-2K^d (Biolegend), IgE (R35–72: BD Pharmingen), CD138 (281–2 : BD Pharmingen), and FasL (MFL3 : Biolegend) when removing feeder cells expressing FasL. Purified naïve B cells were cultured on a feeder layer of irradiated 40 LB cells with IL-4 and IL-21, sequentially, to generate iGB cells, as described previously [17]. The purified iGB cells were used for the adoptive transfer into non-irradiated recipient mice, as described below.

Ag-specific iGB Cell Selection System

The iGB cell culture [17] was performed with the primary culture with IL-4 (1 ng/mL) for 3 days and the secondary culture with IL-21 (10 ng/mL) for 2 days. The following culture was done with IL-21 alone throughout. From the cultured cells, IgE⁻ CD138⁻ iGB cells were purified as described above and seeded onto a feeder layer of 40 LB-mHEL cells (2×10^7 cells/dish) and cultured for 6 hours. Then the iGB cells were purified again, seeded onto a feeder layer of 40 LB-mHEL-FasL (2×10^7 cells/dish) and cultured for 8 hours. Finally, surviving iGB cells were purified with an iMag system using MoAbs against H-2K^d and FasL and seeded onto a feeder layer of 40 LB cells and cultured for 120 hours. As a control, iGB cells were replated on the feeder layers of 40 LB with the same timing as in the selection protocol.

Flow Cytometry

Single cell suspensions were treated with anti-CD16/32 Ab to block FcγRII/III before staining as described previously [17], and stained with various combinations of the following Abs: FITC-, PE-, biotin-, PE-Cy7-, allophycocyanin (APC)-, or Brilliant Violet 421^{TM}-conjugated Abs against IgM, IgG1, IgG2b, IgG2c, IgG3 (Southern Biotechnology), IgA, IgM, IgE, CD19, CD45.1, CD138 (BioLegend), IgE, and CD138 (BD Pharmingen), or biotinylated HEL. Cells were stained with propidium iodide (PI) just before analysis to eliminate dead cells in the data analyses. When the iGB cells were analyzed, 40 LB feeder cells were gated out based on FSC versus SSC. All samples were analyzed using a FACSCalibur or FACSCanto II (BD Biosciences). The data were analyzed using FlowJo (Tree Star, Inc.).

Adoptive Transfer of iGB Cells

iGB cells after the secondary culture with IL-21, derived from Hy10 or WT mice of C57BL/6-CD45.1 background, were injected i.v. into non-irradiated C57BL/6-CD45.2 mice (2×10^7 cells/mouse). HEL-specific Ab forming cells (AFCs) in spleen and BM of the recipient mice were detected by ELISPOT assay 4 weeks after the transfer. HEL-specific Abs in the sera of the recipients were measured by ELISA. ELISPOT and ELISA were performed as described previously [17,36]. As a cancer therapy model, non-irradiated C57BL/6 mice were transferred i.v. with B16-mHEL or B16-mHEL-GFP cells (2×10^5 cells/mouse) and, 24 hours later, with iGB cells (2×10^7 cells/mouse) derived from the Hy10 or WT mice. Survival of the recipient mice was checked daily in the mornings and evenings. Where indicated, lungs of the recipient mice were excised 3 weeks after the tumor transfer and photographed. To examine Ab binding to the tumor cells in vivo, the lungs of the mice transferred with B16-mHEL-GFP and Hy10 iGB cells were excised 3 weeks after the transfer and digested using Collagenase Type1 (GIBCO), and then the single cell suspension was stained with anti-mouse IgG1-APC and analyzed by flow cytometry.

Statistical Analysis

Statistical analysis was performed using the Student's t test as appropriate. To assess survival rate, the Kaplan-Mayer model was used and comparison of survival between groups was performed using the LogRank test with XLSTAT software (Addinsoft SARL, Paris, France).

Acknowledgments

We thank Moeko Matsudaira for contributing in a primary stage of this work, Robert Brink for pcDNA3-mHEL plasmid, Jason G. Cyster and Takaharu Okada for Hy10 mice, Akikazu Murakami, Toshihiro Suzuki, Shinya Hidano, Yasuhiro Kawai, Ryo Goitsuka and the other members of RIBS for technical advice, and Peter D. Burrows for critical comments on the manuscript.

Author Contributions

Conceived and designed the experiments: TM TN DK. Performed the experiments: TM HY TN. Analyzed the data: TM TN. Wrote the paper: TM DK.

References

1. Restifo NP, Dudley ME, Rosenberg SA (2012) Adoptive immunotherapy for cancer: harnessing the T cell response. Nat Rev Immunol 12: 269–281.
2. Lee S, Margolin K (2012) Tumor-infiltrating lymphocytes in melanoma. Curr Oncol Rep 14: 468–474.
3. Schadendorf D, Algarra SM, Bastholt L, Cinat G, Dreno B, et al. (2009) Immunotherapy of distant metastatic disease. Ann Oncol 20 Suppl 6: vi41–50.
4. Vivier E, Ugolini S, Blaise D, Chabannon C, Brossay L (2012) Targeting natural killer cells and natural killer T cells in cancer. Nat Rev Immunol 12: 239–252.
5. Palucka K, Banchereau J (2012) Cancer immunotherapy via dendritic cells. Nat Rev Cancer 12: 265–277.
6. Motz GT, Coukos G (2013) Deciphering and reversing tumor immune suppression. Immunity 39: 61–73.
7. Palucka K, Banchereau J (2013) Dendritic-cell-based therapeutic cancer vaccines. Immunity 39: 38–48.
8. Sliwkowski MX, Mellman I (2013) Antibody therapeutics in cancer. Science 341: 1192–1198.
9. Scott AM, Allison JP, Wolchok JD (2012) Monoclonal antibodies in cancer therapy. Cancer Immun 12: 14.
10. Weiner LM, Surana R, Wang S (2010) Monoclonal antibodies: versatile platforms for cancer immunotherapy. Nat Rev Immunol 10: 317–327.
11. Kubota T, Niwa R, Satoh M, Akinaga S, Shitara K, et al. (2009) Engineered therapeutic antibodies with improved effector functions. Cancer Sci 100: 1566–1572.
12. Iannello A, Ahmad A (2005) Role of antibody-dependent cell-mediated cytotoxicity in the efficacy of therapeutic anti-cancer monoclonal antibodies. Cancer Metastasis Rev 24: 487–499.
13. Chames P, Van Regenmortel M, Weiss E, Baty D (2009) Therapeutic antibodies: successes, limitations and hopes for the future. Br J Pharmacol 157: 220–233.
14. Klee GG (2000) Human anti-mouse antibodies. Arch Pathol Lab Med 124: 921–923.
15. Shlomchik MJ, Weisel F (2012) Germinal center selection and the development of memory B and plasma cells. Immunol Rev 247: 52–63.
16. McHeyzer-Williams M, Okitsu S, Wang N, McHeyzer-Williams L (2012) Molecular programming of B cell memory. Nat Rev Immunol 12: 24–34.
17. Nojima T, Haniuda K, Moutai T, Matsudaira M, Mizokawa S, et al. (2011) In-vitro derived germinal centre B cells differentially generate memory B or plasma cells in vivo. Nat Commun 2: 465.
18. Allen CD, Okada T, Tang HL, Cyster JG (2007) Imaging of germinal center selection events during affinity maturation. Science 315: 528–531.
19. Hartley SB, Crosbie J, Brink R, Kantor AB, Basten A, et al. (1991) Elimination from peripheral lymphoid tissues of self-reactive B lymphocytes recognizing membrane-bound antigens. Nature 353: 765–769.
20. Rothstein TL, Wang JK, Panka DJ, Foote LC, Wang Z, et al. (1995) Protection against Fas-dependent Th1-mediated apoptosis by antigen receptor engagement in B cells. Nature 374: 163–165.
21. Herlyn D, Koprowski H (1982) IgG2a monoclonal antibodies inhibit human tumor growth through interaction with effector cells. Proc Natl Acad Sci U S A 79: 4761–4765.
22. Kaminski MS, Kitamura K, Maloney DG, Campbell MJ, Levy R (1986) Importance of antibody isotype in monoclonal anti-idiotype therapy of a murine B cell lymphoma. A study of hybridoma class switch variants. J Immunol 136: 1123–1130.
23. Seto M, Takahashi T, Nakamura S, Matsudaira Y, Nishizuka Y (1983) In vivo antitumor effects of monoclonal antibodies with different immunoglobulin classes. Cancer Res 43: 4768–4773.
24. Denkers EY, Badger CC, Ledbetter JA, Bernstein ID (1985) Influence of antibody isotype on passive serotherapy of lymphoma. J Immunol 135: 2183–2186.
25. Marks JD, Hoogenboom HR, Bonnert TP, McCafferty J, Griffiths AD, et al. (1991) By-passing immunization. Human antibodies from V-gene libraries displayed on phage. J Mol Biol 222: 581–597.
26. McCafferty J, Griffiths AD, Winter G, Chiswell DJ (1990) Phage antibodies: filamentous phage displaying antibody variable domains. Nature 348: 552–554.
27. Love JC, Ronan JL, Grotenbreg GM, van der Veen AG, Ploegh HL (2006) A microengraving method for rapid selection of single cells producing antigen-specific antibodies. Nat Biotechnol 24: 703–707.
28. Reddy ST, Ge X, Miklos AE, Hughes RA, Kang SH, et al. (2010) Monoclonal antibodies isolated without screening by analyzing the variable-gene repertoire of plasma cells. Nat Biotechnol 28: 965–969.
29. Jin A, Ozawa T, Tajiri K, Obata T, Kondo S, et al. (2009) A rapid and efficient single-cell manipulation method for screening antigen-specific antibody-secreting cells from human peripheral blood. Nat Med 15: 1088–1092.
30. Scheeren FA, van Geelen CM, Yasuda E, Spits H, Beaumont T (2011) Antigen-specific monoclonal antibodies isolated from B cells expressing constitutively active STAT5. PLoS One 6: e17189.
31. Becker PD, Legrand N, van Geelen CM, Noerder M, Huntington ND, et al. (2010) Generation of human antigen-specific monoclonal IgM antibodies using vaccinated "human immune system" mice. PLoS One 5.
32. Kwakkenbos MJ, Diehl SA, Yasuda E, Bakker AQ, van Geelen CM, et al. (2010) Generation of stable monoclonal antibody-producing B cell receptor-positive human memory B cells by genetic programming. Nat Med 16: 123–128.

33. Phan TG, Green JA, Gray EE, Xu Y, Cyster JG (2009) Immune complex relay by subcapsular sinus macrophages and noncognate B cells drives antibody affinity maturation. Nat Immunol 10: 786–793.

34. Nosaka T, Kawashima T, Misawa K, Ikuta K, Mui AL, et al. (1999) STAT5 as a molecular regulator of proliferation, differentiation and apoptosis in hematopoietic cells. EMBO J 18: 4754–4765.

35. Hu F, Lesney PF (1964) The isolation and cytology of two pigmented cell strains from B16 mouse melanomas. Cancer Res 24: 1634–1643.

36. Oda M, Kitai A, Murakami A, Nishimura M, Ohkuri T, et al. (2010) Evaluation of the conformational equilibrium of reduced hen egg lysozyme by antibodies to the native form. Arch Biochem Biophys 494: 145–150.

6

Primary Human Ovarian Epithelial Cancer Cells Broadly Express HER2 at Immunologically-Detectable Levels

Evripidis Lanitis[1,2], Denarda Dangaj[1,2], Ian S. Hagemann[3], De-Gang Song[1], Andrew Best[1], Raphael Sandaltzopoulos[2], George Coukos[1], Daniel J. Powell, Jr.[1,3]*

1 Ovarian Cancer Research Center, Department of Obstetrics and Gynecology, University of Pennsylvania, Philadelphia, Pennsylvania, United States of America, **2** Department of Molecular Biology and Genetics, Democritus University of Thrace, Alexandroupolis, Greece, **3** Abramson Cancer Center, Department of Pathology and Laboratory Medicine, University of Pennsylvania, Philadelphia, Pennsylvania, United States of America

Abstract

The breadth of HER2 expression by primary human ovarian cancers remains controversial, which questions its suitability as a universal antigen in this malignancy. To address these issues, we performed extensive HER2 expression analysis on a wide panel of primary tumors as well as established and short-term human ovarian cancer cell lines. Conventional immunohistochemical (IHC) analysis of multiple tumor sites in 50 cases of high-grade ovarian serous carcinomas revealed HER2 overexpression in 29% of evaluated sites. However, more sensitive detection methods including flow cytometry, western blot analysis and q-PCR revealed HER2 expression in all fresh tumor cells derived from primary ascites or solid tumors as well as all established and short-term cultured cancer cell lines. Cancer cells generally expressed HER2 at higher levels than that found in normal ovarian surface epithelial (OSE) cells. Accordingly, genetically-engineered human T cells expressing an HER2-specific chimeric antigen receptor (CAR) recognized and reacted against all established or primary ovarian cancer cells tested with minimal or no reactivity against normal OSE cells. In conclusion, all human ovarian cancers express immunologically-detectable levels of HER2, indicating that IHC measurement underestimates the true frequency of HER2-expressing ovarian cancers and may limit patient access to otherwise clinically meaningful HER2-targeted therapies.

Editor: Shannon M. Hawkins, Baylor College of Medicine, United States of America

Funding: Ovarian Cancer Research Fund, Sandy Rollman Ovarian Cancer Foundation, National Institutes of Health (1R21CA152540) and the Joint Fox Chase Cancer Center and University of Pennsylvania Ovarian Cancer SPORE (P50 CA083638). The funders had no role in study design, data collection and analysis, decision to publish, or preparation of the manuscript.

Competing Interests: The authors have declared that no competing interests exist.

* E-mail: poda@mail.med.upenn.edu

Introduction

The *ERBB2* proto-oncogene encodes a transmembrane protein tyrosine kinase receptor involved in the development and progression of many cancers including ovarian cancer [1,2]. Dysregulated HER2 signaling in ovarian cancer (OvCa) results from either gene amplification or overexpression and leads to faster cell growth [3], improved DNA repair [4] and increased colony formation [5]. HER2 overexpression is associated with an increased risk of progression and death especially among women with FIGO stage I and II OvCa [6]. However, no correlation has been found between the presence of HER2 overexpression and FIGO stage, suggesting that activation of HER2 overexpression is broad and can occur both in early and late stages of disease [7]. These qualities would appear to make HER2 an attractive molecule for targeted immunotherapies in women with HER2-positive ovarian cancer, where naturally-occurring CD4+ and CD8+ T cell responses have been observed [8].

HER2 protein expression is most commonly detected via semi-quantitative IHC analysis on paraffin embedded tissues using established protocols employed for the assessment of breast cancer patients being considered for anti-HER2 Herceptin (trastuzumab) treatment [9]. The extent to which HER2 is expressed by OvCas remains controversial, as the rate of HER2-positive OvCas reported in the literature ranges from 4.9% to 52.5%

[6,7,10,11,12,13,14,15]. However, in a single study performed by Hellstrom et al., all tumor cell lines that were established *in vitro* from solid tumor or ascites expressed HER2 suggesting a selective growth advantage for HER2-positive cancer cells in culture [16]. One established cell line was shown to be sensitive to HER2-directed antibody-dependent cellular cytotoxicity (ADCC), however, HER2 expression and ADCC sensitivity was not assessed on cells derived from physiological ovaries. Additionally, HER2 expression analysis utilized flow cytometry as the sole detection method and was limited to a relatively small number of cases, relying heavily upon in vitro cell culture.

In the current study, established ovarian cancer cell lines, primary short-term cultured cell lines and fresh ovarian cancer cells derived from ascites and solid tumor specimens were evaluated for HER2 expression utilizing various detection methods, including quantitative PCR (q-PCR), western blot analysis and flow cytometry, and expression levels were compared to corresponding levels in normal ovarian surface epithelium cells. Further, immunologically-active levels of HER2 were measured using human T cells that were genetically engineered to express an HER2-specific chimeric antigen receptor (CAR). Anti-HER2 CAR T cells were evaluated for their capacity to recognize HER2-expressing OvCas and normal cells. Our results demon-

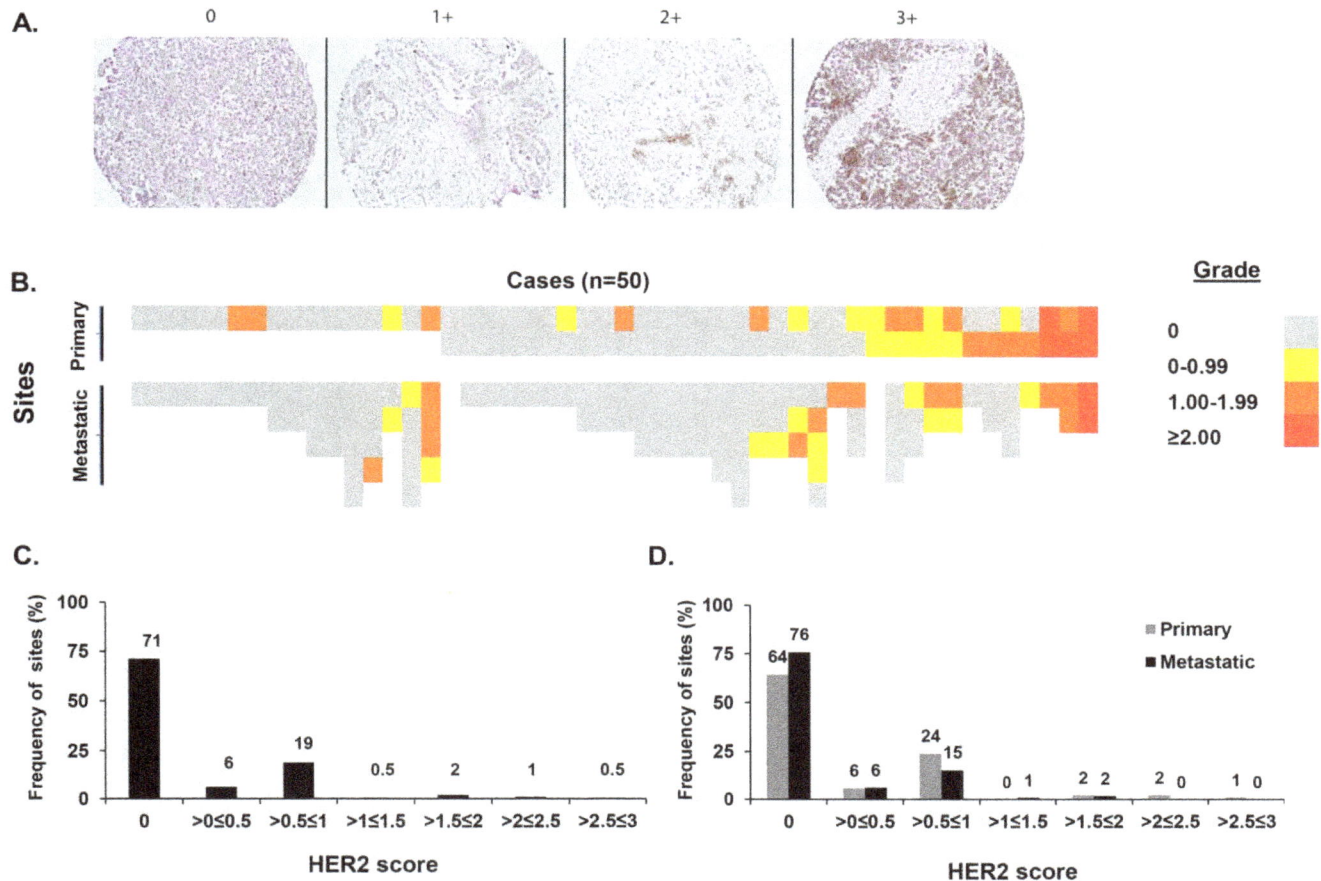

Figure 1. Immunohistochemical detection of HER2 in ovarian cancer. *A.* Immunostaining showing regional diversity of HER2 expression in high-grade papillary serous ovarian adenocarcinoma. HER2 expression levels were graded in a 0–3 scale (score 0 = undetectable, score 3 = strong staining). Original magnification was 200×. *B.* Heatmap illustration of HER2 expression level in 50 primary and metastatic ovarian carcinoma cases, as scored by IHC staining. *C.* Frequency distribution of sites expressing HER2 at levels ranging from score 0 to 3. The mean number of evaluated sites for cases with undetectable or detectable HER2 expression was similar (4.2 vs. 3.7 respectively; $P = 0.19$). *D.* Frequency distribution of either primary or metastatic sites expressing HER2 at levels ranging from score 0 to 3. A greater frequency of primary tumor sites expressed HER2 (36%; 30/84) compared to metastatic sites (24%; 27/111) and had a higher mean HER2 expression score (0.37 vs. 0.21, $P = 0.04$). No statistically significant difference was observed comparing the expression levels among the primary and metastatic sites that expressed HER2 at any level (1.03 vs. 0.86, $P = 0.26$). P values were calculated using unpaired student's t-test analysis.

strate that all OvCa samples express HER2, and that this level of expression is sufficient to elicit immune recognition.

Materials and Methods

Cancer Cells and Lines

Donors entered into a University of Pennsylvania Institutional Review Board (IRB)-approved clinical protocol and signed an informed consent prior to tumor or blood collection. For solid tumors or normal ovarian samples, specimen was diced in RPMI-1640, washed and centrifuged (800 rpm, 5 minutes, 15–22°C), and resuspended in enzymatic digestion buffer (0.2 mg/ml collagenase and 30units/ml DNase in RPMI-1640) for overnight rotation at room temperature. Ascites collections were washed and cryopreserved before study. Short-term cultured primary lines were kindly provided by Dr. Richard Carroll at the University of Pennsylvania [17]. Established human ovarian and breast cancer cell lines, the CEM human T cell lymphoblast-like cell line and the 293T cell line were purchased (ATCC). Normal IOSE-4 and IOSE-6 cell lines were kindly provided by Dr. Birrer from Dana-Farber/Harvard Cancer Center [18] and the 398 cell line was a gift from

Dr. Lin Zhang at the University of Pennsylvania [19]. 293T cells and tumor cell lines were maintained in complete medium; RPMI-1640 (Invitrogen) supplemented with 10% (v/v) heat-inactivated FBS, 2 mM L-glutamine, and 100 µg/mL penicillin and 100 U/mL streptomycin.

Immunohistochemistry

Institutional review board approval was obtained. We retrieved records from 50 consecutive patients with metastatic papillary serous ovarian cancer (FIGO stage IIB and above) undergoing primary resection at our institution between 2005 and 2008. Slides were reviewed and annotated and paraffin-embedded tissue blocks were selected to construct a tissue microarray of primary and metastatic tumors. 206 total tumor deposits (primary sites and metastases) were represented on the array. A mean of 3.7 sites were included per patient. The most common metastatic sites included omentum, peritoneum (e.g., cul-de-sac), uterine serosa, and bowel wall. For each block, triplicate 0.6 mm cores of tumor were placed on a tissue microarray. 5 µm paraffin sections were stained with rabbit anti-human HER2 antibody (Dako) according

A.

B.

C.

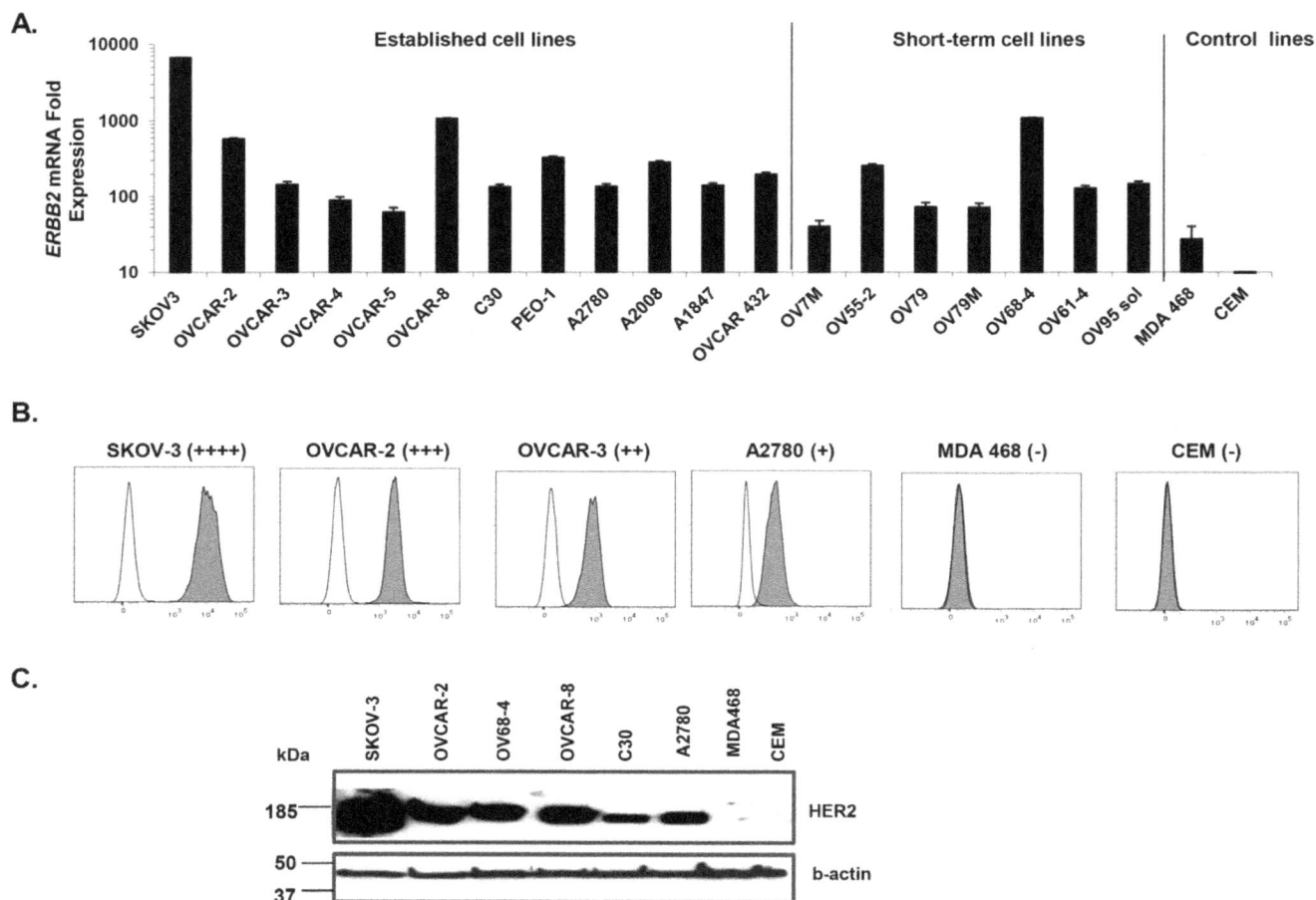

Figure 2. Ubiquitous HER2 expression in ovarian cancer cell lines. *A. ERBB2* mRNA levels in ovarian cancer cell lines by q-PCR. *ERBB2* mRNA levels of ovarian cancer cell lines are relative to that of ErbB2-negative CEM cells. All ovarian cancer cell lines express *ERBB2* mRNA. B-actin was used as an endogenous gene control. Results depict the mean ± SD of triplicate wells. Mean relative *ERBB2* mRNA expression amongst established and short-term OvCa cell lines was not statistically different ($P = 0.45$). *P* value was calculated using unpaired student's t-test analysis. *B.* Detection of surface HER2 protein expression (filled histograms) by human ovarian cancer cell lines by flow cytometry; isotype antibody control (open histograms). *C.* Western blot analysis of HER2 protein expression in representative cell lines expressing differential amounts of HER2. HER2 protein is expressed at variable levels in all the ovarian cell lines tested. B-actin was used as control.

to standard protocols. HER2 expression in each core was scored by light microscopy at 200× magnification using a semiquantitative scale ranging from 0 to 3. Cores showing less than 10% tumor were not scored. For each tumor site, the final score was the mean of the scores for all evaluable cores.

Quantitative PCR

RNA was isolated using RNA easy kit (Qiagen). cDNA was generated from 1 ug of RNA using First Strand Ready-To-Go beads (GE Healthcare). Real-time PCR was performed in triplicates using Applied Biosystem's primers for *ERBB2* and B-actin. *ERBB2* mRNA levels in cancer cells were normalized to B-actin, and compared to those in CEM, and are presented as fold *ERBB2* mRNA level. Data acquisition and analysis was performed according Applied Biosystem's instructions.

Flow Cytometry

Mouse anti-human CD3, CD4, CD8, CD45, CD69, CD107a and CD107b mAbs *(BD Biosciences)* were used for phenotypic analysis. 7-AAD was used for viability staining. HER2 surface expression was evaluated using biotin-conjugated anti-HER2

affibody (Abcam) followed by PE-labeled streptavidin. Anti-HER2 CAR surface expression was evaluated using recombinant human HER2 Fc chimera followed by PE-conjugated anti-huIgG. Acquisition and analysis was performed using a BD FACS CANTO II with DIVA software.

Western Blotting

Cell monolayers were washed with phosphate-buffered saline (PBS) and lysed in RIPA buffer (50 mM Tris-HCl (pH 7.0), 1.0% NP-40, 0.1% deoxycholic acid, 30 mM Na_3VO_4, 1 mM PMSF). Lysates were cleared by centrifugation and quantified using a Nanoorange Kit (Invitrogen). 15 ug total protein per lane was resolved by sodium dodecyl polyacrylamide gel electrophoresis (SDS–PAGE) in pre-cast gradient (4–15%) gels (Bio-Rad) at 120V for 60 minutes. Protein was transferred from gel to Immobilon-P transfer membrane for 30 minutes, blocked overnight with 5% milk/PBST and blotted using 1 ug/ml of mouse anti-human HER2 mAb (clone 3B5, BD biosciences). Membranes were washed 3× with PBST and blotted with HRP-conjugated anti-mouse secondary antibody for 1 h at room temperature. B-actin was detected using anti-human B-actin-HRP (1:30,000). Mem-

Table 1. HER2 surface protein expression in established and primary ovarian cell lines.

Established ovarian cell lines			Short-term ovarian cell lines		
Tumor ID	Specific HER2 MFI	% HER2 positive cells	Tumor ID	Specific HER2 MFI	% HER2 positive cells
SKOV-3	15123	99.7	OV68-4	1261	99.6
OVCAR-2	2946	100	OV55-2	1130	84
OVCAR-3	932	99.6	OV61-4	644	98.8
PEO-1	726	99.9	OV7M	367	96.9
OVCAR-8	616	99.8	OV79	298	94.7
A2008	604	98.9	OV95 Sol	270	83.3
A1847	563	97.5	OV79M	190	64.7
OVCAR-4	475	99	Negative control cell lines		
OVCAR-5	275	98.6	MDA 468	8	1
OVCAR 432	235	98.9	CEM	8	1.9
C30	210	96.1			
A2780	161	84.1			

HER2 is expressed in the cell surface of all ascites and solid tumor-derived tumor cells. HER2 expression was assessed using flow cytometry in a large panel of clinical ascites and solid tumor specimens. A breast cancer cell line (MDA 468) and a leukemia cell line (CEM) which do not express any HER2 were used as negative controls. HER2 was found to be expressed in all tested ascites and solid tumor specimens albeit at different levels. HER2 cell surface levels are expressed as specific MFI. $P = 0.03$ when comparing percentage of HER2 protein-expressing cells in established vs. short-term lines. $P = 0.43$ when comparing MFI of HER2 protein detection in established vs. to short-term cell lines. P values were calculated using student's unpaired t-test analysis.

branes were incubated with ECL Plus (GE Healthcare) for 5 minutes and exposed to films for 15–30 sec.

Anti-HER2 CAR Construction

PCR products containing the C6.5Y100KA HER2 scFv [20] were kindly provided by Silvana Canevari (Instituto Nazionale dei Tumori, Italy) and then cloned into the pCR2.1-TOPO vector using the Topo TA Cloning Kit (Invitrogen). The C6.5 scFv [21] DNA sequence was developed from the above plasmid using QuikChange Multi Site-directed Mutagenesis Kit (Stratagene). The final plasmid was used as a template for PCR amplification of a 795-bp C6.5 scFv fragment using the following primers: 5'-GCGGGATCCATGGCCCAGGTGCAGCTGTTG-CAGTCTGGGGCA-3' (BamHI is underlined) and 5'-GCGGCTAGCCGCACCTAGGACGGT-CAGCTTGGTCCCTCCGCC-3' (NheI is underlined). The resulting PCR product was digested with BamHI and NheI and ligated into the third generation self-inactivating lentiviral expression vector pCLPS containing a CD3ζ signaling CAR sequence, with transgene expression driven by the CMV promoter. The resulting construct was designated pCLPS-C6.5-z.

Recombinant Lentivirus Production

High-titer replication-defective lentiviral vectors were produced and concentrated as previously described [22]. Briefly, 293T cells were transfected with 7 ug pVSV-G plasmid, 18 ug pRSV.REV plasmid, 18 ug pMDLg/p.RRE plasmid, and 15 ug pCLPS-C6.5-z transfer plasmid using Express In (Open Biosytems). Viral supernatant was harvested at 24 h and 48 h post-transfection. Viral particles were concentrated by ultracentrifugation for 3 h at 25,000 rpm with a Beckman SW28 rotor (Beckman Coulter) and resuspended in 0.4 ml RPMI.

T Cell Transduction

Primary human T cells purchased from the Human Immunology Core at University of Pennsylvania were isolated from healthy volunteer donors following leukapheresis by negative selection. All specimens were collected under a University Institutional Review Board-approved protocol, and written informed consent was obtained from each donor. T cells were stimulated in complete media with anti-CD3 and anti-CD28 mAb coated beads (Invitrogen) and transduced with recombinant CAR-encoding lentivirus at MOI of ∼5–10 as described [22].

Cytokine Release Assays

1×10^5 T cells were co-cultured with 1×10^5 target cells per well in triplicate in 96-well round-bottom plates in a final volume of 200 ul of complete media. After 20∼24 hr, cell-free supernatants were assayed for presence of IFN-γ using either an ELISA Kit (Biolegend) or Cytokine Bead Array (BD Biosciences), according to manufacturers' instructions.

Degranulation Assay

Assay was performed as described [23] with minor modifications. 1×10^5 T cells were co-cultured with 1×10^5 target cells in 100 ul media per well in a 96-well plate in triplicate. Control cultures contained T cells alone. Anti-CD107a and Anti-CD107b Ab (10 ul/well) or IgG1 conjugated to FITC (BD Biosciences), and 1 ul/sample of monensin (BD Biosciences) were added to culture and incubated for 5 h at 37°C. Cells were washed twice with PBS, stained for expression of CAR, CD8 and CD69 and analyzed by flow cytometry as described above.

Chromium Release Assay

^{51}Cr release assays were performed as described [24]. Target cells were labeled with 100 uCi ^{51}Cr at 37°C for 1.5 hours. Target cells were washed three times in PBS, resuspended in culture medium at 1×10^5 viable cells/ml and 100 ul added per well of a 96-well V-bottom plate. Effector cells were washed twice in culture medium and added to wells at the given ratios. Plates were quickly centrifuged to settle cells, and incubated at 37°C in a 5% CO_2 incubator for 18 hours after which time the supernatants were

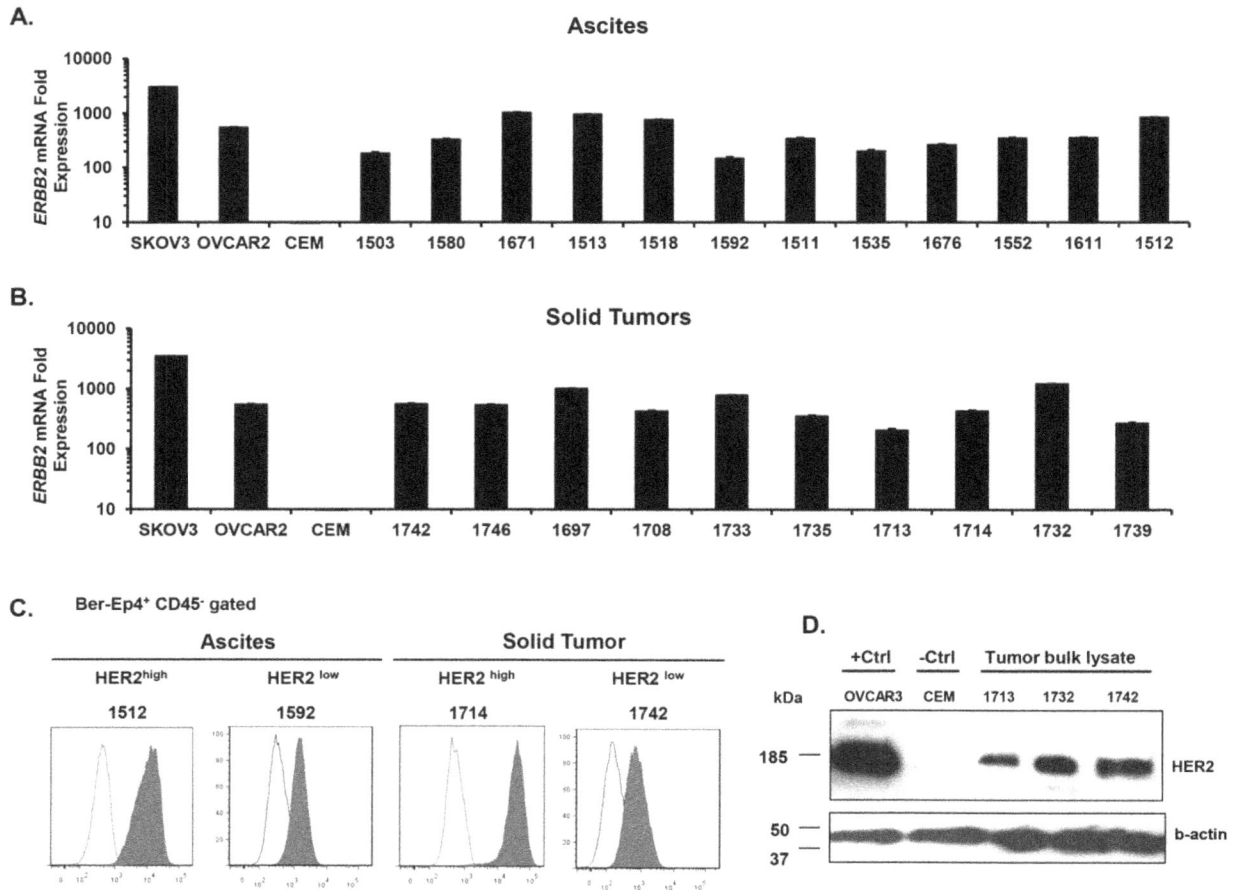

Figure 3. All primary cancers express HER2 protein and *ERBB2* mRNA. *A*. *ERBB2* mRNA quantitation in CD45-depleted primary ascites cancer cells. SKOV-3 and CEM were used as positive and negative HER2-expressing cell line controls respectively. Bars depict the mean ± SD values of triplicate wells. ***B.*** *ERBB2* mRNA quantitation in CD45-depleted primary solid tumor cells. No significant difference in mean *ERBB2* mRNA level was observed between ascites and solid tumors (*P* = 0.46).***C.*** Surface HER2 expression (solid histograms) by representative Ber-Ep4⁺ CD45⁻ gated ascites and solid tumor-derived cancer cells monitored by flow cytometry; isotype antibody control (open histograms). No significant difference in HER2 protein level was observed between ascites or solid tumors derived cells (*P* = 0.95). ***D.*** Western blot analysis of HER2 protein expression in bulk solid tumor lysates. B-actin was used as endogenous gene control. OVCAR-3 and CEM were used as positive and negative controls for HER2 expression. P values were calculated using unpaired student's t-test analysis.

harvested, transferred to a lumar-plate (Packard) and counted using a 1450 Microbeta Liquid Scintillation Counter (Perkin-Elmer). Spontaneous ^{51}Cr release was evaluated in target cells incubated with medium alone. Maximal ^{51}Cr release was measured in target cells incubated with SDS at a final concentration of 2% (v/v). Percent specific lysis was calculated as (experimental - spontaneous lysis/maximal - spontaneous lysis) times 100.

Statistical Analysis

GraphPad Prism 4.0 (GraphPad Software) was used for the statistical calculations. *P*<0.05 values were considered significant. R-squared values (R^2) were calculated using linear regression via Microsoft Excel.

Results

Immunohistochemical Detection of HER2 Expression in Ovarian Cancer

HER2 expression was evaluated in 50 cases of high-grade ovarian serous carcinomas using immunohistochemical (IHC)

analysis in a tissue microarray (TMA). Individual cases varied with respect to the number of tumor sites available for analysis. All cases contained at least one primary lesion site while the majority of cases (96%) had both primary and ≥1 metastatic site available. For many samples, there were ≥2 (62%) or ≥3 (42%) metastatic sites available on the TMA. According to IHC scoring, HER2 was expressed at various levels among the 50 cases ranging from undetectable (score 0) to strong staining (score 3+; **Figure 1A**). Positive HER2 expression at any level was detected in 26 cases (52%) while no HER2 was detectable at any site in 24 cases (**Figure 1B**). Out of the 26 cases expressing HER2 at one or more sites, only 6 (23%) expressed HER2 at all sites by IHC; such cases were weighted toward higher HER2 expression. Most cases that expressed HER2 at any site (20/26) exhibited discordant expression (detectable versus undetectable) at one or more tumor sites. The mean number of evaluated sites was similar amongst the 26 cases with detectable HER2 and the 24 cases with no detectable HER2 (4.2 vs. 3.7, respectively; culture medium *P* = 0.19). Heterogeneity in the patterning of HER2 protein expression among the different sites in individual cases was present with multiple patterns: detectable in all (6/50);

Table 2. HER2 surface protein expression in fresh primary ovarian ascites, solid tumor and normal OSE.

Primary Ascites			Solid Tumors		
Tumor ID	Specific HER2 MFI	% HER2 positive cells	Tumor ID	Specific HER2 MFI	% HER2 positive cells
734	23566	92	1714	22760	98.2
1512	15510	85.8	1735	17824	96.9
1680	13570	76.6	1708	15084	97.7
1565	13099	69.2	1733	4445	72.6
1665	13000	86.4	1697	4318	50.3
1511	10917	93.7	1713	3805	55.3
1671	8769	87.5	1746	2023	59
1515	7359	72.7	1732	1726	64.5
1518	6911	88.7	1742	1044	17.5
1513	6094	91.1	1739	1041	57.8
1659	5128	69.5	Control cell lines		
1611	4776	73.3	SKOV-3	22935	100
1552	4210	67.6	OVCAR-2	7206	100
1676	3996	64.1	OVCAR-3	2267	99.4
1667	3959	61.7	A2780	1750	99.2
736	3939	51	CEM	19	1.3
1689	3697	81.1	Normal controls		
1535	2926	48.5	IOSE-4	1687	100
1503	2401	82.1	IOSE-6	1668	100
1580	1866	67.1	398	1382	94
1592	1530	71.7	1744	1232	42
1637	1365	64.3			

HER2 is expressed in the cell surface of all ascites and solid tumor-derived tumor cells. HER2 expression was assessed using flow cytometry in a large panel of clinical ascites and solid tumor specimens. A breast cancer cell line (MDA 468) and a leukemia cell line (CEM) which do not express any HER2 were used as negative controls. HER2 was found to be expressed in all tested ascites and solid tumor specimens albeit at different levels. HER2 cell surface levels are expressed as specific MFI.

detectable in primary but undetectable in metastatic tumor (8/ 50); detectable in metastatic but undetectable in primary tumor (5/50); detectable in at least one primary and one metastatic sites (7/50). Of 195 tumor sites evaluated, 138 (71%) showed no detectable HER2 expression (**Figure 1C**). Fifty-seven (29%) had positive HER2 expression; 25% (49/195) with a $>0 \leq 1$ HER2 score; 2.5% (5/195) with a $>1 \leq 2$ HER2 score; and 1.5% (3/ 195) with a $>2 \leq 3$ HER2 score. A greater frequency of primary tumor sites expressed HER2 (36%; 30/84) compared to metastatic sites (24%; 27/111) and had a higher mean HER2 expression score (0.37 vs. 0.21, $P = 0.04$; **Figure 1D**). Among primary and metastatic sites that expressed HER2 at any level, there was no statistically significant difference in expression level (1.03 vs. 0.86, $P = 0.26$). In conclusion, IHC allows for the detection of HER2 expression in 29% of all sites and approximately half of all advanced OvCa cases tested.

HER2 is Expressed by All Ovarian Cancer Cell Lines

The relatively low sensitivity of IHC analysis can influence the detection of low abundance proteins and therefore misrepresent the true frequency of cancers that express HER2. To better evaluate HER2 expression in OvCa, 12 established and 7 short-term OvCa cell lines were measured for *ERBB2* mRNA levels by q-PCR, and compared to that detected from CEM, a human T cell lymphoblast-like cell line that lacks HER2 expression [25]. All OvCa cell lines expressed *ERBB2*

mRNA, albeit at various levels (**Figure 2A**). Increased *ERBB2* mRNA expression, relative to the CEM control, ranged from 63- to 6614-fold in established lines and from 40- to 1088-fold in short-term primary cell lines. Mean relative *ERBB2* mRNA expression amongst established (815-fold) and short-term OvCa cell lines (372-fold) was not statistically different from one another ($P = 0.45$). *ERBB2* mRNA was not detected in the CEM control line, but was detectable at low levels in the control breast cancer line, MDA468, which expresses *ERBB2* mRNA but not surface HER2 protein [25].

HER2 protein expression was examined on established and short-term primary tumor cell lines by staining non-permeabilized cells with a highly sensitive anti-HER2 affibody [25], a high affinity ligand against the extracellular domain of HER2, followed by flow cytometric analysis. Representative histograms show established OvCa cell lines expressing high, intermediate or low surface levels of HER2 protein, and negative control cell lines with no detectable HER2 expression (**Figure 2B**). All established (n = 12) and short-term (n = 7) OvCa cell lines tested showed HER2 protein surface expression (**Table 1**). Most cells in established (97.7±1.3%) and short-term lines (88.9±4.8%) expressed HER2 protein, with a higher percentage in the established lines ($P = 0.03$) (**Table 1**). Mean HER2 protein levels measured by specific mean fluorescence intensity (MFI) trended towards being higher in established cell lines (1906±1221 FIU; fluorescence intensity units) compared to short-term cell lines (594±165 FIU) but were not significantly

A.

B.

C.

D.

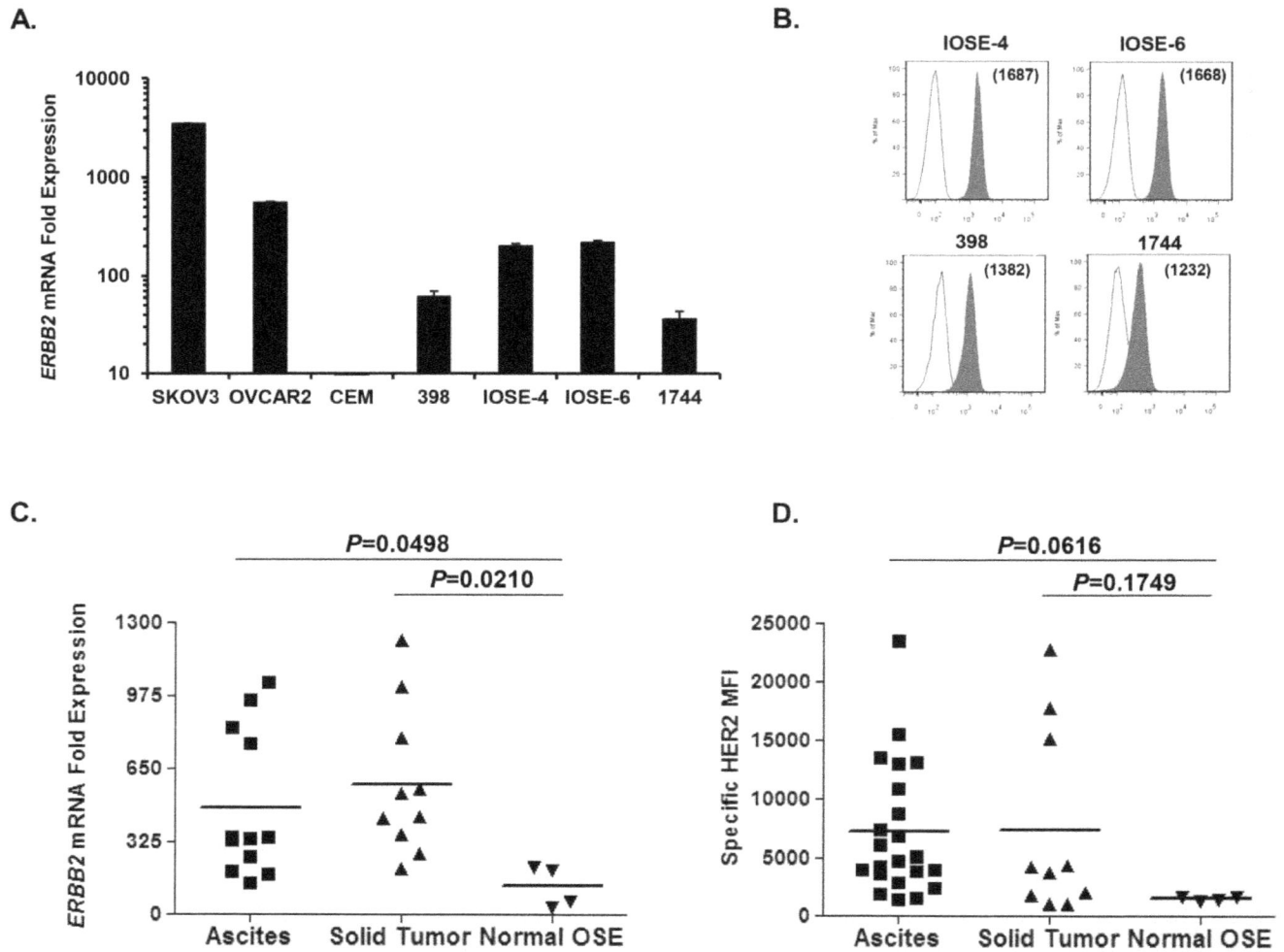

Figure 4. Normal established and primary ovarian surface epithelial cells (OSE) express HER2 protein and *ERBB2* mRNA. *A. ERBB2* mRNA quantitation in normal OSE cells (398, IOSE-4, IOSE-6 and 1744) by q-PCR. SKOV-3 and CEM were used as positive and negative HER2 expressing cell lines respectively. Bars show the mean ± SD value of triplicate wells. *B.* Surface HER2 protein expression (solid histograms) by normal ovarian epithelial cells by flow cytometry; isotype antibody control (open histograms). *C–D.* Comparison of the *ERBB2* mRNA and protein levels between ovarian cancer ascites, solid tumor and normal OSE cells. (*C*) Vertical scatter plots of the *ERBB2* mRNA in ascites, solid tumor and normal OSE determined by q-PCR. The mean of each group is indicated by the horizontal line. *P* = 0.0498 when comparing *ERBB2* mRNA in ascites vs normal OSE cells; *P* = 0.0210 when comparing *ERBB2* mRNA in solid tumors vs normal OSE cells. (*D*) Vertical scatter plots of the protein levels in ascites, solid tumor and normal OSE determined by flow cytometry. The mean of each group is indicated by the horizontal line *P* = 0.0616 when comparing HER2 protein in ascites vs normal OSE cells; *P* = 0.1749 when comparing HER2 protein in solid tumors vs normal OSE cells. *P* values were calculated using unpaired student's t-test analysis.

different (*P* = 0.43) (**Table 1**), consistent with mRNA results. HER2 protein and *ERBB2* mRNA expression levels from all OvCa cell lines were significantly correlated (R^2 = 0.83; calculated using linear regression). Cellular HER2 protein expression was confirmed by western blot analysis (representative samples shown; **Figure 2C**).

Broad HER2 Expression in Primary Ovarian Cancer Specimens

Since *in vitro* culture may selectively enrich for HER2-expressing OvCa cells [16], we measured HER2 expression in uncultured tumor cells derived directly from primary peritoneal OvCa ascites or freshly resected solid tumors. Tumor cells from ascites or solid tumor specimens were enriched by magnetic depletion of CD45+ leukocytes and assessed for relative *ERBB2* mRNA levels via q-PCR (**Figure 3A, B**). All primary

uncultured tumor cells tested (n = 22) expressed *ERBB2* mRNA at levels ranging from 35- to 1225-fold higher than CEM cells. No significant difference in mean *ERBB2* mRNA level was observed between ascites and solid tumors (477 *vs.* 583, respectively; *P* = 0.46). Flow cytometry performed using anti-HER2 affibody showed that non-permeabilized tumor cells (BerEp4+ CD45−) in all primary ascites (n = 22) and solid tumor samples (n = 10) expressed surface HER2 protein, albeit at variable levels, in agreement with the detection of *ERBB2* mRNA by q-PCR (**Table 2**; representative data shown in **Figure 3C**). No significant difference in HER2 protein level was observed between ascites or solid tumors derived cells (7209±1197 FIU *vs.* 7407±2531 FIU, respectively; *P* = 0.95), in agreement with mRNA results. Western blot analysis performed on whole tumor lysates also showed ubiquitous expression of

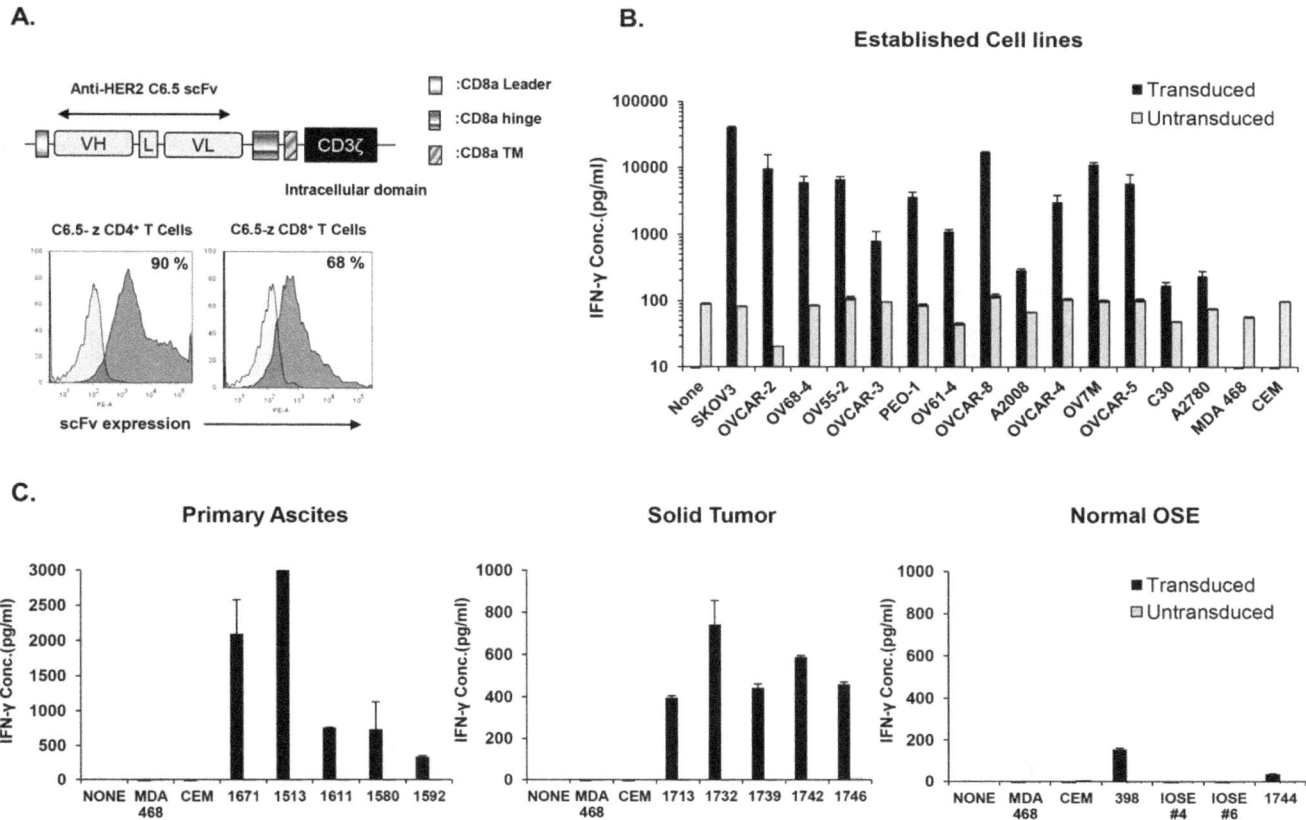

Figure 5. Anti-HER2 CAR-transduced T cells recognize all primary and established ovarian cancer cells. A. Schematic representation of Anti-HER2 Chimeric Antigen Receptor (CAR) construct containing the CD3ζ cytosolic domain alone (C6.5-z). C6.5, anti-HER2 scFv; VL, variable light chain; L, Linker; VH, variable heavy chain; TM, transmembrane region. C6.5 scFv CAR expression (gray histograms) was detected on human CD4$^+$ and CD8$^+$-gated T cells using recombinant human HER2-Fc chimeric protein 10 days after transduction, compared to untransduced T cells (open histograms). Percentage of CAR transduction is indicated. **B.** Anti-HER2 CAR transduced T cells produce IFN-γ specifically after stimulation with human ovarian cancer cell lines. CAR transduced or untransduced T cells were cultured alone (none) or stimulated overnight with human HER2$^+$ established and short-term ovarian cancer cell lines or HER2$^-$ control lines CEM and MDA468. IFN-γ was quantified from cell-free supernatants by ELISA. **C.** Anti-HER2 CAR T cells secrete IFN-γ after stimulation by HER2$^+$ primary ascites (left) or solid ovarian (middle) tumor cells. Minimal amounts of IFN-γ were detected after stimulation with the normal ovarian surface epithelial cells 398, IOSE-4, IOSE-6 or 1744 (right). Cytokine concentrations (pg/ml) are reported as the mean ± SEM of triplicate wells.

HER2 in primary solid tumors (representative samples shown in **Figure 3D**).

Detectable HER2 Expression in Normal Ovarian Epithelial Cells

Three immortalized ovarian surface epithelium cell lines (OSE) and one primary uncultured cell specimen (1744) derived from normal ovaries were tested for HER2 expression. All normal OSE cells expressed low levels of *ERBB2* mRNA that ranged from 35-fold to 217-fold higher than CEM control cells (128±5.5; **Figure 4A**). Flow cytometry (**Figure 4B**) and western blot analysis (not shown) indicated that all normal OSE cells express low yet detectable levels of HER2 protein. IOSE-6 and IOSE-4 cell lines expressed higher protein levels than the 398 line and 1744 normal ovary specimen, in accordance with mRNA results.

Next we compared the *ERBB2* mRNA and protein levels in normal OSE cells, malignant primary ascites and solid tumor-derived tumor cells (**Figures 4C–D**). Ascites and solid tumor samples generally expressed higher levels of *ERBB2* mRNA and protein compared to OSE cells, though an overlap in expression level did exist among groups. Ascites and solid tumors expressed

significantly more *ERBB2* mRNA than OSE cells (Ascites, 483±319-fold, $P = 0.0498$; Solid tumor, 583±330-fold, $P = 0.0210$; OSE, 128±93-fold). HER2 protein levels tended to be higher in ascites (5825±1202-fold) and solid tumor samples (7407±2531-fold) compared to normal OSE (1429±111-fold), but to a low statistical significance (Ascites *vs.* OSE $P = 0.0616$; Solid *vs.* OSE $P = 0.1749$). Variation in HER2 expression levels in OSE samples was limited, allowing a reliable discrimination of tumor samples that overexpress HER2. By comparison, 75% (9/12) of ascites and 90% (9/10) solid tumors expressed higher levels of HER2 compared to OSE, and 91% (20/22) of ascites and 80% (8/10) solid tumors had higher HER2 protein levels than normal OSE cells.

HER2-specific T Cells Recognize All Ovarian Carcinoma Cell Lines

Chimeric antigen receptors (CARs) combine antibody specificity for a surface antigen with the effector activity of T lymphocytes [26]. HER2-specific CAR-expressing T cells can exert potent, dose-dependent *in vitro* anti-tumor activity against HER2-positive target cells [20,25]. To investigate the extent to which broad

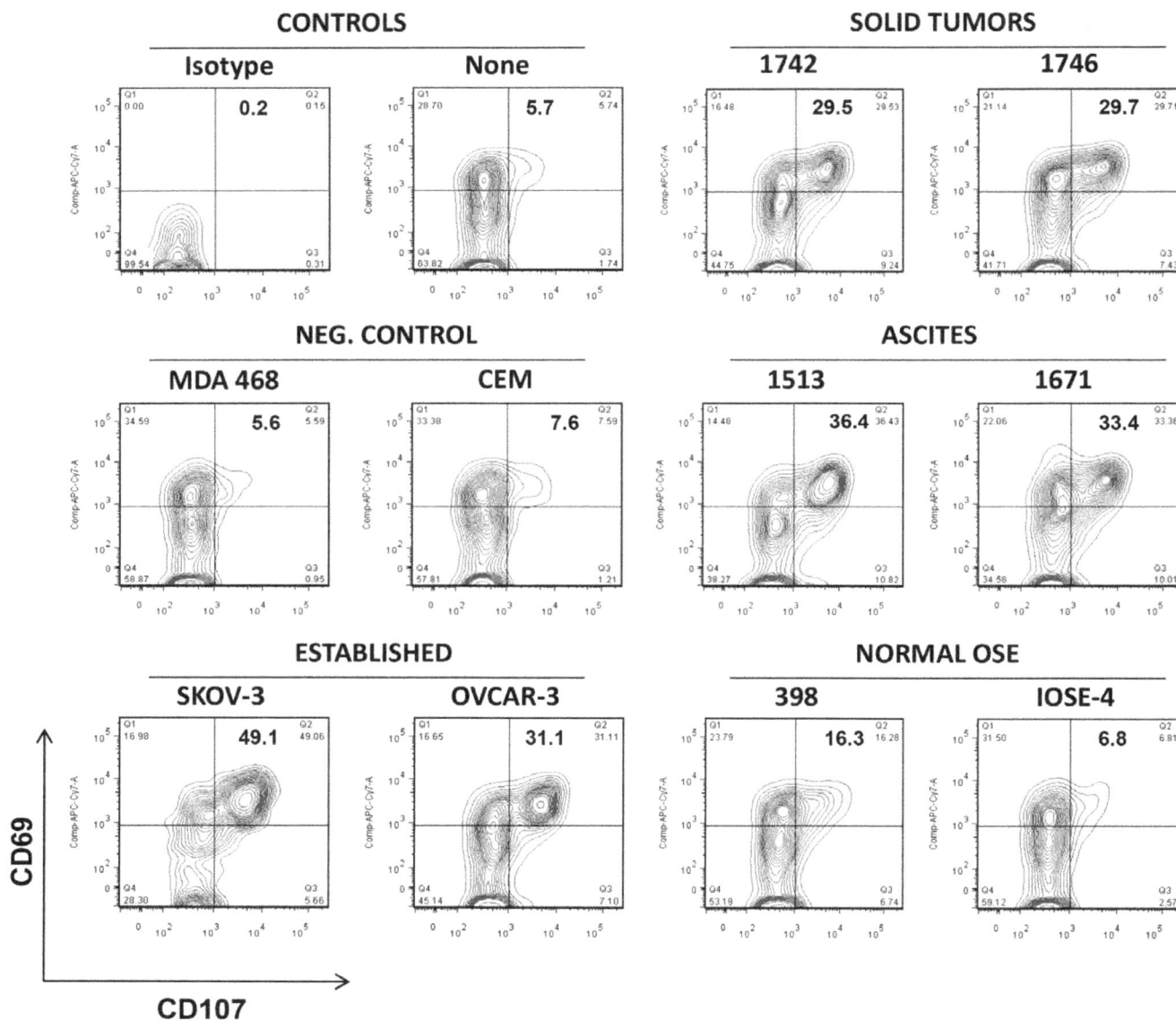

Figure 6. Ovarian cancer cells stimulate a cytolytic phenotype of anti-HER2 CAR T cells. C6.5 CAR T cells degranulate and express T cell activation markers in response to HER2-specific stimulation. C6.5 CAR T cells were cultured without target cells (none) or with the indicated HER2-negative or -positive established and primary tumor cell targets or normal OSE cells for 5 h while being stained by an anti-CD107a, b antibody conjugated with FITC. After the incubation period, T cells were stained for CD8 and CD69 and analyzed by flow cytometry.

HER2 expression by OvCa confers sensitivity to HER2-targeted immunotherapy, human donor T cells were genetically modified to express an anti-HER2 CAR (C6.5) [27], thereby redirecting them against surface HER2, and tested for specific activity against OvCas. The C6.5 CAR construct is comprised of the C6.5 scFv linked to a CD8α hinge and transmembrane region, followed by an intracellular CD3ζ signaling domain (C6.5-z; **Figure 5A**). Primary human CD4$^+$ and CD8$^+$ T cells were efficiently transduced with CAR using lentiviral vectors with transduction efficiencies reproducibly >60% (**Figure 5A**). In co-culture, anti-HER2 CAR T cells recognized and responded to stimulation by all established (n = 10) or short-term (n = 4) human OvCa cells, but not against CEM and MDA-468 cell lines lacking HER2 expression (**Figure 5B**). The amount of IFN-γ secreted was associated with the level of HER2 protein expressed by tumor cells

(R^2 = 0.8064; calculated using linear regression). Untransduced T cells did not produce cytokines upon tumor stimulation, demonstrating the requirement for antigen-specificity. This was confirmed using control anti-mesothelin CAR transduced T cells [22] which did not recognize tumors that express HER2 but lack mesothelin (**Figure S1**).

Importantly, anti-HER2 CAR T cells were also capable of specific recognition and IFN-γ secretion upon stimulation with Ber-Ep4-enriched, primary cancer cells derived from any ascites (n = 5) or solid tumor tested (n = 5; **Figure 5C**). In contrast, anti-HER2 CAR T cells secreted little to no significant amounts of IFN-γ when cultured with normal OSE cells expressing low levels of HER2 antigen (**Figure 5C**). Anti-HER2 CAR T cell effector function was confirmed by monitoring degranulation as a quantitative indicator of T cell cytotoxic activity [23]. Anti-

HER2 CAR-expressing T cells exhibited a cytolytic phenotype in response to all established and primary HER2$^+$ OvCa cells, while minimal degranulation was observed against normal OSE cells (**Figure 6**). Furthermore C6.5 CAR T cells directly and efficiently lysed representative HER2$^+$ human established ovarian cancer cells (OVCAR-3) and primary human solid tumor (1513) or ascites (1742) cancer cells during an 18 hour chromium release assay. C6.5 CAR T cells did not lyse HER2$^-$ tumor cell lines or normal IOSE-4 cells (**Figure S2**).

Discussion

ERBB2 gene amplification and/or overexpression has been reported in a subset of OvCas [6,7,10,11,12,13,14,15] and is associated with poor clinical outcome [10,28]. In these studies, detection relied largely upon IHC analysis to monitor protein over-expression or fluorescence *in situ* hybridization (FISH) to assess gene amplification. In IHC, the amount of protein on the cell surface is determined in a semi-quantitative manner. Samples are scored in a four-tiered scoring system from 0 to 3+ [9]. In FISH, *ERBB2* gene copy number is determined using locus-specific DNA probes [29]. IHC results correlate with FISH results for score 1+ and 3+ samples, but only a limited correlation has been reported for score 2+ samples [30]. Based on these analyses, a subset of patients with clearly positive HER2-expressing tumor may be eligible for HER2-directed treatment using Herceptin. Although Herceptin can mobilize antitumor immune mechanisms, it functions primarily by disrupting HER2 signaling, and therefore its therapeutic efficacy requires overexpression and constitutive activation of HER2 [31]. However, alternate HER2-targeted therapies may be effective even at low levels of surface HER2 expression.

In our study, positive *ERBB2* mRNA and protein expression was found in all established and short-term cultured OvCa cell lines tested as well as in fresh tumor cells derived from ascites or solid tumor utilizing RT-PCR, flow cytometry and western blot analyses. Detection of ubiquitous expression may be explained by the use of these techniques, which are more sensitive than IHC and FISH for measuring HER2 protein and *ERBB2* mRNA levels [32,33]. Indeed, IHC is often applied on fixed tissue where the fixation methods may adversely influence the specificity and sensitivity of the applied antibodies [34]. HER2 testing via IHC on frozen material is less prone to false results but frozen material is rarely available [35,36]. In contrast, surface HER2 protein expression can be detected on cells with high sensitivity via flow cytometry [16]. Despite its merits, FISH-based detection does not assess gene expression and cannot identify gene product overexpression in the absence of gene amplification. However, *ERBB2* mRNA expression can be measured via q-PCR, a fast, reliable and cost-effective alternative to the combination of IHC and FISH procedures, and also correlates with overall and disease-free survival [37].

Our results expand upon those reported by Hellstrom et al. [16], where broad HER2 expression was observed principally on in vitro cultured cell lines established from stage II and IV OvCa via flow cytometry. Binding of the Herceptin antibody inhibited [^{3}H]-thymidine incorporation by two established primary OvCa cell lines, and facilitated antibody-dependent cell-mediated cyto-toxicity (ADCC) by allogeneic immune cells against one cell line [16]. This study was limited by the postulated enhancement of HER2 expression via extended cell culture, use of a single methodology for expression analysis against the established cell panel, and limited numbers of samples tested for HER2-specific immune recognition by Herceptin. In our study, we show positive HER2 expression in both established and short-term cultured lines at both the mRNA and protein level via three independent techniques. Strikingly, broad HER2 expression by ovarian cancer cells is not restricted to established cell lines but was found in all fresh solid tumor and ascites-derived cancer cells in the absence of extended cell culture or manipulation. HER2 expression was generally higher than that detected in normal OSE, suggesting a window of opportunity for cancer targeting. Accordingly, HER2-redirected T cell responses, including proinflammatory cytokine secretion and degranulation, were detected following stimulation with a wide variety of established tumor cells or fresh resected solid tumor or ascites samples, indicating the HER2 is expressed by all OvCa samples at an immunologically active level. Hence, immune recognition was not a phenomenon observed exclusively against established OvCa cell lines which might have undergone *in vitro* selection for high HER2 expression. Lastly, immune recognition against immortalized or primary normal OSE cells was limited or absent, consistent with lower HER2 expression by these cells.

The anti-HER2 CAR used in our study contains the C6.5 scFv with an affinity (1.6×10^{-8}M) above the threshold required to confer reactivity to primary T cells against HER2-expressing tumor cells [27]. Others have shown that T cells bearing a lower affinity C6.5-derivative CAR (C6.5G98A; $Kd > 10^{-8}$M) are exclusively activated by high HER2-expressing tumor cells, and that C6.5-derived CAR T cells of any affinity had no reactivity against cells from normal tissues [27]. In our study, C6.5 CAR-grafted T cells reacted against all established or primary OvCa cells and exhibited minimal or no reactivity against normal OSE, which generally express lower levels of HER2 than malignant ovarian cells. In another study, Zhao and coworkers, constructed an anti-HER2 CAR comprised of a Herceptin-derived scFv (4D5), where the affinity of the scFv (3×10^{-10} M) is approximately two orders of magnitude higher than that of the C6.5 scFv and recognizes a different epitope [25,38]. 4D5 CAR T cells reacted against a panel of tumor cells of different origin expressing even low levels of HER2, as well as multiple normal cells [25,39]. Administration of high numbers of T cells expressing the 4D5 CAR encompassing CD28 and CD137 costimulatory domains following lymphodepletion resulted in an assumed response against lung epithelial cells expressing low levels of HER2, leading to cytokine storm, respiratory distress and ultimately patient death [39]. The impact of high anti-HER2 CAR affinity and epitope specificity on immune recognition and response to normal cells in patients, resulting in the development of toxicity, remains unresolved.

The breadth of HER2 expression among OvCas has a direct implication on determining patients' access to various HER2-targeting therapeutic strategies and drug delivery systems. In contrast to breast cancer, trastuzumab (Herceptin) targeting of HER2 mediated limited responses (7%) in patients with advanced OvCa [12] despite the paradoxical finding of ubiquitous HER2 expression. The mechanisms accounting for the poor response to trastuzumab in OvCa patients remain unknown. Resistance of tumors to trastuzumab might arise through alternative signaling and survival pathways induced as a consequence of a marked inhibition of HER2 [40]. Alternatively, since the activity of trastuzumab is partially mediated through ADCC and is dependent upon a functional immune system [41], it remains possible that administration of chemotherapy prior to trastuzumab treatment, as performed above [12], may hamper overall immune function and ADCC activity. Further complicating effective therapy is the finding that ovarian cancers are prone to harbor an immunosuppressive microenvironment with a limited effective innate compartment necessary for mediating ADCC [42]. HER2-

specific peptide and DNA vaccines that induce T cell responses against HER2 represent alternative treatment strategies, however these approaches have not evolved beyond phase I/II studies due to limited clinical efficacy [43,44,45]. However, T cells engineered to express a HER2-specific CAR have the capacity to recognize HER2 on the surface of all ovarian cancer cells, and thus represent an attractive option for therapy. Despite their potential for toxicity [39], CARs against HER2 have been well characterized, have high *in vitro* and *in vivo* potential, and remain under clinical investigation [27,46,47,48,49].

We conclude that HER2 is broadly expressed in established and primary ovarian carcinomas. Despite the wide range of HER2 expression, all OvCas were sensitive to recognition by genetically modified T cells bearing an anti-HER2 CAR indicating that the surface expression of HER2 is sufficient for the induction of potent immune responses. We postulate that HER2-directed immuno-therapeutic strategies may have beneficial effects in patients with ovarian carcinoma, including many of those who are negative according to routinely applied immunohistochemistry on tumors resected at primary surgery. However, careful design and testing is needed to understand how to safely apply HER2 targeted approaches for the treatment of patients with HER2-expressing ovarian carcinomas.

Supporting Information

Figure S1   Specific HER2 CAR-redirected recognition of HER2-expressing tumor cells. C6.5-z anti-HER2 or P4-z anti-mesothelin CAR T cells were co-cultured with tumor cells expressing both HER2 and mesothelin or only HER2 or lacking both antigens. Cell-free supernatant from three independent cultures was harvested and pooled after ~20 hours of incubation and the IFN-γ secretion was quantified using cytometric bead array technology. Values represent cytokine concentration (pg/ml).

Figure S2   Direct lytic activity of anti-HER2 lentiviral vector-engineered T cells. Antigen-specific killing of HER2$^+$ tumor cells by C6.5 CAR T cells. Primary human T cells transduced to express the C6.5 CAR (~30% expression) were co-cultured with ^{51}Cr-labeled HER2 positive or negative tumor cells or normal OSE for 18 hrs at the indicated effector to target ratio. Percent specific target cell lysis was calculated as (experimental - spontaneous release) ÷ (maximal - spontaneous release)×100. Results are graphed with respect to effective E/T ratio and represent mean (±SEM) cytotoxicity of triplicate wells.

Acknowledgments

The authors gratefully acknowledge Silvana Canevari, Mariangela Figini, Richard Carroll, Lin Zhang, Michael Kalos and Carl June for reagents and discussions.

Author Contributions

Conceived and designed the experiments: EL GC DP. Performed the experiments: EL DD ISH. Analyzed the data: EL DD ISH. Contributed reagents/materials/analysis tools: DS AB. Wrote the paper: EL DD RS DP.

References

1. Engel RH, Kaklamani VG (2007) HER2-positive breast cancer: current and future treatment strategies. Drugs 67: 1329–1341.
2. Wong YF, Cheung TH, Lam SK, Lu HJ, Zhuang YL, et al. (1995) Prevalence and significance of HER-2/neu amplification in epithelial ovarian cancer. Gynecol Obstet Invest 40: 209–212.
3. Juhl H, Downing SG, Wellstein A, Czubayko F (1997) HER-2/neu is rate-limiting for ovarian cancer growth. Conditional depletion of HER-2/neu by ribozyme targeting. J Biol Chem 272: 29482–29486.
4. Pietras RJ, Fendly BM, Chazin VR, Pegram MD, Howell SB, et al. (1994) Antibody to HER-2/neu receptor blocks DNA repair after cisplatin in human breast and ovarian cancer cells. Oncogene 9: 1829–1838.
5. Bartsch R, Wenzel C, Zielinski CC, Steger GG (2007) HER-2-positive breast cancer: hope beyond trastuzumab. BioDrugs 21: 69–77.
6. Verri E, Guglielmini P, Puntoni M, Perdelli L, Papadia A, et al. (2005) HER2/neu oncoprotein overexpression in epithelial ovarian cancer: evaluation of its prevalence and prognostic significance. Clinical study. Oncology 68: 154–161.
7. Hogdall EV, Christensen L, Kjaer SK, Blaakaer J, Bock JE, et al. (2003) Distribution of HER-2 overexpression in ovarian carcinoma tissue and its prognostic value in patients with ovarian carcinoma: from the Danish MALOVA Ovarian Cancer Study. Cancer 98: 66–73.
8. Ioannides CG, Fisk B, Fan D, Biddison WE, Wharton JT, et al. (1993) Cytotoxic T cells isolated from ovarian malignant ascites recognize a peptide derived from the HER-2/neu proto-oncogene. Cell Immunol 151: 225–234.
9. Wolff AC, Hammond ME, Schwartz JN, Hagerty KL, Allred DC, et al. (2007) American Society of Clinical Oncology/College of American Pathologists guideline recommendations for human epidermal growth factor receptor 2 testing in breast cancer. J Clin Oncol 25: 118–145.
10. Felip E, Del Campo JM, Rubio D, Vidal MT, Colomer R, et al. (1995) Overexpression of c-erbB-2 in epithelial ovarian cancer. Prognostic value and relationship with response to chemotherapy. Cancer 75: 2147–2152.
11. Fajac A, Benard J, Lhomme C, Rey A, Duvillard P, et al. (1995) c-erbB2 gene amplification and protein expression in ovarian epithelial tumors: evaluation of their respective prognostic significance by multivariate analysis. Int J Cancer 64: 146–151.
12. Bookman MA, Darcy KM, Clarke-Pearson D, Boothby RA, Horowitz IR (2003) Evaluation of monoclonal humanized anti-HER2 antibody, trastuzumab, in patients with recurrent or refractory ovarian or primary peritoneal carcinoma with overexpression of HER2: a phase II trial of the Gynecologic Oncology Group. J Clin Oncol 21: 283–290.
13. Nielsen JS, Jakobsen E, Holund B, Bertelsen K, Jakobsen A (2004) Prognostic significance of p53, Her-2, and EGFR overexpression in borderline and epithelial ovarian cancer. Int J Gynecol Cancer 14: 1086–1096.
14. Lee CH, Huntsman DG, Cheang MC, Parker RL, Brown L, et al. (2005) Assessment of Her-1, Her-2, And Her-3 expression and Her-2 amplification in advanced stage ovarian carcinoma. Int J Gynecol Pathol 24: 147–152.
15. Mayr D, Kanitz V, Amann G, Engel J, Burges A, et al. (2006) HER-2/neu gene amplification in ovarian tumours: a comprehensive immunohistochemical and FISH analysis on tissue microarrays. Histopathology 48: 149–156.
16. Hellstrom I, Goodman G, Pullman J, Yang Y, Hellstrom KE (2001) Overexpression of HER-2 in ovarian carcinomas. Cancer Res 61: 2420–2423.
17. Bertozzi CC, Chang CY, Jairaj S, Shan X, Huang J, et al. (2006) Multiple initial culture conditions enhance the establishment of cell lines from primary ovarian cancer specimens. In Vitro Cell Dev Biol Anim 42: 58–62.
18. Zorn KK, Jazaeri AA, Awtrey CS, Gardner GJ, Mok SC, et al. (2003) Choice of normal ovarian control influences determination of differentially expressed genes in ovarian cancer expression profiling studies. Clin Cancer Res 9: 4811–4818.
19. Maines-Bandiera SL, Kruk PA, Auersperg N (1992) Simian virus 40-transformed human ovarian surface epithelial cells escape normal growth controls but retain morphogenetic responses to extracellular matrix. Am J Obstet Gynecol 167: 729–735.
20. Turatti F, Figini M, Alberti P, Willemsen RA, Canevari S, et al. (2005) Highly efficient redirected anti-tumor activity of human lymphocytes transduced with a completely human chimeric immune receptor. J Gene Med 7: 158–170.
21. Schier R, Marks JD, Wolf EJ, Apell G, Wong C, et al. (1995) In vitro and in vivo characterization of a human anti-c-erbB-2 single-chain Fv isolated from a filamentous phage antibody library. Immunotechnology 1: 73–81.
22. Lanitis E, Poussin M, Hagemann IS, Coukos G, Sandaltzopoulos R, et al. (2012) Redirected Antitumor Activity of Primary Human Lymphocytes Transduced With a Fully Human Anti-mesothelin Chimeric Receptor. Mol Ther 20: 633–643.
23. Betts MR, Brenchley JM, Price DA, De Rosa SC, Douek DC, et al. (2003) Sensitive and viable identification of antigen-specific CD8+ T cells by a flow cytometric assay for degranulation. J Immunol Methods 281: 65–78.
24. Johnson LA, Heemskerk B, Powell DJ, Jr., Cohen CJ, Morgan RA, et al. (2006) Gene transfer of tumor-reactive TCR confers both high avidity and tumor reactivity to nonreactive peripheral blood mononuclear cells and tumor-infiltrating lymphocytes. J Immunol 177: 6548–6559.
25. Zhao Y, Wang QJ, Yang S, Kochenderfer JN, Zheng Z, et al. (2009) A herceptin-based chimeric antigen receptor with modified signaling domains leads to enhanced survival of transduced T lymphocytes and antitumor activity. J Immunol 183: 5563–5574.
26. Gross G, Waks T, Eshhar Z (1989) Expression of immunoglobulin-T-cell receptor chimeric molecules as functional receptors with antibody-type specificity. Proc Natl Acad Sci U S A 86: 10024–10028.

27. Chmielewski M, Hombach A, Heuser C, Adams GP, Abken H (2004) T cell activation by antibody-like immunoreceptors: increase in affinity of the single-chain fragment domain above threshold does not increase T cell activation against antigen-positive target cells but decreases selectivity. J Immunol 173: 7647–7653.

28. Camilleri-Broët SH-BA, Le Tourneau A, Paraiso D, Levrel O, Leduc B, et al. (2005) Retraction of "The prognostic and predictive value of immunohisto-chemically detected HER-2/neu overexpression in 361 patients with ovarian cancer: a multicenter study" [Gynecol Oncol 2004;95: 89–94]. Gynecol Oncol 96: 1021.

29. Kallioniemi OP, Kallioniemi A, Kurisu W, Thor A, Chen LC, et al. (1992) ERBB2 amplification in breast cancer analyzed by fluorescence in situ hybridization. Proc Natl Acad Sci U S A 89: 5321–5325.

30. Perez EA, Roche PC, Jenkins RB, Reynolds CA, Halling KC, et al. (2002) HER2 testing in patients with breast cancer: poor correlation between weak positivity by immunohistochemistry and gene amplification by fluorescence in situ hybridization. Mayo Clin Proc 77: 148–154.

31. Baselga J, Albanell J, Molina MA, Arribas J (2001) Mechanism of action of trastuzumab and scientific update. Semin Oncol 28: 4–11.

32. Lal G, Padmanabha L, Nicholson R, Smith BJ, Zhang L, et al. (2008) ECM1 expression in thyroid tumors–a comparison of real-time RT-PCR and IHC. J Surg Res 149: 62–68.

33. Diederichsen AC, Hansen TP, Nielsen O, Fenger C, Jensenius JC, et al. (1998) A comparison of flow cytometry and immunohistochemistry in human colorectal cancers. APMIS 106: 562–570.

34. Penault-Llorca F, Adelaide J, Houvenaeghel G, Hassoun J, Birnbaum D, et al. (1994) Optimization of immunohistochemical detection of ERBB2 in human breast cancer: impact of fixation. J Pathol 173: 65–75.

35. Pauletti G, Dandekar S, Rong H, Ramos L, Peng H, et al. (2000) Assessment of methods for tissue-based detection of the HER-2/neu alteration in human breast cancer: a direct comparison of fluorescence in situ hybridization and immunohistochemistry. J Clin Oncol 18: 3651–3664.

36. Pauletti G, Godolphin W, Press MF, Slamon DJ (1996) Detection and quantitation of HER-2/neu gene amplification in human breast cancer archival material using fluorescence in situ hybridization. Oncogene 13: 63–72.

37. Vinatzer U, Dampier B, Streubel B, Pacher M, Seewald MJ, et al. (2005) Expression of HER2 and the coamplified genes GRB7 and MLN64 in human breast cancer: quantitative real-time reverse transcription-PCR as a diagnostic alternative to immunohistochemistry and fluorescence in situ hybridization. Clin Cancer Res 11: 8348–8357.

38. Tang Y, Lou J, Alpaugh RK, Robinson MK, Marks JD, et al. (2007) Regulation of antibody-dependent cellular cytotoxicity by IgG intrinsic and apparent affinity for target antigen. J Immunol 179: 2815–2823.

39. Morgan RA, Yang JC, Kitano M, Dudley ME, Laurencot CM, et al. (2010) Case report of a serious adverse event following the administration of T cells transduced with a chimeric antigen receptor recognizing ERBB2. Mol Ther 18: 843–851.

40. Arteaga CL, Sliwkowski MX, Osborne CK, Perez EA, Puglisi F, et al. (2012) Treatment of HER2-positive breast cancer: current status and future perspectives. Nat Rev Clin Oncol 9: 16–32.

41. Musolino A, Naldi N, Bortesi B, Pezzuolo D, Capelletti M, et al. (2008) Immunoglobulin G fragment C receptor polymorphisms and clinical efficacy of trastuzumab-based therapy in patients with HER-2/neu-positive metastatic breast cancer. J Clin Oncol 26: 1789–1796.

42. Vaughan S, Coward JI, Bast RC, Jr., Berchuck A, Berek JS, et al. (2011) Rethinking ovarian cancer: recommendations for improving outcomes. Nat Rev Cancer 11: 719–725.

43. Brossart P, Wirths S, Stuhler G, Reichardt VL, Kanz L, et al. (2000) Induction of cytotoxic T-lymphocyte responses in vivo after vaccinations with peptide-pulsed dendritic cells. Blood 96: 3102–3108.

44. Scardino A, Alimandi M, Correale P, Smith SG, Bei R, et al. (2007) A polyepitope DNA vaccine targeted to Her-2/ErbB-2 elicits a broad range of human and murine CTL effectors to protect against tumor challenge. Cancer Res 67: 7028–7036.

45. Chu CS, Boyer J, Schullery DS, Gimotty PA, Gamerman V, et al. (2011) Phase I/II randomized trial of dendritic cell vaccination with or without cyclophos-phamide for consolidation therapy of advanced ovarian cancer in first or second remission. Cancer Immunol Immunother.

46. Stancovski I, Schindler DG, Waks T, Yarden Y, Sela M, et al. (1993) Targeting of T lymphocytes to Neu/HER2-expressing cells using chimeric single chain Fv receptors. J Immunol 151: 6577–6582.

47. Pinthus JH, Waks T, Kaufman-Francis K, Schindler DG, Harmelin A, et al. (2003) Immuno-gene therapy of established prostate tumors using chimeric receptor-redirected human lymphocytes. Cancer Res 63: 2470–2476.

48. Moritz D, Wels W, Mattern J, Groner B (1994) Cytotoxic T lymphocytes with a grafted recognition specificity for ERBB2-expressing tumor cells. Proc Natl Acad Sci U S A 91: 4318–4322.

49. Kershaw MH, Jackson JT, Haynes NM, Teng MW, Moeller M, et al. (2004) Gene-engineered T cells as a superior adjuvant therapy for metastatic cancer. J Immunol 173: 2143–2150.

7

Control of Established Colon Cancer Xenografts using a Novel Humanized Single Chain Antibody-Streptococcal Superantigen Fusion Protein Targeting the 5T4 Oncofetal Antigen

Kelcey G. Patterson[1], Jennifer L. Dixon Pittaro[1], Peter S. Bastedo[1], David A. Hess[3,4], S. M. Mansour Haeryfar[1,2,5], John K. McCormick[1,2,5]*

1 Department of Microbiology and Immunology, Western University, London, Ontario, Canada, **2** Centre for Human Immunology, Western University, London, Ontario, Canada, **3** Department of Physiology and Pharmacology, Western University, London Ontario, Canada, **4** Vascular Biology Research Group, Robarts Research Institute, London, Ontario, Canada, **5** Lawson Health Research Institute, London, Ontario, Canada

Abstract

Superantigens (SAgs) are microbial toxins that cross-link T cell receptors with major histocompatibility class II (MHC-II) molecules leading to the activation of large numbers of T cells. Herein, we describe the development and preclinical testing of a novel tumor-targeted SAg (TTS) therapeutic built using the streptococcal pyrogenic exotoxin C (SpeC) SAg and targeting cancer cells expressing the 5T4 tumor-associated antigen (TAA). To inhibit potentially harmful widespread immune cell activation, a SpeC mutation within the high-affinity MHC-II binding interface was generated (SpeC$_{D203A}$) that demonstrated a pronounced reduction in mitogenic activity, yet this mutant could still induce immune cell-mediated cancer cell death *in vitro*. To target 5T4$^+$ cancer cells, we engineered a humanized single chain variable fragment (scFv) antibody to recognize 5T4 (scFv5T4). Specific targeting of scFv5T4 was verified. SpeC$_{D203A}$ fused to scFv5T4 maintained the ability to activate and induce immune cell-mediated cytotoxicity of colorectal cancer cells. Using a xenograft model of established human colon cancer, we demonstrated that the SpeC-based TTS was able to control the growth and spread of large tumors *in vivo*. This required both TAA targeting by scFv5T4 and functional SAg activity. These studies lay the foundation for the development of streptococcal SAgs as 'next-generation' TTSs for cancer immunotherapy.

Editor: Michael P. Bachmann, Carl-Gustav Carus Technical University-Dresden, Germany

Funding: This work was supported by Canadian Institutes of Health Research (CIHR) operating grant to JKM (MOP-64176). SMMH holds a Canada Research Chair in Viral Immunity and Pathogenesis and JKM was the recipient of a New Investigator Award from the CIHR. The funders had no role in study design, data collection and analysis, decision to publish, or preparation of the manuscript.

Competing Interests: The authors have declared that no competing interests exist.

* E-mail: john.mccormick@uwo.ca

Introduction

Superantigens (SAgs) are microbial toxins that function as potent T cell activators and are mediators of the toxic shock syndrome [1]. These molecules function by binding to lateral surfaces of major histocompatibility class II (MHC-II) molecules [2–5], while simultaneously engaging germline-encoded regions within the variable region of the T cell receptor (TCR) β-chain (Vβ) [6–9]. Since there are ~50 functional Vβ genes in humans [10,11], and because different SAgs can often target multiple Vβs [12], these toxins stimulate a very large percentage of exposed T cells leading to the subsequent release of pro-inflammatory cytokines (e.g. IL-2, IFN-γ, and TNF-α) [1]. Although SAgs do not engage MHC I molecules, these toxins do activate both CD4$^+$ and CD8$^+$ T cells [13], and this can subsequently lead to bystander activation of accessory cells including NK cells [14]. In specific cases, SAg can also activate unconventional T cell subsets such as invariant natural killer T (iNKT) cells [15] and γδ T cells [16].

The ultimate goal of cancer immunotherapy is to harness immune-mediated mechanisms to specifically target and eradicate tumor cells. There have been significant efforts to design SAg-based immunotoxins, also known as tumor-targeted superantigens (TTS), in order to artificially 'force' T cells to recognize tumor-associated antigens (TAAs) in a non-HLA-restricted manner. The initial TTS represented the fusion of a mouse antibody fragment (Fab) targeting a colorectal cancer antigen, to the wild-type staphylococcal enterotoxin A (SEA) SAg. In this pioneering work, the Fab::SEA TTS demonstrated a substantial reduction in tumor burden and mortality using a B16 mouse metastasis model [17]. Later studies utilized the fusion of a mouse Fab to target the 5T4 oncofetal antigen with a mutated version of SEA (designed to reduce MHC-II binding) and this resulted in ~95% reduction of tumor mass in a non-small cell lung cancer (NSCLC) model [18]. Furthermore, combination therapies with TTSs have also shown promise in preclinical models in conjunction with cytokine therapies (e.g. IFN-α) [19] and blockade of CTLA-4 [20]. These and other studies have clearly demonstrated the potential of TTSs for cancer immunotherapy. Nonetheless, the TTSs have so far been built exclusively using members of the SE class of SAg, and SEs are also agents of staphylococcal food-borne illness, an activity that is thought to be independent of the ability to activate T cells [21]. Although manageable, some of the side effects seen in TTS Phase I and Phase II clinical trials included nausea, vomiting and diarrhea [22–24], and may have been related to the emetic properties of SEA [25]. Additionally, many patients had pre-existing antibodies to SEA which required individualized TTS dosing [26]. In order to reduce the antigenicity of the TTS therapeutic, anti-5T4 Fab was linked to an engineered SEA/SEE fusion (called Naptumomab estafenatox; ABR-217620) [27]. This latest TTS therapeutic has undergone a Phase I clinical trial as a monotherapy in patients with advanced NSCLC, pancreatic cancer and renal cell carcinoma (RCC), and as a combination therapy with Docetaxel in patients with NSCLC, demonstrating that ABR-217620 was well tolerated with some evidence of anti-tumor activity [24]. Early information from a recently completed Phase II/III trial with ABR-217620 in patients with RCC comparing ABR-217620 and interferon-α, to interferon-α alone, did not reach the primary endpoint of overall survival; however, it appears that many patients had higher than expected baseline levels of anti-SEA/SEE antibodies, which may have contributed to suboptimal therapy [28].

Bacterial genomic sequencing efforts over the last decade have now revealed an extensive 'family' of SAg exotoxins in both *Staphylococcus aureus* and *Streptococcus pyogenes*. A general feature of these toxins is that genetically distinct SAgs are also antigenically distinct, and furthermore, distinct SAgs also typically display unique Vβ activation profiles [12]. Thus, *S. aureus* and *S. pyogenes* have provided an abundance of T cell mitogens that could potentially be engineered as TTSs for cancer therapy. In the current work, we sought to expand the repertoire of TTSs to include the first streptococcal SAg using streptococcal pyrogenic exotoxin C (SpeC) as the prototype. A potential advantage of engineering a streptococcal SAg as a TTS is that these toxins lack bona fide emetic activity [29], which may result in fewer side effects. Also, SpeC is very well studied in terms of both structure [4,30,31] and function [9,32–35] for engagement of host receptors, providing a platform for tailoring activity. Herein, we demonstrate that SpeC mutagenized within the zinc-dependent, high-affinity MHC-II binding domain (SpeC$_{D203A}$) has reduced superantigenicity while retaining tumoricidal properties. We generated a SpeC$_{D203A}$-based TTS fusion protein using an engineered human scFv that specifically targets human 5T4 (scFv5T4). In a humanized mouse model of colon cancer, we demonstrate that the scFv5T4::SpeC$_{D203A}$ TTS controls the growth and metastatic potential of an established colon cancer tumor, and that this anti-tumor activity requires both specific targeting by the scFv5T4 moiety, as well as SAg function.

Materials and Methods

Ethics statements

Experiments using primary human lymphocytes were reviewed and approved by Western University's Research Ethics Board for Health Sciences Research Involving Human Subjects. Informed written consent was obtained from all blood donors. All animal experiments were in accordance with the Canadian Council on Animal Care Guide to the Care and Use of Experimental Animals, and the protocol was approved by the Animal Use Subcommittee at Western University (London, Ontario).

Antibodies and dyes

The following monoclonal antibodies and dyes were used: PE anti-human CD4 (clone RPA-T4; BD Pharmingen); Alexa-Fluor700 anti-human CD8 (clone RPA-T8; BD Pharmingen); APC anti-human CD3 (Clone UCHT1; BD Pharmingen); CellTrace CFSE (carboxyfluorescein diacetate; Molecular Probes); 7-AAD (7-aminoactinomycin D; Molecular Probes); anti-human 5T4 (ab88091; Abcam); IgG2b isotype (eBioscience); FITC anti-mouse IgG (eBioscience); strepavidin-IRDye800 (Rockland Immunochemicals); streptavidin-FITC (Rockland Immunochemicals).

Bacterial strains

Escherichia coli XL1-Blue (Stratagene) or DH5α (Invitrogen) were used for cloning purposes and *E. coli* BL21 (DE3) (Novagen) was used as the protein expression host. *E. coli* strains were grown aerobically at 37°C in Luria broth (LB) containing kanamycin (50 μg/ml), ampicillin (200 μg/ml) or chloramphenicol (10 μg/ml) to maintain plasmids.

Cloning procedures

Plasmid constructs were either previously published [34,35] or generated by standard cloning techniques [36], in either pET-41a (Novagen) or pET-32a (Novagen) and are summarized in **Table S1**. All plasmid inserts were sequenced at the Robarts Research Institute Sequencing Facility (London, Ontario, Canada). Protein expression clones in pET-32a or pET-41a were altered such that the enterokinase cleavage site (DDDDK ↓ X) was replaced with a Tobacco Etch Virus (TEV) protease cleavage site (ENLYFQ ↓ S). Transfection vectors pCMV6-XL5, pCMV6-XL5::5T4 and pEGFP-N1 were purchased from Origene Technologies, and Clonetech Laboratories, respectively. All other transfection plasmids were generated by standard cloning techniques. The murine scFv5T4 cDNA [37] was recoded and then manufactured by GenScript Inc. to generate a humanized sequence. Amino acid substitutions were made in the backbone sequence of scFv5T4 from the original mouse scFv sequence, determined by aligning with a human consensus sequence. The CDR loops specific for 5T4 [37], and the immediate amino acids flanking the predicted loops were not altered to maintain antibody specificity.

Protein expression

Recombinant proteins were produced using an *E. coli* BL21 (DE3) expression system containing the pBirACm plasmid. Cells were grown aerobically at 37°C in LB medium to OD$_{600}$ = 0.5 and protein expression was induced overnight (18–24 h) at room temperature (RT) with 0.2 mM isopropyl-D-thiogalactopyranoside (IPTG; BioBasic Inc.) and biotinylated with the addition of 50 μM D-biotin (BioBasic Inc.). Cells were pelleted at 4°C and resuspended in cold 20 mM Tris-HCl, pH 7.4, 200 mM NaCl containing 0.25 mg/ml lysozyme (Sigma-Aldrich) and 0.02 mg/ml DNase I (Sigma-Aldrich). Cells were incubated on ice for 1 h prior to lysis with a continuous head flow cell disruptor (Constant Systems Ltd.) at 25 psi, followed by sonication with output 4, 1 pulse/ml. Cellular debris was pelleted at 4°C at 10000×g. Supernatants were applied to a charged Ni-NTA affinity column (Novagen) and increasing concentration of imidazole was used to elute the purified protein. Purified fractions were dialyzed 3× against 20 mM Tris-HCl, pH 7.4, 200 mM NaCl buffer and the N-terminal tags were cleaved by autoinactivation-resistant His$_7$::TEV [38], as described [39]. Cleaved proteins were applied and eluted from a second Ni-NTA affinity column to remove TEV protease and obtain a pure protein. Proteins were dialyzed 3×

against 20 mM Tris-HCl, pH 7.4, 200 mM NaCl buffer or 0.9% NaCl (saline) and assessed for homogeneity by SDS-PAGE and quantified (BCA Protein Assay, Pierce).

Cell lines

Human colorectal adenocarcinoma cell lines (HT-29 and WiDr) were cultured in complete Dulbecco's Modified Eagle Medium (cDMEM; Gibco) and HEK293 cells were cultured in complete Minimum Essential Media (cMEM; Gibco). All culture media were supplemented with 10% fetal bovine serum (FBS; Sigma-Aldrich), 10 mM HEPES, pH 7.4 (Gibco), 2 mM L-Glutamine (Gibco), 1 mM sodium pyruvate (Gibco), 100 μM non-essential amino acids (Gibco), 100 μg/ml streptomycin (Gibco), and 100 U/ml penicillin (Gibco).

scFv5T4 specificity assays

HEK293 cells (1×10^5) were seeded into 24-well plates (Corning) with 500 μl cMEM and allowed to grow overnight (24 h) at 37°C with 5% CO_2. Liposome:DNA complexes were formed using Lipofectamine2000 (Invitrogen) and plasmid DNA of choice as per the manufacture's protocol. Complexes were formed in cMEM without FBS or antibiotics. Transfection of cells occurred in the same media for 4 h at 37°C with 5% CO_2, after which the media was removed and replaced with cMEM for plasmid expression over 24 h. Once expressed, scFv5T4::mRFP1 (1:100; 2 mg/ml) was incubated with the cells for 1 h at RT and subsequently washed and viewed with fluorescence microscopy using an Olympus IX71 fluorescent microscope. Alternatively, transfected HEK293 cells (as above) or HT-29 cells (1.0×10^6) were incubated for 1 h with mAb5T4 (1:200) or scFv5T4-biotin (1:100; 2 mg/ml), followed by anti-mouse IgG-FITC (1:1000) or streptavidin-FITC (1:1000), respectively, for 1 h at 4°C and viewed with fluorescence microscopy or FACS (BD FACSCanto II), respectively. Microscopy images were taken using ImagePro Plus Software, and FACS analysis was completed using Flowjo Software.

Proliferation assays

Human peripheral blood mononuclear cells (PBMCs) were prepared from the whole blood of healthy donors and isolated by density centrifugation over Ficoll-Paque Plus (GE Healthcare Life Sciences). Human lymphocytes were cultured in RPMI-1640 (Gibco) with 10% FBS and supplemented as above (cRPMI). All tissue culture cells were maintained at 37°C with 5% CO_2. Human PBMCs were labeled with CellTrace CFSE (Molecular Probes) as per manufacturer's instructions. Cells (0.8×10^6– 1.0×10^6) were cultured in cRPMI containing 2 μg/ml Polymyxin B (ICN Biomedicals Inc.) and treated with either wild-type SpeC (SpeC$_{WT}$) or variants SpeC$_{Y15A}$, SpeC$_{D203A}$ or SpeC$_{Y15A/D203A}$ (1 μg/ml) and incubated for 5 days at 37°C with 5% CO_2. Cells were then washed and stained with anti-human CD3 (1:200), anti-human CD4 (1:200) and anti-human CD8 (1:200) antibodies for 30 min on ice and analyzed by FACS (BD Canto II), using FlowJo software. For radioactive proliferation assays, human PBMCs (2.0×10^5) were cultured in cRPMI containing 2 μg/ml Polymyxin B (ICN Biomedicals Inc.) with titrating SpeC variants, scFv5T4, scFv5T4::SpeC$_{D203A}$ or scFv5T4::SpeC$_{Y15A/D203A}$ in U-bottom 96-well microtitre plates (BD Biosciences). Cells were incubated for 72 h and subsequently labeled with ^{3}H-thymidine (Perkin Elmer Inc.) for 18 h at 37°C with 5% CO_2. Cells were harvested onto glass-fibre filters and DNA-incorporated ^{3}H-thymidine was measured in a beta scintillation counter (Wallac 1450 Microbeta Counter).

Cytotoxicity assays

Two assays were used to measure the ability of the various proteins to induce PBMC-mediated killing of cancer cells. First, *in vitro* killing was evaluated by co-culturing human PBMCs with either WiDr cells or HT-29 at a ratio of 10:1 and titrating SAgs including SpeC$_{WT}$, SpeC$_{Y15A}$, SpeC$_{D203A}$, or SpeC$_{Y15A/D203A}$ for 48 h. Cells were labeled with 7-AAD following the manufacturer's protocol and analyzed by FACS (BD Canto II). Using FlowJo software, the WiDr or HT-29 populations were gated upon by comparison of human PBMC alone samples and subsequently assessed for presence or absence of 7-AAD. Second, human PBMCs were treated with SAg, scFv5T4 or fusion proteins as in the FACS assay for 48 h in a U-bottom microtitre plate (BD Biosciences). Target HT-29 cells were labeled with $(Na)_2{}^{51}CrO_4$ (Perkin Elmer Inc.) in cRPMI. PBMCs were added at effector:-target cell ratios of either 1:1, 5:1 or 10:1 against HT-29. Cytotoxicity was measured after 4–6 h incubation at 37°C with 5% CO_2 in a standard chromium release assay measuring the ^{51}Cr content of culture supernatants using a gamma-counter (Wallac Wizard 1470 Automatic Counter). Total release control was obtained by exposing target cells to 1% sodium dodecyl sulfate (EMD Millipore). The specific lysis was calculated according to the formula:

$$\% \text{ specific lysis} = \frac{\text{experimental release} - \text{spontaneous release}}{\text{total release} - \text{spontaneous release}} x100$$

Evaluation of tumor burden and metastases

Immunodeficient NOD.Cg-Prkdc^{scid} Il2rgt^{m1Wjl}/SzJ (NSG) mice were bred in an animal barrier facility, and housed under sterile conditions with food and water ad libitum. Based on a previously developed protocol [18,40], 13-week old mice were injected intraperitoneally with 3×10^6 HT-29 cells in 0.2 mL vehicle (PBS). Three weeks later, after tumors were palpable, the mice were injected intraperitoneally with either vehicle alone (n = 3) or 1×10^6 human PBMCs in 0.2 mL vehicle (n = 20). PBMC-treated mice were grouped (n = 4) with a random number generator to receive either scFv5T4::SpeC$_{D203A}$, or controls SpeC$_{D203A}$, scFv5T4, scFv5T4::SpeC$_{Y15A/D203A}$, or vehicle alone. Two hours after receiving PBMCs, 2 μM/kg of treatment, controls, or vehicle alone was injected intravenously. Mice with no PBMCs received vehicle alone. Intravenous treatment injections were given daily for 7 additional days. After 4 weeks, the mice were sacrificed and the total tumor volume was determined. The mice were also examined visually for macro-metastases and scored accordingly based on the degree of regional spread distant from the primary tumor site. All tumors were excised, size- and weight-measured in a blinded fashion.

Statistical analysis

Statistical comparisons were performed using an unpaired Student t test or by 2-way ANOVA with Bonferroni multiple comparison test (GraphPad Prism). Differences were considered significant when $p < 0.05$.

Results

Generation of a SpeC-based TTS

SpeC is a potent and well-characterized streptococcal SAg known to target primarily Vβ2$^+$ human T cells [32] which

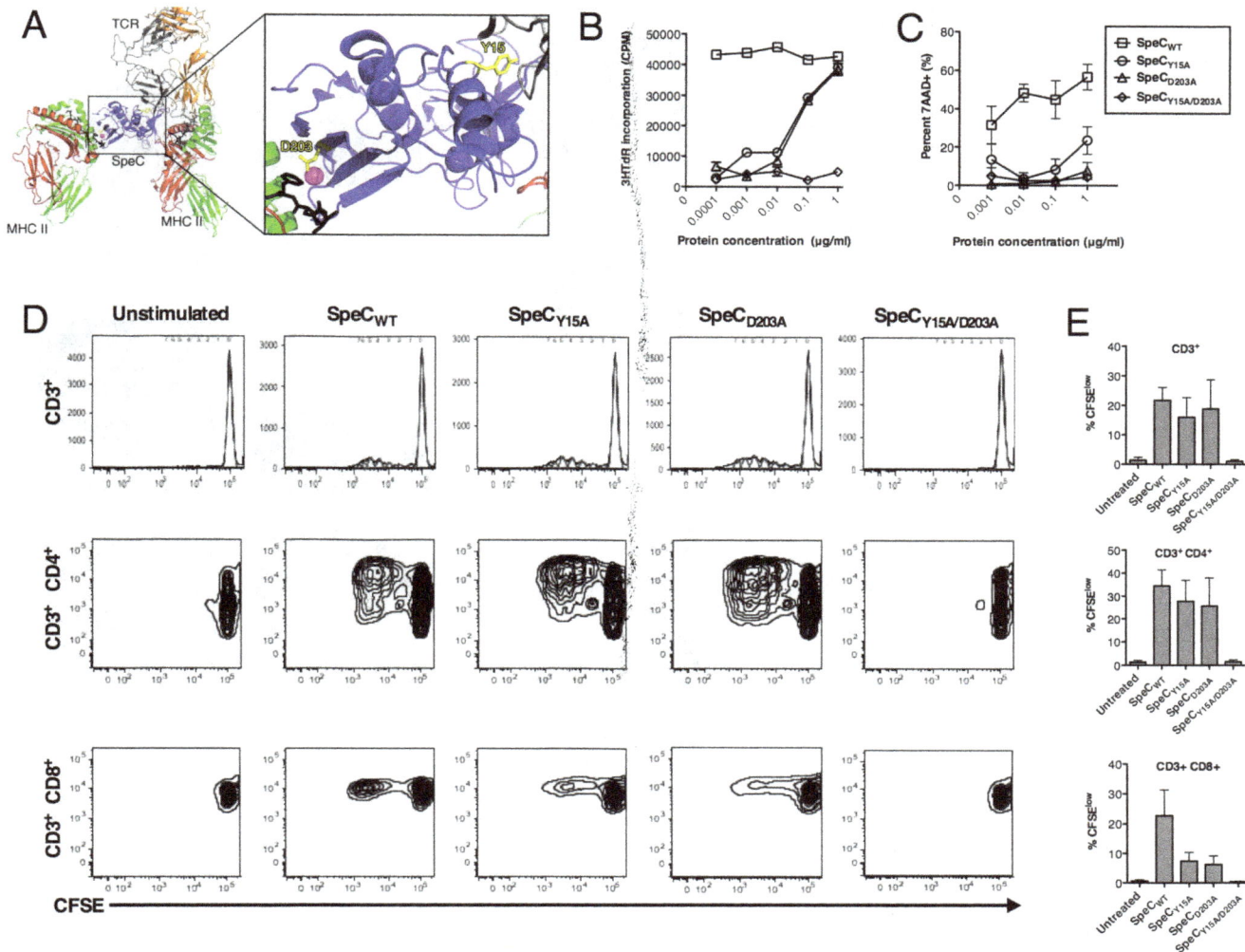

Figure 1. Overview of the SpeC-mediated T cell activation complex and mutations to reduce systemic toxicity. A) Structural overview of SpeC in complex with TCR and MHC-II. TCR Vα chain is colored orange, TCR Vβ chain is colored grey, MHCα-chains are colored red, MHCβ-chains are colored green, antigenic peptides are colored black, and the zinc atom is colored magenta. SpeC is colored blue with important interface residues Y15 and D203 highlighted in yellow. The ternary model of TCR-SpeC-(MHC)$_2$ was produced as described previously [9] and the ribbon diagram was generated using PyMOL (http://www.pymol.org). B) Proliferation of human PBMCs mediated by $SpeC_{WT}$ or proteins containing mutated residues Y15A (TCR-binding mutant), D203A (MHC-II-binding mutant) or Y15A/D203A was determined by the uptake of ^{3}H-thymidine after 72 h post-stimulation (n = 5 in triplicate; data representative of one individual). C) Dose-dependent cytotoxicity of 7-AAD$^+$ WiDr cells after 48 h incubation with human PBMCs and either $SpeC_{WT}$, $SpeC_{Y15A}$, $SpeC_{D203A}$, or $SpeC_{Y15A/D203A}$ (n = 3–6 per group). (D–E) Proliferation of CFSE labeled-human PBMCs mediated by $SpeC_{WT}$ or proteins containing mutated residues was determined by FACS five days post-stimulation, specifically measuring total CD3$^+$ T cell population, CD3$^+$CD4$^+$ T cells and, CD3$^+$CD8$^+$ T cells (n = 4; FACS data representative of one individual).

represent ~7% of the approximately 25 million distinct TCRs [41]. Prior work indicates that Tyr[15] is a critical residue for this SAg to engage the TCR [34], and Asp[203] is necessary to co-ordinate a zinc-mediated high-affinity interface with the β-chain of MHC-II [4,35,42] (**Figure 1A**). Indeed, the single Asp[203]→Ala mutation in SpeC has been demonstrated to dramatically reduce toxicity in a lethal model of toxic shock syndrome [42]. We first evaluated the ability of wild-type SpeC ($SpeC_{WT}$), $SpeC_{Y15A}$, $SpeC_{D203A}$, and $SpeC_{Y15A/D203A}$ to activate human PBMCs and induce PBMC-mediated killing of cancer cells. Both $SpeC_{Y15A}$ and $SpeC_{D203A}$ were impaired for the ability to expand PBMCS by ~100-fold compared with $SpeC_{WT}$, and the $SpeC_{Y15A/D203A}$ double mutant was unable to induce PBMC proliferation (**Figure 1B**). Next, PBMC-dependent killing of the human

colorectal cancer cell line WiDr was evaluated. $SpeC_{Y15A}$ caused a significant reduction in WiDr cytotoxicity compared with $SpeC_{WT}$, and both the $SpeC_{D203A}$ and $SpeC_{Y15A/D203A}$ mutants failed to induce WiDr cytotoxicity (**Figure 1C**). We also assessed the ability of the recombinant proteins to specifically induce proliferation of human CD3$^+$CD4$^+$ and CD3$^+$CD8$^+$ T cell populations at 1 µg/ml. $SpeC_{WT}$ and each of the single mutants were able to induce proliferation of both subsets, while the double mutant failed to induce proliferation of either subset (**Figure 1D and 1E**). These data indicate that TCR and MHC-II engagement are important for induction of immune cell-mediated killing by $SpeC_{WT}$, and that $SpeC_{D203A}$ may be a suitable mutant to reduce or prevent systemic immune cell activation while maintaining full engagement with the TCR.

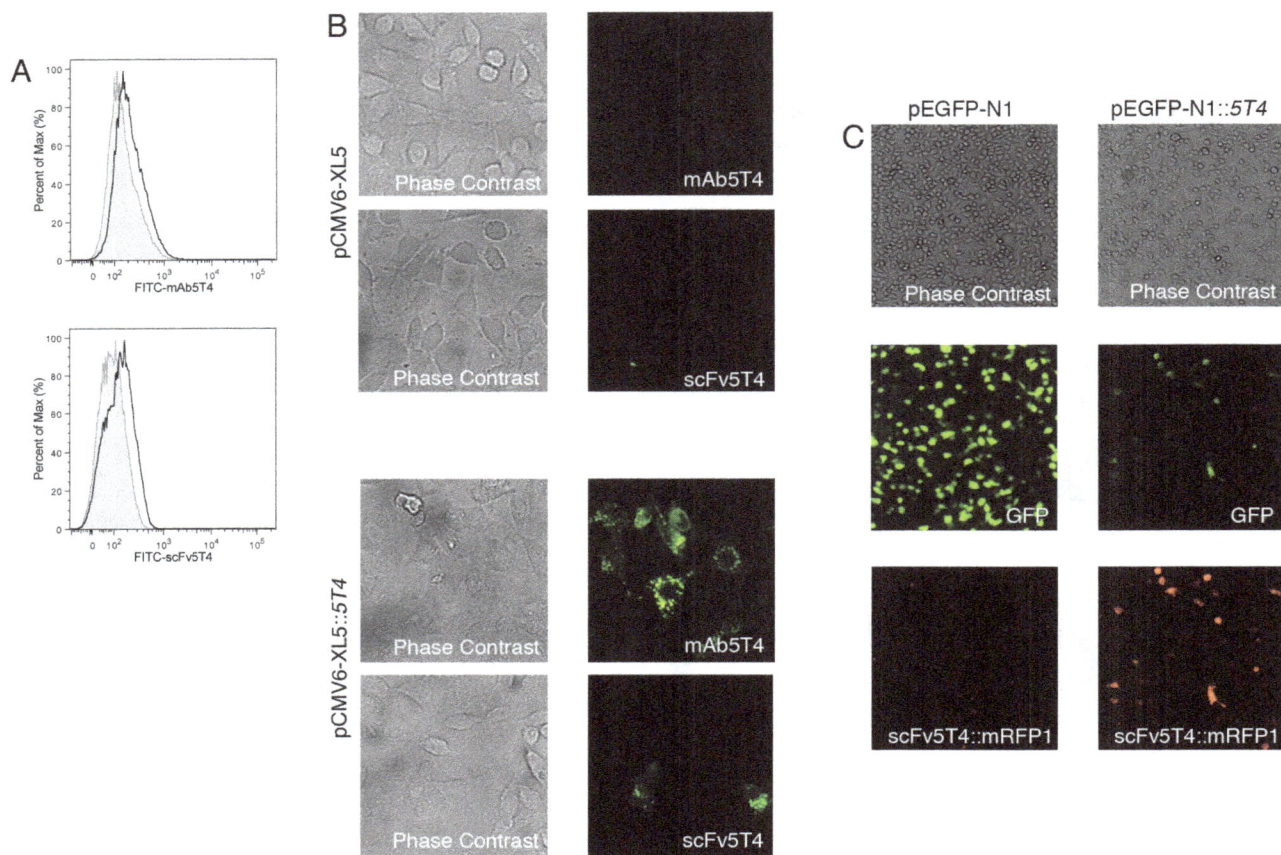

Figure 2. Specific targeting of scFv5T4. A) Histograms demonstrating surface binding of the indicated antibodies, either commercial mAb5T4 or generated scFv5T4 (empty curves), to 5T4 TAA on colorectal cancer cell line HT-29 measured by FACS. The shaded curves show the IgG2b isotype control (top panel) or streptavidin-FITC alone (bottom panel). B) Visualization of commercial mAb5T4, or scFv5T4, targeting of HEK293 cells transfected with empty vector (pCMV6-XL5) or pCMV6-XL5::5T4 by fluorescence microscopy. Representative images taken at 400× magnification. C) Visualization of HEK293 transfected with pEGFP-N1 or pEGFP-N1::5T4 and incubated with scFv5T4::mRFP1. Same field of view photographs were taken under phase contrast, and green and red fluorescent filters at 100× magnification.

Engineered human scFv5T4 specifically targets the 5T4 tumor-associated antigen

In order to develop a specific targeting mechanism for $SpeC_{D203A}$, we generated a humanized scFv based on the complementarity determining regions (CDRs) of the characterized mouse scFv specific for the human 5T4 TAA [37]. The cDNA sequence was designed to incorporate a 'humanized' backbone sequence, with the CDRs remaining specific for human 5T4. Amino acid substitutions were determined by aligning the previously described mouse scFv5T4 with 10 human scFv sequences generating a consensus sequence. This cDNA sequence was codon optimized for *E. coli* and synthesized, and was subsequently used for the generation of a number of recombinant proteins (**Table S1**).

To first examine the specificity of the humanized scFv5T4 for binding to human 5T4, the scFv5T4 cDNA was engineered to contain a C-terminal biotin tag, or genetically fused to monomeric red fluorescent protein 1 (mRFP1) [43]. Upon incubation with the human HT-29 colorectal cancer cells known to express 5T4 [44], from which WiDr cells are derived [45], scFv5T4 bound to the surface of these cells comparably to commercial anti-human 5T4 mAb (**Figure 2A**). HEK293 cells engineered to express the 5T4 antigen bound both the mAb5T4 as well as the scFv5T4 fragment as shown by immunofluorescence microscopy, whereas control

HEK293 cells that contain only the vector did not stain with either antibody (**Figure 2B**). scFv5T4 specificity for 5T4 was also determined by incubation of scFv5T4::mRFP1 with HEK293 cells transfected with pEGFP-N1::5T4, or control vector pEGFP-N1. Microscopic analysis of GFP::5T4-expressing HEK293 cells demonstrated that scFv5T4 bound only to those cells expressing the 5T4::GFP fusion, but not to control transfected cells (**Figure 2C**). Together, these data indicate that the humanized scFv5T4 can bind specifically to human 5T4.

Generation of scFv5T4::SpeC$_{D203A}$

In order to target SpeC to 5T4, SpeC was translationally fused to scFv5T4 and recombinant scFv5T4::SpeC$_{D203A}$ was expressed from *E. coli* BL21(DE3) and purified (**Figure 3**). In addition, control reagents were generated including scFv5T4 alone, and a non-functional fusion protein containing SpeC$_{Y15A/D203A}$, each as soluble proteins containing C-terminal biotin tags (**Figure 3**).

Human T-cell proliferation and cytotoxicity induced by scFv5T4::SpeC$_{D203A}$

We first tested scFv5T4::SpeC$_{D203A}$ and the control proteins for the ability to proliferate induced human PBMCs. scFv5T4::SpeC$_{D203A}$ induced a dose-dependent proliferative

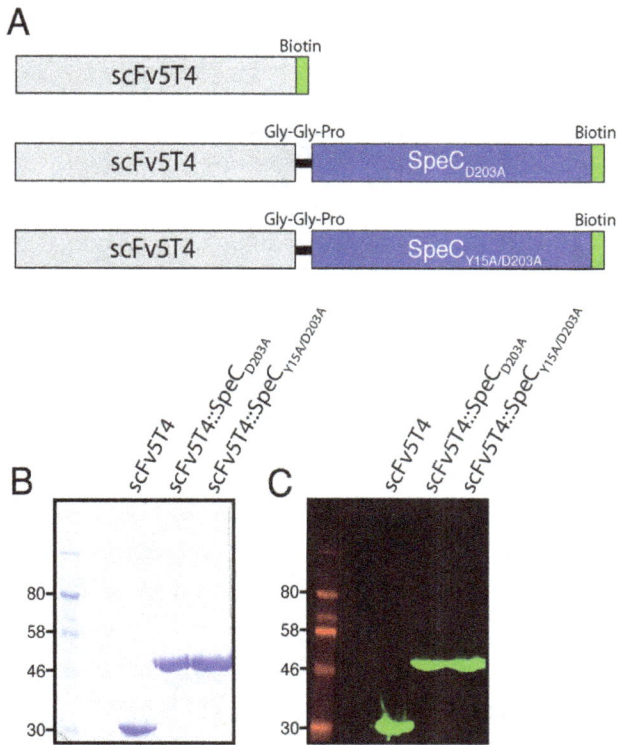

Figure 3. Generation of the scFv5T4::SpeC$_{D203A}$ fusion protein and control reagents. A) Schematic illustration representing the components of the generated fusion protein constructs. The protein consists of the generated 5T4-targeted humanized single chain variable fragments, V$_H$ and V$_L$ (grey bar), genetically fused to streptococcal superantigen SpeC (blue bar) either containing an alanine substitution at residue D203 or an additional alanine substitution at residue Y15. All constructs were generated to contain a C-terminal biotin tag. The purified recombinant proteins are shown by SDS-PAGE (panel B), and detected by Western blot analysis by streptavidin-IRDye800 (panel C).

response of human lymphocytes that was comparable to SpeC$_{D203A}$ (**Figure 4A**). Importantly, the scFv5T4 antibody fragment alone and the double mutant fusion (scFv5T4::SpeC$_{Y15A/D203A}$) did not induce significant proliferative responses. This indicates that the SpeC$_{D203A}$ portion of the fusion is responsible for inducing PBMC activation. The immunotherapeutic agent was then evaluated for the ability to mediate tumor cell killing by human SpeC-reactive PBMCs in two assays. First, the human colorectal cancer cell line WiDr was used as the target in a 7-AAD-based killing assay. Efficient cell killing was observed after human PBMCs were stimulated with 200 nM of the agent for 48 hours, compared to wild-type SpeC and unstimulated controls (**Figure 4B**). Second, HT-29 cells labeled with ^{51}Cr were used as targets. Efficient cell killing was observed in a dose-dependent manner after human PBMCs were stimulated with the agent for 48 hours, and subsequently added to tumor cells with increasing effector to target (E:T) ratios (**Figure 4C**). Furthermore, the single mutant fusion (scFv5T4::SpeC$_{D203A}$) was more efficient than that of the similar double mutant fusion (scFv5T4::SpeC$_{Y15A/D203A}$) or antibody alone, but was reduced when compared with SpeC$_{WT}$. These data indicate that scFv5T4::SpeC$_{D203A}$ is functional for inducing immune cell-mediated cancer cell death and that SpeC$_{D203A}$, scFv5T4, and scFv5T4::SpeC$_{Y15A/D203A}$ proteins can function as precise controls to evaluate the requirement for targeting and SAg activity *in vivo*.

Immunotherapy of established colon cancer using scFv5T4::SpeC$_{D203A}$

SpeC is specific for human Vβ2$^+$ T cells, but this SAg does not recognize mouse T cells [32]. Thus, testing the SpeC-based TTS required a model utilizing human lymphocytes. Furthermore, the human 5T4 targeting scFv has minimal cross-reactivity with murine 5T4 [37]. Therefore, human tumor cells expressing human 5T4 were necessary for the experiments. Based on a previously developed model [18,40], we employed immunodeficient NOD SCID IL2Rγ$^{-/-}$ (NSG) mice for the engraftment of 5T4$^+$ human HT-29 colorectal adenocarcinoma cells. NSG mice lack T, B and NK cells [46] and represent an optimum mouse strain for human tumor engraftment [47]. Furthermore, these mice permit the survival of transferred human immune cells [46,48]. HT-29 cells were injected intraperitoneally into NSG mice and once solid tumors were palpable (at 3 weeks post-injection), treatments were initiated with intraperitoneal injection of human PBMCs, followed by 8 daily intravenous injections of scFv5T4::SpeC$_{D203A}$ (**Figure 5A**). Control NSG mice did not receive PBMCs, or received PBMCs without additional treatments. Additional groups included the scFv5T4 alone, SpeC$_{D203A}$ alone, or inactive scFv5T4::SpeC$_{Y15A/D203A}$. Tumor surface area was monitored using caliper measurement throughout the experiment and demonstrated little to no growth of the tumors in the scFv5T4::SpeC$_{D203A}$ treatment group, while growth was observed in all other groups (**Figure 5B**). Mice were sacrificed at week 8 of the experiment and tumors were evaluated in a blinded fashion. This experiment demonstrated a dramatic reduction in the total tumor volume after treatment with scFv5T4::SpeC$_{D203A}$ that was significantly different from mice that did not received PBMCs, sham treated mice (saline), and mice treated SpeC$_{D203A}$ or scFv5T4::SpeC$_{Y15A/D203A}$ (**Figure 5C**). Importantly, the scFv5T4::SpeC$_{D203A}$ treatment group also demonstrated a significant reduction in the total metastases score compared with all other groups (**Figure 5D and 5E**). There were no differences in tumor volumes or number of metastases between mice that did not receive PBMCs and the different control reagents (**Figure 5D**).

Discussion

T lymphocytes are recognized as one of the most important immune cells involved in tumor regression in cancer immunotherapy, and bacterial SAgs are among the most potent naturally occurring specific activators of T cells. Thus, the appropriation of SAgs to target cancer cells [17] has received significant attention, and TTS therapeutics have now been evaluated in human clinical trials [22–24,26,49,50].

In the current study, we describe the development of a "next generation" TTS composed of the streptococcal T cell activating toxin SpeC and a humanized scFv targeting the 5T4 TAA. In this work, we focused on colorectal cancer as this carcinoma is difficult to diagnose with few symptoms until the onset of stage III or IV, and ~20% of patients will present with inoperable colorectal cancer [51]. The expression of the 5T4 TAA is restricted on normal adult tissues but is found on an array of carcinomas [52] and has been associated with metastasis in colorectal cancer [53]. This work provides further preclinical evidence for 5T4 as a potential TAA for targeted colorectal cancer immunotherapy, and that TTSs may be useful to inhibit or prevent further metastatic disease. As monoclonal antibodies that target vascular endothelial growth factor (VEGF) (e.g. Bevacizumab) and epidermal growth factor receptor (EGFR) (e.g. Cetuximab or Panitumumab) have shown benefit in patients with metastatic colorectal cancer [54–

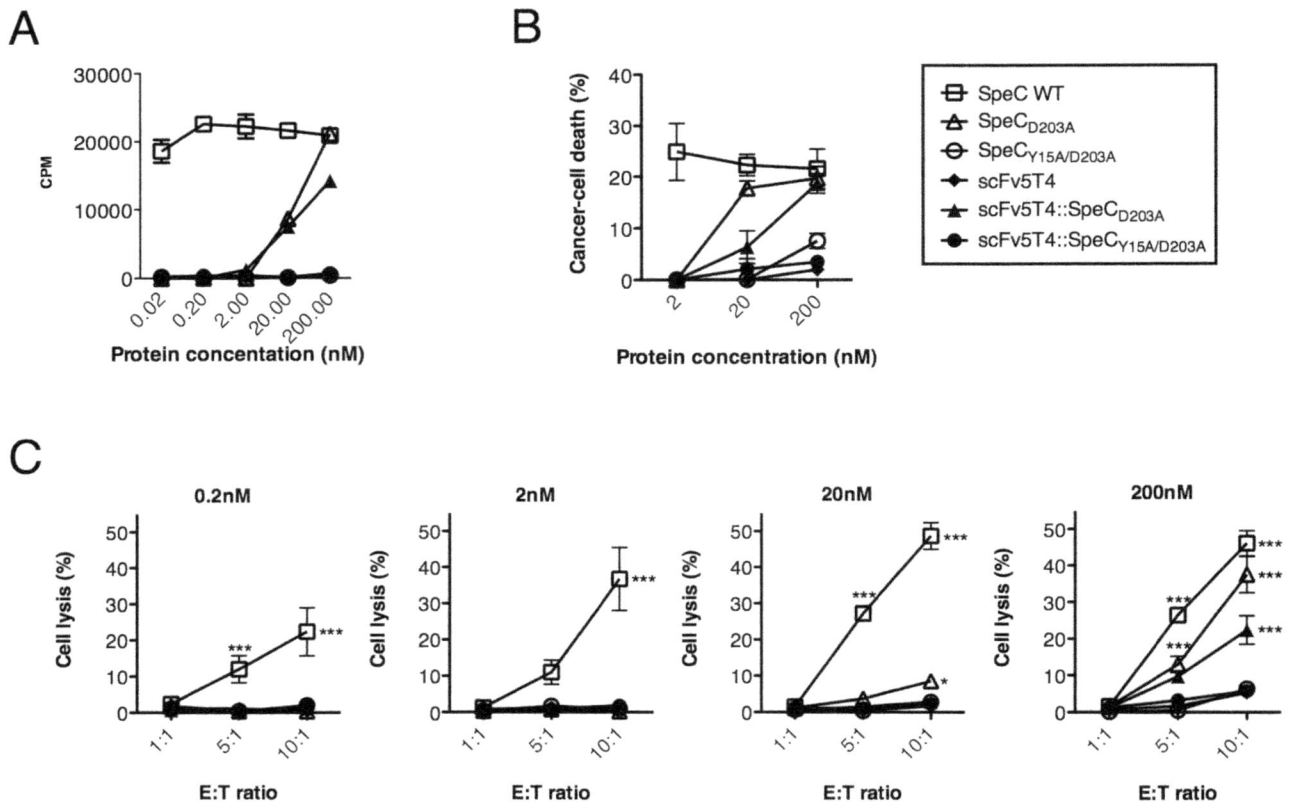

Figure 4. Functionality of SpeC mutants and fusion proteins for human PBMC proliferation and cytotoxicity *in vitro*. A) SpeC proteins were used to compare scFv5T4 alone, scFv5T4::SpeC$_{Y15A/D203A}$ and subsequently scFv5T4::SpeC$_{D203A}$ in the uptake of ^{3}H-thymidine as a measure of PBMC proliferation after 4 day incubation (n = 5). B–C) Dose-dependent SpeC-mediated PBMC cytotoxicity of scFv5T4::SpeC$_{D203A}$ was determined by comparing SpeC controls, scFv5T4 alone and scFv5T4::SpeC$_{Y15A/D203A}$ after 48 h incubation by using FACS analysis of WiDr (panel B), measuring percent cancer cell death with 7AAD-exclusion staining (n = 3) and ^{51}Cr-release to measure the specific cytotoxic potential (panel C) when incubated with increasing effector:target ratios and ^{51}Cr-labeled HT-29 cancer cells. Data shown (mean ±SEM) is from four independent human donors each done in triplicate. *p<0.05, ***p<0.001, compared to the inactive SpeC$_{Y15A/D203A}$ control protein.

56], a future area of interest would be to evaluate TTS combination therapies with these more established treatments.

This work demonstrated that the soluble recombinant fusion protein scFv5T4::SpeC$_{D203A}$ was able to specifically target 5T4 to elicit a T cell response that substantially reduced tumor burden *in vivo*. Importantly, we used a model of large and established tumors in order to robustly test the SpeC-based TTS. Although the tumors did not appear to regress, the data clearly demonstrates that scFv5T4::SpeC$_{D203A}$ was able to prevent further tumor growth as well as the development of peritoneal metastases. As scFv5T4::SpeC$_{D203A}$ and SpeC$_{D203A}$ showed similar activity *in vitro* (**Figure 4a**), the inability of SpeC$_{D203A}$ to impact tumor size or metastatic disease indicates that the scFv5T4 moiety of the fusion protein was required for *in vivo* targeting of 5T4$^+$ HT-29 cells (**Figures 2A, 5C and 5D**). Likewise, the inability of scFv5T4 alone, or the inactive scFv5T4::SpeC$_{Y15A/D203A}$ fusion to show any measurable impact (**Figure 5C and 5D**) demonstrates that T cell-dependent SAg activity was also required for tumor cell killing. Although the SpeC$_{D203A}$ mutant was designed to reduce systemic T cell activation, the mouse Fab moiety in the 5T4Fab-SEA/E-120 TTS has been shown to effectively replace the MHC-II binding domain such that T cells are efficiently activated when artificially 'presented' by the tumor [57]. We suspect that the humanized scFv5T4 moiety here played a similar role contributing to the dramatic reduction in tumor volume and metastatic disease.

There are some potential advantages, and disadvantages, in using TTSs for tumor immunotherapy that require further consideration. The use of a mouse derived antibody as a targeting motif may result in human anti-mouse antibody (HAMA) responses since murine mAbs are highly immunogenic [58]. This may limit the utility of subsequent treatments and thus the use of a humanized scFv containing TTS as developed in this work may provide clinical benefit. Second, bacterial SAgs are produced by bacteria that are often frequent colonizers in humans and thus many individuals will have pre-existing and neutralizing antibodies to many streptococcal and staphylococcal SAgs [59,60]. To overcome this issue, we foresee the future generation of 'combinatorial' TTSs with different SAgs such that individual patients could be screened for SAg neutralizing antibodies and then treated with an appropriate TTS. Early work in this area demonstrated that multiple SEs are capable of inducing T cell-mediated cytotoxicity against cancer cells [61]; however, we envision the SAg panel would include members from the Group IV and Group V subclass of SAgs [1,39,62], as these subclasses contain only streptococcal SAgs and staphylococcal enterotoxin-like (SEl) SAgs, that collectively lack the emetic properties of the bona fide SEs [62]. Indeed, the SEl-M, SEl-N and SEl-O SAgs from the staphylococcal 'enterotoxin gene cluster' (*egc*) have recently been demonstrated to induce T cell dependent killing of a broad panel of human tumor cells *in vitro* [63]. Also, human

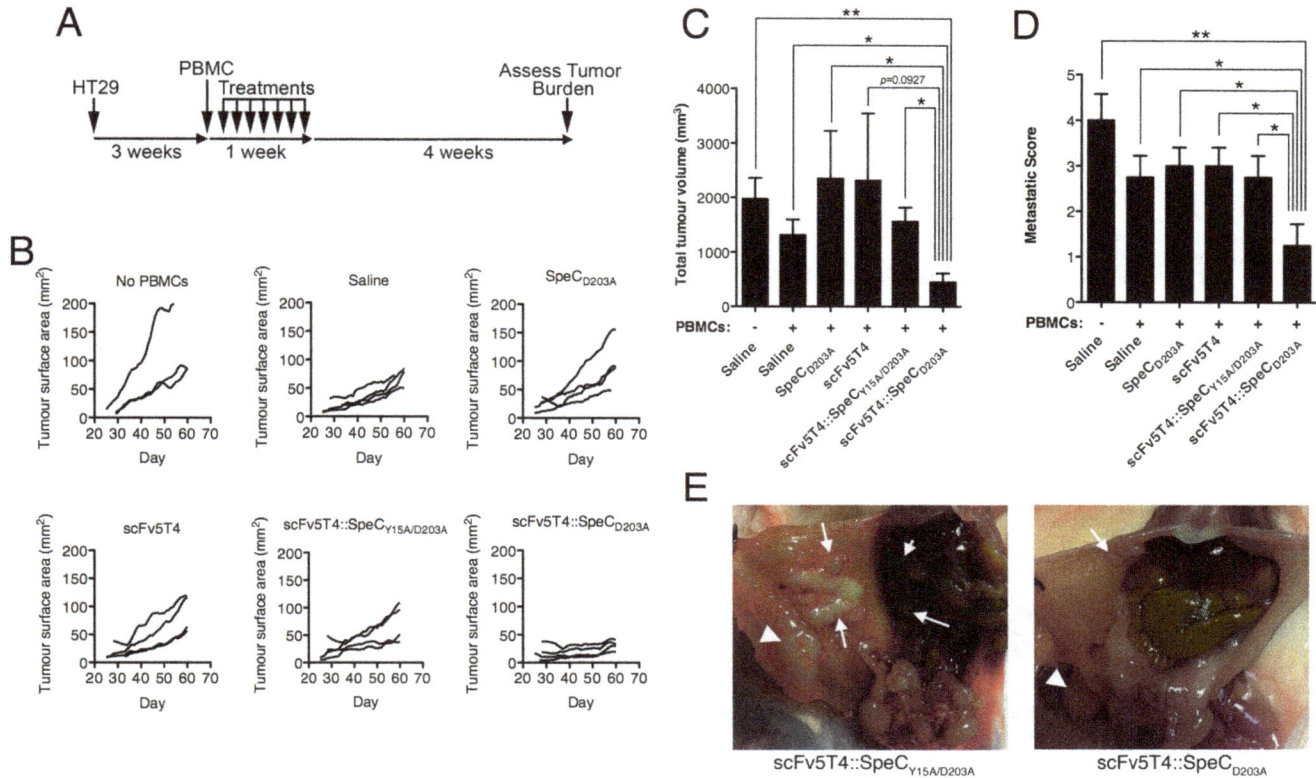

Figure 5. SpeC-based TTS therapy of established HT-29 colon cancer. A) Schematic illustration of the xenograft solid tumor model experimental timeline. NSG mice with established (3 week) intraperitoneal human HT-29 tumors were injected once with human PBMC intraperitoneally, followed by 8 daily intravenous injections of scFv5T4::SpeC$_{D203A}$, or individual controls (2 µM/kg/injection). B) Primary tumor size was evaluated throughout the experimental timeline by external caliper measurements. Twenty-eight days post-final injection, final tumor volume was measured (panel C) and metastatic score (panel D) evaluated. All groups contained n = 4, with exception of saline alone control (n = 3). *p<0.05, **p<0.005. Gross pathology and metastases in representative NSG mice with HT-29 tumors treated with scFv5T4::SpeC$_{Y15A/D203A}$ or scFv5T4::SpeC$_{D203A}$. The primary tumor is labeled with a triangle and metastases are labeled with arrows.

serum levels of neutralizing antibodies against the *egc* SEs have been shown to be lower than those directed against the 'classic' SEs [64]. In addition, each of the Group IV and V SAgs have a well defined zinc-binding motif [1] involved in high-affinity MHC-II binding [4,5] that can be targeted for appropriate mutagenesis to prevent systemic immune activation as shown here and previously for SEA [65]. A third important limitation to TTS immunotherapy is that bacterial SAgs are well known to induce Vβ-specific T cell deletion or anergy [66], which includes CD8$^+$ T cells [67]. Thus, repeated administration of the same TTS in humans may result in populations of non-responsive T cells. However, using the B16 model of melanoma, a sufficient resting period between treatments did restore immune responsiveness resulting in prolonged survival with repeated cycles of therapy [68]. Nevertheless, this limitation could potentially be circumvented by the use of multiple SAgs with different Vβ profiles. A remaining and important issue with TTS immunotherapy is the targeting of a single TAA. An effective TTS would likely invoke a form of cancer immunoediting [69], and simple down regulation of the TAA may provide a means of escape. The TTS immunotherapy platform offers an approach for targeting a number of different TAAs, and it will be of future interest to engineer and combine TTSs that utilize SAgs with different Vβ profiles.

Immunotherapies such as the chimeric antigen receptors (CARs) targeting CD19 have now demonstrated some extraordinary clinical outcomes in patients with advanced B cell leukemia [70–73]. In addition, blocking immune system regulatory checkpoints with antibodies (e.g. anti-CTLA-4 or anti-PD-1) is providing additional avenues for cancer immunotherapy [74]. TTSs may represent a additional 'off-the-shelf' therapy to harness Vβ-specific T cell subsets without the requirement for manipulation of autologous T cells. This work may help to guide the 'next generation' of TTSs for tailored cancer immunotherapy.

Acknowledgments

This work is dedicated to the memory of Alison Look (nee Poon) (1969–2005). We thank members of the McCormick laboratory for helpful discussions and assistance, and Dr. Roger Tsein (University of California, San Diego) for providing the initial mRFP1 gene.

Author Contributions

Conceived and designed the experiments: KGP JLDP PSB SMMH JKM. Performed the experiments: KGP JLDP PSB. Analyzed the data: KGP JKM. Contributed reagents/materials/analysis tools: DAH SMMH. Wrote the paper: KGP JKM.

References

1. McCormick JK, Yarwood JM, Schlievert PM (2001) Toxic shock syndrome and bacterial superantigens: an update. Annu Rev Microbiol 55: 77–104.
2. Jardetzky TS, Brown JH, Gorga JC, Stern LJ, Urban RG, et al. (1994) Three-dimensional structure of a human class II histocompatibility molecule complexed with superantigen. Nature 368: 711–718.
3. Kim J, Urban RG, Strominger JL, Wiley DC (1994) Toxic shock syndrome toxin-1 complexed with a class II major histocompatibility molecule HLA-DR1. Science 266: 1870–1874.
4. Li Y, Li H, Dimasi N, McCormick JK, Martin R, et al. (2001) Crystal structure of a superantigen bound to the high-affinity, zinc-dependent site on MHC class II. Immunity 14: 93–104.
5. Petersson K, Hakansson M, Nilsson H, Forsberg G, Svensson LA, et al. (2001) Crystal structure of a superantigen bound to MHC class II displays zinc and peptide dependence. EMBO J 20: 3306–3312.
6. Fields BA, Malchiodi EL, Li H, Ysern X, Stauffacher CV, et al. (1996) Crystal structure of a T-cell receptor beta-chain complexed with a superantigen. Nature 384: 188–192.
7. Li H, Llera A, Tsuchiya D, Leder L, Ysern X, et al. (1998) Three-dimensional structure of the complex between a T cell receptor beta chain and the superantigen staphylococcal enterotoxin B. Immunity 9: 807–816.
8. Andersen PS, Schuck P, Sundberg EJ, Geisler C, Karjalainen K, et al. (2002) Quantifying the energetics of cooperativity in a ternary protein complex. Biochemistry 41: 5177–5184.
9. Nur-ur Rahman AK, Bonsor DA, Herfst CA, Pollard F, Peirce M, et al. (2011) The T cell receptor beta-chain second complementarity determining region loop (CDR2beta) governs T cell activation and Vbeta specificity by bacterial superantigens. J Biol Chem 286: 4871–4881.
10. Arden B, Clark SP, Kabelitz D, Mak TW (1995) Human T-cell receptor variable gene segment families. Immunogenetics 42: 455–500.
11. Wei S, Charmley P, Robinson MA, Concannon P (1994) The extent of the human germline T-cell receptor V beta gene segment repertoire. Immunogenetics 40: 27–36.
12. Fleischer B, Necker A, Leget C, Malissen B, Romagne F (1996) Reactivity of mouse T-cell hybridomas expressing human Vbeta gene segments with staphylococcal and streptococcal superantigens. Infect Immun 64: 987–994.
13. Herrmann T, Baschieri S, Lees RK, MacDonald HR (1992) In vivo responses of CD4+ and CD8+ cells to bacterial superantigens. Eur J Immunol 22: 1935–1938.
14. Ami K, Ohkawa T, Koike Y, Sato K, Habu Y, et al. (2002) Activation of human T cells with NK cell markers by staphylococcal enterotoxin A via IL-12 but not via IL-18. Clin Exp Immunol 128: 453–459.
15. Hayworth JL, Mazzuca DM, Maleki Vareki S, Welch I, McCormick JK, et al. (2012) CD1d-independent activation of mouse and human iNKT cells by bacterial superantigens. Immunol Cell Biol 90: 699–709.
16. Morita CT, Li H, Lamphear JG, Rich RR, Fraser JD, et al. (2001) Superantigen recognition by gammadelta T cells: SEA recognition site for human Vgamma2 T cell receptors. Immunity 14: 331–344.
17. Dohlsten M, Abrahmsen L, Bjork P, Lando PA, Hedlund G, et al. (1994) Monoclonal antibody-superantigen fusion proteins: tumor-specific agents for T-cell-based tumor therapy. Proc Natl Acad Sci U S A 91: 8945–8949.
18. Forsberg G, Ohlsson L, Brodin T, Bjork P, Lando PA, et al. (2001) Therapy of human non-small-cell lung carcinoma using antibody targeting of a modified superantigen. Br J Cancer 85: 129–136.
19. Sundstedt A, Celander M, Hedlund G (2008) Combining tumor-targeted superantigens with interferon-alpha results in synergistic anti-tumor effects. Int Immunopharmacol 8: 442–452.
20. Sundstedt A, Celander M, Eriksson H, Torngren M, Hedlund G (2012) Monotherapeutically nonactive CTLA-4 blockade results in greatly enhanced antitumor effects when combined with tumor-targeted superantigens in a B16 melanoma model. J Immunother 35: 344–353.
21. Dinges MM, Orwin PM, Schlievert PM (2000) Exotoxins of *Staphylococcus aureus*. Clin Microbiol Rev 13: 16–34.
22. Nielsen SE, Zeuthen J, Lund B, Persson B, Alenfall J, et al. (2000) Phase I study of single, escalating doses of a superantigen-antibody fusion protein (PNU-214565) in patients with advanced colorectal or pancreatic carcinoma. J Immunother 23: 146–153.
23. Shaw DM, Connolly NB, Patel PM, Kilany S, Hedlund G, et al. (2007) A phase II study of a 5T4 oncofoetal antigen tumour-targeted superantigen (ABR-214936) therapy in patients with advanced renal cell carcinoma. Br J Cancer 96: 567–574.
24. Borghaei H, Alpaugh K, Hedlund G, Forsberg G, Langer C, et al. (2009) Phase I dose escalation, pharmacokinetic and pharmacodynamic study of naptumomab estafenatox alone in patients with advanced cancer and with docetaxel in patients with advanced non-small-cell lung cancer. J Clin Oncol 27: 4116–4123.
25. Hu DL, Zhu G, Mori F, Omoe K, Okada M, et al. (2007) Staphylococcal enterotoxin induces emesis through increasing serotonin release in intestine and it is downregulated by cannabinoid receptor 1. Cell Microbiol 9: 2267–2277.
26. Cheng JD, Babb JS, Langer C, Aamdal S, Robert F, et al. (2004) Individualized patient dosing in phase I clinical trials: the role of escalation with overdose control in PNU-214936. J Clin Oncol 22: 602–609.
27. Erlandsson E, Andersson K, Cavallin A, Nilsson A, Larsson-Lorek U, et al. (2003) Identification of the antigenic epitopes in staphylococcal enterotoxins A and E and design of a superantigen for human cancer therapy. J Mol Biol 333: 893–905.
28. Eisen T, Hedlund G, Forsberg G, Hawkins R (2014) Naptumomab estafenatox: targeted immunotherapy with a novel immunotoxin. Curr Oncol Rep 16: 370.
29. Schlievert PM, Jablonski LM, Roggiani M, Sadler I, Callantine S, et al. (2000) Pyrogenic toxin superantigen site specificity in toxic shock syndrome and food poisoning in animals. Infect Immun 68: 3630–3634.
30. Sundberg EJ, Li H, Llera AS, McCormick JK, Tormo J, et al. (2002) Structures of two streptococcal superantigens bound to TCR beta chains reveal diversity in the architecture of T cell signaling complexes. Structure 10: 687–699.
31. Roussel A, Anderson BF, Baker HM, Fraser JD (1997) Crystal structure of the streptococcal superantigen SPE-C: dimerization and zinc binding suggest a novel mode of interaction with MHC class II molecules. Nat Struct Biol 4: 635–643.
32. Li PL, Tiedemann RE, Moffat SL, Fraser JD (1997) The superantigen streptococcal pyrogenic exotoxin C (SPE-C) exhibits a novel mode of action. J Exp Med 186: 375–383.
33. McCormick JK, Tripp TJ, Olmsted SB, Matsuka YV, Gahr PJ, et al. (2000) Development of streptococcal pyrogenic exotoxin C vaccine toxoids that are protective in the rabbit model of toxic shock syndrome. J Immunol 165: 2306–2312.
34. Rahman AK, Herfst CA, Moza B, Shames SR, Chau LA, et al. (2006) Molecular basis of TCR selectivity, cross-reactivity, and allelic discrimination by a bacterial superantigen: integrative functional and energetic mapping of the SpeC-Vbeta2.1 molecular interface. J Immunol 177: 8595–8603.
35. Kasper KJ, Xi W, Nur-Ur Rahman AK, Nooh MM, Kotb M, et al. (2008) Molecular requirements for MHC class II alpha-chain engagement and allelic discrimination by the bacterial superantigen streptococcal pyrogenic exotoxin C. J Immunol 181: 3384–3392.
36. Sambrook J, Russell DW (2001) Molecular Cloning: A Laboratory Manual: Cold Spring Harbor Laboratory Press, Cold Spring Harbor, N. Y.
37. Shaw DM, Embleton MJ, Westwater C, Ryan MG, Myers KA, et al. (2000) Isolation of a high affinity scFv from a monoclonal antibody recognising the oncofoetal antigen 5T4. Biochim Biophys Acta 1524: 238–246.
38. Kapust RB, Tozzer J, Fox JD, Anderson DE, Cherry S, et al. (2001) Tobacco etch virus protease: mechanism of autolysis and rational design of stable mutants with wild-type catalytic proficiency. Protein Eng 14: 993–1000.
39. Brouillard JN, Gunther S, Varma AK, Gryski I, Herfst CA, et al. (2007) Crystal structure of the streptococcal superantigen SpeI and functional role of a novel loop domain in T cell activation by group V superantigens. J Mol Biol 367: 925–934.
40. Forsberg G, Skartved NJ, Wallen-Ohman M, Nyhlen HC, Behm K, et al. (2010) Naptumomab estafenatox, an engineered antibody-superantigen fusion protein with low toxicity and reduced antigenicity. J Immunother 33: 492–499.
41. Arstila TP, Casrouge A, Baron V, Even J, Kanellopoulos J, et al. (1999) A direct estimate of the human alphabeta T cell receptor diversity. Science 286: 958–961.
42. Tripp TJ, McCormick JK, Webb JM, Schlievert PM (2003) The zinc-dependent major histocompatibility complex class II binding site of streptococcal pyrogenic exotoxin C is critical for maximal superantigen function and toxic activity. Infect Immun 71: 1548–1550.
43. Campbell RE, Tour O, Palmer AE, Steinbach PA, Baird GS, et al. (2002) A monomeric red fluorescent protein. Proc Natl Acad Sci U S A 99: 7877–7882.
44. Hole N, Stern PL (1988) A 72 kD trophoblast glycoprotein defined by a monoclonal antibody. Br J Cancer 57: 239–246.
45. Chen TR, Drabkowski D, Hay RJ, Macy M, Peterson W, Jr. (1987) WiDr is a derivative of another colon adenocarcinoma cell line, HT-29. Cancer Genet Cytogenet 27: 125–134.
46. Shultz LD, Lyons BL, Burzenski LM, Gott B, Chen X, et al. (2005) Human lymphoid and myeloid cell development in NOD/LtSz-scid IL2R gamma null mice engrafted with mobilized human hemopoietic stem cells. J Immunol 174: 6477–6489.
47. Carreno BM, Garbow JR, Kolar GR, Jackson EN, Engelbach JA, et al. (2009) Immunodeficient mouse strains display marked variability in growth of human melanoma lung metastases. Clin Can Res 15: 3277–3286.
48. Ishikawa F, Yasukawa M, Lyons B, Yoshida S, Miyamoto T, et al. (2005) Development of functional human blood and immune systems in NOD/SCID/IL2 receptor {gamma} chain(null) mice. Blood 106: 1565–1573.
49. Alpaugh RK, Schultz J, McAleer C, Giantonio BJ, Persson R, et al. (1998) Superantigen-targeted therapy: phase I escalating repeat dose trial of the fusion protein PNU-214565 in patients with advanced gastrointestinal malignancies. Clin Cancer Res 4: 1903–1914.
50. Giantonio BJ, Alpaugh RK, Schultz J, McAleer C, Newton DW, et al. (1997) Superantigen-based immunotherapy: a phase I trial of PNU-214565, a monoclonal antibody-staphylococcal enterotoxin A recombinant fusion protein, in advanced pancreatic and colorectal cancer. J Clin Oncol 15: 1994–2007.
51. Jemal A, Siegel R, Ward E, Hao Y, Xu J, et al. (2008) Cancer statistics, 2008. CA Cancer J Clin 58: 71–96.
52. Southall PJ, Boxer GM, Bagshawe KD, Hole N, Bromley M, et al. (1990) Immunohistological distribution of 5T4 antigen in normal and malignant tissues. Br J Cancer 61: 89–95.

53. Starzynska T, Marsh PJ, Schofield PF, Roberts SA, Myers KA, et al. (1994) Prognostic significance of 5T4 oncofetal antigen expression in colorectal carcinoma. Br J Cancer 69: 899–902.
54. Karapetis CS, Khambata-Ford S, Jonker DJ, O'Callaghan CJ, Tu D, et al. (2008) K-ras mutations and benefit from cetuximab in advanced colorectal cancer. N Engl J Med 359: 1757–1765.
55. Van Cutsem E, Kohne CH, Hitre E, Zaluski J, Chang Chien CR, et al. (2009) Cetuximab and chemotherapy as initial treatment for metastatic colorectal cancer. N Engl J Med 360: 1408–1417.
56. Hurwitz H, Fehrenbacher L, Novotny W, Cartwright T, Hainsworth J, et al. (2004) Bevacizumab plus irinotecan, fluorouracil, and leucovorin for metastatic colorectal cancer. N Engl J Med 350: 2335–2342.
57. Hedlund G, Eriksson H, Sundstedt A, Forsberg G, Jakobsen BK, et al. (2013) The tumor targeted superantigen ABR-217620 selectively engages TRBV7-9 and exploits TCR-pMHC affinity mimicry in mediating T cell cytotoxicity. PLoS ONE 8: e79082.
58. Swann PG, Tolnay M, Muthukkumar S, Shapiro MA, Rellahan BL, et al. (2008) Considerations for the development of therapeutic monoclonal antibodies. Curr Opin Immunol 20: 493–499.
59. Basma H, Norrby-Teglund A, Guedez Y, McGeer A, Low DE, et al. (1999) Risk factors in the pathogenesis of invasive group A streptococcal infections: role of protective humoral immunity. Infect Immun 67: 1871–1877.
60. Holtfreter S, Roschack K, Eichler P, Eske K, Holtfreter B, et al. (2006) Staphylococcus aureus carriers neutralize superantigens by antibodies specific for their colonizing strain: a potential explanation for their improved prognosis in severe sepsis. J Infect Dis 193: 1275–1278.
61. Dohlsten M, Lando PA, Hedlund G, Trowsdale J, Kalland T (1990) Targeting of human cytotoxic T lymphocytes to MHC class II-expressing cells by staphylococcal enterotoxins. Immunology 71: 96–100.
62. Xu SX, McCormick JK (2012) Staphylococcal superantigens in colonization and disease. Front Cell Infect Microbiol 2: 52.
63. Terman DS, Serier A, Dauwalder O, Badiou C, Dutour A, et al. (2013) Staphylococcal entertotoxins of the enterotoxin gene cluster (egcSEs) induce nitrous oxide- and cytokine dependent tumor cell apoptosis in a broad panel of human tumor cells. Front Cell Infect Microbiol 3: 38.
64. Holtfreter S, Bauer K, Thomas D, Feig C, Lorenz V, et al. (2004) egc-Encoded superantigens from Staphylococcus aureus are neutralized by human sera much less efficiently than are classical staphylococcal enterotoxins or toxic shock syndrome toxin. Infect Immun 72: 4061–4071.
65. Abrahmsen L, Dohlsten M, Segren S, Bjork P, Jonsson E, et al. (1995) Characterization of two distinct MHC class II binding sites in the superantigen staphylococcal enterotoxin A. EMBO J 14: 2978–2986.
66. Kawabe Y, Ochi A (1990) Selective anergy of V beta 8+,CD4+ T cells in Staphylococcus enterotoxin B-primed mice. J Exp Med 172: 1065–1070.
67. Sundstedt A, Hoiden I, Hansson J, Hedlund G, Kalland T, et al. (1995) Superantigen-induced anergy in cytotoxic CD8+ T cells. J Immunol 154: 6306–6313.
68. Rosendahl A, Kristensson K, Hansson J, Ohlsson L, Kalland T, et al. (1998) Repeated treatment with antibody-targeted superantigens strongly inhibits tumor growth. Int J Cancer 76: 274–283.
69. Vesely MD, Schreiber RD (2013) Cancer immunoediting: antigens, mechanisms, and implications to cancer immunotherapy. Ann N Y Acad Sci 1284: 1–5.
70. Kalos M, Levine BL, Porter DL, Katz S, Grupp SA, et al. (2011) T cells with chimeric antigen receptors have potent antitumor effects and can establish memory in patients with advanced leukemia. Sci Transl Med 3: 95ra73.
71. Porter DL, Levine BL, Kalos M, Bagg A, June CH (2011) Chimeric antigen receptor-modified T cells in chronic lymphoid leukemia. N Engl J Med 365: 725–733.
72. Kochenderfer JN, Wilson WH, Janik JE, Dudley ME, Stetler-Stevenson M, et al. (2010) Eradication of B-lineage cells and regression of lymphoma in a patient treated with autologous T cells genetically engineered to recognize CD19. Blood 116: 4099–4102.
73. Kochenderfer JN, Dudley ME, Feldman SA, Wilson WH, Spaner DE, et al. (2012) B-cell depletion and remissions of malignancy along with cytokine-associated toxicity in a clinical trial of anti-CD19 chimeric-antigen-receptor-transduced T cells. Blood 119: 2709–2720.
74. Pardoll DM (2012) The blockade of immune checkpoints in cancer immunotherapy. Nat Rev Cancer 12: 252–264.

8

Inter- and Intra-Patient Heterogeneity of Response and Progression to Targeted Therapy in Metastatic Melanoma

Alexander M. Menzies[1,2]*, Lauren E. Haydu[1,2], Matteo S. Carlino[1,2,3,5], Mary W. F. Azer[3], Peter J. A. Carr[2,4], Richard F. Kefford[1,2,3,5], Georgina V. Long[1,2]

1 Melanoma Institute Australia, Sydney, Australia, 2 The University of Sydney, Sydney, Australia, 3 Westmead Hospital, Crown Princess Mary Cancer Centre, Sydney, Australia, 4 Westmead Hospital, Department of Radiology, Sydney, Australia, 5 Westmead Institute for Cancer Research, Westmead, Australia

Abstract

Background: MAPK inhibitors (MAPKi) are active in *BRAF*-mutant metastatic melanoma patients, but the extent of response and progression-free survival (PFS) is variable, and complete responses are rare. We sought to examine the patterns of response and progression in patients treated with targeted therapy.

Methods: MAPKi-naïve patients treated with combined dabrafenib and trametinib had all metastases ≥ 5 mm (lymph nodes ≥ 15 mm in short axis) visible on computed tomography measured at baseline and throughout treatment.

Results: 24 patients had 135 measured metastases (median 4.5/patient, median diameter 16 mm). Time to best response (median 5.5 mo, range 1.7–20.1 mo), and the degree of best response (median −70%, range +9 to −100%) varied amongst patients. 17% of patients achieved complete response (CR), whereas 53% of metastases underwent CR, including 42% ≥ 10 mm. Metastases that underwent CR were smaller than non-CR metastases (median 11 vs 20 mm, $P<0.001$). PFS was variable among patients (median 8.2 mo, range 2.6–18.3 mo), and 50% of patients had disease progression in new metastases only. Only 1% (1/71) of CR-metastases subsequently progressed. Twelve-month overall survival was poorer in those with a more heterogeneous initial response to therapy than less heterogeneous (67% vs 93%, $P=0.009$).

Conclusion: Melanoma response and progression with MAPKi displays marked inter- and intra-patient heterogeneity. Most metastases undergo complete response, yet only a small proportion of patients achieve an overall complete response. Similarly, disease progression often occurs only in a subset of the tumor burden, and often in new metastases alone. Clinical heterogeneity, likely reflecting molecular heterogeneity, remains a barrier to the effective treatment of melanoma patients.

Editor: Keiran Smalley, The Moffitt Cancer Center & Research Institute, United States of America

Funding: This work was supported by Program Grants from the National Health and Medical Research Council of Australia (NHMRC), Cancer Institute NSW, Australian Cancer Research Foundation, the Melanoma Foundation of the University of Sydney and Melanoma Institute Australia. GlaxoSmithKline funded the clinical trial from which these data were obtained. The funders had no role in study design, data collection and analysis, decision to publish, or preparation of the manuscript.

Competing Interests: The authors have read the journal's policy and have the following conflicts: AMM – Roche (H & T), GlaxoSmithKline (T). RFK – Roche (C), GlaxoSmithKline (C), Novartis (C). GVL – Roche (C, T & H), GlaxoSmithKline (C), Novartis (C). None to declare for the remaining authors. There are no employment or leadership positions, no stock ownership, no expert testimony. Note: (C) = Consultant advisor, (H) Honoraria and (T) Travel support for conference attendance.

* E-mail: alexander.menzies@sydney.edu.au

Introduction

Molecular heterogeneity exists in all cancers [1,2], particularly melanoma [3–5]. Genetic divergence occurs during clonal evolution, resulting in inter- and intra-tumoral molecular heterogeneity within patients [3,6,7]. Certain driver genetic aberrations exist in all tumor cells within an individual, but several others exist in subclones, conferring varying degrees of drug resistance [2]. Intrinsic resistance mechanisms present in subclones of the overall tumor burden diminish the initial response to systemic treatment, and these and acquired mechanisms result in disease progression. Ultimately the presence or development of these mechanisms influence the initial response to systemic treatment, time to progression, and overall survival. The influence and heterogeneity

of the tumor micro-environment is also increasingly understood to play a role in tumor cell heterogeneity and treatment outcome [8].

Clinically, inter- and intra-patient molecular heterogeneity is manifest by the variable responses observed between and within patients treated with targeted therapies. BRAF inhibitors, used as single agents or in combination with MEK inhibitors, are active in most patients with metastatic melanoma, but the extent of response and time to progression are variable between patients, and complete responses are uncommon [9–11]. Patterns of disease progression are also variable, with existing metastases progressing or new metastases developing at the same time as ongoing response in other metastases [12,13]. The terms "mixed response" and "isolated progression" are now used commonly, however these terms have not yet been accurately defined, and there is little known as to the prevalence or predictors of these phenomena, nor the clinical outcomes of patients with these patterns of response and progression.

We therefore sought to examine the patterns of response and progression to targeted therapy by measuring every metastasis ≥5 mm via computed tomography (CT) in a cohort of patients with metastatic melanoma treated with combined BRAF and MEK inhibitors.

Patients and Methods

Patients and Treatment

All MAPK inhibitor naïve BRAF-mutant metastatic melanoma patients treated with dabrafenib and trametinib (CombiDT) on parts B–D of the BRF113220 Phase 1/2 [11] trial (NCT01072175) at Westmead Hospital in association with Melanoma Institute Australia were included for analysis. The collection and analysis of clinical data was approved by the Westmead and Royal Prince Alfred Hospitals Human Research Ethics Committees (Protocol No. X11-0023 and HREC/11/RPAH/32) and written informed consent was obtained from each patient. Patients received a range of doses of dabrafenib and trametinib. Patient demographic and disease characteristic data at trial entry were collected.

Disease Assessments

CT scans of 3 mm slice thickness were performed at baseline and then every 8 weeks as per the clinical trial protocol. In

Table 1. Patient demographics and clinical characteristics.

Feature	All patients		Uniform Response at First Scan*		Mixed Response at First Scan*		P-value#
	N	%	N	%	N	%	
Number of patients	24	100	15	62	9	38	–
Age (years)							
Median	51	–	57	–	42	–	0.290
Range	29–78	–	28–77	–	38–74	–	
Sex							
Male	13	54	8	53	5	56	0.625
Female	11	46	7	47	4	44	
BRAF genotype							
V600E	20	85	13	87	7	78	0.486
V600K	4	15	2	13	2	22	
ECOG PS							
0	19	79	11	73	8	89	0.360
1	5	21	4	27	1	11	
AJCC Stage							
M1a	5	21	3	20	2	22	0.418^
M1b	5	21	4	27	1	11	
M1c	14	58	8	53	6	67	
Baseline LDH							
<1×ULN	19	79	13	87	6	67	0.255
>1×ULN	5	21	2	13	3	33	
Drug doses (Dab/Tra)							
300/2	8	33	6	40	2	22	Not Tested
300/1.5	1	4	0	0	1	11	
300/1	4	17	2	13	2	22	
300/0 then 300/2 at PD	2	8	2	13	0	0	
150~/2	8	33	4	27	4	44	
300~/2	1	4	1	7	0	0	
Dab with 2 mg Tra	17	71	11	73	6	67	0.539
Dab with <2 mg Tra	7	29	4	27	3	33	

Abbreviations: ECOG PS, Eastern Cooperative Oncology Group Performance Status; AJCC, American Joint Committee on Cancer; LDH, lactate dehydrogenase; ULN, upper limit of normal; Dab, dabrafenib total daily dose; Tra, trametinib daily dose; PD, progressive disease.
~hydroxymethylcellulose dabrafenib preparation.
^testing M1a & M1b versus M1c.
*Uniform response: ≥80% of metastases with a complete or partial response and no progressing or new metastases. Mixed response: <80% of metastases with a complete or partial response, or the presence of any progressing or new metastases.
#testing uniform versus mixed response cohorts.

Table 2. Baseline disease assessments by examining RECIST targets versus ALL metastases.

	RECIST targets	ALL metastases
Total	**56**	**135**
Diameter (mm)		
Median	16	16
Range	10–108	5–108
Number ≥10 mm	56	102
Number per patient		
Median	2	4.5
Range	1–5	1–18
Sum of Diameters (mm)		
Median	48	100
Range	10–174	11–317
Site of metastases (n, %)		
SQ	13, 23%	43, 32%
Lymph node	10, 18%	15, 11%
Lung	16, 29%	48, 36%
Liver	12, 21%	24, 18%
Gastrointestinal*	5, 9%	5, 4%

Abbreviations: SQ, subcutaneous and soft tissue.
*Gastrointestinal sites include adrenal ($N = 3$), small bowel ($N = 1$), pancreas ($N = 1$).

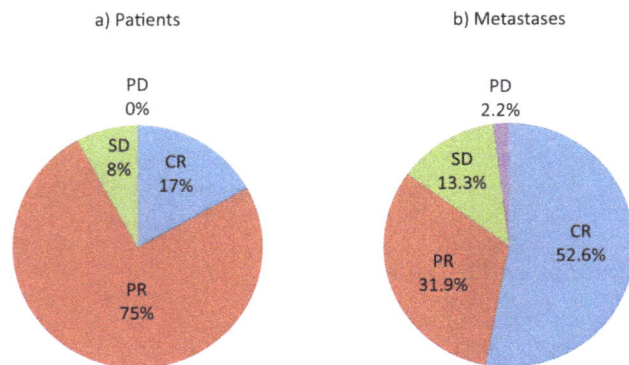

Figure 1. The proportions of categories of response a) by patients ($N = 24$), b) by metastases ($N = 135$). Abbreviations: CR, complete response; PR, partial response; SD, stable disease; PD, progressive disease.

addition to the RECIST v1.1 assessments [14] conducted prospectively as part of the clinical trial, a more detailed radiologic assessment of every metastasis ≥5 mm diameter in long axis (lymph nodes ≥15 mm in short axis) visible on CT was performed on every scan. This was referred to as the "ALL metastasis" assessment, and was conducted retrospectively, blinded to the RECIST assessment and clinical data. Measurements were made on each scan to the nearest millimeter using the IntelePACS© computer software program.

RECIST data were used only as a comparison to the ALL metastasis assessment data to assess for concordance of these measures for best overall response, time to best response (TTBR), and progression-free survival (PFS) (see supplementary methods).

The patient's overall response at each time point was determined using similar criteria as RECIST [14], but included all metastases ≥5 mm to calculate the sum of diameters (SoD). Disease progression was defined as the development of new metastases and/or a ≥20% and ≥5 mm increase in the sum of diameters of all metastases from nadir.

In addition, a response was recorded for each individual measured metastasis at each time point and classified as complete response (CR, disappearance or to less than 10 mm for a lymph node), partial response (PR, ≥30% reduction), stable disease (SD, neither CR/PR/PD) or progressive disease (PD, ≥5 mm and ≥20% growth).

At first radiologic assessment, for this study, a uniform response was predefined as ≥80% of metastases having a complete or partial response with no progressing or new metastases. A mixed response was defined as <80% of metastases having a complete or partial response, or the presence of any progressing or new metastases.

Statistical Analysis

Patient demographic and clinical features were tested for association with uniform versus mixed response at first scan using the Fisher's Exact Test, Pearson's χ^2, and/or the Mann Whitney U test as appropriate. Overall survival (OS) and PFS were calculated from the date of commencement of targeted therapies to the date of last follow-up or date of progression, respectively. Univariate time to event analyses were conducted with the Kaplan-Meier method together with the Log Rank test for comparison of categorical covariates, and with the Cox proportional hazards method for continuous covariates. Multivariate overall survival was conducted with the Cox proportional hazards method. When comparing the two assessment methods (RECIST and ALL metastasis), best overall response was deemed concordant if there was ≤10% difference in the percentage degree of best response and also within the same response category. Time to best response and progression-free survival were concordant if they occurred at the same time (on the same scan) by both measures. All statistical analyses were conducted with IBM SPSS Statistic v21.

Results

Patient Demographics and Disease Characteristics

Twenty-four patients were included for analysis. The patient population was typical for patients with BRAF-mutant metastatic melanoma; the median age of patients was 51 years, 54% of patients were men, 85% of patients had the V600E genotype, and 58% of patients had stage M1c melanoma (Table 1). All patients were MAPK inhibitor naïve. Although several dosing regimens were administered, 71% of patients were treated with trametinib at the recommended part two dose of 2 mg daily in combination with dabrafenib from trial commencement (Table 1). Two patients received dabrafenib monotherapy until disease progression, after which 2 mg daily trametinib was added.

Baseline Disease Assessments

135 metastases from the 24 patients were included for assessment (median 4.5 per patient, range 1–18), substantially more than included as RECIST targets ($N = 56$, median 2 per patient, range 1–5) (Table 2). The median diameter of metastases was the same as RECIST targets (16 mm), but ranged from a minimum 5 mm rather than 10 mm. Seventy-six percent ($N = 102$) of metastases were ≥10 mm, and 46 (45%) of these had not been

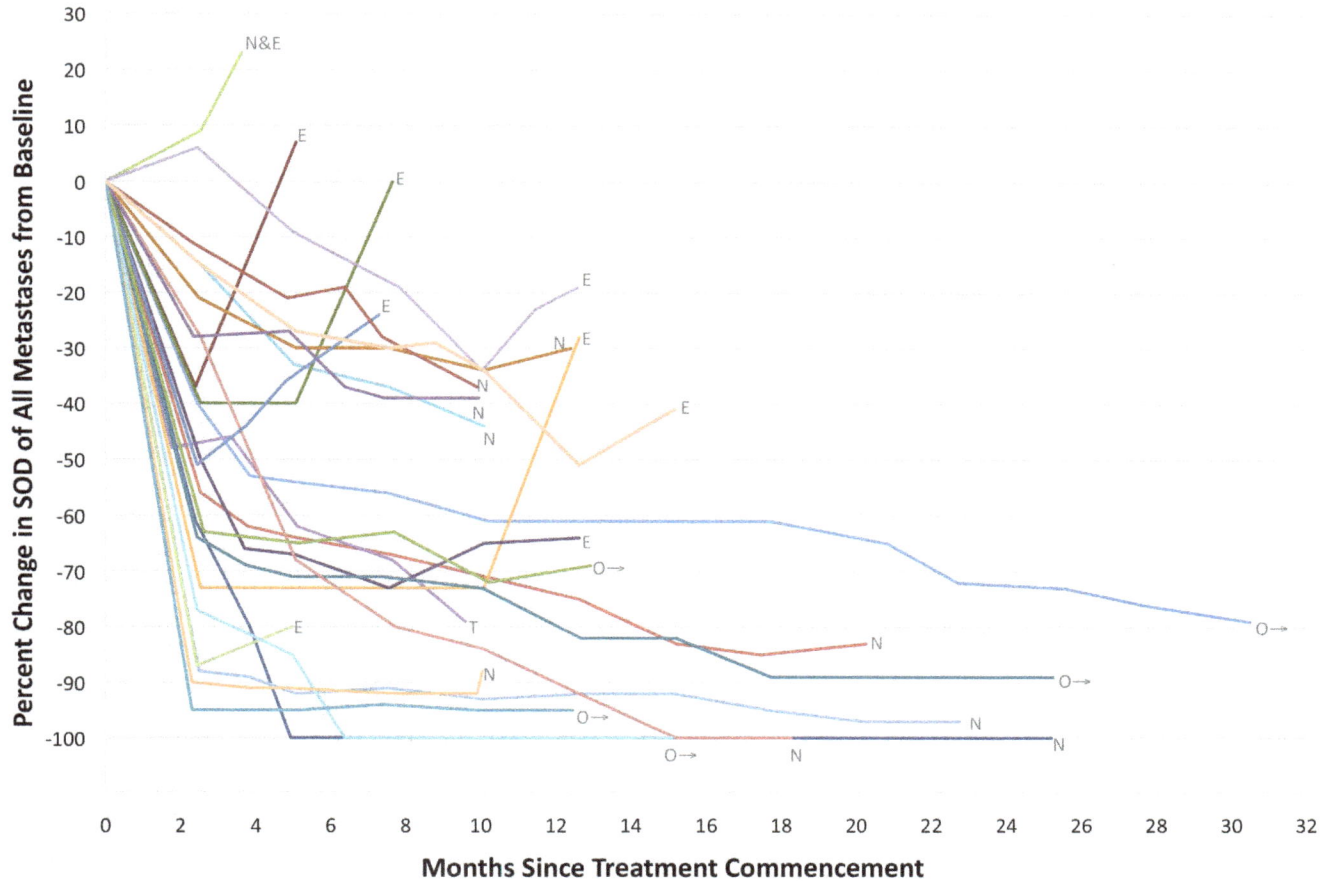

Figure 2. Inter-patient heterogeneity of response and progression with CombiDT. Plot of the percent change in the sum of diameters of all metastases ≥5 mm within an individual patient compared to baseline at various time points during treatment with CombiDT until disease progression. Each line represents an individual patient. Abbreviations: E, disease progressing due to existing lesions; N, new lesions; N+E, new and existing lesions; O→, ongoing response without progression; T, treatment ceased due to toxicity.

included as RECIST targets. Most frequent sites of disease included lung and subcutaneous/soft tissue (SQ) (36% and 32% respectively) (Table 2).

Overall Patient Response

The majority of patients had a response to treatment. When all metastases ≥5 mm were measured, 17% ($N = 4$) of patients had a complete response and 75% ($N = 18$) had a partial response to treatment (Figure 1a). No patients had progressive disease as best response. The median time to best response was diverse (median 5.5 months, range 1.7 to 20.1 months), and there was variability in the degree of response at first assessment (median change −49%, range +9 to −95%), the kinetics of response (% change over time), and the degree of best response (median change −70%, range +9 to −100) within the patient population (Figure 2). The degree of best overall response by ALL metastasis and RECIST assessment measures was concordant in 19/24 (79%) patients (Figure 3), the category of response was concordant in 20/24 (83%) patients, and TTBR was concordant in 17/24 (71%) patients.

Individual Metastasis Response

Ninety-three percent (126/135) of metastases had some reduction in size with treatment and 84.5% (114/135) had either a complete or partial response. Only 2.2% (3/135) of metastases demonstrated progressive disease at first assessment, all within the

same patient. Importantly, 52.6% ($N = 71$) of metastases had a complete response (Figure 1b, Figure 4). Of 102 metastases ≥10 mm diameter, 42% (43/102) had a complete response, and 41% (23/56) RECIST target metastases had complete response.

The median TTBR for all metastases was 12.1 weeks (range 7.3–87.6 weeks) (Table 3). Compared with subcutaneous and soft tissue metastases (median 8.3 weeks), median TTBR was significantly longer for lymph nodes (30.3 weeks, $P = 0.009$) and liver metastases (31.7 weeks, $P = 0.038$), but not significantly different for lung metastases (8.0 weeks, $P = 0.076$). TTBR was significantly shorter as metastases decreased in size (HR = 0.98, 95% CI 0.96–0.998, $P = 0.030$), and the degree of response at first scan correlated with the degree of best response ($R^2 = 0.6613$, p<0.001) (Figure 5).

There was no significant difference in the rate of complete response by disease site ($P > 0.05$) (Table 3). Metastases that had a complete response were significantly smaller compared with metastases that had PD/SD/PR (median 11 mm vs 20 mm, $P < 0.001$). This factor remained significant when stratifying by disease sites for lung, liver, and SQ metastases (all $P < 0.05$), but not for lymph nodes ($N = 15$).

Plots of the response of individual metastases over time within individual patients (Figure 6) demonstrated the marked variability in the degree of first response and best response, the kinetics of

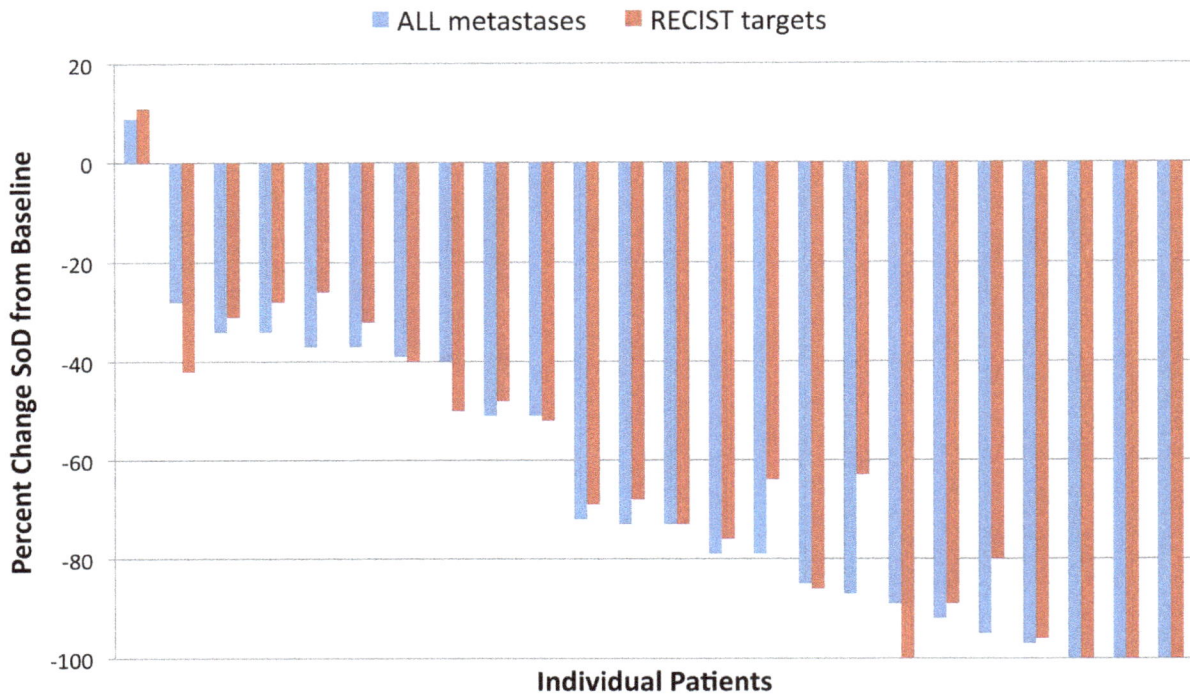

Figure 3. The degree of overall best response for each patient by RECIST and ALL metastasis disease assessments.

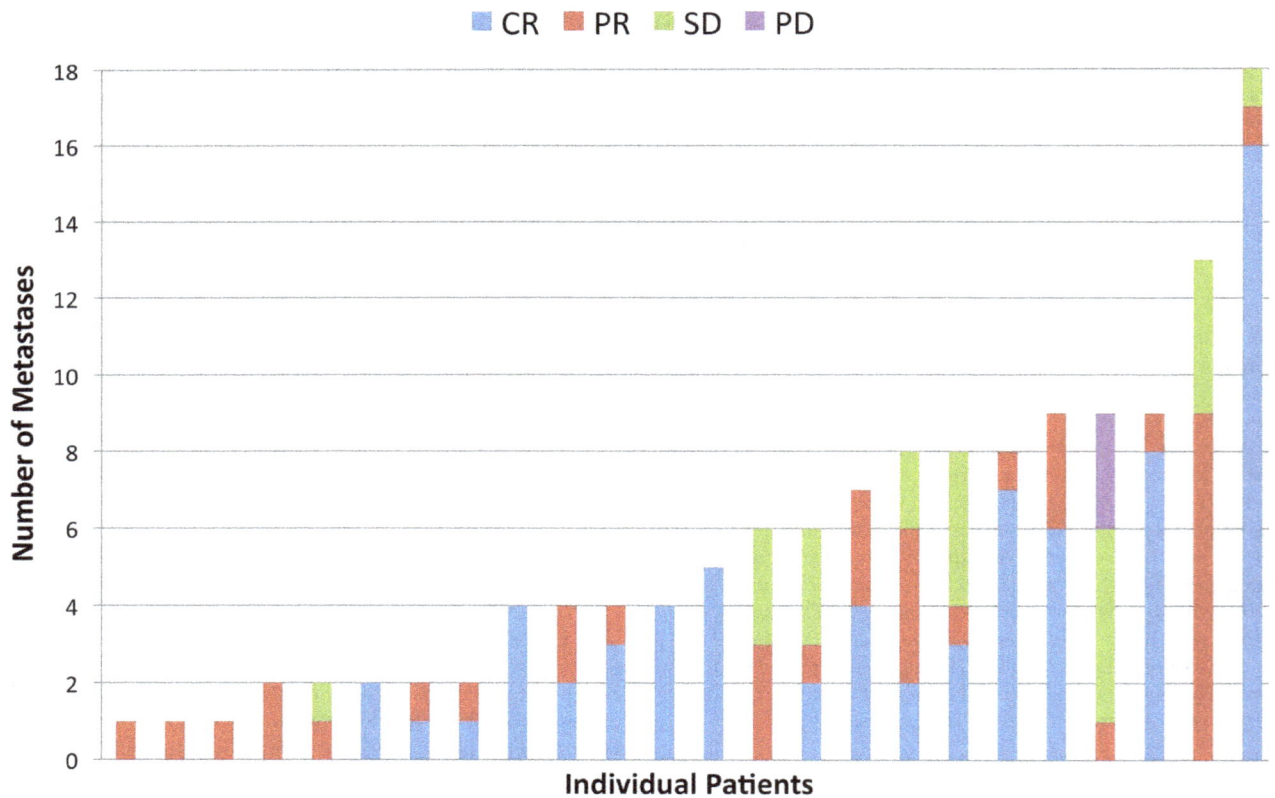

Figure 4. The best response of each individual metastasis within each patient. Abbrevations: CR, complete response; PR, partial response; SD, stable disease; PD, progressive disease.

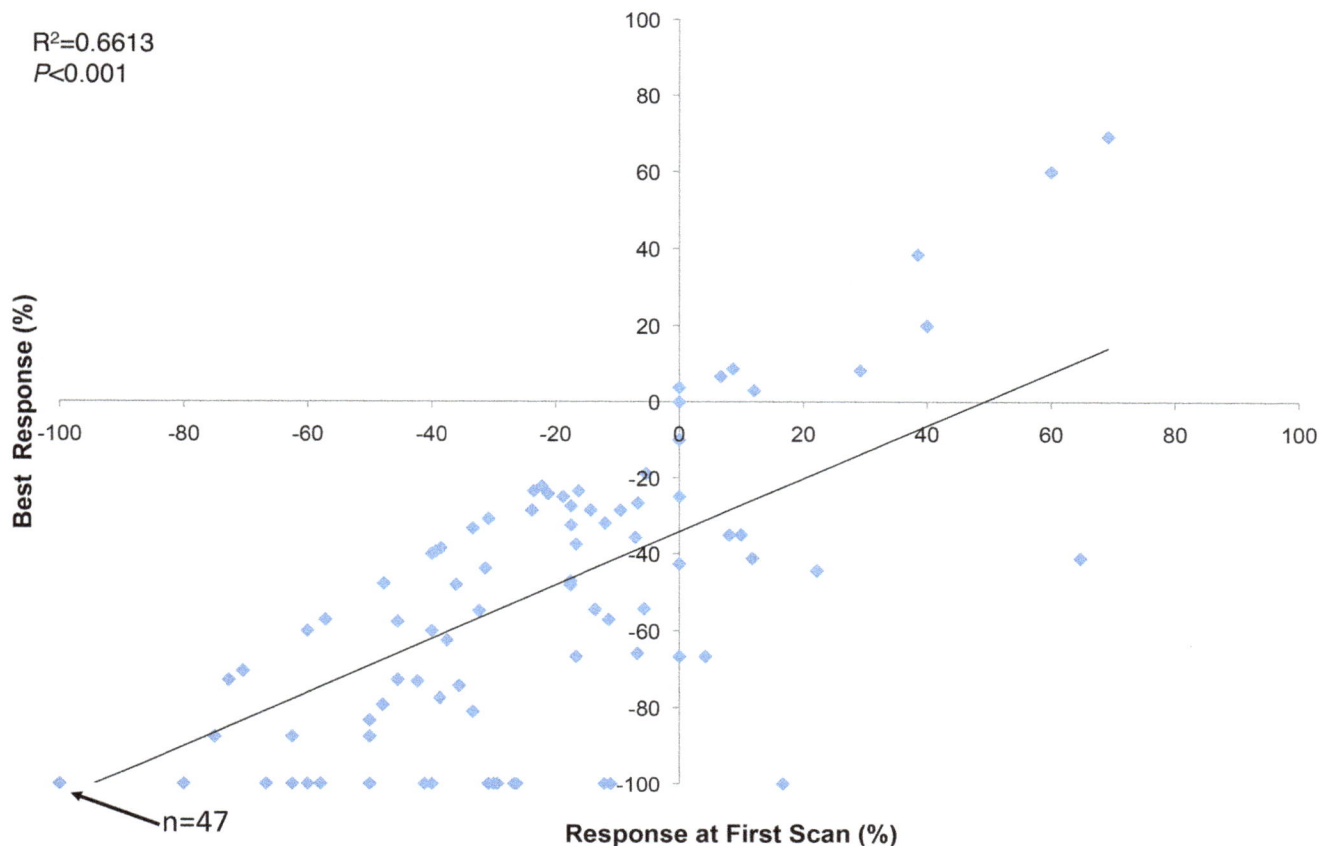

Figure 5. Correlation of the response of individual metastases at first scan versus best response (*N*= 135).

response, and the time to best response for each individual metastasis.

Sixty-two percent (15/24) of patients had a uniform response at first assessment, and 38% (9/24) of patients had a mixed response. Patient demographics, disease characteristics and CombiDT doses received were similar in the two groups (Table 1). The two patients that received dabrafenib monotherapy until disease progression had a uniform response to treatment.

Patterns of Disease Progression

At the time of analysis 18 (75%) patients had disease progression (PD) (Figure 2). Median PFS was 8.2 months (range 2.6 to 18.3 months). PFS was highly concordant by ALL metastasis and RECIST assessment methods (14/18, 77% of patients). Fifty percent of patients progressed in new metastases only, 44% in existing metastases only, and 6% in both new and existing metastases simultaneously. There was no dominant site of disease progression, but four (22%) patients with no prior history of brain metastases progressed in new metastases in the brain. At time of

Table 3. Factors influencing individual metastasis response to treament; time to best response by metastasis site, and the effect of metastasis site and size on response.

Site of metastasis	Median Time to Best Response (Range) Weeks	CR		PR/SD/PD		P-value*
		N	Median Size (Range) mm	N	Median Size (Range) mm	
All	12.1 (7.3–87.6)	71	11 (5–44)	64	20 (5–108)	<0.001
SQ	8.3 (7.6–56.3)	24	10 (7–30)	19	20 (10–98)	<0.001
LN	30.3 (7.7–87.6)	7	22 (15–31)	8	21 (17–48)	0.38
Lung	8.0 (7.3–63.9)	27	9 (5–44)	21	15 (5–44)	0.036
Liver	31.7 (7.7–56.0)	10	18 (7–27)	14	31 (16–47)	0.006

*P-value for comparison of median size of lesions with CR versus non-CR, Mann Whitney U test.
Abbreviations: CR, complete response; PR, partial response; SD, stable disease; PD, progressive disease; SQ, subcutaneous and soft tissue; LN, lymph node.

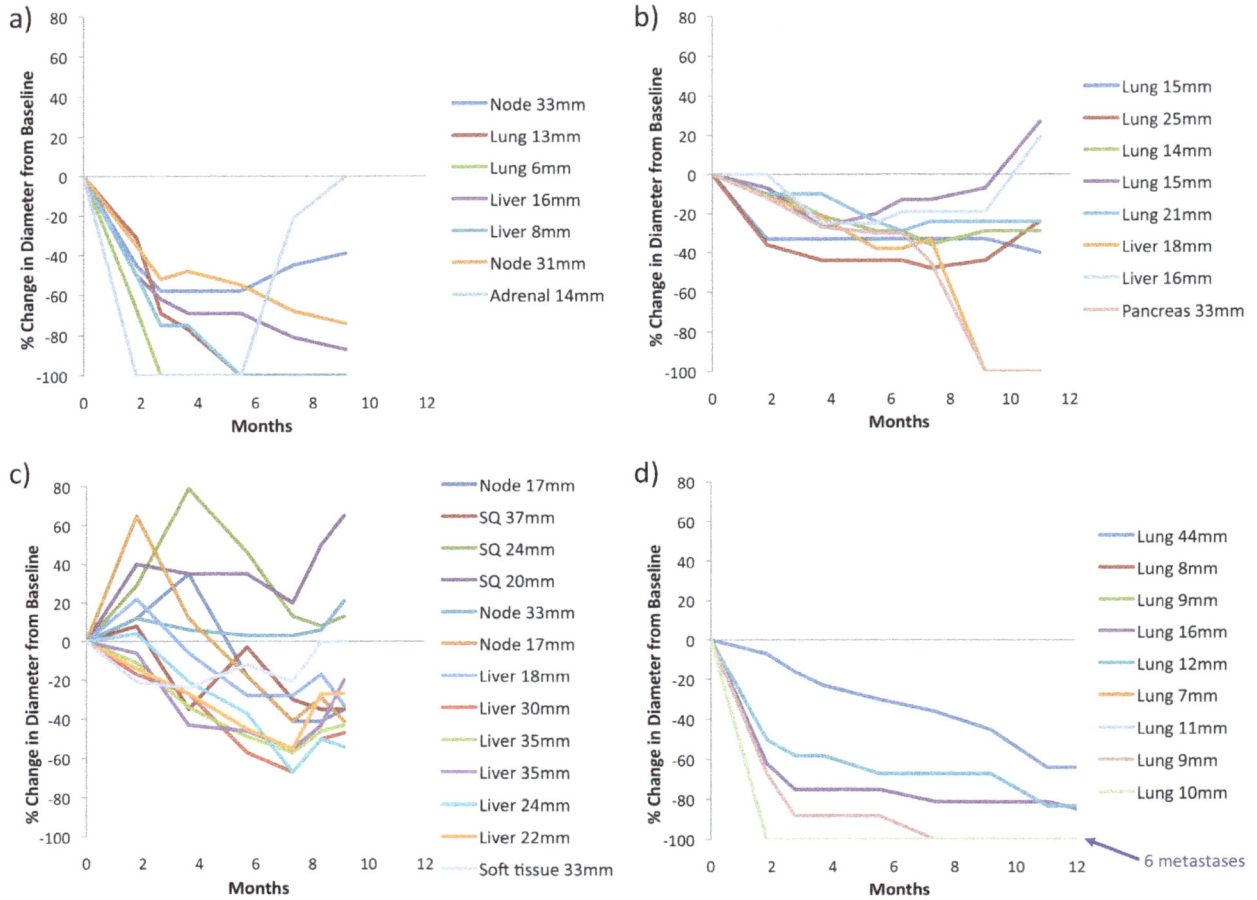

Figure 6. Intra-patient heterogeneneity of response and progression with CombiDT. Example plots of the percent change in the diameter of individual metastases within four patients (a-d) compared to baseline at various time points during treatment until overall disease progression. The degree and kinetics of response of individual metastases vary within a patient. Similarly, progression often occurs only in a subset of the overall tumour burden. Patient D had disease progression in new lesions only.

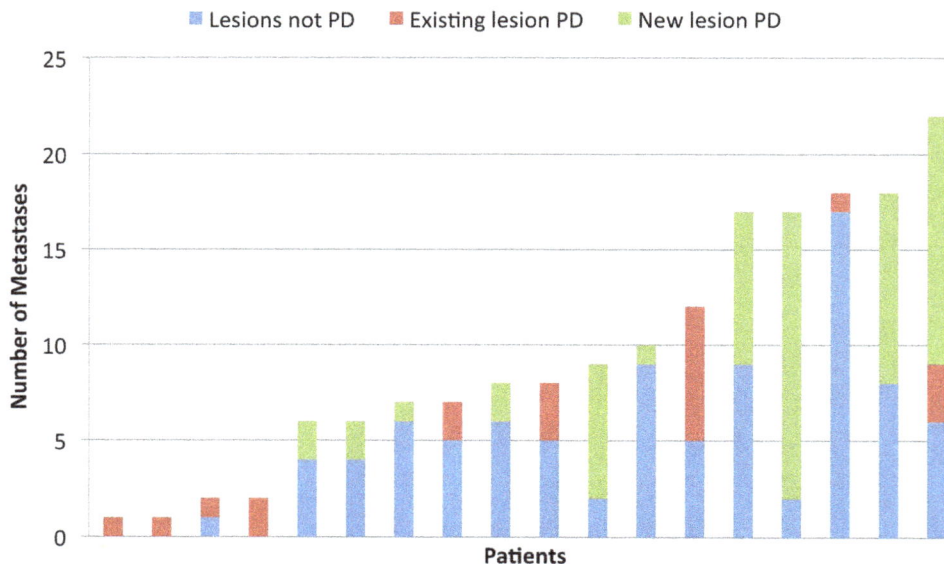

Figure 7. Intra-patient heterogeneity of disease progression. The number and type of metastases progressing at time of disease progression.

Table 4. Univariate progression-free and overall survival.

Outcome	Factor	P-value
PFS	Baseline SoD	0.101
	Percent Response at First Scan	0.084
	Uniform versus Mixed Response at First Scan*	0.124
OS	Baseline SoD	0.349
	Percent Response at First Scan	0.105
	Uniform versus Mixed Response at First Scan*	0.009

Abbreviations: SoD, sum of diameters.
*Uniform response: ≥80% of metastases with a complete or partial response and no progressing or new metastases. Mixed response: <80% of metastases with a complete or partial response, or the presence of any progressing or new metastases.

PD, the median proportion of metastases progressing in an individual compared to the total tumor burden ever (including all metastases at baseline and new metastases) was 49% (range 6 to 100%) (Figure 7). Only one metastasis that underwent complete response subsequently progressed (1.4%, 1/71).

Survival Analyses

The burden of disease at baseline (SoD of ALL metastasis) and the degree of overall response at first scan did not correlate with PFS, 12-month survival or OS (Table 4). The type of initial response (uniform versus mixed) similarly did not correlate with PFS. 12-month and OS, however was significantly inferior for mixed responders (67% and median 14.2 months) compared with uniform responders (93% and median not reached, $P = 0.009$), a result which remained significant when adjusting for baseline disease burden (HR = 5.1, 95% CI: 1.2–21.1, $P = 0.025$).

Discussion

This is the first systematic study of patterns of clinical response and progression to MAPK targeted therapy in all assessable individual metastases in patients with metastatic melanoma, demonstrating that melanoma response and progression is heterogeneous between and within patients. Most individual metastases undergo a complete response to treatment, yet only a small proportion of patients achieve an overall complete response. Disease progression is similarly heterogeneous, both in timing and nature. Many patients have disease progression in a subset of their overall tumor burden, and often in new metastases only. Metastases that initially undergo complete response with treatment seldom subsequently progress, and a more heterogeneous initial response to treatment is associated with shorter overall survival.

Results of this study are strengthened by the detailed clinical assessment of patients on the most highly active targeted therapy in melanoma [11], the use of a standard modality for disease assessment (3 mm slice thickness CT) at predetermined specified time points, inclusion of every metastasis visible and measurable on CT scan (≥5 mm or ≥15 for lymph nodes), and an assessment of every individual metastasis across every time point from baseline prior to treatment until disease progression. The inclusion of all metastases as targets for assessment, as opposed to the maximum 5 target metastases for RECIST (and maximum 2 in any one organ) provided a more detailed assessment, with increased ability to assess for intra-patient heterogeneity. This question has been previously addressed in studies of ^{18}F-labelled fluorodeoxyglucose positron emission tomography (PET) metabolic response to single

agent BRAF inhibitors at day 15, with varying results, one study examining 5 target metastases and observing a homogeneous response [15], while the other examined every metastasis and observed heterogeneity [16].

In this study, most metastases achieved a complete response with treatment. These metastases were located at any body site, and tended to be smaller than those that did not undergo complete response, however, some metastases several centimeters in diameter still had complete response. The reasons why smaller metastases have a higher complete response rate may be because they have to shrink less to become clinically occult, however, the observation that these metastases seldom subsequently progress perhaps supports alternative hypotheses, for example, they undergo a more effective secondary immune response [17,18], or contain less molecular or microenvironmental heterogeneity, with less resistant tumor subclones. This observation warrants further research, particularly as larger metastases may be amenable for resection prior to therapy, and adjuvant trials for occult metastatic disease are in progress.

Despite heterogeneity observed in the degree and timing of best overall response amongst patients, most metastases undergo the majority of tumor shrinkage by 3 months of treatment. Metastases that have not undergone meaningful initial clinical response (e.g. persisting local symptoms) by 3 months may therefore warrant treatment with local therapy (surgery, radiotherapy). Furthermore, in selected patients where the vast majority of metastases have undergone complete response, remaining metastases could be treated locally to render the patient free of overt disease. The observation that the majority of tumor response occurs early during treatment also suggests that additional systemic therapies (e.g. immunotherapy) should be incorporated early in the course of MAPK inhibitor treatment. Translational data demonstrating early immune cell infiltration into tumors soon after treatment commencement (as early as day 3) further supports this, and may indicate that immunotherapies should be combined from the start of MAPK inhibitor treatment [17,18].

Disease progression occurred at varying time points among the patient cohort, and there was a high rate of disease progression due to the emergence of new metastases. Often, patients progressed in only a few metastases, with the remainder of disease under treatment control. In this instance, disease progression may therefore not equate to overt treatment failure, and local treatment (e.g. surgery, radiotherapy) may be delivered to progressing metastases with systemic treatment continued for ongoing clinical benefit to the remainder of drug-sensitive disease [12,13,19]. This approach may be more beneficial than a switch to immunotherapy (e.g. ipilimumab), as little efficacy has been observed in this setting [20,21], likely at least in part due to the release of MAPK inhibition, whereas relative ongoing MAPK inhibition still occurs in resistant tumors with continued MAPK inhibitor treatment [22].

In this study cohort, a mixed response at first assessment correlated with shorter overall survival, but not progression-free survival. This result was likely influenced by small number of patients, the doses of therapy received, and the fact that many patients progressed in new metastases alone. Subsequent treatments may have also influenced overall survival. Despite this, however, this finding warrants validation in future studies, as biomarkers to predict treatment outcome are scant, and the method of categorizing response in this study could be reproduced without additional procedures such as PET.

The clinical heterogeneity of tumor response and progression demonstrated in this study likely reflects underlying molecular heterogeneity. The majority of the melanoma burden in patients is sensitive to MAPK inhibition, however, a varying proportion of primarily resistant subclones exist at baseline, and resistance may also be acquired during treatment. This heterogeneity complicates clinical management, confounds biopsy driven biomarker research, and remains a barrier to the effective treatment of melanoma patients, including the deployment of biopsy-driven adaptive clinical trial design. A broader multi-targeted treatment approach from the outset (e.g, MAPK and PI3K inhibitors) may improve response rates and prolong survival, but will likely face the same problem of clonal drug resistance and treatment failure. Combinations of MAPK inhibitors and novel immunotherapies (e.g. PD-1 antibodies) may provide more complete and durable responses.

Acknowledgments

We acknowledge the assistance of Arthur Clements, Clara Lee, Matthew Chan, Vicky Wegener, Rebecca Hinshelwood, Amie Cho, Katherine Carson, Joanna Jackson, Andrea Del Pilar Forero Velandia, Jacob Cunningham, and Kiran Patel (GSK).

Author Contributions

Conceived and designed the experiments: AMM GVL. Performed the experiments: AMM. Analyzed the data: AMM LEH GVL. Contributed reagents/materials/analysis tools: PJAC RFK GVL. Wrote the paper: AMM LEH MSC MWFA PJAC RFK GVL.

References

1. Meacham CE, Morrison SJ (2013) Tumour heterogeneity and cancer cell plasticity. Nature 501: 328–337.
2. Vogelstein B, Papadopoulos N, Velculescu VE, Zhou S, Diaz LA Jr, et al. (2013) Cancer genome landscapes. Science 339: 1546–1558.
3. Yancovitz M, Litterman A, Yoon J, Ng E, Shapiro RL, et al. (2012) Intra- and inter-tumor heterogeneity of BRAF(V600E))mutations in primary and metastatic melanoma. PLoS ONE 7: e29336.
4. Takata M, Morita R, Takehara K (2000) Clonal heterogeneity in sporadic melanomas as revealed by loss-of-heterozygosity analysis. Int J Cancer 85: 492–497.
5. Lin J, Goto Y, Murata H, Sakaizawa K, Uchiyama A, et al. (2011) Polyclonality of BRAF mutations in primary melanoma and the selection of mutant alleles during progression. British Journal of Cancer 104: 464–468.
6. Katona TM, Jones TD, Wang M, Eble JN, Billings SD, et al. (2007) Genetically heterogeneous and clonally unrelated metastases may arise in patients with cutaneous melanoma. Am J Surg Pathol 31: 1029–1037.
7. Wilmott JS, Tembe V, Howle JR, Sharma R, Thompson JF, et al. (2012) Intratumoral Molecular Heterogeneity in a BRAF-Mutant, BRAF Inhibitor-Resistant Melanoma: A Case Illustrating the Challenges for Personalized Medicine. Molecular Cancer Therapeutics 11: 2704–2708.
8. Junttila MR, de Sauvage FJ (2013) Influence of tumour micro-environment heterogeneity on therapeutic response. Nature 501: 346–354.
9. Chapman PB, Hauschild A, Robert C, Haanen JB, Ascierto P, et al. (2011) Improved survival with vemurafenib in melanoma with BRAF V600E mutation. New England Journal of Medicine 364: 2507–2516.
10. Hauschild A, Grob JJ, Demidov LV, Jouary T, Gutzmer R, et al. (2012) Dabrafenib in BRAF-mutated metastatic melanoma: a multicentre, open-label, phase 3 randomised controlled trial. Lancet 380: 358–365.
11. Flaherty KT, Infante JR, Daud A, Gonzalez R, Kefford RF, et al. (2012) Combined BRAF and MEK inhibition in melanoma with BRAF V600 mutations. New England Journal of Medicine 367: 1694–1703.
12. Kim KB, Flaherty KT, Chapman PB, Sosman JA, Ribas A, et al. (2011) Pattern and outcome of disease progression in phase I study of vemurafenib in patients with metastatic melanoma (MM). Journal of Clinical Oncology 29: (abstract 8519).

13. Azer MF, Menzies AM, Haydu LE, Kefford RF, Long GV (2013) Patterns of Response and Progression in Patients with BRAF-mutant Melanoma Metastatic to the Brain treated with Dabrafenib. Cancer: in press.
14. Eisenhauer EA, Therasse P, Bogaerts J, Schwartz LH, Sargent D, et al. (2009) New response evaluation criteria in solid tumours: revised RECIST guideline (version 1.1). European Journal of Cancer 45: 228–247.
15. McArthur GA, Puzanov I, Amaravadi R, Ribas A, Chapman P, et al. (2012) Marked, homogeneous, and early [18F]fluorodeoxyglucose-positron emission tomography responses to vemurafenib in BRAF-mutant advanced melanoma. Journal of Clinical Oncology 30: 1628–1634.
16. Carlino MS, Saunders CA, Haydu LE, Menzies AM, Martin Curtis C Jr, et al. (2013) (18)F-labelled fluorodeoxyglucose-positron emission tomography (FDG-PET) heterogeneity of response is prognostic in dabrafenib treated BRAF mutant metastatic melanoma. European Journal of Cancer 49: 395–402.
17. Wilmott JS, Long GV, Howle JR, Haydu LE, Sharma RN, et al. (2012) Selective BRAF inhibitors induce marked T-cell infiltration into human metastatic melanoma. Clinical Cancer Research 18: 1386–1394.
18. Frederick DT, Piris A, Cogdill AP, Cooper ZA, Lezcano C, et al. (2013) BRAF Inhibition Is Associated with Enhanced Melanoma Antigen Expression and a More Favorable Tumor Microenvironment in Patients with Metastatic Melanoma. Clinical Cancer Research 19: 1225–1231.
19. Chan M, Haydu L, Menzies AM, Azer MWF, Klein O, et al. (2013) Clinical characteristics and survival of BRAF-mutant metastatic melanoma patients treated with BRAF inhibitor dabrafenib or vemurafenib beyond disease progression. Journal of Clinical Oncology 31: (abstract 9062).
20. Ackerman A, Klein O, McDermott DF, Lawrence DP, Gunturi A, et al. (2013) Outcomes of patients with metastatic melanoma treated with immunotherapy prior to or after BRAF inhibitors. Cancer: in press.
21. Ascierto PA, Simeone E, Giannarelli D, Grimaldi AM, Romano A, et al. (2012) Sequencing of BRAF inhibitors and ipilimumab in patients with metastatic melanoma: a possible algorithm for clinical use. Journal of Translational Medicine 10: 107.
22. Carlino MS, Gowrishankar K, Saunders CA, Pupo GM, Snoyman S, et al. (2013) Antiproliferative effects of continued mitogen-activated protein kinase pathway inhibition following acquired resistance to BRAF and/or MEK inhibition in melanoma. Molecular Cancer Therapeutics 12: 1332–1342.

9

Bystander Activation and Anti-Tumor Effects of CD8+ T Cells Following Interleukin-2 based Immunotherapy is Independent of CD4+ T Cell Help

Arta M. Monjazeb[1,9], Julia K. Tietze[2,9], Steven K. Grossenbacher[2], Hui-Hua Hsiao[2], Anthony E. Zamora[2], Annie Mirsoian[2], Brent Koehn[3], Bruce R. Blazar[3], Jonathan M. Weiss[4], Robert H. Wiltrout[4], Gail D. Sckisel[2], William J. Murphy[2,5]*

1 Department of Radiation Oncology School of Medicine, University of California Davis, Sacramento, California, United States of America, 2 Department of Dermatology, School of Medicine, University of California Davis, Sacramento, California, United States of America, 3 Department of Pediatrics, Division of Blood and Marrow Transplantation and Masonic Cancer Center, University of Minnesota, Minneapolis, Massachusetts, United States of America, 4 Cancer and Inflammation Program, National Cancer Institute, Frederick, Maryland, United States of America, 5 Department of Internal Medicine, School of Medicine, University of California, Davis, Sacramento, California, United States of America

Abstract

We have previously demonstrated that immunotherapy combining agonistic anti-CD40 and IL-2 (IT) results in synergistic anti-tumor effects. IT induces expansion of highly cytolytic, antigen-independent "bystander-activated" (CD8$^+$CD44^{high}) T cells displaying a CD25$^-$NKG2D$^+$ phenotype in a cytokine dependent manner, which were responsible for the anti-tumor effects. While much attention has focused on CD4+ T cell help for antigen-specific CD8+ T cell expansion, little is known regarding the role of CD4+ T cells in antigen-nonspecific bystander-memory CD8+ T cell expansion. Utilizing CD4 deficient mouse models, we observed a significant expansion of bystander-memory T cells following IT which was similar to the non-CD4 depleted mice. Expanded bystander-memory CD8+ T cells upregulated PD-1 in the absence of CD4+ T cells which has been published as a hallmark of exhaustion and dysfunction in helpless CD8+ T cells. Interestingly, compared to CD8+ T cells from CD4 replete hosts, these bystander expanded cells displayed comparable (or enhanced) cytokine production, lytic ability, and in vivo anti-tumor effects suggesting no functional impairment or exhaustion and were enriched in an effector phenotype. There was no acceleration of the post-IT contraction phase of the bystander memory CD8+ response in CD4-depleted mice. The response was independent of IL-21 signaling. These results suggest that, in contrast to antigen-specific CD8+ T cell expansion, CD4+ T cell help is not necessary for expansion and activation of antigen-nonspecific bystander-memory CD8+ T cells following IT, but may play a role in regulating conversion of these cells from a central memory to effector phenotype. Additionally, the expression of PD-1 in this model appears to be a marker of effector function and not exhaustion.

Editor: Natalia Lapteva, Baylor College of Medicine, United States of America

Funding: This work was supported by a grant from the NIH R01 CA095572. The funders had no role in study design, data collection and analysis, decision to publish, or preparation of the manuscript.

Competing Interests: The authors have declared that no competing interests exist.

* Email: wmjmurphy@ucdavis.edu

⑨ These authors contributed equally to this work.

Introduction

Classically, naïve and memory T cell activating signals include engagement of T-cell receptor (TCR) by cognate antigen in the setting of MHC. In a phenomenon termed "bystander activation" memory T-cells can proliferate and activate without the need for antigen specific TCR engagement [1,2,3]. These "bystander cells" proliferate and gain effector functions in response to the highly stimulatory local cytokine milieu produced during the course of viral and bacterial infections in mice and humans [4,5,6]. The function and regulation of these bystander activated T cells is unclear but they likely play a role in viral clearance [4,5,6].

Based on promising results in recent pilot clinical trials for cancer there has been a renewed interest in IL-2 based immunotherapy [7] as well as in agonistic CD40 antibodies [8].

We previously described that a combination immunotherapy consisting of agonist CD40 antibody and high dose systemic IL-2 (IT) resulted in synergistic antitumor effects which were CD8$^+$ T-cell dependent [9]. Recently we demonstrated that IT and other strong immunostimulatory therapies can overcome the need for antigen specificity for cytotoxic T lymphocyte (CTL) expansion and tumor cell killing [3]. Such regimens resulted in a massive expansion of CD44^{high} memory, but not naïve, CD8+ T-cells. This "bystander expansion" may play an important role in tumor immunity as it does in viral and bacterial infections. IT-induced bystander CD8+ T cells have a distinct phenotype (CD25$^-$NKG2D$^+$CD44^{high}) from CD8+ T cells activated via T-cell receptor (TCR) engagement and have the ability to initiate effector functions and cell killing independent of TCR engagement. IT-induced CD8+ T cells express NKG2D and provide anti-tumor killing in part due to NKG2D expression [3]. The anti-tumor effects of IT have been observed in a number of murine tumor models but whether this therapy would be effective against a tumor type completely devoid of NKG2D ligands remains unresolved.Further, in models of influenza infection, bystander CD8+ T cells (CD25⁻NKG2D⁺CD44ʰⁱᵍʰ) also acutely expand and play an important role in controlling early viral infection in an antigen nonspecific manner [10]. These findings demonstrate that during conditions of strong immunostimulation, such as viral infection or cancer immunotherapy, there is a massive expansion of cytolytic bystander activated memory phenotype CD8+ T cells which play a critical role in controlling viral infection or tumor in an antigen nonspecific manner.

IT can lead to loss of peripheral CD4+ T cells due to activation-induced cell death [11]. Little is known regarding the role of CD4+ T cells in regulating the expansion and function of bystander activated memory CD8+ T cells. The critical role of CD4+ T cell help in antigen-specific CD8+ T lymphocyte and general immune function is well illustrated by the sequelae suffered by patients suffering from AIDS. The need for CD4+ T-lymphocyte help in the function of both primary and memory CD8+ T lymphocyte responses is well established [12,13]. It has been demonstrated that the presence of CD4+ help during antigen-specific CD8+ cytotoxic T lymphocyte (CTL) priming is necessary for clonal expansion upon re-encountering antigen, since otherwise the restimulated CD8+ cells undergo TRAIL mediated cell death [14,15]. Furthermore, despite having been primed in the presence of CD4+ cells, memory CD8+ T cells can become functionally impaired if lacking CD4+ help [16]. Upregulation of PD-1 has become an important hallmark of the exhaustion and dysfunction of "helpless" CD8+ T cells [17,18]. The importance of CD4+ help has also been demonstrated for the recruitment, proliferation, and effector function of CTLs in the tumor microenvironment [19] and studies demonstrated increased tumor growth after CD4 depletion [20,21,22,23].

To further characterize the immunologic mechanisms behind the anti-tumor effects of IL-2-based immunotherapy and the role of CD4+ T cells in antigen non-specific bystander expansion, we analyzed the phenotype and function of the proliferating CD8+ cells after IT in the absence of CD4+ T cells. We observed that IT induces a massive expansion of CD25⁻NKG2D⁺ bystander memory CD8+ T cells and that the anti-tumor effects are CD8+ dependent. With both the in vivo depletion of CD4+ T cells or the use of CD4 KO mice we observed no change in the function or extent of expansion of CD44ʰⁱᵍʰ CD8+ T cells displaying a CD25⁻NKG2D⁺ bystander phenotype following immunotherapy compared to IT treated CD4 replete mice. Interestingly, in the absence of CD4+ T cells, the expanded bystander activated CD8+ T cell population upregulated PD-1 had an increased effector memory phenotype and did not have any functional evidence of exhaustion. These results suggest that, although antigen non-specific bystander expansion of memory CD8+ T-cells does not require CD4+ help in the same way as antigen specific CD8+ T cell expansion, there is a role for CD4+ help in regulating the conversion of these bystander cells from a central memory to effector memory/effector phenotype.

Materials and Methods

Ethics Statement

Mouse studies were performed with the approval of the University of California, Davis and University of Minnesota Institutional Animal Care and Use Committees (IACUC). For survival studies mice were sacrificed at humane endpoints as specified by IACUC guidelines using CO2 overdose. Humane endpoints included, but were not limited to, tumor burden greater than or equal to 10% of the animal's normal body weight, tumors exceeding 2 cm in size in, a 20% decrease in body weight, inability to reach food or water, or a body condition score less than 2 on a 5 point scale. Mice were monitored twice daily during the study period. No anesthesia or analgesia was used.

Mice

C57BL/6, CD4 knockout (B6.129S2-CD4ᵗᵐ¹ᴹᵃᵏ/J), and control mice were purchased from the animal production area of the National Cancer Institute (NCI) or The Jackson Laboratory. IL-21 receptor knockout mice (RKO) were generated as previously described [24]. Mice were 8 to 16 weeks old in all studies. Mice were housed in a specific pathogen free facility, four mice per cage, in micro-isolation cages, with a 12 hour light/dark cycle, and free access to food and water.

IT and depletion regimens

Mice were assigned to treatment or control groups randomly on a cage by cage basis. C57BL/6 mice were treated with agonistic anti-CD40 antibody and recombinant human IL-2 (rhIL-2) or IgG and PBS in the control groups as previously described [9]. The treatment schema is outlined in Fig. S1a. Briefly, anti-CD40 was administered daily for a total of 5 consecutive days (Days: 0, 1, 2, 3 and 4) and IL-2 was administered twice a day for a total of 4 days (Days: 1,4, 8 and 12). Control mice received rat-IgG (rIgG, Jackson ImmunoResearch Laboratories, Inc.) and PBS (Cellgro). Mice received 80 ug of agonist anti-CD40 and 1×10⁶ IU of IL-2 in 0.2 ml PBS i.p. Control mice received 80 ug of rIgG in PBS. The anti-mouse CD40 antibody (clone FGK115B3) was generated via ascites production, as previously described [9]. Recombinant human IL-2 (IL-2; TECIN Teceleukin) was provided by the National Cancer Institute repository (Frederick, MD). For in vivo depletion studies CD4⁺ T cells were depleted with i.p. injections of anti-CD4 antibody at 500 µg (clone GK1.5; gift from G.B. Huffnagle, University of Michigan, Ann Arbor, MI) (Fig. S1a). In short term depletion experiments mice received i.p. injections on days 0, 4, and 8. In long term depletion experiments mice received i.p. injections twice weekly for four weeks. CD8⁺ cells were depleted in vivo by i.p. injection of anti-mouse CD8 (clone 19–178). Two doses of Ab (163 µg/dose) were administered before the beginning of therapy and were continued three times weekly during the course of immunotherapy (>90% depletion). All treatments were performed in the vivarium in the housing cages.

Bromodeoxyuridine (BrdU) was purchased from BD Bioscience (San Jose, CA) and was used per the manufacturer's instructions. In experiments involving BrdU, 1 mg BrdU in 0.1 mL D-PBS was injected intraperitoneally 24 hours prior to harvest.

The 3LL cell line (ATCC) was maintained in RF10 complete media (RF10c). For *in vivo* tumor studies one million 3LL cells were administered by s.c. injection into the flank of C57BL/6 mice. Tumor volume was measured biweekly. All tumor survival experiments contained 8–15 mice/treatment group. In all experiments immunotherapy was initiated 7–10 days after tumor implantation when tumors were roughly 6×6 mm in size.

Flow cytometry and antibodies

Single cell suspensions were labeled with Fc Block (BD Bioscience) and antibodies for 20 minutes, and then washed twice with staining buffer consisting of DPBS (Mediatech, Herndon, VA) and 1% FBS (Gemini Bio-Products, Sacramento, CA). Samples were analyzed using a custom-configured LSRII with FACSDiva software (Becton Dickinson, San Jose, CA). The IntraPrep kit

(Beckman Coulter, Brea, CA) was used for granzyme staining, per manufacturer's instructions. Interferon gamma production was assayed by restimulating splenocytes with PMA/Ionomycin (0.16/1.6 ug/ml) for 4 hours in vitro. Golgi stop (0.7 ug/ml, BD Bioscience) was added following 1 hr of stimulation. Following stimulation, staining and analysis by flow cytometry was performed. Data were analyzed using FlowJo, Version 8 software (TreeStar, Ashland, OR). Antibodies included: PE-Cy7–conjugated anti-CD62L, FITC, PE, PE-Cy5, or APC-conjugated anti-CD25, APC-conjugated anti-CD44, PE or PE-Cy7–conjugated anti-NKG2D, FITC or PE-conjugated anti–PD-1, PE-conjugated anti-Vα2, APC-Cy7–conjugated anti-CD122 (eBioscience, San Diego, CA) FITC or APC-conjugated antiBrdU, APC-conjugated anti-CD8, and APC-Cy7–conjugated anti-CD25 (BD Pharmingen). Pacific Blue–conjugated anti-CD44 (BioLegend, San Diego, CA), PE-TexasRed–conjugated anti-CD8, and PE-conjugated anti–human Granzyme B (Invitrogen, Grand Island, NY). Intracellular staining was performed using staining kits for FoxP3 (eBioscience) and intra-cellular cytokines (BD biosciences) per manufacturer's instructions.

Antibody-redirected lysis assay

Splenic CD8+ T cells were serially diluted in 96-well U bottom plates in RF10c media. P815 (ATCC) cells were labeled with 100uCi ^{51}Cr (NEZ030S; Perkin Elmer) per 10^6 cells and incubated for 30 minutes with 10 ug/mL anti-CD3e (eBiosciences). P815 targets (10^4) were added to each well and incubated at 37°C for 4 hours. Supernatants were removed, mixed 1:1 with scintillation fluid, and analyzed on a Wallac scintillation counter (Wallac, Ramsey, MN). Total release was determined by adding 100 uL of 1× Triton X-100 detergent (Sigma-Aldrich, St. Louis, MO) to target cells. Specific release was calculated as: % lysis = 100% ×(Experimental-Spontaneous)/(Maximum–Spontaneous).

Tissue collection and processing

Lymph nodes including the cervical, scapular, axillary, and inguinal nodes were collected at day 11 or day 15 after the initiation of IT. Lymph nodes and spleens were crushed, filtered, and counted in DPBS. Prior to counting, red blood cells were lysed and cells counted using a Z1 Particle Counter (Beckman Coulter).

Statistics

Statistical analysis was performed using Prism Version 4 (GraphPad Software, Location). For analysis of 3 or more groups, the nonparametric ANOVA test was performed with the Bonferroni post-test. Analysis of differences between 2 normally distributed groups was performed using the Student's t test. Nonparametric groups were analyzed with the Mann-Whitney test. Welch's correction was applied to Student's t test datasets with significant differences in variance. Data were tested for normality and variance. A P value of <0.05 was considered significant (*P<0.05, **P<0.01, ***P<0.001).

Results

Expansion of bystander activated CD8+ T cells after systemic immunotherapy (IT)

The IT treatment schema for high dose IL-2 and agonist anti-CD40 is outlined in Figure S1a. Mice were harvested 11 days after the initiation of therapy to examine immune parameters. IT induced marked expansion of the CD8+ T-cell compartment that was predominately accounted for by the expansion of bystander activated CD8+ T cells with a CD44^{high} NKG2D+ CD25- phenotype (Fig. 1). The population of CD44^{high} T cells in these

naïve mice could result from homeostatic expansion or due to encountering cognate antigen in the environment or gut microflora. We have not distinguished between the two and this population which expands in response to therapy could be bonafide memory or memory-like cells (henceforth referred to simply as memory). The expanded cells are not CD8+ NK cells as they also express CD3 (data not shown) and this phenotype has also been seen on bystander activated OT-1 CD8+ T cells [3]. The number of these bystander activated cells was increased by greater than 30 fold in both the spleen and lymph nodes (Fig. 1b–c, p<0.05). In both the spleen and lymph nodes (LNs) these bystander activated memory cells became a significant portion of the CD8+ T-cell compartment with over 40% of splenic CD8+ T-cells displaying this phenotype after IT (Fig. 1d–e, p<0.05). Additionally, in a 3LL tumor model we found that the anti-tumor effects of IT were abrogated by CD8 depletion illustrating the critical role of CD8+ T-cells in the effectiveness of this therapy. Although IT was able to eradicate tumor growth (Fig. 1f) and lead to long term survival (Fig. 1g), in the absence of CD8+ cells there was no significant difference between untreated and IT treated mice. These effects are likely due to the absence of CD8+ T-cells and not CD8+ NK or DC cells as similar outcomes are seen in SCID mice which lack T-cells but have normal NK and DC cells [9].

Expansion of bystander activated CD8+ T-cells after IT is independent of CD4+ help

To elucidate the role of CD4+ T cell help in the expansion of bystander activated CD8+ T cells we employed multiple models in which CD4 T cells were absent. A short term (2 week) CD4 depletion model (Figure S1a) was used as the primary model for the majority of experiments. The long term depletion (6 weeks) model was used to confirm our results as it has been suggested that CD8+ T cell dysfunction only occurs after longer periods of lack of CD4 help [16]. Finally, CD4 knockout (CD4 KO) mice were used to validate our results in a model where complete absence of the cells occurs. The number of CD4+ T cells in the spleens and LNs of mice in our short term depletion model, long term depletion model and CD4 KO mice were >95% reduced in comparison to control CD4+ replete (CD4+ CTRL) mice (p<0.001, Figure S1b,c). Immunotherapy increased the expansion of the CD4+ T cells but CD4 depleted mice still had a significant reduction (p< 0.001) in the number of CD4+ T cells after IT (Figure S1b,c).

As demonstrated above, expansion of bystander activated memory CD8+ T cells is observed after treatment of CD4+ CTRL mice with IT (Fig. 1). This expansion can be accompanied by loss of CD4+ T cell help due to activation induced cell death [9,11]. We questioned whether CD4 depletion may influence the expansion of this antigen-nonspecific bystander memory compartment after IT. The IT induced increase of CD8+ T cells or CD44^{high} memory CD8+ cells in the LNs and spleens of CD4 depleted animals was maintained. In all cases, 11 days after the initiation of therapy IT induced a sizeable and statistically significant increase in cell numbers compared to untreated CD4+ CTRL mice regardless of CD4+ cell status (Fig. 2a–d). Similarly, the percentage of CD8+ or memory CD44^{high} CD8+ T cells after IT was increased in the spleens and LNs of both CD4+ CTRL and CD4 depleted mice compared to vehicle treated mice (data not shown). Additionally, assessment of proliferation by BrdU incorporation demonstrated that the memory CD8+ cells were expanding after IT in both CD4+ CTRL and CD4 depleted mice (Fig. 2e). CD44^{high} CD8+ cells were previously observed to proliferate after IT, and this is also the population seen to expand after IT in the setting of CD4 depletion.

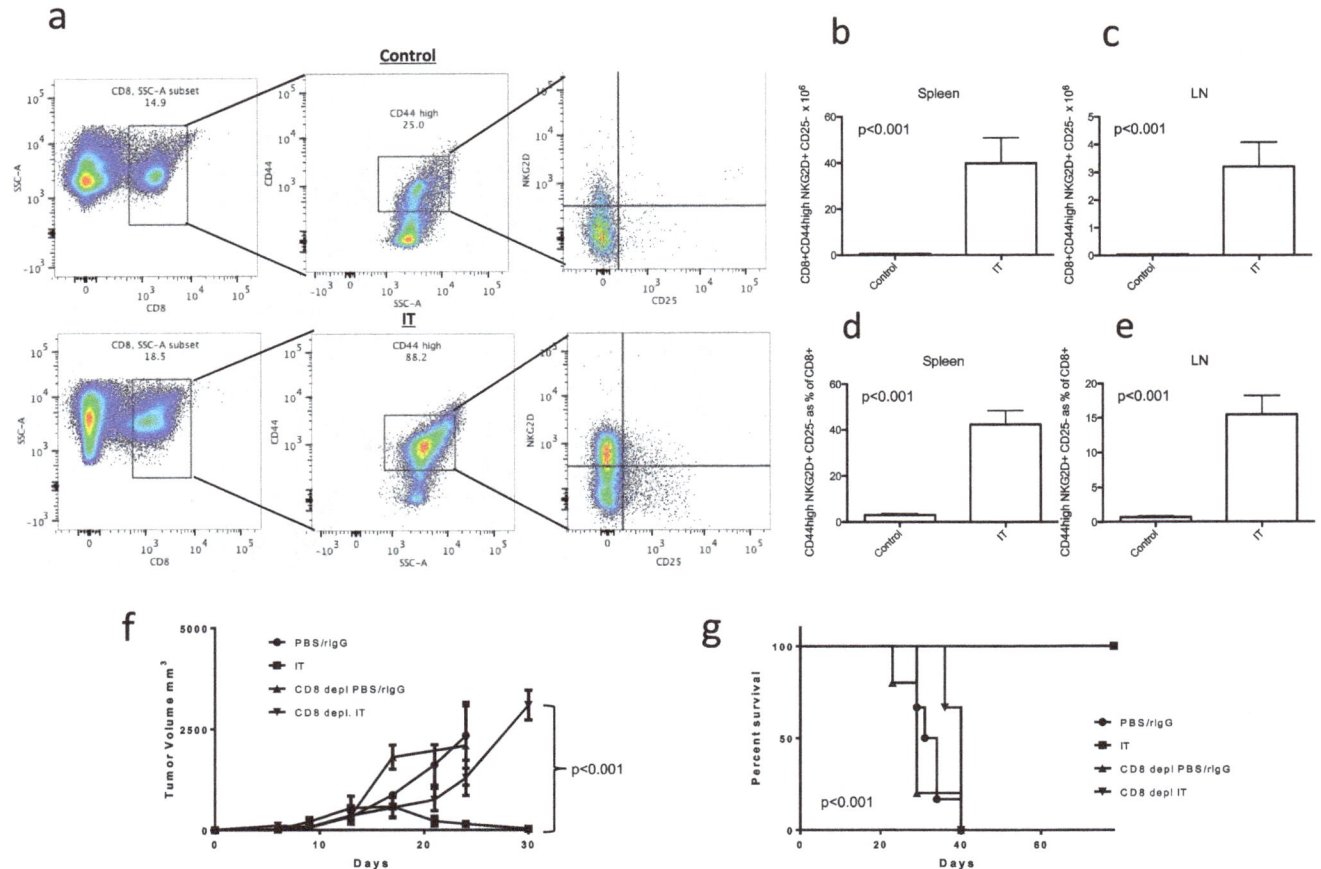

Figure 1. CD40/IL-2 Immunotherapy induces massive expansion of bystander memory CD8+ cells and anti-tumor effects are CD8 dependent. Three C57BL/6 mice per group were treated with IT or PBS/rIgG (control) and effects on CD8+ T cell expansion were quantified by flow cytometric analysis 11 days after the initiation of therapy. For *in vivo* tumor studies one million 3LL cells were administered by s.c. injection into the flank of C57BL/6 mice seven days prior to initiation of therapy. Six to eight 3LL bearing mice were treated with IT and/or CD8+ T cell depletion to examine CD8 dependence of anti-tumor effects. (**a**) Gating strategy for bystander memory CD8+ CD44^high NKG2D+ CD25− cells. (**b–e**) Expansion of bystander memory CD8+ T cells in the spleen and lymph nodes of IT or vehicle treated mice expressed as total numbers (**b,c**) or as a percentage of total CD8+ T cells (**d,e**). Effects of IT and/or CD8 depletion on tumor growth (**f**) and survival (**g**).

The effects of long term CD4 depletion on the memory CD8+ compartment after IT were examined using mice with long term depletion of CD4+ cells starting 30 days prior to treatment, or genetic disruption of CD4, using CD4 KO mice. Mirroring the above results, neither long-term depletion of CD4 (Figure S2) nor CD4 KO mice (Fig. 2f–i) demonstrated a reduction in the IT induced expansion of CD8+ cells or memory CD44^high CD8+ cells. Hence, in each of our models, that lack of CD4+ cells caused no reduction in the expansion of memory CD8+ T cells in response to IT. Surprisingly, in most instances, regardless of the model examined, the lack of CD4+ T-cells resulted in a trend or a statistically significant increase in the IT-induced expansion of memory CD8+ T cells compared to IT-treated CD4+ CTRL mice (Fig. 2a–d,f–i).

"Helpless" bystander activated memory CD8+ cells increase expression of PD-1 after IT but do not display functional characteristics of exhaustion and maintain anti-tumor effects in-vivo

It has been demonstrated in models of viral infection that lack of CD4+ help can upregulate PD-1 expression on CD8+ T cells leading to diminished anti-viral responses and a decrease in central

memory CD8+ cells [18,25]. PD-1 upregulation on CD8+ cells in chronic infections, such as HIV, has been associated with exhaustion of antigen specific CD8 +cells [26]. As demonstrated above, we observed no change in CD8+ T cell expansion after IT despite lack of CD4+ help. We further investigated the role of PD-1 expression after IT in mice lacking CD4 help. Interestingly, we found that, 11 days after the initiation of IT PD-1 expression was increased on memory CD8+ T cells in mice lacking CD4+ T cells compared to IT treated CD4+ CTRL mice (Fig. 3a–e). In CD4+ CTRL, CD4 depleted, and CD4 KO mice the levels of PD-1+ memory CD8+ T cells was minimal at baseline (Fig. 3a–e). IT induced a statistically significant increase in both the percentage (Fig. 3a) and total numbers of PD-1+ memory CD8+ T cells in both CD4+ CTRL and CD4 depleted or KO mice (Fig. 3b–e). Although PD-1 was increased in both the CD4+ CTRL and CD4 deficient models, the increase was most pronounced and significantly higher in the IT-treated CD4 depleted or KO mice when compared to IT treated CD4+ CTRL mice (Fig. 3a–e). For example, the levels of PD-1+ memory CD8+ T cells in the LNs of IT treated CD4 depleted mice were about 3-fold higher than IT-treated control mice (Fig. 3c,p<0.01). Similar results were observed in our long term depletion model (Figure S2).

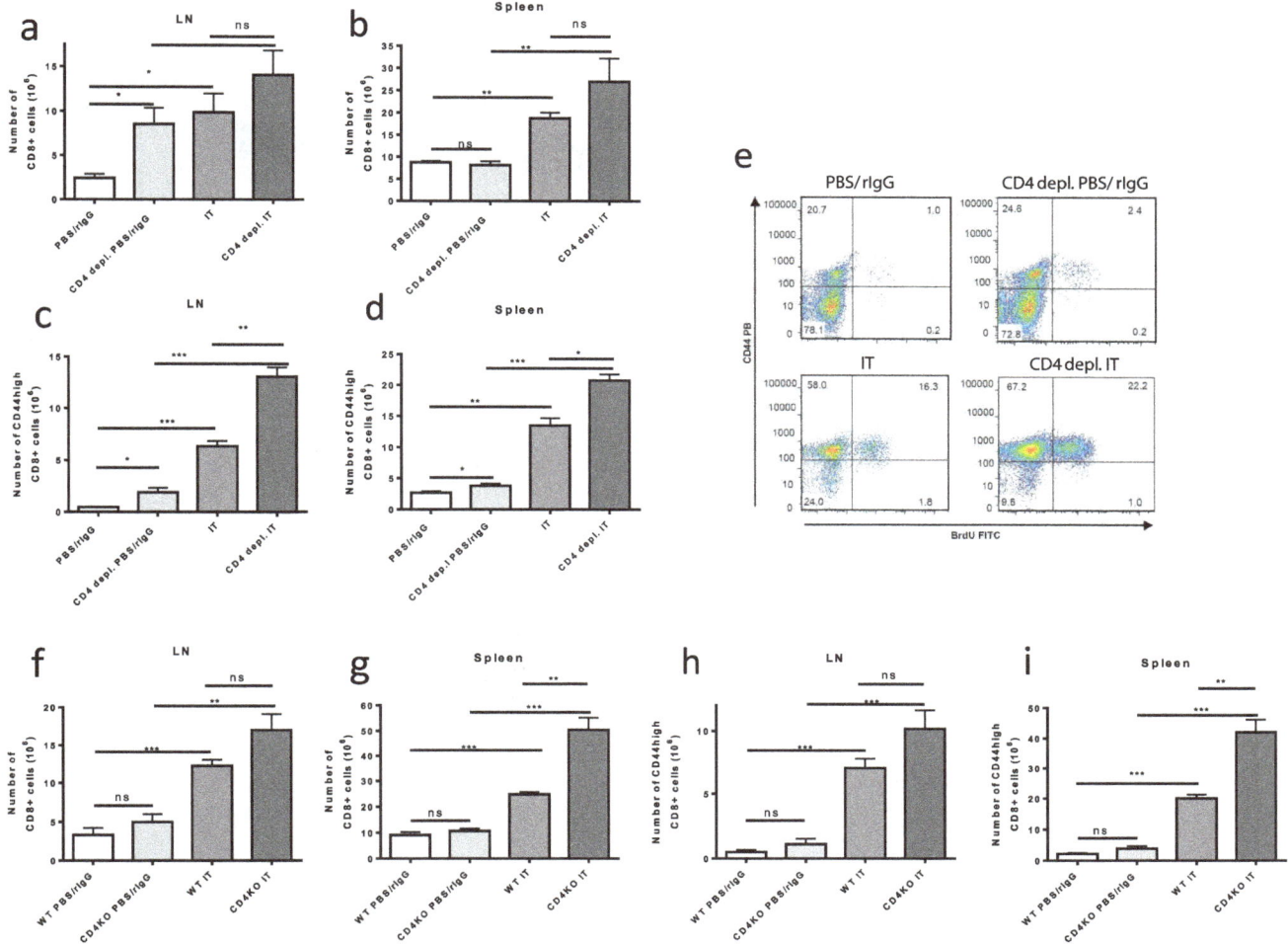

Figure 2. IT induced expansion of memory CD8+ T cells in CD4+ T cell deficient models. Control or CD4 deficient (depleted or knockout) C57BL/6 mice were treated with IT or PBS/rIgG (control) and effects on CD8+ T cell expansion were quantified by flow cytometric analysis 11 days after the initiation of IT. CD8+ (**a,b**) and memory CD8+ (**c,d**) T cell numbers in the LNs (**a,c**) and spleens (**b,d**) of control or CD4+ T cell depleted mice treated with vehicle or IT. (**e**) BrdU incorporation in CD8+ T cells from spleens of control or CD4+ T cell depleted mice treated with vehicle or IT. CD8+ (**f,g**) and memory CD8+ (**h,i**) T cell numbers in the LNs (**f,h**) and spleens (**g,i**) of wild-type or CD4 knockout mice treated with vehicle or IT. Results are representative of two (CD4 knockout) or three (CD4 depletion) independent experiments with a minimum of three mice per group. ($*P<.05$, $**P<.01$, $***P<.001$).

Given the intact expansion, but increased exhaustion phenotype of memory CD8+ T cells after IT in CD4 deficient mice we hypothesized that CD4+ help is required for the proper function but not expansion of the bystander memory CD8+ T-cells in response to IL-2 based immunotherapy. To test this hypothesis the phenotype, function, activation and *in-vivo* anti-tumor effects of CD8+ T-cells after IT in the absence of CD4+ cells was investigated. No differences in NKG2D upregulation after IT, which defines the IT induced bystander memory phenotype (CD8+ CD44^{high} NKG2D+ CD25−), was observed between CD4+ CTRL and CD4 depleted (Fig. 4a) or CD4 KO (Fig. 4f) mice 11 days after the initiation of IT. Despite the upregulation of PD-1 in the CD4 deficient models after IT, there was no functional impairment or dysfunction. The ability to produce cytokines was analyzed by assaying the percentage of memory CD8+ T-cells producing IFNγ after *in vitro* stimulation with PMA/Ionomycin. Again, IT significantly increased IFNγ production with no differences between IT treated CD4+ CTRL and CD4 depleted (Fig. 4c) or CD4 KO (Fig. 4g) mice. Likewise,

expression of granzyme B, a marker of CD8+ T cell activation, was increased after IT treatment with no differences between IT treated CD4+ CTRL and CD4 depleted (Fig. 4e) or CD4 KO (Fig. 4h) mice. Using *ex vivo* killing assays, we also observed that IT increased the lytic capacity of splenic CD8+ T cells across all groups (Fig. 4i,j). Not only was there no detriment in the killing function of the CD4 depleted (Fig. 4i) or CD4 KO (Fig. 4j) mice but they displayed a statistically significant improvement in killing function in comparison to IT-treated CD4+ CTRL mice. Similar results in regards to expression of NKG2D, IFNγ, and granzyme B as well as in vitro killing were observed in our long term CD4 depletion model (Figure S2).

Importantly, the *in vivo* anti-tumor effects of IT were also not diminished in CD4 deficient mice. IT conferred long term survival to both CD4+ CTRL and CD4 KO mice bearing 3LL tumors whereas the median survival for untreated mice ranged from 41–44 days (Fig. 5a). Likewise, all tumor growth was abrogated in IT treated CD4+ CTRL and CD4 KO mice whereas most tumors displayed progressive outgrowth in vehicle treated mice (Fig. 5b–f).

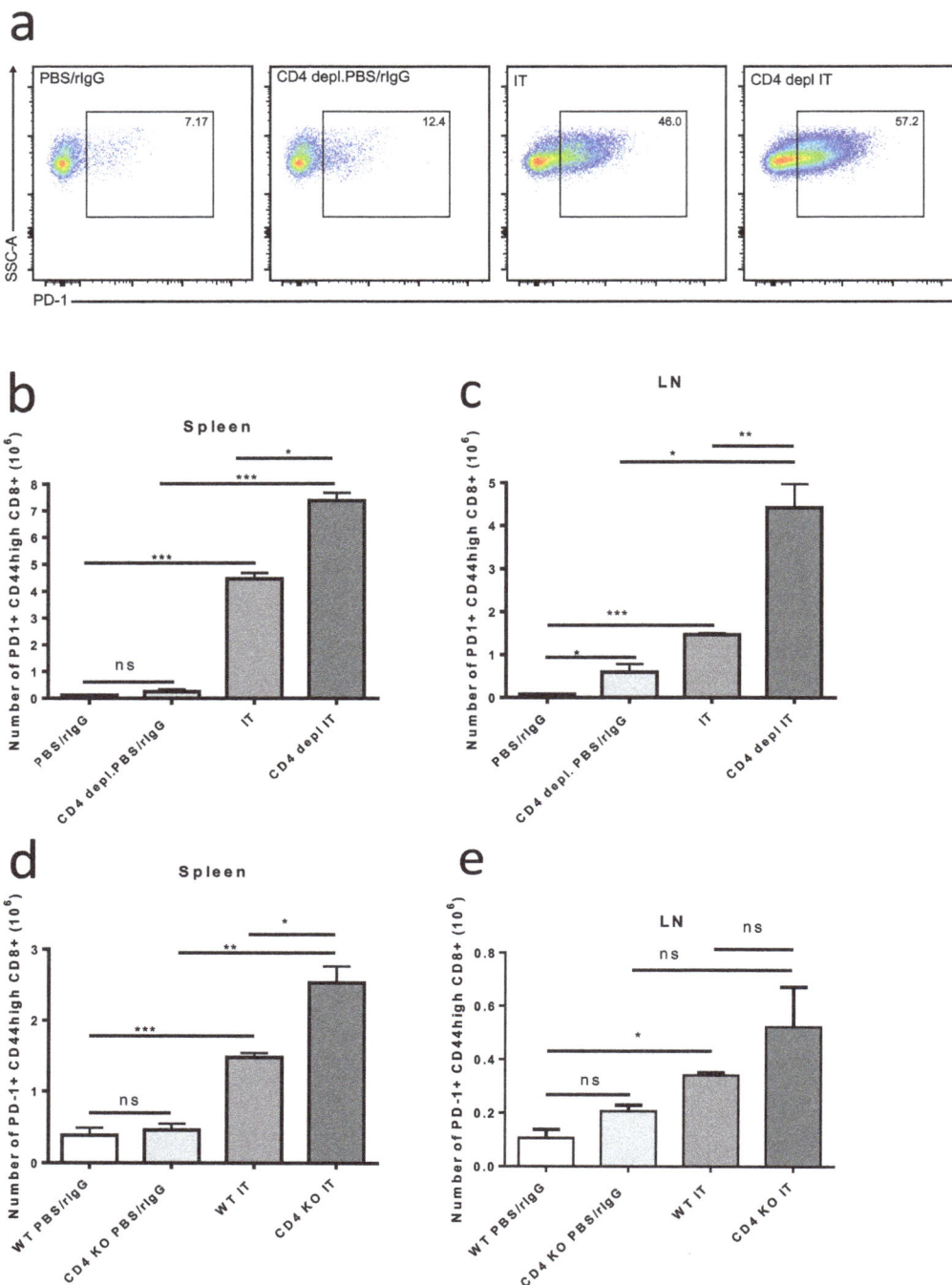

Figure 3. Increased number of PD-1+ memory CD8+ T cells after IT in CD4+ T cell deficient mice. Control or CD4 deficient (depleted or knockout) C57BL/6 mice were treated with IT or PBS/rIgG (control) and PD-1 expression on memory T-cells was quantified by flow cytometric analysis 11 days after the initiation of IT. (a) Representative dot plots for PD-1+ gating on CD8+ CD44high cells in the spleens of CD4+ depletion model mice. Number of PD-1+ memory (CD44high) CD8+ T cells in spleens (b,d) and LNs+ (c,e) of IT or vehicle treated mice in CD4+ depletion (b,c) or CD4 knockout (d,e) models. Results are representative of two (CD4 knockout) or three (CD4 depletion) independent experiments with a minimum of three mice per group. (*$P<.05$, **$P<.01$, ***$P<.001$).

Similar results were seen in tumor-bearing mice in our CD4 depletion model (data not shown). Taken together with our data above, these results clearly indicate that, despite upregulation of exhaustion markers, the expansion, function, and anti-tumor effects of the bystander memory CD8+ T cells induced by IT are independent of CD4 help and in some aspects, possibly enhanced by CD4 deficiency.

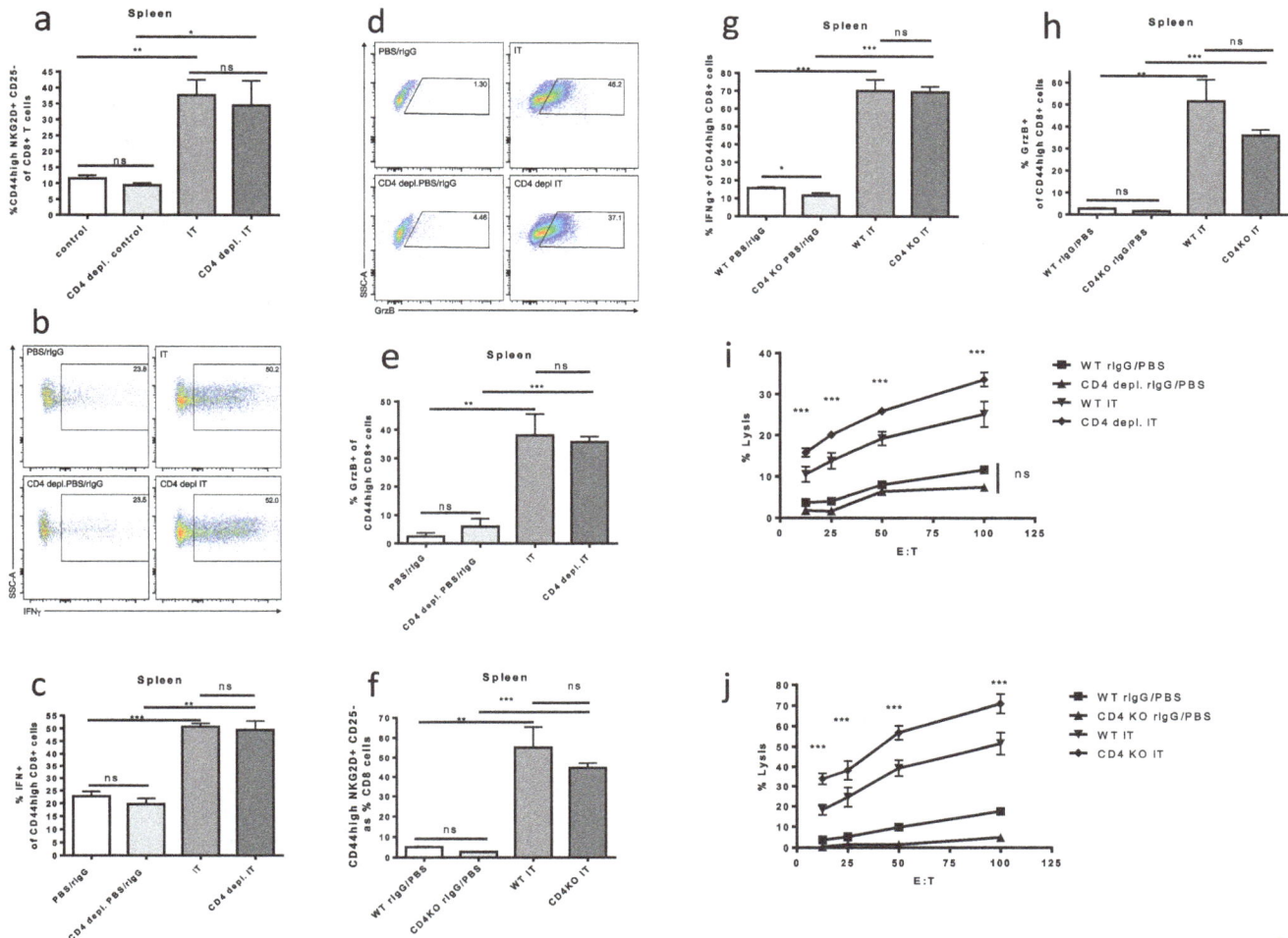

Figure 4. Memory CD8+ T cell function after IT in CD4+ T cell deficient models. Control or CD4 deficient (depleted or knockout) C57BL/6 mice were treated with IT or PBS/rIgG (control) and assessed for function of memory CD8+ T cells 11 days after the initiation of IT. NKG2D and granzyme B expression were quantified by flow cytometric analysis. Interferon gamma production was quantified by flow cytometric analysis after *in vitro* restimulation of splenocytes with PMA/Ionomycin (0.16/1.6 ug/ml) for one hour followed by incubation with golgi stop (0.7 ug/ml) for three hours. CD8+ T cell killing function was assayed by scintillation counting using an *in vitro* redirected lysis assay with ^{51}Cr labeled P815 target cells incubated for 30 minutes with 10 ug/mL anti-CD3e. (**a,f**) NKG2D expression on memory CD8+ T cells in CD4 depletion (**a**) and knockout (**f**) models. Representative dot plots for NKG2D+ CD25− gating are presented in Figure 1. (**b**) Representative dot plots for IFNγ+ gating on CD8+ CD44^{high} cells in the spleens of CD4+ depletion model mice. (**c,g**) Interferon gamma production by memory CD8+ T cells in CD4 depletion (**c**) and knockout (**g**) models. (**d**) Representative dot plots for Granzyme B+ gating on CD8+ CD44^{high} cells in the spleens of CD4+ depletion model mice. (**e,h**) Granzyme B expression by memory CD8+ T cells in CD4 depletion (**e**) and knockout (**h**) models. Killing function of splenocytes from CD4 depleted (**i**) or CD knockout (**j**) mice expressed as percentage of maximal lysis. Results are representative of two (CD4 knockout) or three (CD4 depletion) independent experiments with a minimum of three mice per group. (*P<.05, **P<.01, ***P<.001).

IL-21 signaling is not required for bystander memory CD8+ T cell expansion

IL-21 is able to sustain T cell responsiveness in chronic viral infections [27]. Other studies have found that a "helper-independent" phenotype of CTLs in cancer immunotherapy is due to IL-21 at the time of priming [28] and IL-21 has also been demonstrated to upregulate PD-1 [29]. Thus, IL-21 signaling could explain the phenotype and function of the expanded memory CD8 cells. Using mice lacking the receptor for IL-21 (IL-21rKO) the importance of IL-21 signaling on the IT induced function and expansion of bystander memory CD8+ T cells was examined. The lack of IL-21 signaling did not abrogate the IT induced proliferation of total CD8+ or CD44^{high} CD8+ memory cells in our models 11 days after the initiation of IT (Figure S3a,b). We also observed no differences in the expression of activation

(NKG2D) or exhaustion (PD-1) markers on the CD44^{high} memory CD8 T cells (Figure S3c,d). These results demonstrate that bystander memory CD8+ T cell expansion and function does not require IL-21 signaling.

Lack of CD4+ T cell help does not accelerate acute contraction of IT induced bystander memory CD8+ cells

It has been reported that CD4 help is required for the maintenance and survival of memory CD8+ T cells [16]. Although lack of CD4 help does not appear to adversely affect the acute phase of the IT induced response, it is possible that the magnitude or duration of IT effects on bystander memory CD8+ T cells would be adversely affected leading to accelerated contraction or dysfunction. To answer this question we used our long term CD4 depletion model (Figure S1a) and examined the immune response

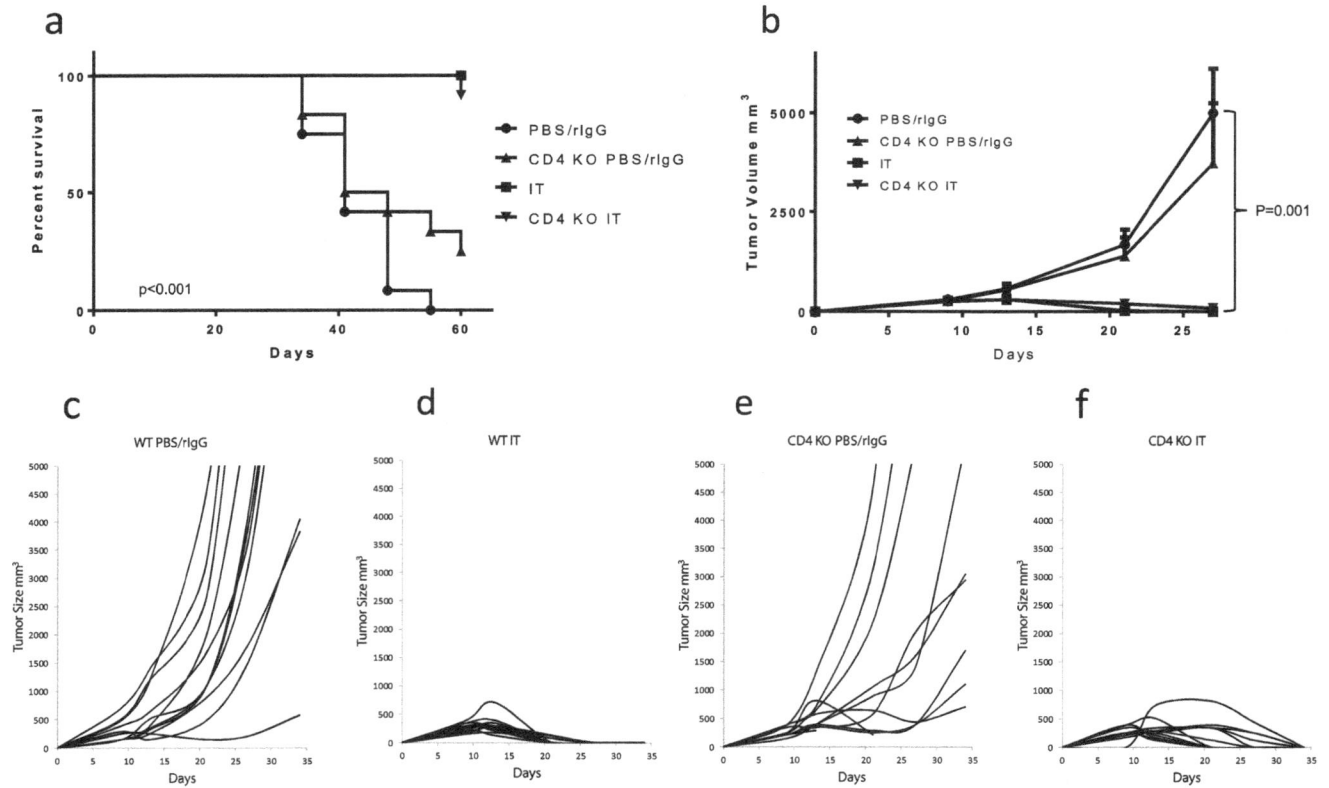

Figure 5. Anti-tumor effects of IT in CD4 knockout mice. 3LL tumor bearing WT or CD4 knockout (B6.129S2-CD4^{tm1Mak}/J) mice were treated with IT or PBS/rIgG (control) and survival and tumor growth were measured. For *in vivo* tumor studies one million 3LL cells were administered by s.c. injection into the flank of C57BL/6 mice seven days prior to initiation of therapy. (**a**) Survival. (**b**) Mean tumor volume with SEM. (**c–f**) Growth plots of individual tumors in each group. N = 12 mice per group. (*$P<.05$, **$P<.01$, ***$P<.001$).

at day 15 after the initiation of IT, as opposed to day 11 used above. Even at this later time point we see that the IT induced increase in bystander memory CD8+ T cells (CD25$^-$NKG2D$^+$CD44^{high}) is maintained in CD4 depleted mice (Fig. 6a,b) as is the increase in PD-1 expression (Fig. 6c,d). Furthermore, the functionality of these cells as assayed by IFNγ (Fig. 6e), granzyme b (Fig. 6f), and *in vitro* killing (Fig. 6g) was also maintained at this time point despite lack of CD4+ help. This does not rule out the possibility that there could be increased contraction or dysfunction, at later time points, in CD4 deficient mice.

CD4 depletion increases expression of PD-1 and conversion to effector phenotype on bystander memory CD8+ T cells after IT

Based on the lack of functional exhaustion above, we hypothesized that upregulation of PD-1 corresponded with another defined role as a marker of effector T cells [30,31]. Using CD62L to further characterize the bystander memory cells into central memory (CM) and effector/effector memory (EM) cells we investigated the expansion of these compartments and PD-1 expression 11 days after IT in CD4+ CTRL and CD4 deficient mice (Fig. 7a–c). In all cohorts of mice there was a significantly larger proportion of PD-1 expression on the EM CD62L^{low}CD44^{high}CD8+ cells than the CM CD62L^{high}CD44^{high}CD8+ cells (26–59% vs. 5–13%; Fig. 7a–c). IT treated mice had a statistically significant increase in PD-1 expression of both CM and EM cells whereas CD4+ depletion did not effect PD-1 expression (Fig. 7c). There was also a shift in the

composition of the memory compartment in IT treated mice from predominately CM to predominately EM with no more than 25% of memory cells displaying the EM phenotype in untreated mice and up to 75% after IT (Fig. 7d). Interestingly, in the setting of CD4 depletion, the IT induced shift to the EM phenotype was even more pronounced with 66% of memory cells from CD4+ CTRL mice displaying an EM phenotype compared to 83% in CD4 depleted mice (Fig. 7d, p = 0.07). Thus, IT increased PD-1 expression in the memory CD8+ T cells both by upregulating PD-1 expression on all memory cells and also by increasing the EM:CM ratio. This effectively increased PD-1 expression since PD-1 expression was in general higher on EM cells (Fig. 7a–d). In contrast, CD4 depletion did not increase PD-1 expression outright on EM or CM cells (Fig. 7c) but further increased the EM:CM ratio (Fig. 7d) thereby leading to the observed increase in PD-1 expression in the memory CD8+ T-cell compartment as a whole (Fig. 3). This notion, that PD-1 was predominately expressed on the EM cells and that lack of CD4 help increased the conversion of bystander cells from a central to effector memory phenotype, is further supported by examining PD-1 expression in the memory compartment as a whole. Neither IT nor CD4 depletion increased the subset of memory CD8+ T cells with a CM PD-1+ phenotype (Fig. 7e). Although IT did increase the percentage of PD-1+ CM cells (Fig. 7c), this was counterbalanced by the decrease of total CM cells in the memory CD8+ T cell compartment (Fig. 7d) leading to overall stability of CM PD-1+ cells as a percentage of total memory CD8+ T-cells. In contrast, the percentage of EM PD-1+ cells as a subset of total memory CD8+ T cells increased from 6% in CD4+ CTRL mice to 34% in IT treated

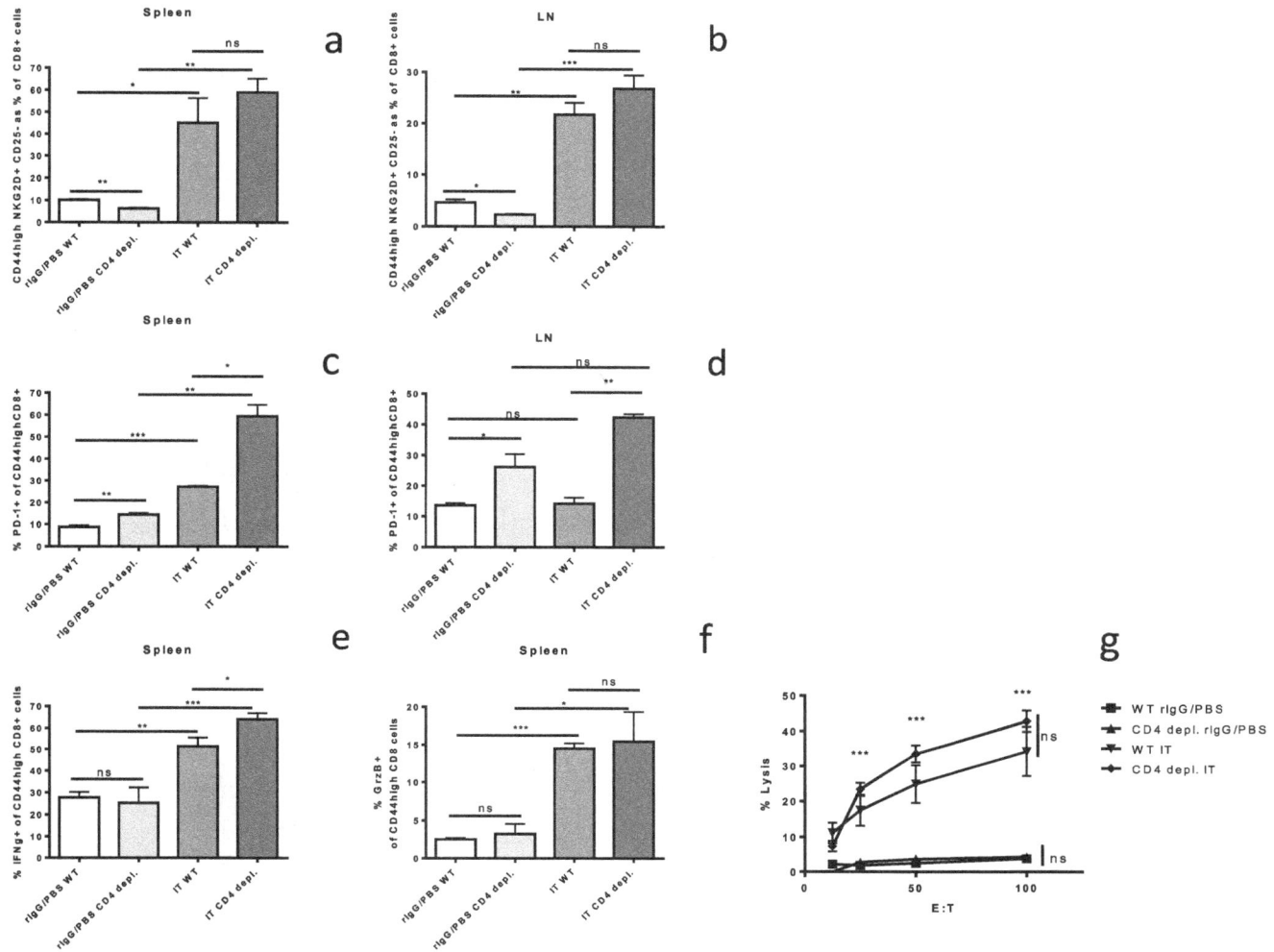

Figure 6. CD4 independence of IT induced bystander activated memory CD8+ T cells persists at longer time points. Control or long term CD4+ depleted C57BL/6 mice were treated with IT or PBS/rIgG (control) and harvested at Day 15 after the initiation of therapy. Bystander memory CD8+ T cells, PD-1 expression, interferon gamma production, and granzyme B production were quantified by flow cytometric analysis. Cytotoxic effector function was assayed by a redirected lysis assay. The percentage of CD8+ T cells with the CD44^{high} NKG2D+ CD25− bystander memory phenotype in the spleen (**a**) and LNs (**b**). PD-1 expression on the memory CD8+ T cells in the spleen (**c**) and LNs (**d**). Interferon gamma production (**e**) and granzyme B expression (**f**) in splenic memory CD8+ T cells. (**g**) Killing function of splenocytes from long term CD4 depleted mice expressed as percentage of maximal lysis. N = 3 mice per group (*P<.05, **P<.01, ***P<.001).

CD4+ CTRL mice (Fig. 7f, p<0.01). CD4 depletion further increased this to 49% which was significantly more than IT treated CD4+ CTRL mice (Fig. 7f, p<0.05). It, therefore, seems likely that PD-1 upregulation in CD4 depleted mice is not a result of increased exhaustion as we previously suspected but rather due to differential regulation of the conversion of CM to EM in the absence of CD4 T cell help.

Discussion

It has been demonstrated across different models that CD4+ help is needed to raise an efficient antigen specific CD8+ T cell response and for proper functioning of CD8+ memory cells. In general CD4+ T cell help can take many forms including activation of antigen presenting cells [32,33], direct CD40-CD40L interactions [34], maintenance [14,35] or mobilization of CD8+ cells [36]. In certain infections or inflammatory insults the initiation of CD8+ effector function may bypass the need for

CD4+ help [35,37,38]. Even in these instances the central role of CD4+ help has been demonstrated for maintenance and memory functions [35,38]. Some groups have demonstrated that CD4+ help is not required during priming but is mandatory for long term maintenance of the CD8+ cells [16] and protection from TRAIL induced death [15], while others have shown that CD8+ cells primed in the absence of CD4+ help may have an intact primary response but have a defective recall response even in the presence of CD4+ help [12]. The critical role of CD4+ T cell help in proper immune functioning is most clearly demonstrated in HIV+ patients suffering from AIDS. In models of viral infection including HIV it has been demonstrated that "helpless" CD8+ T cells upregulate PD-1 that diminishes the anti-viral response [17,18]. In this setting PD-1 expression is associated with T cell exhaustion and disease progression [17]. Although the critical nature of CD4+ help in primary and memory CD8+ responses is well examined the nature and necessity of CD4+ help in bystander generated memory T-cell responses is less well defined.

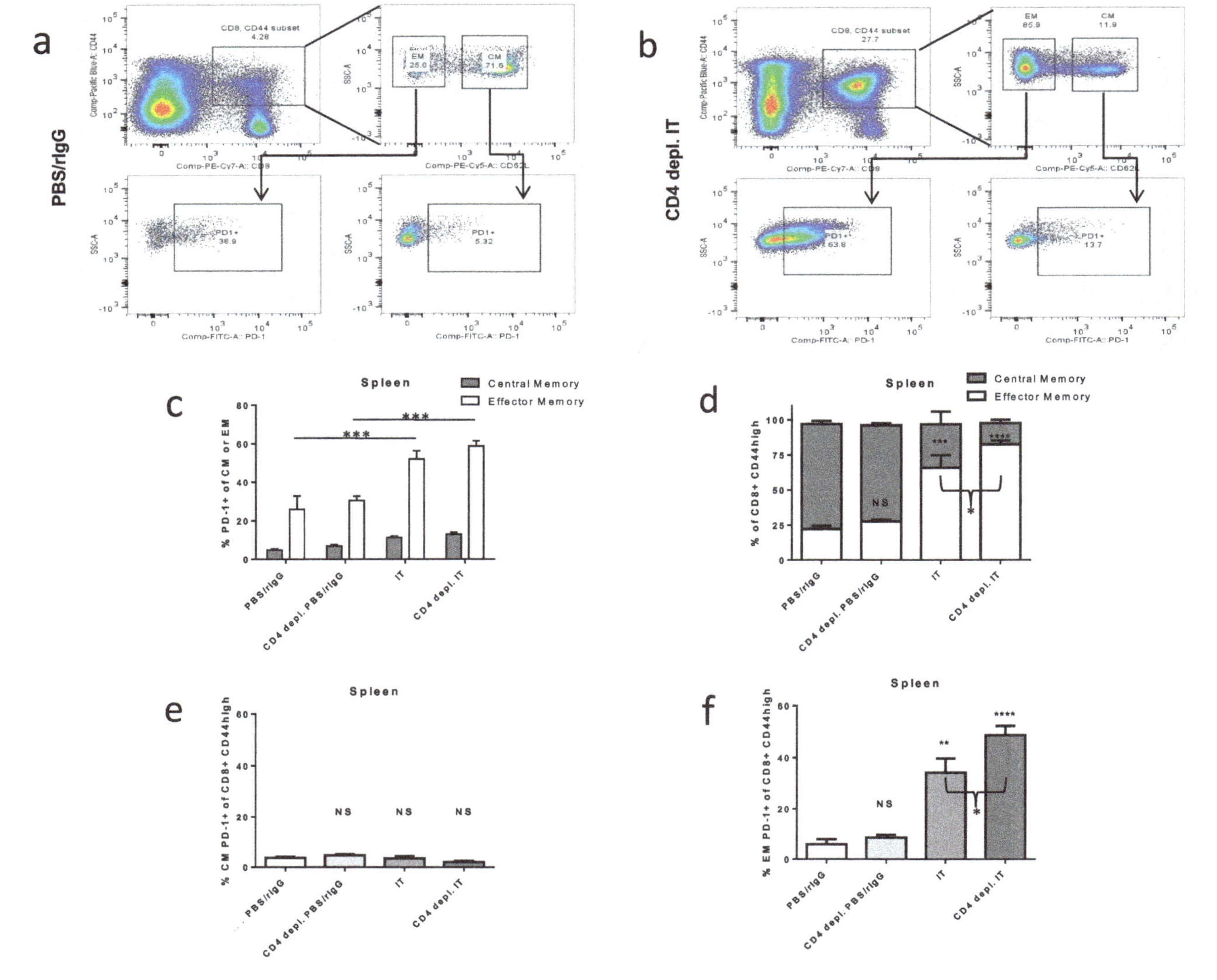

Figure 7. PD-1 expression on central and effector memory CD8+ T cells after IT in CD4+ T cell depleted mice. Control or CD4+ depleted C57BL/6 mice were treated with IT or PBS/rIgG (control). CD62L and PD-1 expression on memory T-cells was quantified by flow cytometric analysis 11 days after the initiation of IT. (**a,b**) Examples of the gating strategy for PD-1 expression on the CM and EM components of the memory CD8+ T cell compartment. The majority of cells in the memory compartment are CM in untreated mice (**a**) and EM in IT treated mice (**b**). (**c**) PD-1 expression on CM and EM cells. (**d**) The composition of the memory CD8+ T cell compartment in control or CD4 depleted mice treated with IT or PBS/rIgG. PD-1+ CM cells (**e**) and PD-1+ EM cells (**f**) as a percentage of the total memory CD8+ T cell compartment. Results are representative of two to three independent experiments with 3 mice per group (*$P<.05$, **$P<.01$, ***$P<.001$, ****$P<.0001$).

We have previously demonstrated that IL-2 based immunotherapy, in combination with CD40 agonist, results in synergistic anti-tumor effects which are CD8+ T-cell dependent but not antigen restricted [3,9] and (Fig. 1). There is a massive expansion of bystander (CD25−NKG2D+CD44^{high}) memory CD8+ T-cells (Fig. 1) similar to "bystander expansion" that is seen after viral or bacterial infections [2,3,4,10]. We have also demonstrated that IT can lead to progressive loss of CD4+ T cells by activation induced cell death [11]. Interestingly in our models of influenza infection these same bystander activated memory CD8+ T cells (CD25−NKG2D+CD44^{high}) acutely expand and play an important role in controlling early viral infection in an antigen nonspecific manner [10]. Thus, understanding the role of CD4+ help in the expansion and effector function of these bystander cells

has important implications for both cancer immunotherapy and viral immunity.

In this study we observed that lack of CD4+ cells causes homeostatic proliferation in the CD8+ T cell compartment of mice with increased numbers of CD8+ and CD44^{high}CD8+ T cells in spleens and LNs of CD4 deficient non-IT treated mice compared to CD4 replete non-IT treated mice (Fig. 2a–d). This is in agreement with other studies of homeostatic expansion of CD8+ T-cells in CD4 deficiency. Using IT in models of CD4 deficient mice we found that surface expression of exhaustion marker PD-1 was upregulated (Fig. 3). However, in contrast to other settings of CD4 deficiency, the lack of CD4+ T cell help did not appear to have any implications on the expansion or function of bystander memory CD8+ T cells induced by IT. We found that neither the expansion of memory CD8+ T cells nor of the CD8+ T cell compartment in general was adversely affected by depletion or genetic disruption of CD4+ help (Fig. 2). Likewise, when analyzing the functional characteristics of these IT induced bystander memory cells, such as upregulation of NKG2D, increased production of granzyme b and interferon gamma, and *in vitro* killing, we observed no detrimental effects of CD4+ deficiency (Fig. 4). Importantly, the in vivo anti-tumor effects of IT also remained intact in CD4+ deficient models (Fig. 5). Although some of the phenotypic CD8+ T cell changes observed in other "helpless" models, such as upregulation of PD-1, were expressed, it appears that in our models the cells are not exhausted and that their functional effector capabilities remain intact. The long term consequences of IT in the setting of CD4 depletion on the function of CD8+ T-cells and response to tumor re-challenge have not been explored, however, we have previously demonstrated that even in the presence of CD4+ T-cell help secondary responses after immunotherapy can become impaired due to activation induced cell death after strong cytokine stimulation [11].

In some aspects the expansion and effector function of CD8+ T cells after IT was enhanced in our CD4 deficient models. Whether our results are due to lack of helper CD4+ T cells or other CD4 expressing cells such as regulatory T cells or natural killer-T cells is unclear. Indeed one general shortcoming of our models is that they fail to distinguish between CD4+ helper T-cells and other CD4+ cell types. These findings could be attributed to lack of CD4+ CD25+FoxP3+ regulatory T cells (Tregs) in the CD4 deficient models. However, the effects of IT in CD25 deficient mouse models (data not shown) were similar to that observed in control mice and did not mirror the enhanced effects in CD4 deficient models. This would argue against lack of Tregs as the mechanism for enhanced response seen in CD4 deficient models although further study in other models is needed. Likewise, the increased expression of PD-1 seen after IT (Fig. 3) in our CD4 deficient mice was not mirrored in our CD25 deficient mouse models (data not shown) also arguing against lack of Tregs as the underlying mechanism for this finding. The increased shift from CM to EM phenotype in CD4 deficient models (Fig. 7) could explain the increased killing function after IT but does not explain the increased expansion. As previously mentioned, there is increased baseline homeostatic expansion of the CD8+ compartment even in the absence of IT and it is reasonable to presume that this could contribute to the increased expansion seen with IT.

Although PD-1 is generally considered an exhaustion marker, other functions have also described. For example PD-1 has been shown to be upregulated during activation it can have a role in stimulating CD8+ cells during a primary response, and it can be a marker of cytotoxic effector function [30,31]. The exact reason for the discrepancy between the need for CD4+ help and the role of PD-1 in our models versus much of the published literature is unresolved. A few possibilities might explain this discrepancy: 1) IL-21 in the setting of IT and anti-tumor responses bypasses the need for CD4+ help; 2) the effects of our highly stimulatory IT are such that they "rescue" the "helpless" CD8+ cells from exhaustion; or 3) the regulation of bystander activated memory CD8+ T-cells is different than the regulation of antigen specific CD8+ T-cells. Further study is needed to resolve these possibilities although our current findings, highlighted below, suggest that these last two possibilities are most likely.

PD-1 has been described to be inducible on many subsets of immune cells [26] and on CD8+ T cells can occur as early as 24 hours after stimulation [39]. The role of early PD-1 upregulation is not yet completely defined, but it is likely that it dampens CD8+ effector responses to control the immune response. Prolonged upregulation of PD-1 is associated with exhaustion

[17]. Thus, the CD4+ independent effects of IT may be an artifact of our model and at longer time points there could be increased exhaustion and dysfunction or acceleration in the contraction phase post-IT. To address this possibility we examined the effects of long term depletion of CD4+ T cells on IT and also analyzed later time points after the completion of IT. 15 days after the initation of IT there was no deterioration of the numbers or function of the bystander memory CD8+ T cells in CD4 depleted mice as compared to IT treated CD4+ CTRL mice (Fig. 6). This does not rule out the possibility that there could be increased contraction or dysfunction, at even later time points, in CD4 deficient mice. We have previously observed that there are negative long-term consequences after IT even in the presence of CD4+ T-cell help [11].

Others have also reported CD4 helper independent CD8+ T-cell anti-tumor activity. In a report by Adam et al. [40] they find that in certain settings NK cells can activate DCs and IL-12 production bypassing the need for CD4 help in the activation of anti-tumor CD8+ T-cells. We have previously demonstrated that depletion of NK cells does not abrogate the efficacy of our IT making it unlikely that this mechanism is responsible for our findings [9]. Another possibility is that the CD40 agonist anti-body and may bypass the need for CD4+ help by directly activating APCs [41] which seems plausible. It has also been demonstrated in cancer immunotherapy models that there can be a "helper-independent" phenotype of CTLs after immunotherapy that is due to IL-21 at the time of priming [28]. IL-21 has been described to be predominately produced by CD4 T cells and natural killer cells [42]. It promotes CD8 cell activation and has been proposed to act as a third signal [27,43]. IL-21 has also been demonstrated to upregulate PD-1 [29]. Thus, it is possible that IL-21 present in the setting of immunotherapy, but perhaps lacking in antigen specific CD8+ T cell expansion models, is circumventing the need for CD4+ help in this setting. Our results, however, demonstrated that genetic abrogation of IL-21 signaling did not disrupt the phenotype of the CD8+ bystander memory cells in our model (Figure S3). This argues against IL-21 signaling as being the sole or predominant mechanism of the "helper-independent" phenotype. This does not discount the possibility of other potential differences between the immune system in IT settings and other settings could be responsible for our findings. The upregulation of PD-1 on "helpless" CD8+ cells has been shown to be marker of the exhaustion and dysfunction of T cells. In our studies, however, we found no evidence of dysfunction or exhaustion in the CD4 deficient setting and found that in some instances there was even upregulation of functional activity. Further examination showed that in the CD8+ memory compartment PD-1 expression was much higher on effector memory than central memory cells. Although PD-1 increased in response to IT, the additional increase in PD-1 seen in CD4 deficient mice was due to an increased shift from the central to effector memory phenotypes compared to CD4 replete mice treated with IT (Fig. 7). This increase in effector memory cells could also explain the enhanced effectiveness of IT in CD4 deficient models seen in some of our studies.

Taken together our results suggest that, in contrast to antigen-specific CD8+ T cell expansion, CD4+ T cell help is not necessary for the expansion and activation of antigen-nonspecific bystander memory CD8+ T cells following immunotherapy, yet may play a role in regulating the conversion of these bystander cells from a central memory to effector phenotype. Further study is needed to clarify whether bystander cells induced by acute viral infections are regulated in a similar manner. Another important consideration, which is a topic of current investigation in our lab, is how the altered function and regulation of bystander activated memory

CD8+ T cells effects the functioning of the rest of the immune system. The strong immunostimulatory conditions, such as IL-2 immunotherapy or viral infection, that induce bystander activated memory CD8+ T cells may allow for expansion and antigen independent effector function of these cells, even in the absence of CD4+ help which is lost via activation induced cell death. What effect these conditions have on the priming of a new response is unknown. However, we could posit, and are currently investigating, that the epitope spreading required for a successful immune response in the setting of viral infection or cancer immunotherapy could be hampered. Also under investigation is the long term effects of IT induced bystander cells on immune function weeks to months after post-IT contraction. These unresolved questions will provide us with greater insight into the functioning, regulation, and consequences of antigen non-specific bystander memory CD8+ T cell responses.

Supporting Information

Figure S1 Depiction of treatment schemas and evaluation of CD4 deficient models. (a) Schema of short-term CD4 depletion, long term CD4 depletion, and immunotherapy protocols. These therapies were administered to naïve or tumor bearing mice depending on the experiment. (b,c) Evaluation of the CD4[+] T-cell compartment in control and CD40 + IL-2 immunotherapy (IT) treated mice in WT or CD4 deficient mice. Lymph nodes (b) and spleens (c) of anti-body depleted or knock out mice were evaluated for CD4+ staining by FACS analysis after treatment with vehicle or IT. Data are results of two to four independent experiments with three mice per group. (*** $P<.001$).

Figure S2 IT induced immunologic effects in the long term CD4 depletion model. Control or long term CD4 depleted C57BL/6 mice were treated with IT or PBS/rIgG (control) and effects on CD8+ T cell expansion, PD-1 expression, and function were quantified by flow cytometric analysis. NKG2D and granzyme B expression were quantified by flow cytometric analysis. Interferon gamma production was quantified by flow cytometric analysis after *in vitro* restimulation of splenocytes with

PMA/Ionomycin (0.16/1.6 ug/ml) for one hour followed by incubation with golgi stop (0.7 ug/ml) for three hours. CD8+ T cell killing function was assayed by scintillation counting using an *in vitro* redirected lysis assay with ^{51}Cr labeled P815 target cells incubated for 30 minutes with 10 ug/mL anti-CD3e. CD8+ (a,b) and memory CD8+ (c,d) T cell numbers in the LNs (a,c) and spleens (b,d) of control or CD4 T cell depleted mice treated with vehicle or IT. Number of PD-1+ memory (CD44^{high}) CD8+ T cells in LNs (e) and spleen (f) of IT or vehicle treated mice. (g) NKG2D expression, (h) Interferon gamma production, and (i) Granzyme B expression by memory CD8+ T cells in long term CD4 depleted mice. (j) Killing function of splenocytes from CD4 depleted mice expressed as percentage of maximal lysis. Results are representative of three independent experiments with a minimum of three mice per group. (*$P<.05$, **$P<.01$, ***$P<.001$).

Figure S3 IT induced function and expansion of bystander memory CD8+ Tcells does not require IL-21 signaling. Wild-type or IL-21 RKO were treated with IT or PBS/rIgG (control) and harvested at Day 11 after the initiation of therapy. CD8+ T cell and memory CD8+ T cell expansion, and NKG2D and PD-1 expression were quantified by flow cytometric analysis. Total number of splenic CD8+ T cells (a) and memory CD8+ T cells (b). The percentage of NKG2D+ (c) or PD-1+ (d) splenic memory CD8+ T cells. Results are representative of three independent experiments with three mice per group. (*$P<.05$, **$P<.01$, ***$P<.001$).

Author Contributions

Conceived and designed the experiments: AMM JKT GDS WJM BRB. Performed the experiments: AMM JKT SKG HH AEZ AM BK GDS. Analyzed the data: AMM JKT SKG GDS BRB JMW RHW GDS WJM. Contributed reagents/materials/analysis tools: AMM BRB JMW RHW WJM. Wrote the paper: AMM JKT. Critical Review of Data: BRB JMW RHW AMM JKT GDS WJM.

References

1. Murali-Krishna K, Altman JD, Suresh M, Sourdive DJ, Zajac AJ, et al. (1998) Counting antigen-specific CD8 T cells: a reevaluation of bystander activation during viral infection. Immunity 8: 177–187.
2. Tough DF, Borrow P, Sprent J (1996) Induction of bystander T cell proliferation by viruses and type I interferon in vivo. Science 272: 1947–1950.
3. Tietze JK, Wilkins DE, Sckisel GD, Bouchlaka MN, Alderson KL, et al. (2012) Delineation of antigen-specific and antigen-nonspecific T-cell responses after cytokine-based cancer immunotherapy. Blood 119: 3073–3083.
4. Belz GT, Doherty PC (2001) Virus-specific and bystander CD8+ T-cell proliferation in the acute and persistent phases of a gammaherpesvirus infection. J Virol 75: 4435–4438.
5. Dhanji S, Teh SJ, Oble D, Priatel JJ, Teh HS (2004) Self-reactive memory-phenotype CD8 T cells exhibit both MHC-restricted and non-MHC-restricted cytotoxicity: a role for the T-cell receptor and natural killer cell receptors. Blood 104: 2116–2123.
6. Ehl S, Hombach J, Aichele P, Hengartner H, Zinkernagel RM (1997) Bystander activation of cytotoxic T cells: studies on the mechanism and evaluation of in vivo significance in a transgenic mouse model. J Exp Med 185: 1241–1251.
7. Seung SK, Curti BD, Crittenden M, Walker E, Coffey T, et al. (2012) Phase 1 study of stereotactic body radiotherapy and interleukin-2–tumor and immunological responses. Sci Transl Med 4: 137ra174.
8. Beatty GL, Chiorean EG, Fishman MP, Saboury B, Teitelbaum UR, et al. (2011) CD40 agonists alter tumor stroma and show efficacy against pancreatic carcinoma in mice and humans. Science 331: 1612–1616.
9. Murphy WJ, Welniak L, Back T, Hixon J, Subleski J, et al. (2003) Synergistic anti-tumor responses after administration of agonistic antibodies to CD40 and IL-2: coordination of dendritic and CD8+ cell responses. J Immunol 170: 2727–2733.
10. Sckisel GD, Tietze JK, Zamora AE, Hsiao HH, Priest SO, et al. (2014) Influenza infection results in local expansion of memory CD8(+) T cells with antigen non-specific phenotype and function. Clin Exp Immunol 175: 79–91.
11. Berner V, Liu H, Zhou Q, Alderson KL, Sun K, et al. (2007) IFN-gamma mediates CD4+ T-cell loss and impairs secondary antitumor responses after successful initial immunotherapy. Nat Med 13: 354–360.
12. Shedlock DJ, Shen H (2003) Requirement for CD4 T cell help in generating functional CD8 T cell memory. Science 300: 337–339.
13. Sun JC, Bevan MJ (2003) Defective CD8 T cell memory following acute infection without CD4 T cell help. Science 300: 339–342.
14. Janssen EM, Lemmens EE, Wolfe T, Christen U, von Herrath MG, et al. (2003) CD4+ T cells are required for secondary expansion and memory in CD8+ T lymphocytes. Nature 421: 852–856.
15. Janssen EM, Droin NM, Lemmens EE, Pinkoski MJ, Bensinger SJ, et al. (2005) CD4+ T-cell help controls CD8+ T-cell memory via TRAIL-mediated activation-induced cell death. Nature 434: 88–93.
16. Sun JC, Williams MA, Bevan MJ (2004) CD4+ T cells are required for the maintenance, not programming, of memory CD8+ T cells after acute infection. Nat Immunol 5: 927–933.
17. Day CL, Kaufmann DE, Kiepiela P, Brown JA, Moodley ES, et al. (2006) PD-1 expression on HIV-specific T cells is associated with T-cell exhaustion and disease progression. Nature 443: 350–354.
18. Fuse S, Tsai CY, Molloy MJ, Allie SR, Zhang W, et al. (2009) Recall responses by helpless memory CD8+ T cells are restricted by the up-regulation of PD-1. J Immunol 182: 4244–4254.
19. Bos R, Sherman LA (2010) CD4+ T-cell help in the tumor milieu is required for recruitment and cytolytic function of CD8+ T lymphocytes. Cancer Res 70: 8368–8377.

20. Hu HM, Winter H, Urba WJ, Fox BA (2000) Divergent roles for CD4+ T cells in the priming and effector/memory phases of adoptive immunotherapy. J Immunol 165: 4246–4253.

21. Marzo AL, Kinnear BF, Lake RA, Frelinger JJ, Collins EJ, et al. (2000) Tumor-specific CD4+ T cells have a major "post-licensing" role in CTL mediated anti-tumor immunity. J Immunol 165: 6047–6055.

22. Lodge A, Yu P, Nicholl MB, Brown IE, Jackson CC, et al. (2006) CD40 ligation restores cytolytic T lymphocyte response and eliminates fibrosarcoma in the peritoneum of mice lacking CD4+ T cells. Cancer Immunol Immunother 55: 1542–1552.

23. Liu Z, Noh HS, Chen J, Kim JH, Falo LD Jr, et al. (2008) Potent tumor-specific protection ignited by adoptively transferred CD4+ T cells. J Immunol 181: 4363–4370.

24. Bucher C, Koch L, Vogtenhuber C, Goren E, Munger M, et al. (2009) IL-21 blockade reduces graft-versus-host disease mortality by supporting inducible T regulatory cell generation. Blood 114: 5375–5384.

25. Allie SR, Zhang W, Fuse S, Usherwood EJ (2011) Programmed Death 1 Regulates Development of Central Memory CD8 T Cells after Acute Viral Infection. J Immunol.

26. Keir ME, Butte MJ, Freeman GJ, Sharpe AH (2008) PD-1 and its ligands in tolerance and immunity. Annu Rev Immunol 26: 677–704.

27. Yi JS, Cox MA, Zajac AJ (2010) Interleukin-21: a multifunctional regulator of immunity to infections. Microbes Infect 12: 1111–1119.

28. Li Y, Bleakley M, Yee C (2005) IL-21 influences the frequency, phenotype, and affinity of the antigen-specific CD8 T cell response. J Immunol 175: 2261–2269.

29. Kinter AL, Godbout EJ, McNally JP, Sereti I, Roby GA, et al. (2008) The common gamma-chain cytokines IL-2, IL-7, IL-15, and IL-21 induce the expression of programmed death-1 and its ligands. J Immunol 181: 6738–6746.

30. Zelinskyy G, Myers L, Dietze KK, Gibbert K, Roggendorf M, et al. (2011) Virus-specific CD8+ T cells upregulate programmed death-1 expression during acute friend retrovirus infection but are highly cytotoxic and control virus replication. J Immunol 187: 3730–3737.

31. Hokey DA, Johnson FB, Smith J, Weber JL, Yan J, et al. (2008) Activation drives PD-1 expression during vaccine-specific proliferation and following lentiviral infection in macaques. Eur J Immunol 38: 1435–1445.

32. Schoenberger SP, Toes RE, van der Voort EI, Offringa R, Melief CJ (1998) T-cell help for cytotoxic T lymphocytes is mediated by CD40-CD40L interactions. Nature 393: 480–483.

33. Ridge JP, Di Rosa F, Matzinger P (1998) A conditioned dendritic cell can be a temporal bridge between a CD4+ T-helper and a T-killer cell. Nature 393: 474–478.

34. Bourgeois C, Rocha B, Tanchot C (2002) A role for CD40 expression on CD8+ T cells in the generation of CD8+ T cell memory. Science 297: 2060–2063.

35. Matloubian M, Concepcion RJ, Ahmed R (1994) CD4+ T cells are required to sustain CD8+ cytotoxic T-cell responses during chronic viral infection. J Virol 68: 8056–8063.

36. Nakanishi Y, Lu B, Gerard C, Iwasaki A (2009) CD8(+) T lymphocyte mobilization to virus-infected tissue requires CD4(+) T-cell help. Nature 462: 510–513.

37. Rahemtulla A, Fung-Leung WP, Schilham MW, Kundig TM, Sambhara SR, et al. (1991) Normal development and function of CD8+ cells but markedly decreased helper cell activity in mice lacking CD4. Nature 353: 180–184.

38. von Herrath MG, Yokoyama M, Dockter J, Oldstone MB, Whitton JL (1996) CD4-deficient mice have reduced levels of memory cytotoxic T lymphocytes after immunization and show diminished resistance to subsequent virus challenge. J Virol 70: 1072–1079.

39. Carreno BM, Collins M (2002) The B7 family of ligands and its receptors: new pathways for costimulation and inhibition of immune responses. Annu Rev Immunol 20: 29–53.

40. Adam C, King S, Allgeier T, Braumuller H, Luking C, et al. (2005) DC-NK cell cross talk as a novel CD4+ T-cell-independent pathway for antitumor CTL induction. Blood 106: 338–344.

41. Sotomayor EM, Borrello I, Tubb E, Rattis FM, Bien H, et al. (1999) Conversion of tumor-specific CD4+ T-cell tolerance to T-cell priming through in vivo ligation of CD40. Nat Med 5: 780–787.

42. Spolski R, Leonard WJ (2010) IL-21 is an immune activator that also mediates suppression via IL-10. Crit Rev Immunol 30: 559–570.

43. Casey KA, Mescher MF (2007) IL-21 promotes differentiation of naive CD8 T cells to a unique effector phenotype. J Immunol 178: 7640–7648.

10

Screening of Multiple Myeloma by Polyclonal Rabbit Anti-Human Plasmacytoma Cell Immunoglobulin

Bo Mu[1,2]*, Huan Zhang[1], Xiaoming Cai[1], Junbao Yang[1], Yuewu Shen[1], Baofeng Chen[1], Suhua Liang[1]

1 The Medical Biology Staff Room of North Sichuan Medical College, Sichuan Nanchong, the People's Republic of China, **2** Sichuan Key Laboratory of Medical Imaging, Affiliated Hospital of North Sichuan Medical College, North Sichuan Medical College, Nanchong, the People's Republic of China

Abstract

Antibody-based immunotherapy has been effectively used for tumor treatment. However, to date, only a few tumor-associated antigens (TAAs) or therapeutic targets have been identified. Identification of more immunogenic antigens is essential for improvements in multiple myeloma (MM) diagnosis and therapy. In this study, we synthesized a polyclonal antibody (PAb) by immunizing rabbits with whole human plasmacytoma ARH-77 cells and identified MM-associated antigens, including enlonase, adipophilin, and HSP90s, among others, via proteomic technologies. 3-(4,5-Dimethylthiazol-2-yl)-2,5-diphenyltetrazolium bromide assay showed that 200 μg/mL PAb inhibits the proliferation of ARH-77 cells by over 50% within 48 h. Flow cytometric assay indicated that PAb treatment significantly increases the number of apoptotic cells compared with other treatments (52.1% vs. NS, 7.3% or control rabbit IgG, 9.9%). In vivo, PAb delayed tumor growth and prolonged the lifespan of mice. Terminal deoxynucleotidyl transferase dUTP nick end labeling assay showed that PAb also induces statistically significant changes in apoptosis compared with other treatments ($P<0.05$). We therefore conclude that PAb could be used for the effective screening and identification of TAA. PAb may have certain anti-tumor functions in vitro and in vivo. As such, its combination with proteomic technologies could be a promising approach for sieving TAA for the diagnosis and therapy of MM.

Editor: Pranela Rameshwar, University of Medicine and Dentistry of New Jersey, United States of America

Funding: This project was supported by National Natural Science Foundation of China, number 81101733 (http://www.nsfc.gov.cn/). The funders had no role in study design, data collection and analysis, decision to publish, or preparation of the manuscript.

Competing Interests: The authors have declared that no competing interests exist.

* E-mail: ppnu2@yahoo.com.cn

Background

Multiple myeloma (MM), which accounts for approximately 10% of all malignant hematologic neoplasms [1], is difficult to cure by conventional chemotherapy, high-dose radiotherapy, autologous stem cell transplantation, and allogeneic transplantation [2,3]. Immunotherapy based on antibodies has achieved significant success for MM treatment [4,5]. Targeting of cell-surface antigens with promising monoclonal antibodies is a very attractive approach for treating MM. Rituximab, Daratumumab, atlezumab, and atlizumab [5–7] have been evaluated in preclinical and clinical studies. However, only a few tumor-associated antigens (TAAs) or therapeutic targets are currently available. Thus, identification of novel antigens is necessary to improve MM immunotherapy.

Over the last 20 years, several approaches have been used for the identification of TAA, among which serological screening of cDNA expression libraries, phage display libraries, and, more recently, proteomics-based approaches have been the most successful. Hundreds of candidate TAAs have been identified in various human cancer types [8], including liver cancer, breast cancer [9], prostate cancer [10], ovarian cancer [11], renal cancer [12], head and neck cancer [13], esophageal cancer [14], lymphoma [15], gastric cancer [16] and leukemia [17].

TAAs have been used mainly to identify tumor-specific overexpressing proteins in patient serum and/or tissue. The amount of certain TAAs in the circulation and/or tumor tissue is usually very low, especially during the early stages of cancer. In addition, antigens that are highly expressed in a tumor from a particular patient may not be overexpressed in a tumor from another patient. An example of such a TAA is CD20, which has been detected only in 13% to 22% of the patients studied [18]. TAA may also display heterogeneity in terms of epitope recognition within a given antigen. Thus, the current methods must be optimized continually to enhance the identification of candidate TAAs.

In the present study, we synthesized a polyclonal antibody (PAb), specifically anti-human MM line ARH-77 cells, and then screened and identified multiple proteins, including enolase, adipophilin (ADPH), and HSP90s, among others, as potential TAAs via proteomics-based approaches. Flow cytometric assay and immunofluorescence staining showed that the antigens are expressed in the ARH-77 cellular membrane. Verification of the antitumor functions of PAb showed the inhibitory effect of PAb on MM growth and its ability to induce apoptosis of myeloma cells in vitro and in vivo. Our results suggest that PAb may be effectively used for screening and identifying TAAs and that the PAb produced by the proposed method could have certain anti-tumor functions.

A

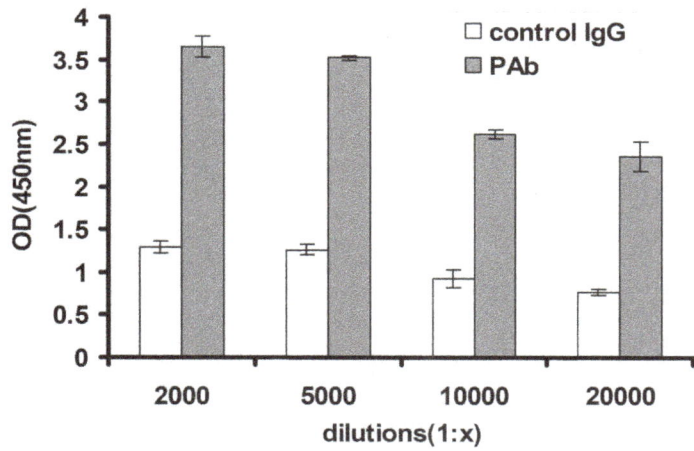

B

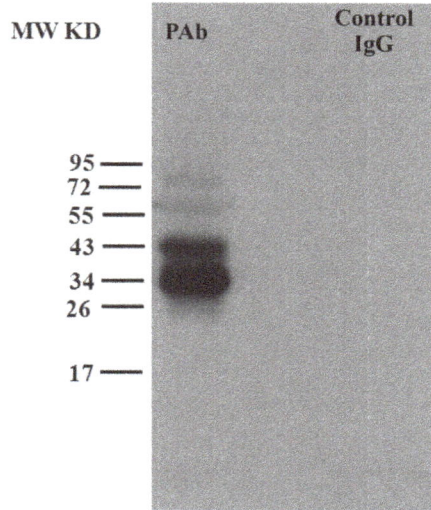

C

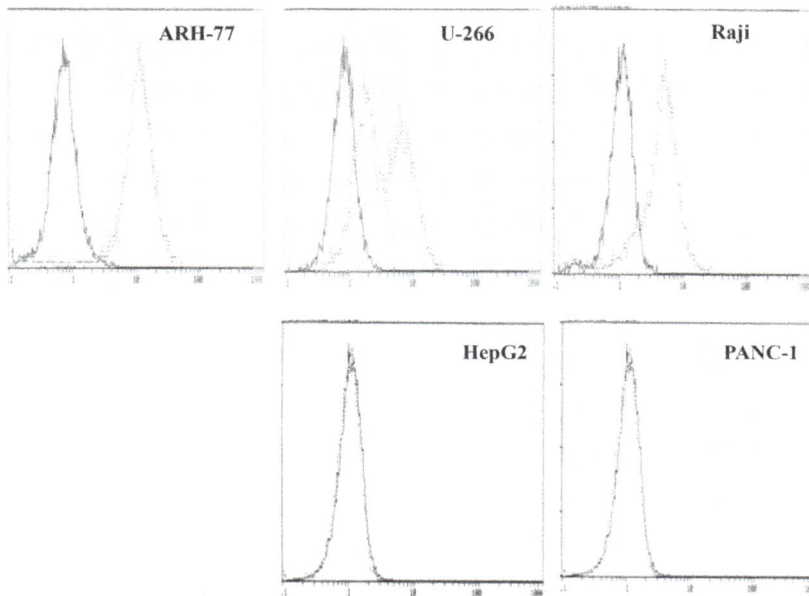

D

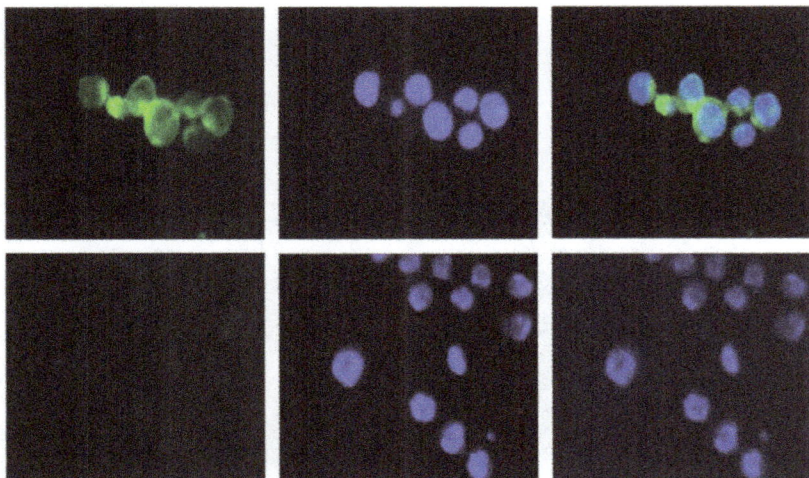

Figure 1. Production and characterization of PAb. (A) ELISA of PAb on ARH-77. Control rabbit IgG and PAb were incubated with ARH-77 at dilutions from 1:2,000 to 1:20,000. After addition of an alkaline phosphatase-conjugated secondary antibody, the absorbance was measured at 450 nm. Represented here is the mean of 4 wells to 6 wells ± standard deviation for every dilution. (B) Western blot showed the multiple protein bands recognized by PAb but not by control IgG. (C) Indirect immunofluorescence assay of PAb on myeloma and non-myeloma cell line by flow cytometry. Gray line represents 1:2,000 PAb dilutions reacted with ARH-77 (left panel), U266 (upper part, middle panel), and Raji (upper part, right panel), human hepatocellular carcinoma cell line HepG2 (lower part, middle panel) and human pancreatic carcinoma cell line Panc-1(lower part, right panel). Black line represents control IgG diluted to 1:2,000 used as a negative control. (D) Indirect immunofluorescence assay of antigens on ARH-77 by fluorescence microscopy with FITC-goat anti-rabbit IgG (left, green fluorescence) and with hoechst33258 (middle, blue fluorescence). Up line represents the treatment group with PAb and down line represents the treatment group with control IgG. Merged images (right) show localization of antigens on ARH-77 cells (400×).

Materials and Methods

Animals and Cell Lines

SCID mice (6 wk to 8 wk old) were purchased from the Model Animal Research Center of Nanjing University. New Zealand white rabbits were purchased from the West China Experimental Animal Center. Animal protocols for the experiments were approved by the West China Hospital Cancer Center's Animal Care. In this study, two human MM ARH-77 and U266 cell lines and one human Burkitt's lymphoma Raji cell line obtained from the American Type Culture Collection were cultured in RPMI-1640 (Gibco BRL) containing 10% heat-inactivated FCS, 100 units/mL penicillin, and 100 units/mL streptomycin in a humid incubator with 5% CO_2 at 37°C.

Rabbit Immunization and PAb Isolation

PAb was generated by immunizing New Zealand white rabbits with ARH-77 cells with densities ranging from 1×10^7 to 5×10^7 cells per injection. The rabbits were then inoculated with Freund's complete adjuvant (Sigma) followed by three booster injections of Freund's incomplete adjuvant (Sigma) once every 10 d to 14 d. Sera were pooled after week administration of the last injection. Blood was allowed to clot overnight at 4°C, after which the serum was removed from the top of the mixture by centrifugation at 12000 g. Immunoglobulin (Ig) was isolated using an affinity chromatography system (AKTA Explore, GE, USA), freeze-dried using a freeze dryer (Rlphr 1–4 LSC, Christ, Germany), and kept frozen at −80°C until use. Control rabbit IgG was similarly purified from whole normal rabbit serum.

Enzyme-linked Immunosorbent Assay (ELISA)

Tumor cells (5×10^3 per well) were grown overnight in a poly-lysine-coated-96-well plate for ELISA. The media were removed and the cells were washed three times with PBS. After washing, the cells were blocked with 5% skim milk in blocking buffer (PBS containing 0.05% Tween-20, PBST) for 1 h at room temperature. The blocking reagent was then removed and cells were washed three times with PBS before addition of PAb. The PAb was diluted from 1:2,000 to 1:20,000 in dilution buffer (5% skim milk in PBST) and incubated for 1 h at room temperature. The antibody was then removed and the cells were washed three times with PBST. A second antibody (goat anti-rabbit linked to alkaline phosphatase, 1:5,000, Sigma) was added to the cells and incubated for 30 min. The cells were then washed three times with PBST. Alkaline phosphatase substrate BCIP/NCP (Sigma) was subsequently added to the cells and the absorbance of the mixtures was measured at 450 nm using a 96-well plate reader (Molecular Device, M5, USA).

Western Blot

Western blot was conducted as described previously [19]. Briefly, ARH-77 cells were lysed in 1 mL of lysis buffer. Proteins (25 μg/lane) were separated by SDS-PAGE and transferred on polyvinylidene fluoride (PVDF) membranes by electroblotting. The membranes were then blocked in 5% (w/v) skim milk, washed, and probed with PAb at 1:20,00 dilution. Blots were washed and incubated with an HRP-conjugated secondary antibody diluted from 1:5,000 to 1:10,000 and visualized with chemiluminescence reagents.

Immunofluorescence Staining of MM Cells

Three myeloma cell lines and two non-myeloma cell lines in the logarithmic phase were harvested and washed with PBS three times. The cells were blocked with 5% skim milk in PBST for 1 h at room temperature, after which the blocking reagent was removed. PAb and control rabbit IgG diluted to 1:1,000 in PBST containing 5% skim milk were added to the cells. Incubation for 30 min followed. The antibody was then removed and the cells

Table 1. Protein spots in GC searched by Peptident software in the SWISS-PROT database.

Spot	Protein name	IPI: ID	Top score	Theoretic pI	Theoretic Mr	Sequence coverd Rate(%)
A1	Heat shock protein HSP 90-alpha (**HSP90A**)	IPI00382470	429	4.94	84607	35
A2	Stress-induced phosphoprotein 1 (**STIP1**)	IPI00013894	179	6.4	62599	23
A3	Bifunctional purine biosynthesis protein PURH (**PUR9**)	IPI00289499	205	6.27	64575	31
A4	Alpha-enolase (**ENO1**)	IPI00465248	1533	7.01	47139	45
A5	Adipophilin (**ADPH**)	IPI00293307	154	6.34	48045	28
A6	Vacuolar protein sorting-associated protein 37B (**VP37B**)	IPI00002926	50	6.78	31287	30
A7	Isocitrate dehydrogenase [NAD] subunit alpha (**IDH3A**)	IPI00030702	638	6.47	39566	26
A8	Phosphoglycerate kinase 1(**PGK1**)	IPI00169383	688	8.3	44586	45
A9	Voltage-dependent anion-selective channel protein 2 (**VDAC2**)	IPI00024145	158	7.49	31547	26

A

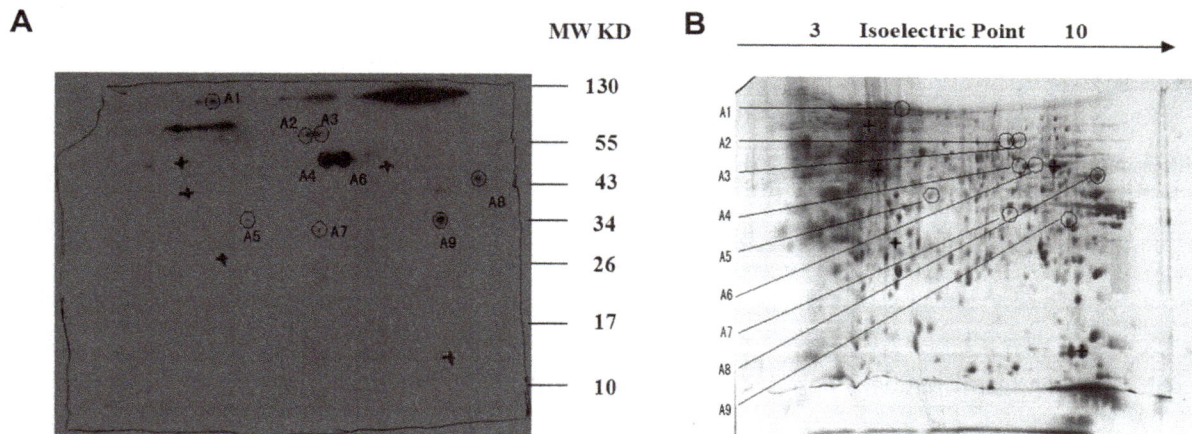

B

C

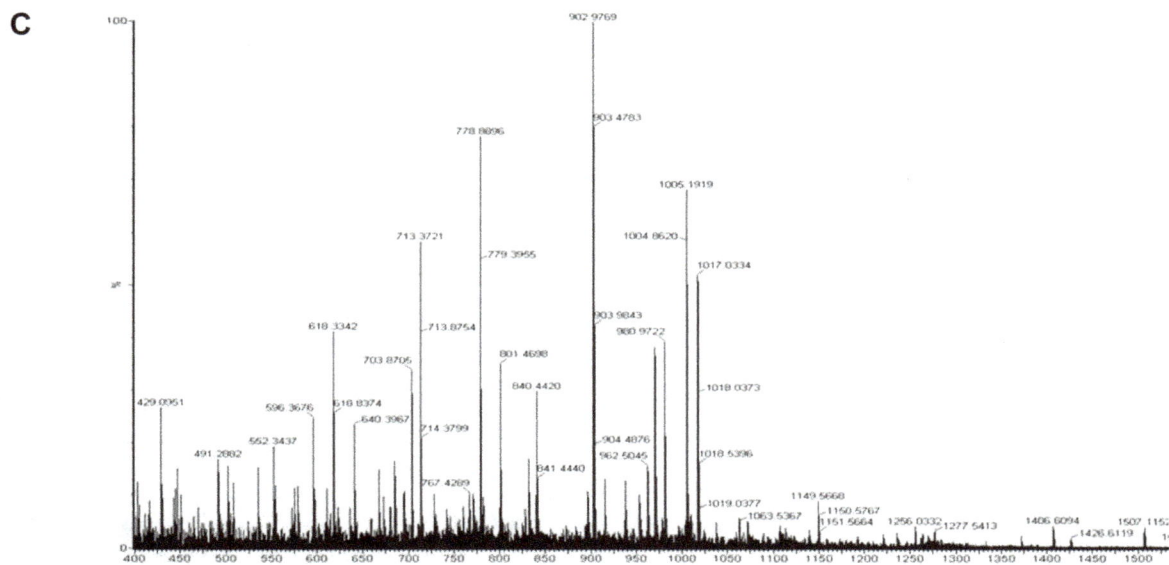

D

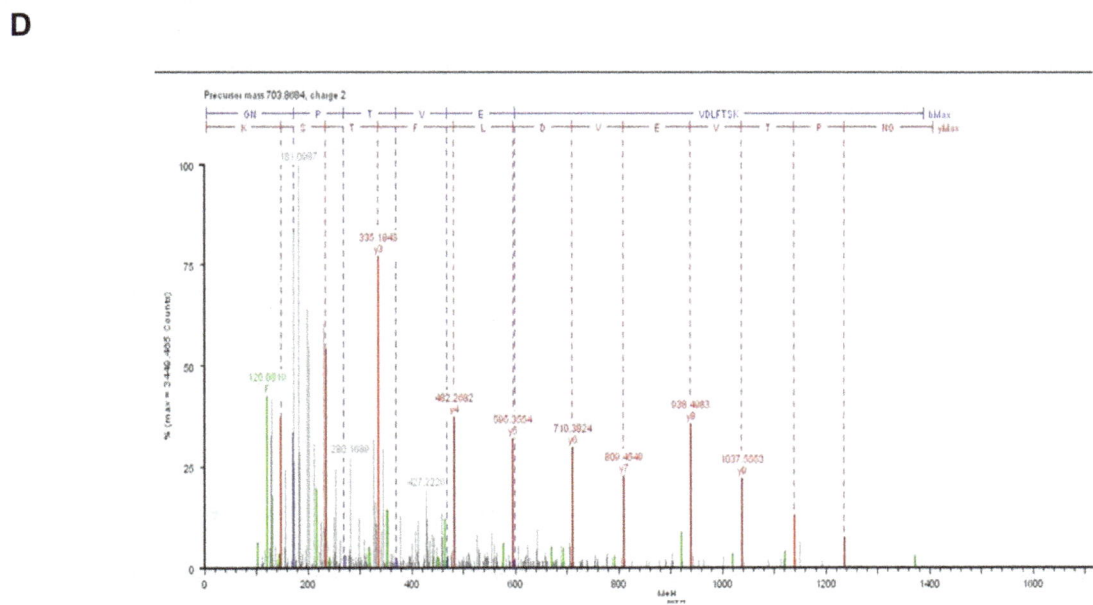

Figure 2. 2-D PAGE and Western blot analysis of ARH-77 cell proteins. (A) Western blot detection of the targeted-protein spot recognized by PAb. (B) 2-D protein pattern of ARH-77 cells after Commassie Blue staining. (C) MALDI-MS spectrum obtained from spot A1 after trypsin digestion and peptide sequences from ENO1 matching peaks obtained from MALDI-MS spectra. (D) The peptide of 703.6864 selected from the PMF of the A1 spot was sequenced by nano-ESI-MS/MS.

were washed three times in PBST. The second antibody (FITC-goat anti-rabbit IgG, 1:500; Beijing Zhong Shan Golden Bridge Biological Technology Co., Ltd., China) was added to the cells. Incubation for 30 min followed. The antibody was then removed and the cells were washed three times in PBST. Up to 10,000 cells were acquired for flow cytometric analysis (Beckman-Coulter, USA).

Localization of PAb Binding with Antigens on MM Cells

About 5×10^6 cells were fixed with 100 μL 4% formaldehyde in PBS for 5 min at pH 7.6, after which 30 μL of the cell suspension was spread on a microscope slide by cell smearing. After drying, the cells were made permeable by treatment for 5 min with 0.5% Triton X-100/10 mM Hepes/300 mM sucrose/3 mM MgCl2/50 mM NaCl (pH 7.4) and incubated with PAb or control IgG (dilution 1:1,000) overnight at 4°C. The antibody was then removed and the cells were washed three times in PBST. A second antibody (FITC-goat anti-rabbit IgG 1:500; Beijing Zhong Shan Golden Bridge Biological Technology Co.) was added to the cells and the cells were incubated in a humidified chamber for 30 min. The antibody was removed and the cells were washed three times in PBST, stained with Hoechst33258 for 5 min, and then washed with PBS. Fluorescent microscopy was performed with a Zeiss Photoscope Imager Z I.

Two-dimensional Electrophoresis (2D–E)

About 2×10^7 ARH-77 cells were solubilized in 1 mL of lysis solution (7 M urea, 2 M thiourea, 4% CHAPS, 2 mmol/L TBP, 0.2% ampholyte, traces of bromophenol blue) at 4°C for 20 min. Insoluble material was removed by centrifugation at 15000 rpm at 4°C for 30 min. Protein concentrations were determined by the Bradford method. Samples were frozen at −70°C and thawed immediately before use. Approximately 1 mg protein was loaded on 17 cm of IPG Ready Strips. After rehydrating the strips for 14 h, IEF was carried out for 1 h at 200 V, 1 h at 500 V, and 1 h at 1000 V. A gradient was then applied from 1,000 to 8,000 for 1 h and finally at 8,000 V for 8 h to reach a total of 72 KVh at 20°C. After IEF separation, the gel strips were incubated first in equilibration buffer (50 mM Tris-HCl, pH 8.8, 6 M urea, 30% glycerol, 2% SDS) with 10 mg/mL DTT and then in equilibration buffer with 25 mg/mL iodoacetamide for 15 min each. The strips were then loaded on 12% SDS-PAGE gel and electrophoresed for 20 min at a constant current of 10 mA and at 30 mA per gel until the bromophenol blue indicator reached the bottom of the gels. One gel was then stained with Coomassie Brilliant Blue R-250 and destained with 40% methanol and 10% acetic acid. Another gel was analyzed by 2D Western blot.

2D Western Blot

The separated proteins were transferred on PVDF membranes and incubated for 2 h at room temperature with a blocking buffer consisting of TBST (Tris-buffered saline +0.01% Tween 20) and 5% skim milk. The PVDF membranes were dyed with Commassie Blue staining solution for 15 min [0.1% Coomassie Brilliant Blue R-250 (w/v) and 50% methanol (v/v)] and outstanding points were marked as landmarks. The membranes were then decolorized for 1 h in destaining solution [40% methanol (v/v) with 10% acetic acid (v/v)], washed, and incubated with PAb for 1 h at

room temperature. After additional washes with TBST, the membranes were incubated with a secondary antibody conjugated with horseradish peroxidase at 1:5,000 dilution for 1 h and transferred to Vectastain ABC (Vector Laboratories, Burlingame, CA, USA). The protein spots on the film were matched with the 2-DE map of the same sample and excised from the 2-DE gel stained with Coomassie Brilliant Blue. The excised proteins were then digested as described previously for protein identification by mass spectrometry using spots from different gel with at least two replicates. The obtained peptide mass fingerprint was used to search through the Swiss-Prot and National Center for Biotechnology Information nonredundant databases by the Mascot search engine (www. matrixscience.co.uk). Protein identification was reconfirmed by an ESI-MS/MS approach. The database search was finished with the Mascot search engine (www.matrixscience.co.uk) using a Mascot MS/MS ion search.

Cell Viability Analysis by 3-(4,5-dimethylthiazol-2-yl)-2, 5-diphenyltetrazolium Bromide (MTT) Assay

Cell growth inhibition was determined by MTT assay (Sigma). Briefly, myeloma cells (2×10^4 cells/well to 3×10^4 cells/well) were seeded on a 96-well plate at a volume of 100 μL per well and incubated for 24 h. The cells were then treated with normal saline (NS), control rabbit IgG, or PAb for 48 h at 37°C and subjected to MTT assay. Cells treated with NS served as the indicator of 100% cell viability.

Apoptosis Analysis by Flow Cytometry Assay

The cells (3×10^5 per well) were plated in 6-well plates and treated with NS, control IgG (200 μg/mL) or PAb (200 μg/mL). After 48 h, flow cytometric analysis was conducted to identify sub-G1 phase cells/apoptotic cells. Briefly, the cells were suspended in 1 mL of hypotonic fluorochrome solution containing 50 μg/mL propidium iodide in 0.1% sodium citrate with 0.1% Triton X-100 and analyzed by a flow cytometer. Apoptotic cells appeared in the cell cycle distribution as cells with DNA content less than that of G1 phase cells.

Antitumor Effect of PAb on Xenograft SCID Mouse Models with ARH-77

Human ARH-77 MM cells (5×10^6) were implanted subcutaneously into the right flanks of female SCID mice. When the tumor nodules were palpable, the mice were divided randomly into three groups with six mice each and treated with NS, control IgG, or PAb via the tail vein. Control IgG and PAb (200 μg/dose, dissolved in NS) were administered seven times every 2 d in a volume of 100 μL along with the control injection in a volume of 100 μL NS. The tumor volume was observed and the tumor size was determined once every 3 d by caliper measurement as described previously [20].

Terminal Deoxynucleotidyl Transferase-mediated dUTP Nick end Labeling (TUNEL) Assay

Cell apoptosis in vivo was examined by TUNEL assay according to the manufacturer's instructions (Promega, USA). Three tumors per group were analyzed 48 h after the last treatment.

A

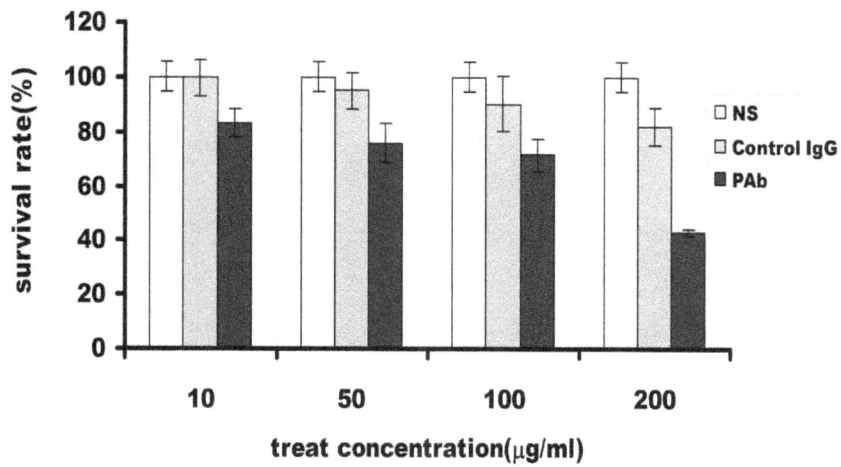

B

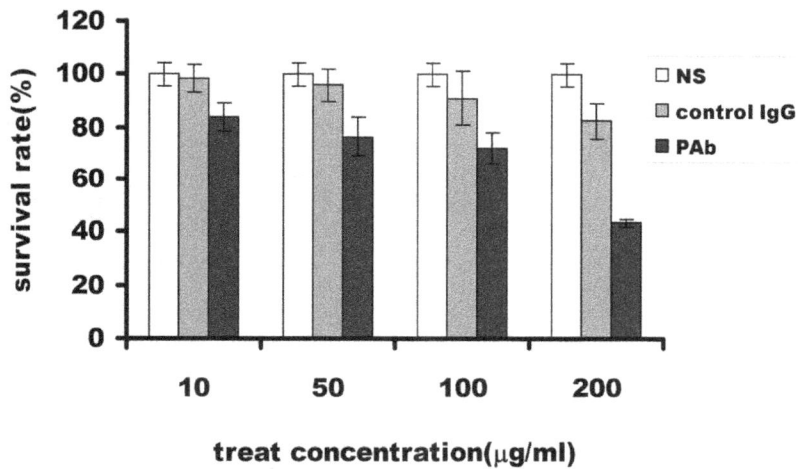

C

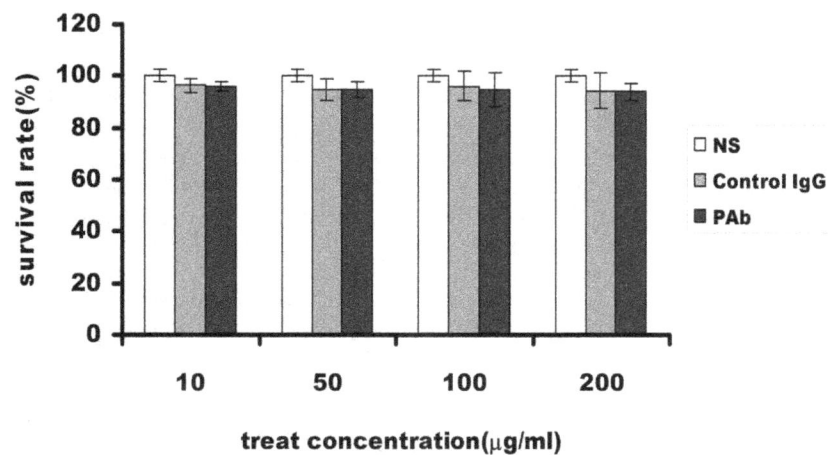

Figure 3. Inhibition of myeloma cells growth in vitro determined by MTT. (A)The growth of PAb-treated cells was significantly inhibited compared with the control IgG and NS groups, and the inhibitory rates on different concentrations on ARH-77 cells after 48 h were 16.7%, 23.98%, 28.47%, and 56.84%. (B)The similar results were shown in U266 cell line. (C) The PAb did not effect growth of HepG2 cell line.

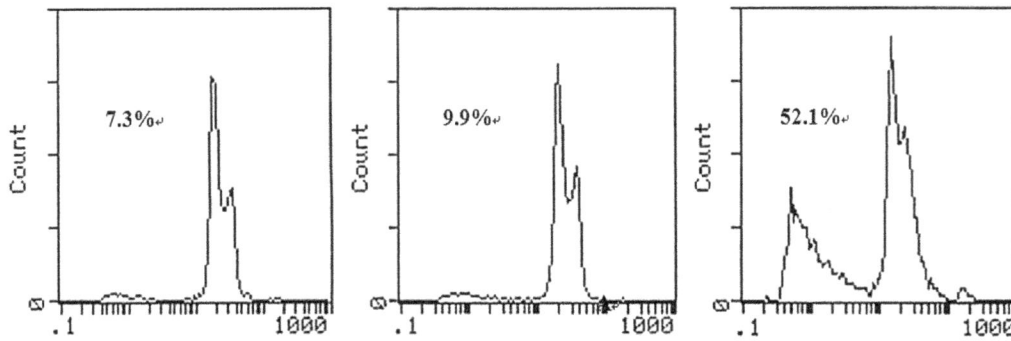

Figure 4. PAb-induced apoptosis in myeloma cell lines. Flow cytometric analysis revealed the proportion of sub-G1 phase cells (apoptotic cells) to be 7.3% (NS), 9.9% (control), and 52.1% (PAb). The experiments were repeated at least three times.

Statistical Analysis

SPSS version 13 was used for statistical analysis. The statistical significance of results in all of the experiments was determined by Student's t-test and analysis of variance. The findings were regarded as significant if $P<0.05$.

Results

Production and Characterization of PAb

To investigate the possibility of vaccination of rabbits with ARH-77, two rabbits were inoculated with ARH-77 cells to produce polyclonal antibody. PAb was tested for its ability to bind MM cell lines (Fig. 1A). The binding of ARH-77 by PAb differed by 3- to 10-fold from control IgG. The binding was dose-dependent, with dilutions of 1:2,000 and 1:5,000 showing greater binding to ARH-77 than dilutions of 1:10,000 or 1:20,000. As to the antigens recognized by PAb, we further performed Western blot, flow cytometric assay, and immunofluorescence studies. ARH-77 cell lysates were probed with either PAb or control IgG on Western blots. Multiple bands (Fig. 1B) were recognized by PAb but not by the control IgG. Immunofluorescence and flow cytometric assay studies to detect the combination between PAb or control IgG and fixed ARH-77cells revealed that PAb significantly binds to the surface of ARH-77 but shows no reactivity to control IgG, as well as in U266 and Raji cells. However, PAb did not bind non-myeloma cell lines, such as the human hepatocellular carcinoma cell line HepG2 and human pancreatic carcinoma cell line Panc-1(Figs. 1C and 1D). These results suggest the synthesis of PAb with high specificity and ability to identify myeloma cell surface antigens.

Antigen Identification of PAb by 2-DE/Western Blot and MALDI-TOF MS/MS Analysis

To recognize the targeted antigens of PAb, 2-DE and Western blot were performed with the ARH-77 cell lysate. Gels (17 cm) (3 to 10 NL) were used for Western blot to determine the PI and MW of the corresponding antigens of PAb (Fig. 2A). The protein spot showing a positive reaction with PAb in X-film was excised from the gel (Fig. 2B). The excised gel piece was destained and trypsinized into peptides for MS and MS/MS analysis. Mass spectra were acquired with a Q-TOF Premier mass spectrometer. MS/MS data, including the mass values, the intensity, and the charge of the precursor ions, were analyzed with a licensed copy of the Mascot 2.0 program against the SWISS-PROT protein database. On the map, nine tumor-specific spots were excised

and subjected to in-gel digestion followed by peptide mass fingerprinting for protein identification. Figure 2C shows the identification of Spot No.1 as an example. The results of antigen identification are summarized in the Appendix, Table 1.

Inhibitory Effect of PAb on ARH-77 Cell Proliferation

Antigens recognized by PAb, such as enolase, ADPH, and HSP90, were correlated closely with cancer cell proliferation, survival, and metastasis. Thus, we hypothesized that PAb could have antitumor functions for blocking these TAAs. The effect of PAb on the proliferation of ARH-77 cells was evaluated by MTT and flow cytometric assay. Compared with the NS and control IgG treated cells, the inhibitory rates of PAb in 10 μg/mL, 50 μg/mL, 100 μg/mL, and 200 μg/mL ARH-77 cells after 48 h were 16.7%, 23.98%, 28.47%, and 56.84%, respectively (Fig. 3A), and similar results were also shown in U266 cell lines (Fig. 3B), but the PAb did not effect the growth of HepG2 cell (Fig. 3C). The results indicate that PAb can decrease the proliferation of ARH-77 cells in vitro. Moreover, flow cytometric assay revealed that PAb treatment significantly increased the number of apoptotic cells compared with the other treatments (52.1% vs. NS, 7.3% or control IgG, 9.9%)($P<0.05$; Fig. 4). These findings suggest that PAb inhibits proliferation and induces apoptosis in cancer cells in vitro.

Inhibition of Tumor Growth in an Animal Model of Myeloma

Based on the findings in vitro, we tested the efficacy of the PAb in an SCID mice model. The results show that PAb treatment significantly regresses the established tumors and prolongs the lifespan of mice compared with the NS or control IgG treatments (Fig. 5). The average tumor volume in the PAb group was stable for most of the experiment after administration of PAb whereas the average tumor volumes in NS and control IgG groups continued to increase. The inhibition rate reached approximately 61.6% in the PAb group. This result supports the hypothesis that PAb displays antitumor activity in vivo. TUNEL assay showed an apparent increase in the number of apoptotic cells and apoptotic index within the residual tumors treated with PAb compared with the NS and control IgG groups ($P<0.05$; Fig. 6). These data suggest that both inhibition of myeloma proliferation and apoptosis-inducing activity are involved in the antitumor effects of PAb.

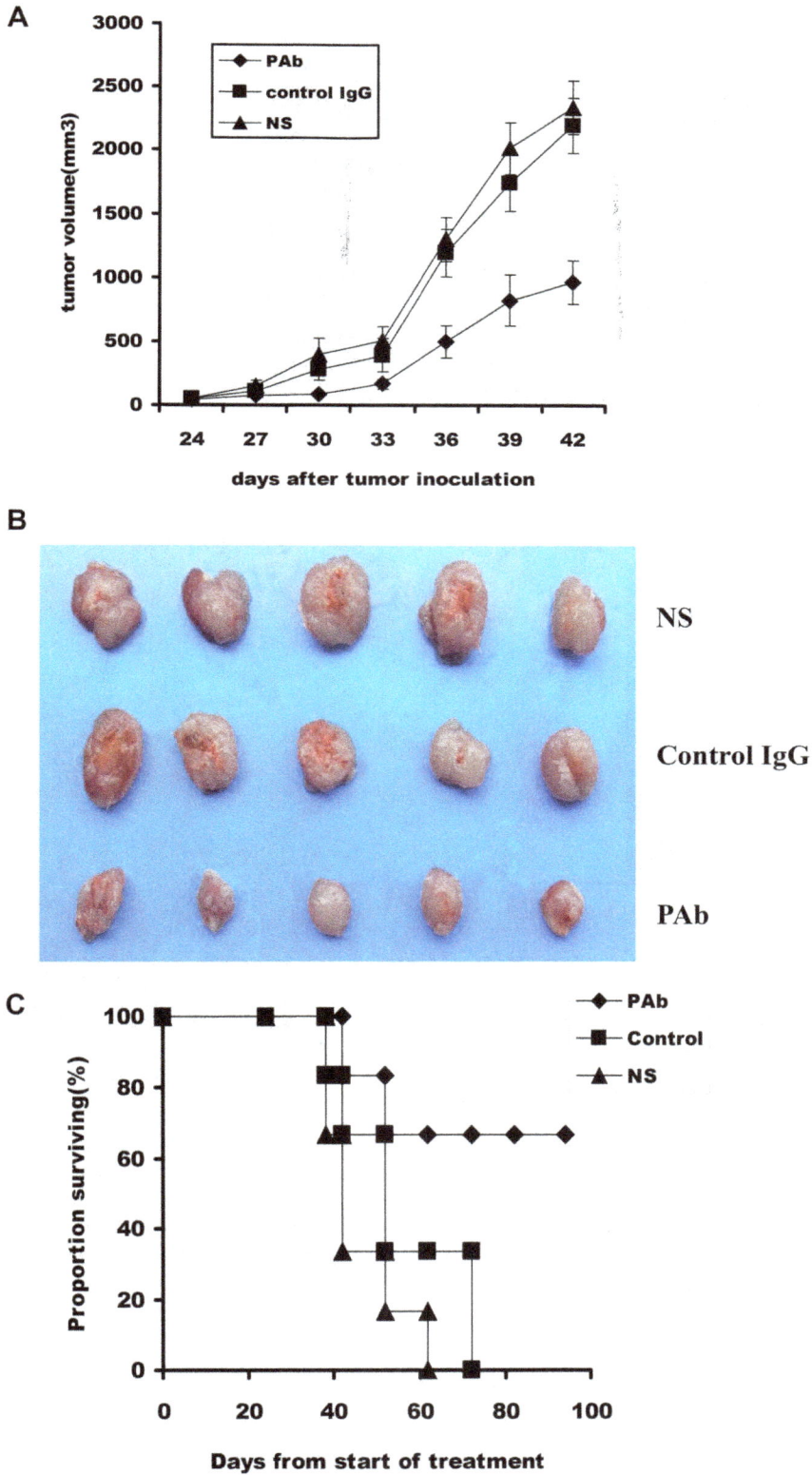

Figure 5. Inhibitory effect of PAb on tumor growth in xenograft SCID mouse models. (A) A significant difference in tumor volume (P<0.05) was observed between PAb-treated mice and other treatment groups. The mean ± standard error of the mean of tumor growth of five mice is shown. (B) Representative picture for tumor volume different groups. (C) A significant increase in survival was observed in PAb-treated mice compared with other treatment groups (P<0.05).

A

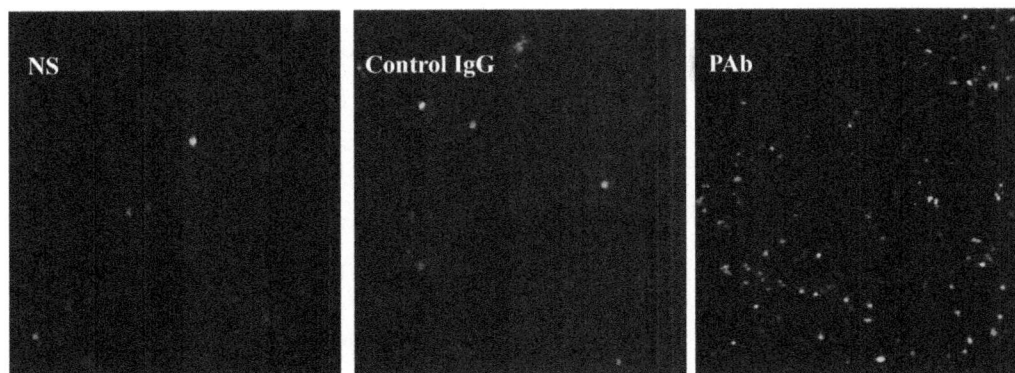

B

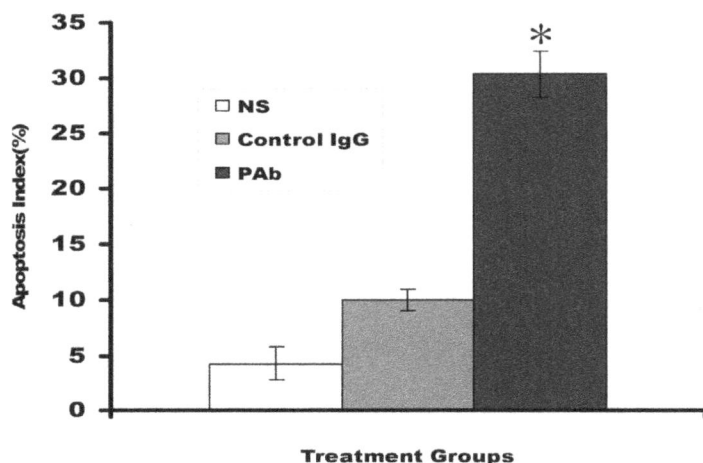

Figure 6. PAb-induced tumor cells apoptosis in vivo by TUNEL assay. (A) Sections from the tumor-bearing mice treated with NS (left panel), control IgG (middle panel), or PAb (right panel) were stained with FITC-dUTP as described in the Materials and Methods section (200×). (B) An apparent increase in the number of apoptotic cells and apoptotic index was observed within residual tumors treated with PAb compared with other treatment groups in the ARH-77 subcutaneous injection tumor models. * represents the PAb group showing significant difference compared with NS and control IgG group mice (P<0.05).

Discussion

The availability of high throughput 2-DE gels and initial screening using automated procedures has made the identification of TAA in the proteome of various tumor cell lines and/or tissues possible. This study was based on PAb combined with proteomic analysis and aimed to screen TAAs in the proteome level to help further improve the diagnosis and immunotherapy of MM. We synthesized a PAb by immunizing rabbits with the human plasmacytoma cell line ARH-77 and identified multiple TAAs of MM, such as enolase, ADPH, and HSP90s, among others, using 2-DE, Western blot, and mass spectrometric techniques.

To validate the MS/MS results, we selected three proteins for examination according to their positions in the Mascot score list, which lists the vital role they play in many cancers. These proteins are discussed below.

α-Enolase

The propensity for glycolysis is enhanced in cancer cells because of increased cell proliferation. Previous studies have indicated that

α-enolase, a key enzyme in the glycolysis pathway, is upregulated in 18 out of 24 types of cancer, as determined by bioinformatics study using gene chips and EST databases [21]. A recent proteomic analysis further revealed that overexpression of α-enolase in hepatitis C virus-related hepatocellular carcinomas is associated with tumor progression [22]. Although the mechanisms of the surface expression and orientation of α-enolase on the membrane have yet to be clearly understood, surface α-enolase is known to act as a strong plasminogen-binding receptor [23]. The binding of plasminogen to the cell surface and its consequent activation to plasmin may play crucial roles in the intravascular and pericellular fibrinolytic systems, cell invasion, tumor cell migration, and metastasis as a plasminogen-binding receptor [24]. Thus, we hypothesize that α-enolase is a diagnostic marker and therapeutic target of MM.

ADPH

ADPH, a member of the perilipin family of lipid droplet-associated proteins, hypothetically mediates milk lipid formation and secretion [25]. Previous studies have indicated that ADPH functions in lipid storage droplets formation [26], fatty acid uptake [27], and milk lipid secretion [28]. In addition, ADPH is reportedly overexpressed in colorectal cancer [29], hepatocellular cancer, renal cell cancer [30]and kidney cancer [31].

To date, the direct interactions of ADPH with cancer cells have yet to be clearly understood. Cellular levels of ADPH are reportedly correlated with lipid accumulation in various cells and tissues [26,32]. Moreover, ADPH is involved in lipid droplet/apical cell surface membrane recognition or interaction because of its interaction with milk lipid globule membranes inner surface coat constituents [33]. The recent discovery of human cancer cells expressing high levels of fatty acid synthase and undergoing significant endogenous fatty-acid synthesis has allowed researchers to perform in-depth reviews of the roles of fatty acids in tumor biology [34,35]. Wright et al. [36] showed that ADPH could induce PPAR-gamma activation, which is a potential path for promoting tumor cell differentiation in malignant melanoma. ADPH can augment tumor-necrosis factor-α (TNF-α), MCP-1, and interleukin-6 (IL-6) expression [37]. However, IL-6 and TNF-α could mediate MM growth, survival, and resistance to apoptosis [38]. Thus, ADPH may be a novel target pathway for tumor therapy because of its interaction with cytokines and fatty acid synthesis.

HSP90

HSP90, one of the most abundant molecular chaperones, is important for the maturation, stability, and activity of numerous cancer-related proteins, such as mutated p53, EarB2/Her2, Raf-1, cyclin-dependent kinases 1 and 4, Akt/PKB, Bcr-Abl, and Hif-1a, which are involved in cell signaling, proliferation, and survival, as well as neoangiogenesis, adhesion, and drug resistance [39,40]. HSP90 is frequently overexpressed and activated in cancer cells, including acute leukemias [41], gastrointestinal cancers [42], glioblastoma [43], cervical cancer [44], lung cancers [45] and human breast cancers [46]. Several studies have shown that HSP90 is localized in the cytoplasm and on the cell surface in certain types of cancer cells [47], including prostate cancer [48], melanomas [49], non-small-cell lung cancer cells [50], fibrosarcoma cells [51], lymphomas [52] and breast cancer cell [53].

The mechanism of HSP90 function has been reviewed in detail [54–57] but knowledge of the function of cell-surface HSP90 in tumor cells is limited. HSP90 has been correlated with cancer metastasis [58]and migration of malignant cells [43]. HSP90 proteins may interact with other cell-surface proteins through transmembrane signaling, thereby triggering intracellular events necessary for cell invasion [47]. In addition, the cancer-specific expression of cell-surface HSP90 has been found to be associated with MHC class I [59] and increases in expression level through

several stages of early and late apoptotic death with immune response activation [60]. Increasing evidence suggests that HSP90 can function as a central regulator of proliferative and anti-apoptotic signal transduction and may be a potential biomarker and therapeutic target for the immunotherapy of tumors like MM.

Other proteins have been implicated in cell proliferation [61], aging [62], multidrug resistance [63,64], and mitochondrial apoptosis [65]. Although the data are preliminary, the antigens detected in this paper may be candidate diagnostic markers and therapy targets in MM. Proteomic technologies provide a powerful tool for identifying TAAs and, especially, verifying cellular membrane antigens.

The PAb produced by our method has certain antitumor functions in vitro and in vivo that may block TAAs correlated with tumor cell proliferation, survival, and apoptosis. We found that PAb induces the apoptosis of various myeloma cell lines, inhibits tumor growth, and prolongs the lifespan of mice. PAb also induces statistically significant apoptosis compared with other treatments, as determined by TUNEL assay in vivo. As such, its combination with polyclonal rabbit anti-human plasmacytoma cell globulins may be a promising approach for sieving TAA for the diagnosis and therapy of MM.

In conclusion, the use of PAb against whole tumor cells coupled with high throughput proteomic technologies could be a potential tool for screening TAAs. The major advantages of this approach are as follows: (1) the isolated antibodies bind to native forms of their antigens or ligands on the cell surface, whereas purified tumor antigens are often recombinant in nature and lack post-translational modification; (2) the antigens are accessible to the isolated antibodies, due to those isolated by using whole tumor cell as antigens could recognize multiple antigens at the same time; and (3) PAb can recognize multiple cell surface proteins correlated with cell death simultaneously. Thus, the approach linking high-throughput proteomic technologies can help discern TAAs efficiently. In the present study, we identified multiple proteins as TAA-presumed potential biomarkers and therapeutic targets for the immunotherapy of MM, including enolase, ADPH, and HSP90s, among others. To explore the function of these proteins and evaluate their clinical applicability and specificity, further studies need to be conducted Integration of PAb with target identification by proteomic technologies may ultimately translate into novel and improved diagnosis and therapy for cancer patients.

Author Contributions

Read and approved of the final manuscript: BM HZ XC JY YS BC SL. Conceived and designed the experiments: BM. Performed the experiments: BM HZ XC JY YS. Analyzed the data: BM BC SL. Wrote the paper: BM.

References

1. Rajkumar SV (2011) Treatment of multiple myeloma. Nature Reviews Clinical Oncology 8: 479–491.

2. Rajkumar S, Gertz M, Kyle R, Greipp P (2002) Current therapy for multiple myeloma. Mayo Clin Proc 77: 813–822.

3. Mahindra A, Laubach J, Raje N, Munshi N, Richardson PG, et al. (2012) Latest advances and current challenges in the treatment of multiple myeloma. Nature Reviews Clinical Oncology 9: 135–143.

4. Roos R, Jansen P (2012) Novel immunotherapy strategies for multiple myeloma and other haematological malignancies. Ned Tijdschr Klin Chem Labgeneesk 37: 38–41.

5. Tai YT, Anderson KC (2011) Antibody-based therapies in multiple myeloma. Bone marrow research 2011. 1–14.

6. de Weers M, Tai YT, van der Veer MS, Bakker JM, Vink T, et al. (2011) Daratumumab, a novel therapeutic human CD38 monoclonal antibody, induces killing of multiple myeloma and other hematological tumors. The Journal of Immunology 186: 1840–1848.

7. Ohno H (2010) Long-term response to maintenance treatment with rituximab in CD20+ multiple myeloma. Leukemia & lymphoma 51: 2144–2146.

8. Tureci O, Usener D, Schneider S, Sahin U (2005) Identification of tumor-associated autoantigens with SEREX. Methods Mol Med 109: 137–154.

9. Qian F, Odunsi K, Blatt L, Scanlan M, Mannan M, et al. (2005) Tumor associated antigen recognition by autologous serum in patients with breast cancer. International journal of molecular medicine 15: 137–144.

10. Kiessling A, Wehner R, Füssel S, Bachmann M, Wirth MP, et al. (2012) Tumor-Associated Antigens for Specific Immunotherapy of Prostate Cancer. Cancers 4: 193–217.

11. Charoenfuprasert S, Yang Y, Lee Y, Chao K, Chu P, et al. (2011) Identification of salt-inducible kinase 3 as a novel tumor antigen associated with tumorigenesis of ovarian cancer. Oncogene 30: 3570–3584.

12. Devitt G, Meyer C, Wiedemann N, Eichmüller S, Kopp-Schneider A, et al. (2005) Serological analysis of human renal cell carcinoma. International Journal of Cancer 118: 2210–2219.

13. Vaughan H, St Clair F, Scanlan M, Chen Y, Maraskovsky E, et al. (2004) The humoral immune response to head and neck cancer antigens as defined by the serological analysis of tumor antigens by recombinant cDNA expression cloning. Cancer Immunity 4: 5–21.

14. Liu W, Zhang G, Wang J, Cao J, Guo X, et al. (2008) Proteomics-based identification of autoantibody against CDC25B as a novel serum marker in esophageal squamous cell carcinoma. Biochemical and biophysical research communications 375: 440–445.

15. Liggins A, Guinn B, Banham A (2005) Identification of lymphoma-associated antigens using SEREX. Methods in molecular medicine 115: 109–128.

16. Tsunemi S, Nakanishi T, Fujita Y, Bouras G, Miyamoto Y, et al. (2010) Proteomics-based identification of a tumor-associated antigen and its corresponding autoantibody in gastric cancer. Oncology reports 23(4): 949–956.

17. Anguille S, Van Tendeloo VF, Berneman Z (2012) Leukemia-associated antigens and their relevance to the immunotherapy of acute myeloid leukemia. Leukemia.26(10): 2186–2196.

18. Adams G, Weiner L (2005) Monoclonal antibody therapy of cancer. Nature biotechnology 23: 1147–1157.

19. Wei Y, Wang Q, Zhao X, Yang L, Tian L, et al. (2000) Immunotherapy of tumors with xenogeneic endothelial cells as a vaccine. Nature medicine 6: 1160–1166.

20. Wang Y, Li D, Shi H, Wen Y, Yang L, et al. (2009) Intratumoral Expression of Mature Human Neutrophil Peptide-1 Mediates Antitumor Immunity in Mice. Clinical Cancer Research 15: 6901–6911.

21. Altenberg B, Greulich K (2004) Genes of glycolysis are ubiquitously overexpressed in 24 cancer classes. Genomics 84: 1014–1020.

22. Takashima M, Kuramitsu Y, Yokoyama Y, Iizuka N, Fujimoto M, et al. (2005) Overexpression of alpha enolase in hepatitis C virus-related hepatocellular carcinoma: association with tumor progression as determined by proteomic analysis. Proteomics 5: 1686–1692.

23. Díaz-Ramos À, Roig-Borrellas A, García-Melero A, López-Alemany R (2012) α-Enolase, a Multifunctional Protein: Its Role on Pathophysiological Situations. BioMed Research International 2012. 1–12.

24. Liu K, Shih N (2007) The Role of Enolase in Tissue Invasion and Metastasis of Pathogens and Tumor Cells. Journal of Cancer Molecules 3: 45–48.

25. Chong BM, Reigan P, Mayle-Combs KD, Orlicky DJ, McManaman JL (2011) Determinants of adipophilin function in milk lipid formation and secretion. Trends in Endocrinology & Metabolism 22: 211–217.

26. Ambrosio MR, Piccaluga PP, Ponzoni M, Rocca BJ, Malagnino V, et al. (2012) The Alteration of Lipid Metabolism in Burkitt Lymphoma Identifies a Novel Marker: Adipophilin. PloS one 7: e44315.

27. McManaman J, Zabaronick W, Schaack J, Orlicky D (2003) Lipid droplet targeting domains of adipophilin. The Journal of Lipid Research 44: 668–673.

28. Mather I, Keenan T (1998) Origin and secretion of milk lipids. Journal of mammary gland biology and neoplasia 3: 259–273.

29. Matsubara J, Honda K, Ono M, Sekine S, Tanaka Y, et al. (2011) Identification of adipophilin as a potential plasma biomarker for colorectal cancer using label-free quantitative mass spectrometry and protein microarray. Cancer Epidemiology Biomarkers & Prevention 20: 2195–2203.

30. Lewandrowski P, Flohr C (2011) Novel formulations of tumour-associated peptides binding to human leukocyte antigen (HLA) class I or II molecules for vaccines. EP Patent 2,111,867.

31. Grebe SK, Erickson LA (2010) Screening for kidney cancer: is there a role for aquaporin-1 and adipophilin? Mayo Foundation. 85(5): 410–412.

32. Russell TD, Schaack J, Orlicky DJ, Palmer C, Chang BHJ, et al. (2011) Adipophilin regulates maturation of cytoplasmic lipid droplets and alveolae in differentiating mammary glands. Journal of cell science 124: 3247–3253.

33. Heid H, Moll R, Schwetlick I, Rackwitz H, Keenan T (1998) Adipophilin is a specific marker of lipid accumulation in diverse cell types and diseases. Cell and tissue research 294: 309–321.

34. Flavin R, Peluso S, Nguyen PL, Loda M (2010) Fatty acid synthase as a potential therapeutic target in cancer. Future Oncology 6: 551–562.

35. R Pandey P, Liu W, Xing F, Fukuda K, Watabe K (2012) Anti-Cancer Drugs Targeting Fatty Acid Synthase (FAS). Recent Patents on Anti-Cancer Drug Discovery 7: 185–197.

36. Wright S, Unfer R, Shellnut J (2006) Adipophilin induction, lipid accumulation, and anti-proliferation through PPAR-gamma activation in malignant melanoma. Proceedings of the American Association for Cancer Research 2006: 320–330.

37. Chen F, Yang Z, Wang X, Liu Y, Yang Y, et al. (2010) Adipophilin affects the expression of TNF-α, MCP-1, and IL-6 in THP-1 macrophages. Molecular and cellular biochemistry 337: 193–199.

38. Hideshima T, Mitsiades C, Tonon G, Richardson P, Anderson K (2007) Understanding multiple myeloma pathogenesis in the bone marrow to identify new therapeutic targets. Nature Reviews Cancer 7: 585–598.

39. Mahalingam D, Swords R, Carew J, Nawrocki S, Bhalla K, et al. (2009) Targeting HSP90 for cancer therapy. British journal of cancer 100: 1523–1529.

40. Trepel J, Mollapour M, Giaccone G, Neckers L (2010) Targeting the dynamic HSP90 complex in cancer. Nature Reviews Cancer 10: 537–549.

41. Zhang F, Lazorchak AS, Liu D, Chen F, Su B (2012) Inhibition of the mTORC2 and chaperone pathways to treat leukemia. blood 119: 6080–6088.

42. Bauer S, Yu L, Demetri G, Fletcher J (2006) Heat shock protein 90 inhibition in imatinib-resistant gastrointestinal stromal tumor. Cancer research 66: 9153–9161.

43. Miekus K, Kijowski J, Sekuła M, Majka M (2012) 17AEP-GA, an HSP90 antagonist, is a potent inhibitor of glioblastoma cell proliferation, survival, migration and invasion. Oncology reports.28(5): 1903–1909.

44. Fu J, Chen D, Zhao B, Zhao Z, Zhou J, et al. (2012) Luteolin Induces Carcinoma Cell Apoptosis through Binding Hsp90 to Suppress Constitutive Activation of STAT3. PloS one 7(11): e49194.

45. Shimamura T, Shapiro G (2008) Heat shock protein 90 inhibition in lung cancer. Journal of Thoracic Oncology 3: S152–S159.

46. Zagouri F, Bournakis E, Koutsoukos K, Papadimitriou CA (2012) Heat Shock Protein 90 (Hsp90) Expression and Breast Cancer. Pharmaceuticals 5: 1008–1020.

47. El Hamidieh A, Grammatikakis N, Patsavoudi E (2012) Cell Surface Cdc37 Participates in Extracellular HSP90 Mediated Cancer Cell Invasion. PloS one 7: e42722.

48. Liu X, Yan Z, Huang L, Guo M, Zhang Z, et al. (2011) Cell surface heat shock protein 90 modulates prostate cancer cell adhesion and invasion through the integrin-β1/focal adhesion kinase/c-Src signaling pathway. Oncology reports 25(5): 1343–1351.

49. Shipp C, Derhovanessian E, Pawelec G (2012) Effect of Culture at Low Oxygen Tension on the Expression of Heat Shock Proteins in a Panel of Melanoma Cell Lines. PloS one 7: e37475.

50. Ferrarini M, Heltai S, Zocchi M, Rugarli C (2006) Unusual expression and localization of heat-shock proteins in human tumor cells. International Journal of Cancer 51: 613–619.

51. Eustace B, Sakurai T, Stewart J, Yimlamai D, Unger C, et al. (2004) Functional proteomic screens reveal an essential extracellular role for hsp90 ¦Å in cancer cell invasiveness. Nature cell biology 6: 507–514.

52. Sapozhnikov A, Ponomarev E, Tarasenko T, Telford W (2007) Spontaneous apoptosis and expression of cell surface heat-shock proteins in cultured EL-4 lymphoma cells. Cell proliferation 32: 363–378.

53. Sims JD, McCready J, Jay DG (2011) Extracellular heat shock protein (Hsp) 70 and Hsp90α assist in matrix metalloproteinase-2 activation and breast cancer cell migration and invasion. PloS one 6: e18848.

54. Hainzl O, Lapina MC, Buchner J, Richter K (2009) The charged linker region is an important regulator of Hsp90 function. Journal of Biological Chemistry 284: 22559–22567.

55. Mollapour M, Tsutsumi S, Neckers L (2010) Hsp90 phosphorylation, Wee1 and the cell cycle. Cell Cycle 9: 2310–2316.

56. Banerji U (2009) Heat shock protein 90 as a drug target: some like it hot. Clinical Cancer Research 15: 9–14.

57. Chiosis G, Dickey CA, Johnson JL (2013) A global view of Hsp90 functions. Nature Structural &Molecular Biology 20: 1–4.

58. Tsutsumi S, Beebe K, Neckers L (2009) Impact of heat-shock protein 90 on cancer metastasis. Future Oncology 5: 679–688.

59. Tsutsumi S, Neckers L (2007) Extracellular heat shock protein 90: a role for a molecular chaperone in cell motility and cancer metastasis. Cancer science 98: 1536–1539.

60. Ferrarini M, Heltai S, Zocchi MR, Rugarli C (2006) Unusual expression and localization of heat-shock proteins in human tumor cells. International Journal of Cancer 51: 613–619.

61. Ho MY, Tang SJ, Ng WV, Yang W, Leu SJJ, et al. (2010) Nucleotide-binding domain of phosphoglycerate kinase 1 reduces tumor growth by suppressing COX-2 expression. Cancer science 101: 2411–2416.

62. Hartmann C, Meyer J, Balss J, Capper D, Mueller W, et al. (2009) Type and frequency of IDH1 and IDH2 mutations are related to astrocytic and oligodendroglial differentiation and age: a study of 1,010 diffuse gliomas. Acta neuropathologica 118: 469–474.

63. Duan Z, Lamendola D, Yusuf R, Penson R, Preffer F, et al. (2002) Overexpression of human phosphoglycerate kinase 1 (PGK1) induces a multidrug resistance phenotype. Anticancer research 22: 1933–1941.

64. Zieker D, Königsrainer I, Tritschler I, Löffler M, Beckert S, et al. (2010) Phosphoglycerate kinase1 a promoting enzyme for peritoneal dissemination in gastric cancer. International Journal of Cancer 126: 1513–1520.

65. Roy SS, Ehrlich AM, Craigen WJ, Hajnóczky G (2009) VDAC2 is required for truncated BID-induced mitochondrial apoptosis by recruiting BAK to the mitochondria. EMBO reports 10: 1341–1347.

11

Focal Radiation Therapy Combined with 4-1BB Activation and CTLA-4 Blockade Yields Long-Term Survival and a Protective Antigen-Specific Memory Response in a Murine Glioma Model

Zineb Belcaid[1], Jillian A. Phallen[1], Jing Zeng[2], Alfred P. See[1], Dimitrios Mathios[1], Chelsea Gottschalk[1], Sarah Nicholas[1], Meghan Kellett[1], Jacob Ruzevick[1], Christopher Jackson[1], Emilia Albesiano[3], Nicholas M. Durham[3], Xiaobu Ye[1], Phuoc T. Tran[2], Betty Tyler[1], John W. Wong[2], Henry Brem[1,4], Drew M. Pardoll[3], Charles G. Drake[3], Michael Lim[1]*

1 Department of Neurosurgery, Johns Hopkins University School of Medicine, Baltimore, Maryland, United States of America, 2 Department of Radiation Oncology and Molecular Radiation Sciences, Johns Hopkins University School of Medicine, Baltimore, Maryland, United States of America, 3 Department of Oncology and Medicine, Johns Hopkins University School of Medicine, Baltimore, Maryland, United States of America, 4 Departments of Oncology, Ophthalmology, and Biomedical Engineering, Johns Hopkins University School of Medicine, Baltimore, Maryland, United States of America

Abstract

Background: Glioblastoma (GBM) is the most common malignant brain tumor in adults and is associated with a poor prognosis. Cytotoxic T lymphocyte antigen -4 (CTLA-4) blocking antibodies have demonstrated an ability to generate robust antitumor immune responses against a variety of solid tumors. 4-1BB (CD137) is expressed by activated T lymphocytes and served as a co-stimulatory signal, which promotes cytotoxic function. Here, we evaluate a combination immunotherapy regimen involving 4-1BB activation, CTLA-4 blockade, and focal radiation therapy in an immune-competent intracranial GBM model.

Methods: GL261-luciferace cells were stereotactically implanted in the striatum of C57BL/6 mice. Mice were treated with a triple therapy regimen consisted of 4-1BB agonist antibodies, CTLA-4 blocking antibodies, and focal radiation therapy using a small animal radiation research platform and mice were followed for survival. Numbers of brain-infiltrating lymphocytes were analyzed by FACS analysis. CD4 or CD8 depleting antibodies were administered to determine the relative contribution of T helper and cytotoxic T cells in this regimen. To evaluate the ability of this immunotherapy to generate an antigen-specific memory response, long-term survivors were re-challenged with GL261 glioma en B16 melanoma flank tumors.

Results: Mice treated with triple therapy had increased survival compared to mice treated with focal radiation therapy and immunotherapy with 4-1BB activation and CTLA-4 blockade. Animals treated with triple therapy exhibited at least 50% long-term tumor free survival. Treatment with triple therapy resulted in a higher density of CD4+ and CD8+ tumor infiltrating lymphocytes. Mechanistically, depletion of CD4+ T cells abrogated the antitumor efficacy of triple therapy, while depletion of CD8+ T cells had no effect on the treatment response.

Conclusion: Combination therapy with 4-1BB activation and CTLA-4 blockade in the setting of focal radiation therapy improves survival in an orthotopic mouse model of glioma by a CD4+ T cell dependent mechanism and generates antigen-specific memory.

Editor: Mike Chen, City of Hope, United States of America

Funding: These authors have no support or funding to report.

Competing Interests: Michael Lim is a PLOS ONE Editorial Board member. This does not alter the authors' adherence to PLOS ONE Editorial policies and criteria. Michael Lim is also a speaker for Accuray and receives research funding from Accuray, Bristol-Meyers Squibb, Celldex and Agenus. Charles Drake is a consultant for Bristol-Meyers Squibb, Compugen, Dendreon, and Roche/Genentech and he is an advisor for Aduro and Bristol-Meyers Squibb. He receives research funding from Bristol-Meyers Squibb, Aduro and Medarex and has stock ownership of Compugen. Drew Pardoll is a consultant/advisor for Jounce Therapeutics, Bristol-Meyers Squibb, ImmuneXcite and Aduro and receives research funding from Bristol-Meyers Squibb. Jing Zeng, Michael Lim, Charles Drake and Drew Pardoll hold a patent for the work related to this study. The authors declare that they have a patent relating to material pertinent to this article; this international patent application PCT/US2012/043124 entitled "Use of Adjuvant Focused Radiation Including Stereotactic Radiosurgery for Augmenting Immune Based Therapies Against Neoplasms" was filed 19 June 2012. This application was subsequently filed on the national stage in the United Stage, Europe, Canada, Australia, India and China. There are no further patents, products in development or marketed products to declare.

* Email: mlim3@jhmi.edu

Introduction

The prognosis for patients with glioblastoma (GBM) remains poor despite treatment with surgical resection followed by adjuvant radiotherapy and the addition of temozolomide [1,2]. Immune checkpoint inhibitors have emerged as a promising strategy in cancer immunotherapy. Immune checkpoints are a class of cell surface molecules expressed by activated T and B lymphocytes. Upon engaging their ligands, immune checkpoints inhibit proliferation and activity of immune cells thereby protecting against autoimmunity [3]. Studies and clinical trials of immunotherapy for GBM pointed out the immunosuppressive influence of the GBM microenvironment as a significant hurdle, however, GBM infiltrating immune cells have been found to express immune checkpoint molecules [4,5]. Blocking these immunosuppressive mechanisms while generating a strong antitumor response is an intuitive strategy for cancer immunotherapy. A variety of tools are now available to test this strategy empirically and move these agents into clinical trials [5].

Our group recently published results demonstrating that PD-1 blockade, in combination with stereotactic radiation therapy resulted in a durable, long-term survival in GL261 bearing mice [6]. Antibodies against co-stimulatory molecules, such as 4-1BB (CD137) and Cytotoxic T-Lymphocyte Antigen 4 (CTLA-4, CD152) have the potential to enhance immune responses and produce anti-tumor immunity [7–10]. 4-1BB is expressed on activated T cells and engagement of 4-1BB with its ligand drives proliferation of $CD8^+$ T cells, increased pro-inflammatory cytokine production and plays an essential role in the formation of long-lived memory cytotoxic T cells [9,11,12]. CTLA-4 signaling impairs the capacity of T cells to proliferate and to produce pro-inflammatory cytokines [13]. Blockade of CTLA-4 removes these suppressive signals and allows antigen-specific T cells to expand and perform their effector functions [7]. Ipilimumab, a human monoclonal antibody that blocks CTLA-4, has been approved by the FDA for first line treatment of advanced melanoma. In phase III trials, ipilimumab improved survival in patients with metastatic melanoma and produced a durable anti-tumor memory response [14,15]. Ipilimumab has also been shown to induce regression of melanoma brain metastases [16] and may be potentiated by radiation therapy [17]. However, some patients treated with ipilimumab suffered from severe immune-related adverse events, which was consistent with the proposed mechanism of CTLA-4 blockade [14]. An approach to overcome this burden is to combine CTLA-4 blockade with 4-1BB activation: both individual antibodies cause inflammation to selective organs, however, a combination of the two antibodies increased cancer immunity while reducing inflammation and autoimmune effects [18].

To bolster the anti-tumor immunity created by the monoclonal antibodies anti-CTLA-4 and anti-4-1BB, our group investigated the effects of radiation on glioma treatment as well. Radiation therapy has the potential to augment immune responses against central nervous system tumors [19,20]. Furthermore, cancer cells destroyed by radiation therapy are considered to be a source of tumor associated antigens that can be processed by professional antigen presenting cells [21].

We investigated the use of focal radiation therapy in addition to anti-4-1BB and anti-CTLA-4 immunotherapy as a combination strategy in an orthotopic, preclinical model of malignant glioma. We hypothesized that radiation therapy followed by 4-1BB activation and CTLA-4 blockade produces an effective and durable anti-tumor response against intracranial GL261 gliomas.

Materials and Methods

Ethics statement

Animal procedures were performed in accordance with institutional protocols and approved by the Johns Hopkins University Animal Care and Use Committee (protocol # MO09M395).

Mice

Six- to eight-week old female C57BL/6 mice (Harlan) were maintained under pathogen-free conditions at Johns Hopkins University.

Cells and reagents

Luciferase-expressing cell lines, GL261-luciferase (GL261-luc) glioma, and B16-luc melanoma cells were produced as previously described [6]. GL261-luc glioma cells and B16-luc melanoma cells were cultured in DMEM supplemented with 10% fetal bovine serum and 1% penicillin-streptomycin at $37°C$ in a 5% CO_2 and 95% humidified air atmosphere. Anti-CTLA-4 mAb producing hybridoma 4F10 was purchased from American Type Culture Collection and the anti-4-1BB hybridoma 2A was kindly provided by Dr. Lieping Chen (Yale University). Both antibodies were purified from supernatant by a protein G column. Hamster and rat IgG to serve as control antibodies were purchased from Rockland Immunochemicals Inc. CD4-FITC and CD8-PE antibodies were used for FACS analysis (BD-Pharmingen). Anti-CD4 and anti-CD8 rat antibodies were used for *in vivo* depletion studies (BioXcell).

Treatment protocol

The orthotopic glioma model was established as previously described [6]. Animals were stratified into treatment groups on day 7 following intracranial implantation based on tumor burden as determined by bioluminescent imaging. For those mice treated with focal radiation therapy, a single fraction of radiation at a dose of 10 Gy was delivered using a 3 mm collimator on day 10 following intracranial implantation using the Small Animal Radiation Research Platform (SARRP) [22]. With the built-in micro-CT scanner we identified the burr hole, which served as the coordinate for delivery of radiation [23]. In those mice treated with anti-4-1BB mAb, 200 µg of anti-4-1BB antibodies was dosed via intra-peritoneal injection on days 11, 14 and 17 following intracranial implantation. In mice treated with anti-CTLA-4 mAb, 800 µg of anti-CTLA-4 antibodies was dosed via intra-peritoneal injection on days 11, 17 and 23. Controls in all treatment groups received rat and hamster IgG. For the pilot experiments in which treatment with a single antibody was compared to combination therapy with SRS and antibody therapy, five animals were used per treatment group and this experiment was performed once. In the CTLA-4 timing experiments, eight animals were used per treatment group and these experiments were repeated twice. The triple therapy experiments were repeated three times and a total of 18 animals per treatment group were used. Animals were observed three times a week for signs of lethargy such as weight loss, hunched position and epilepsy. In order to reduce suffering when these symptoms occurred, animals were euthanized with cervical dislocation after i.p. injections with a ketamine/xylazine anesthetic. Survival time was recorded and long-term survivors were defined as animals surviving longer than 3 times the median survival of non-treated animals.

Analysis of tumor infiltrating CD4$^+$ and CD8$^+$ T cells

Three mice from each treatment group and an additional three naïve mice were randomly selected at day 18 following intracranial implantation and euthanized. Brains and cervical lymph nodes were harvested from each mouse separately and processed into single cell suspensions in RPMI. The cells were filtered through a 40 μm nylon cell strainer, centrifuged at 1000 rpm, and resuspended in 4 mL of 30% Percoll. The cells were overlaid onto a Percoll gradient (30%/37%/60%) and centrifuged at 1200 rpm for 20 minutes. Lymphocytes were collected from the 37%/60% interface and washed twice in PBS. The cells were stained with anti-CD4 and anti-CD8 antibodies and then fixed. Stained cells were analyzed on a FACS Calibur flow cytometer (BD Biosciences) and data analysis was performed with FlowJo software (TreeStar, Ashland OR).

Depletion of CD4$^+$ and CD8+ T cell subsets *in vivo*

Mice were implanted with GL261-luc cells as described above and on day 7 stratified based on bioluminescence into four treatment groups. On days 5, 6 and 7 mice from the CD4 and CD8 depletion groups received 200 μg of anti-CD4 and anti-CD8 antibody respectively in order to achieve *in vivo* depletion. Treatment was administered as described in the triple therapy arm above. Mice received depletion antibodies every 7 days to maintain the depleted condition. Response to *in vivo* depletion of CD4$^+$ and CD8$^+$ T cells was recorded as a change in survival time compared to the non-depleted mice receiving triple therapy.

GL261 and B16 flank tumors

On day 100 after intracranial implantation, long-term survivors from the triple therapy group and naïve (non-tumor bearing) mice were challenged by subcutaneous injection in both hind limbs with 10^6 GL261-luc cells in 100 μL of mixed PBS and Matrigel (BD Biosciences) in a 1:1 ratio. A second set of long-term survivors from both the triple therapy group and double antibody group were challenged subcutaneously with 10^6 GL261-luc cells in the left flank and 10^5 B16-luc cells in the right flank. Tumor growth was measured every 2 to 3 days using calipers and tumor volumes were calculated in three dimensions using the formula: $\frac{4}{3}\pi r^3$. Animals were observed for an additional 50 days or euthanized when tumor volumes reached approximately 1000 mm^3 in each flank.

Statistical analysis

Survival was analyzed with the log-rank Mantel-Cox test. Comparison of infiltrating T cells in the brains and lymph nodes was performed with the Student's t-test. All statistical analyses were performed using GraphPad Prism 5 (GraphPad Software Inc., La Jolla, CA).

Results

Focal radiation therapy combined with CTLA-4 blockade prolonged survival in established intracranial GL261 tumors

Our first aim focused on determining the efficacy of combination therapy with focal RT and 4-1BB activation or CTLA-4 blockade. We proceeded with the treatment protocol shown in Figure 1A. Treatment with 4-1BB agonist antibodies alone did not enhance survival when compared to untreated mice ($p = 0.16$). The addition of 4-1BB agonist antibodies to RT extended survival

significantly compared to untreated mice ($p < 0.05$). However, this combination did not significantly differ from treatment with focal RT alone (Fig. 1B; $p = 0.99$). Combination therapy with RT and CTLA-4 blockade improved survival in our glioma model. Animals treated with anti-CTLA-4 antibodies alone did not extend survival in comparison with untreated animals ($p = 0.11$; one-sided Log-rank test). Combination therapy with RT and CTLA-4 blockade resulted in a significantly prolonged survival time than untreated animals ($p < 0.01$) and when compared with focal RT alone ($p < 0.05$; one-sided Log-rank test). Mice treated with the combination of RT and CTLA-4 blockade had a median survival of 29 days, and 50% of mice treated with this combination where still alive after 30 days whereas all mice from the anti-CTLA-4 antibody alone and focal RT alone group died before day 30 after intracranial implantation (figure 1B). These results show that combination therapy with focal RT and anti-CTLA-4 antibodies prolongs overall survival in treated mice.

Optimal timing of treatment with anti-CTLA-4 antibodies does not influence therapeutic efficacy

We next assessed whether timing of CTLA-4 blockade influenced treatment efficacy (Fig. 2A). Animals treated with focal RT first on day 10 followed with CTLA-4 blockade on days 12, 14 and 15, had a significantly longer survival time of 27.5 days compared to untreated animals (Fig. 2B; $p < 0.01$). When CTLA-4 blockade was administered simultaneously with RT on day 10 followed with injections on days 12 and 14, median survival extended from 21.5 days to 29 days ($p < 0.001$ vs. untreated). CTLA-4 blockade starting two days prior to RT on day 8, and followed with injections on days 10 and 12, resulted in a median survival of 29.5 days ($p < 0.01$ vs. untreated). Survival times of all three RT and CTLA-4 blockade combination groups were comparable. This suggests that the treatment efficacy of the combination treatment (RT and CTLA-4 blockade) is independent of the sequence of the two therapeutic components. Moreover, these results confirm that combination therapy with focal RT and CTLA-4 blockade prolong overall survival resulting in long-term tumor free survival in 25% of treated mice from the earlier time points group (day 8–10–12), 22% long-term survival in treated mice from the middle time points group (day 10–12–14), and 12.5% long-term survival in treated mice from the later time points group (day 12–14–16).

Combining stereotactic radiosurgery with 4-1BB activation and CTLA-4 blockade results in long-term survival

After confirming that combination therapy with RT and 4-1BB activation or CTLA-4 blockade extends median survival, we proceeded with combining all three modalities into a "triple therapy" (Fig. 3A). Immunotherapy with the combination treatment of anti-4-1BB and anti-CTLA-4 antibodies resulted in a significantly higher median survival of 23 days instead of 21.5 days when untreated (Fig. 3B; $p < 0.05$). Furthermore, where treatment with RT failed to produce long-term survival, immunotherapy with anti-4-1BB and anti-CTLA-4 antibodies produced a long-term tumor free survival in 3 out of 18 mice (16.7%). Triple therapy with RT, 4-1BB activation and CTLA-4 blockade extended the median survival from 24 days when treated with focal RT to 67 days ($p < 0.05$ vs. all other treatment modalities) with 50% of the mice going on to become long-term survivors.

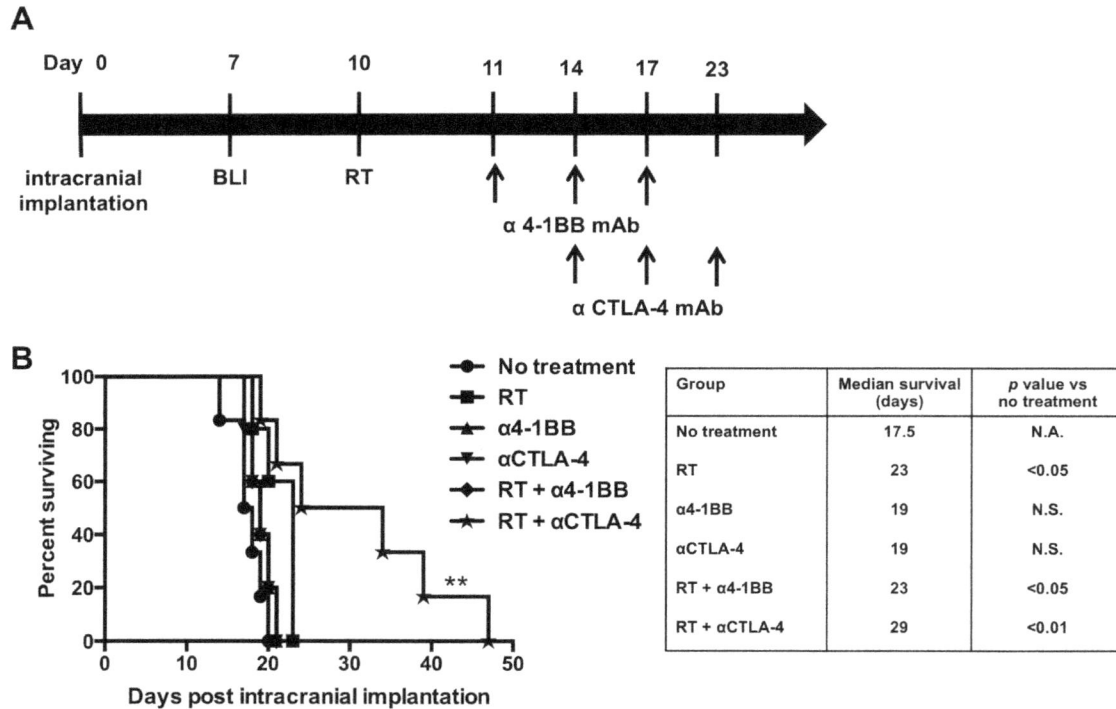

Figure 1. Focal radiation therapy combined with CTLA-4 blockade prolonged survival in established intracranial GL261 tumors. A) Schematic of the treatment protocol for combination therapy with RT and 4-1BB activation or CTLA-4 blockade. B) Kaplan Meier survival curves for single immunotherapy with anti-4-1BB antibodies and combination therapy with RT and 4-1BB activation or CTLA-4 blockade ($n = 5$–6 mice/group). Single immunotherapy with anti-4-1BB antibodies did not extend median survival ($p = 0.16$ vs. untreated mice). Combination treatment with RT and 4-1BB activation extended median survival times significantly ($p < 0.05$ vs. untreated mice), however, this result was not significant when compared to treatment with focal RT alone ($p = 0.99$). CTLA-4 blockade alone did not extend median survival in treated animals, however, trended towards significance ($p = 0.11$ vs. controls). Combination therapy with RT and anti-CTLA-4 antibodies prolonged overall survival significantly compared to either treatment modality alone ($p = 0.045$ vs. RT; one-sided Log-Rank test). P values were calculated with the Log-Rank test.

Triple therapy leads to increased CD4$^+$ and CD8$^+$ infiltrating lymphocytes in the brain

After establishing the significance of the triple therapy regimen *in vivo*, we quantified infiltrating T cells in brains and cervical lymph nodes harvested from animals in each treatment arm. We found significantly higher numbers of infiltrating CD4$^+$ T cells in the brains of mice treated with the combination of anti-4-1BB and anti-CTLA-4 antibodies as well as the mice treated with triple therapy when compared to brains of non-tumor bearing mice (Fig. 4A; $p < 0.05$). We also found similar results when we looked at infiltrating CD8$^+$ T cells; the density of CD8$^+$ T cells from these groups was significantly higher than that of non-tumor bearing mice (Fig. 4B; $p < 0.05$). In order to assess the immune modulation in the periphery, we collected and analyzed CD4$^+$ and CD8$^+$ T lymphocyte populations from the draining (cervical) lymph nodes from mice in each treatment group. We observed no significant differences in the percentages of CD4$^+$ and CD8$^+$ lymphocytes when looking specifically at the cervical lymph nodes (Fig. 4C and 4D). At day 18 post intracranial tumor implantation, we thus did not observe any changes in T cell populations in the periphery for any treatment group, however, the primary tumor site did exhibit significant changes in both CD4$^+$ and CD8$^+$ T cell percentages in the triple treatment group as well as the anti-4-1BB and anti-CTLA-4 double treatment group. These findings indicate that differences in lymphocyte modulation exist between the primary tumor site within the brain and the draining lymph nodes in the periphery.

The anti-tumor activity of triple therapy is CD4$^+$ T cell dependent

To determine which subset of immune cells contributes to the anti-tumor effect elicited by triple therapy, CD4$^+$ and CD8$^+$ T cells were depleted with monoclonal antibodies in mice that subsequently received treatment with triple therapy. Depletion of CD4$^+$ T cells completely abolished the anti-tumor activity of triple therapy ($p < 0.001$) and median survival times were comparable to untreated mice (Fig. 5). In contrast, mice with depleted CD8$^+$ T cells survived significantly longer than untreated mice, as well as significantly longer than mice in the CD4$^+$ depletion group ($p < 0.01$). Moreover, depletion of CD8$^+$ T cells also resulted in 43% of mice exhibiting long-term survival making this group comparable to the non-depleted triple therapy group. These data suggest that long-term survival due to triple therapy is primarily CD4$^+$ T cell dependent.

Treatment with triple therapy results in a glioma-specific protective memory response

To evaluate whether long-term survivors had developed a protective anti-tumor memory response, we challenged them with a subcutaneous flank injection of GL261 cells at day 100 after their first intracranial implantation. Figure 6A displays the tumor growth measurements for each flank tumor ($n = 8$) in naïve animals ($n = 4$); in all four animals, tumors had progressive growth by day 28. However, all of the long-term survivors ($n = 3$; 6 flank tumors), that had successfully rejected the intracranially implanted

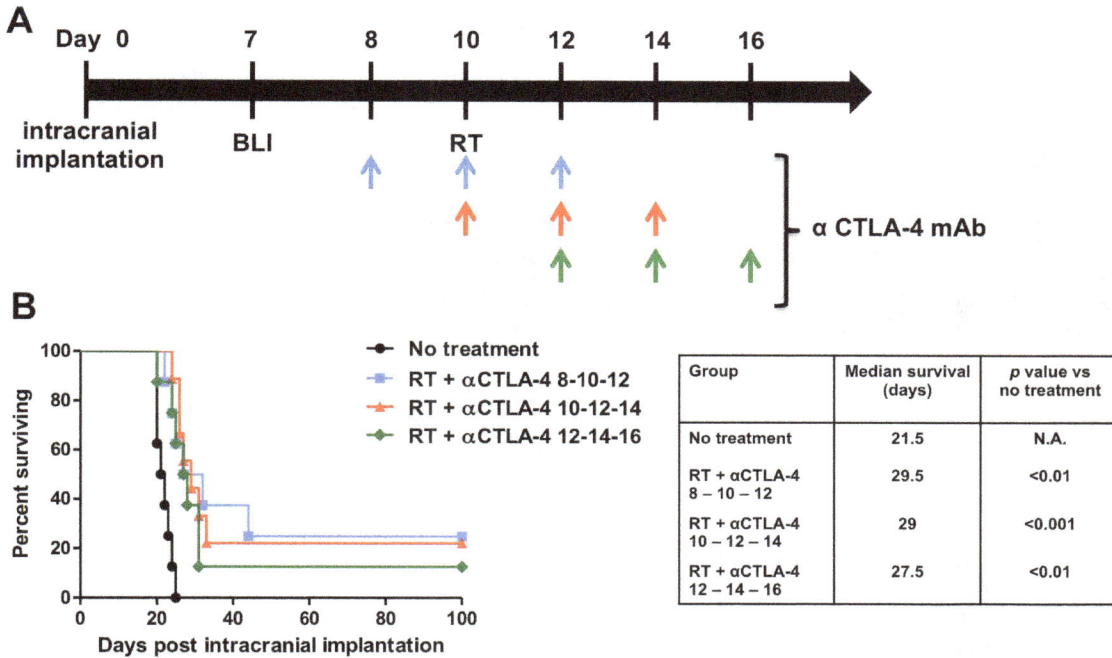

Figure 2. The role of timing in efficacy of anti-CTLA-4 antibody therapy. A) Schematic of the treatment protocol for the CTLA-4 blockade timing experiment. Please note that all treated animals received RT on day 10 and three antibody injections in three different timing schedules (colored arrows). B) Combination therapy with RT and CTLA-4 blockade results in long-term survival compared to controls ($p<0.01$), however, there was no significant difference in treatment efficacy between the three combination therapy groups. P values were calculated with the Log-Rank test.

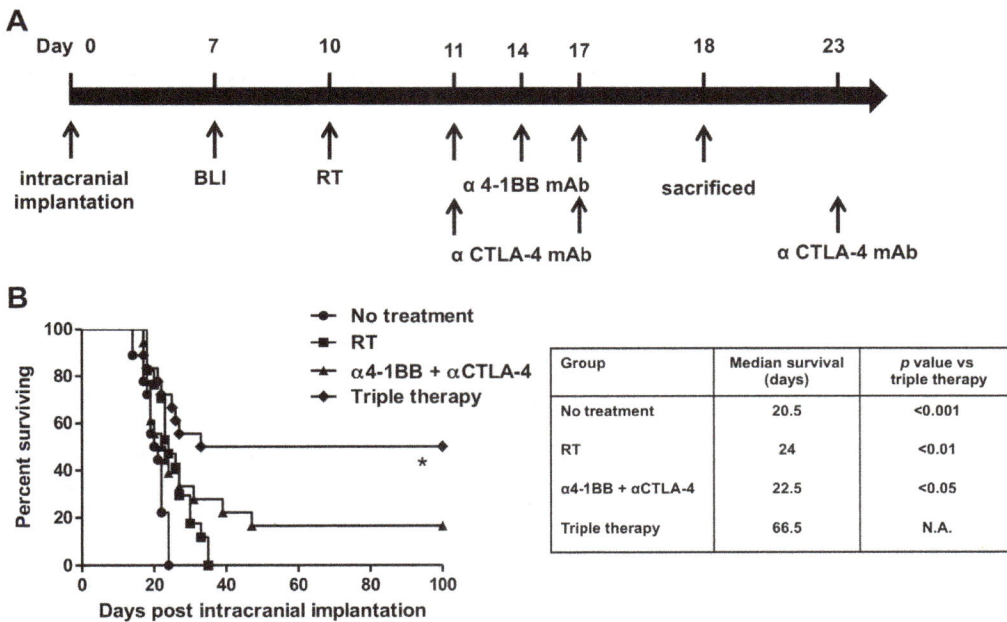

Figure 3. Combining focal radiation therapy with anti-4-1BB and anti-CTLA-4 antibodies results in long-term survival. A) Schematic of the treatment protocol for triple therapy. B) Kaplan Meier survival curves for double immunotherapy and triple therapy ($n=18$/group). Treatment with triple therapy was superior to double immunotherapy with anti-4-1BB and anti-CTLA-4 antibodies ($p<0.05$), focal RT alone ($p<0.01$) and untreated mice ($p<0.001$). Furthermore, triple therapy results in long-term survival in at least 50% of treated animals, whereas immunotherapy with both 4-1BB activation and CTLA-4 blockade produced long-term survival in 3/18 mice (16.7%). Data from three repeated experiments with similar results was pooled into single Kaplan Meier curves. P values were calculated with the Log-Rank test.

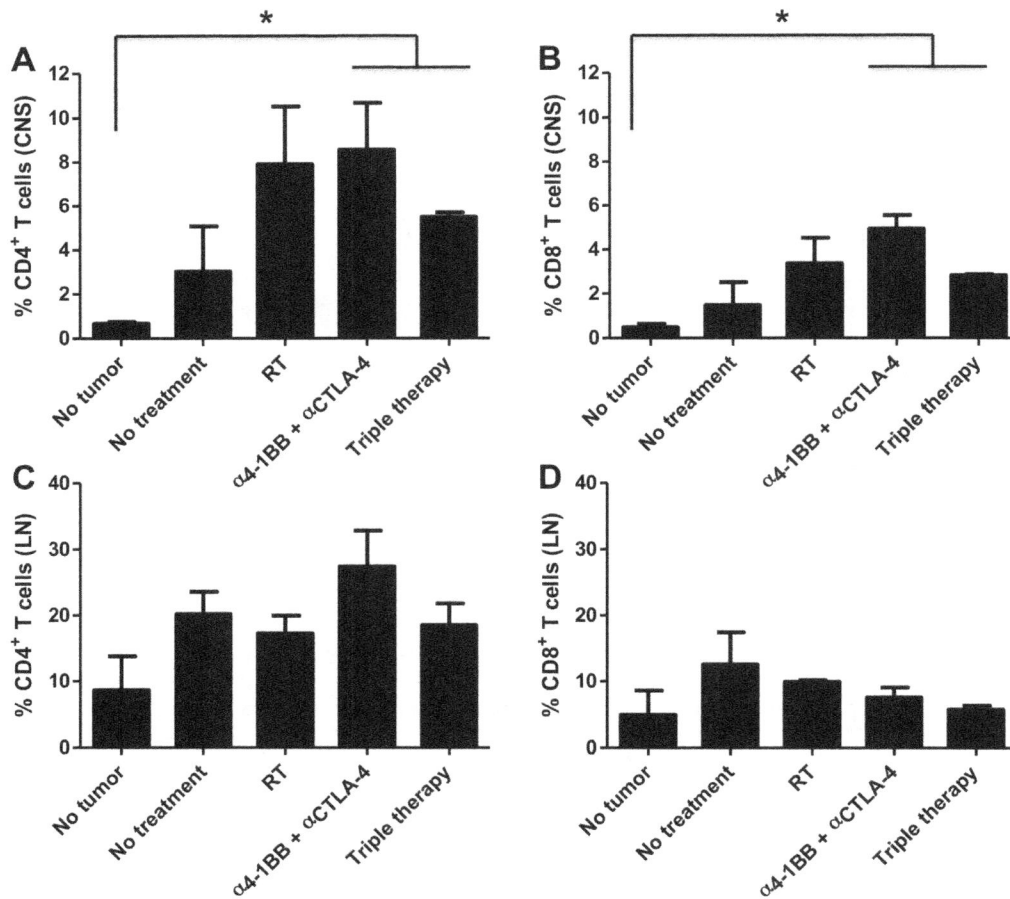

Figure 4. Triple therapy leads to increased CD4$^+$ and CD8$^+$ infiltrating lymphocytes in the brain. A, B) Influx of CD4$^+$ and CD8$^+$ tumor infiltrating lymphocytes respectively was higher in brains of animals treated with immunotherapy with 4-1BB activation and CTLA-4 blockade and triple therapy compared to brains from non-tumor bearing mice ($p<0.05$). C, D) Cervical lymph nodes from naïve mice showed a higher baseline of CD4$^+$ and CD8$^+$ T cells which resulted in comparable densities of T cells between all groups. Error bars represent standard error of the mean (SEM) and p values were calculated with the student t-test.

tumor in the first round of experimentation, did not develop flank tumors (Fig. 6B). Next, we developed a model to determine whether the systemic anti-tumor memory response in long-term

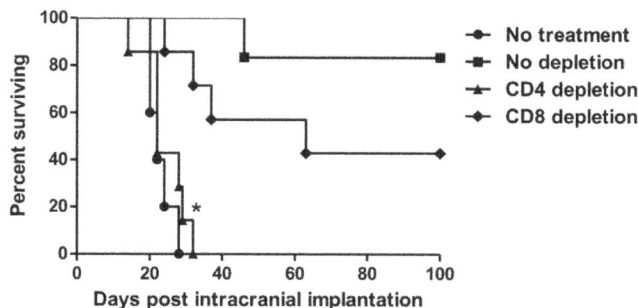

Figure 5. The anti-tumor activity of triple therapy is CD4$^+$ T cell dependent. Kaplan Meier survival curves for untreated animals, triple therapy (no depletion), triple therapy with depleted CD4$^+$ T cells and triple therapy with depleted CD8$^+$ T cells ($n=5-7$ mice/group). CD4$^+$ T cell depletion abolishes the survival benefit of triple therapy ($p<0.001$). Depletion of CD8$^+$ T cells did not interfere with the efficacy of triple therapy and resulted in long-term survival.

survivors is specific for GL261 glioma tumors only or is also responsive to other types of tumors. We compared GL261 glioma and B16 melanoma tumor growth in long-term survivors and in naïve mice. GL261 cells were implanted subcutaneously into the left flank, while B16 cells were implanted into the right flank. Figure 6C shows bioluminescent imaging data on day 21 after GL261 and B16 flank tumor implantation in both naïve mice and long-term survivors. Naïve mice grew both tumor types resulting in palpable nodules on both flanks (Fig. 6D and 6E), whereas long-term survivors grew only B16 tumors with no evidence of palpable GL261 tumors (Fig. 6F and 6G). The observed difference between absent GL261 glioma and active B16 melanoma growth, therefore, indicates a glioma-specific anti-tumor memory response.

Discussion

In our preclinical study, we have shown that triple therapy combining RT with anti-4-1BB and anti-CTLA-4 antibodies confers long-term survival in a murine GL261 glioma model. The long-term survivors exhibit a glioma-specific memory response. Furthermore, we have shown that triple therapy is primarily CD4$^+$ T cell dependent.

Immunotherapy has been widely tested in both pre-clinical studies and clinical trials as a treatment for multiple cancer types.

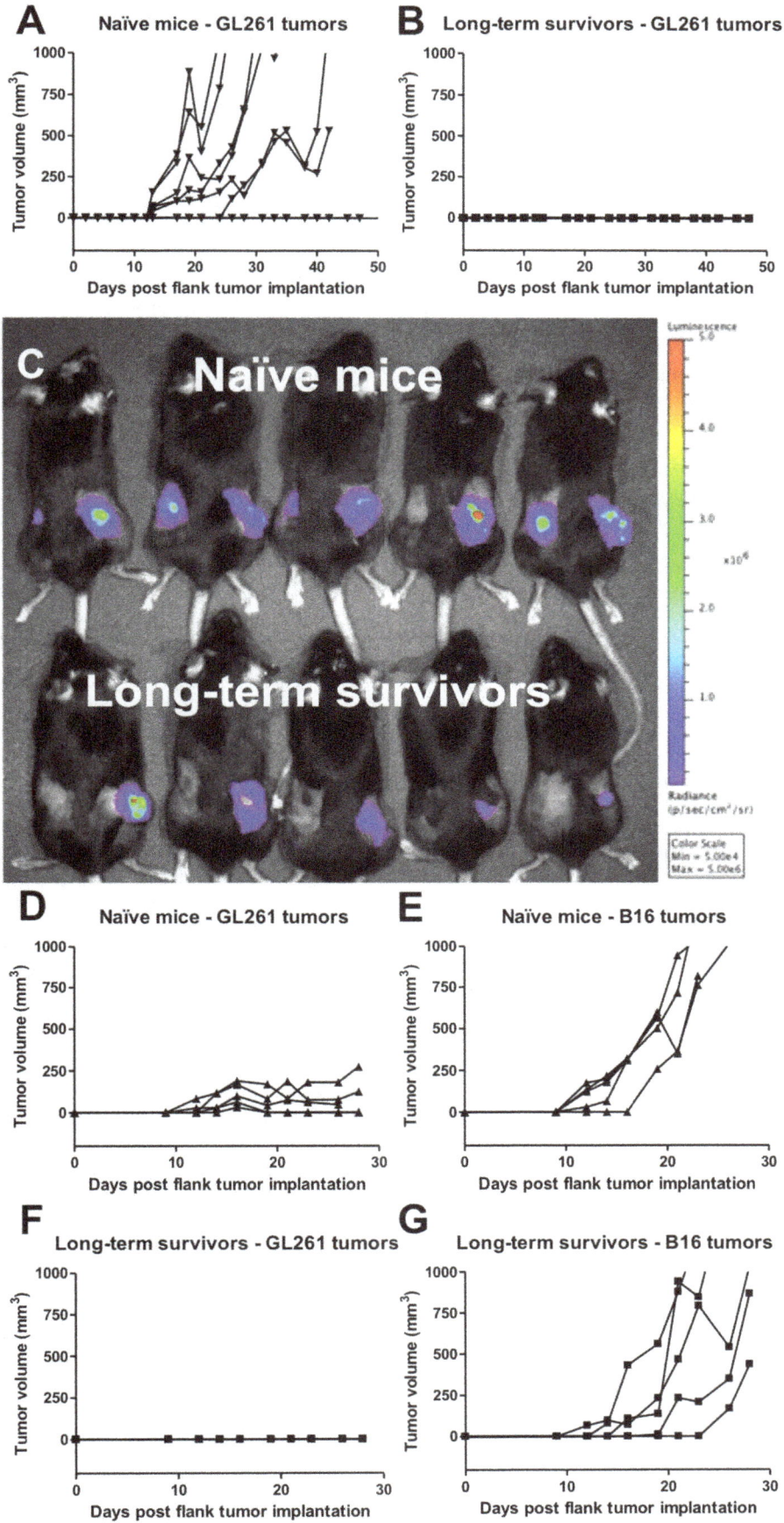

Figure 6. Treatment with triple therapy results in a glioma-specific memory response. A) Naïve mice ($n = 4$/group) challenged with GL261 cells in both flanks formed flank tumors in 6/8 flanks. All control animals formed GL261 flank tumors; two animals formed bilateral flank tumors and two animals formed unilateral flank tumors. B) Long-term survivors ($n = 3$/group) developed long-lasting immunity to GL261 tumors and successfully rejected flank tumor formation in 6/6 flanks. Mice were observed for 50 days. Each line represents tumor growth in one flank. C) Bioluminescent imaging data on day 21 after flank tumor implantation for an experiment where naïve mice (top row) and long-term survivors (bottom row) were inoculated subcutaneously with 10^6 GL261-luc cells in the *left* flank and 10^5 B16-luc cells in the *right* flank. D) Naïve mice had progressive GL261 and E) B16 flank tumor growth. Note that B16 tumors grew faster in comparison to GL261 tumors. F) Long-term survivors established a protective memory response and rejected GL261 flank tumor growth. G) Long-term survivors established a glioma-specific memory response which did not affect the formation of B16 melanoma flank tumors.

These studies have shown promising results when immunotherapy has been tested against less aggressive tumor types, but fail to achieve equally robust anti-tumor responses when utilized against some of the most malignant tumor models. More specifically, immunotherapy combining 4-1BB activation and CTLA-4 blockade resulted in tumor rejection in 100% of treated animals in a murine RM-1 prostate model [24]. This double therapy also resulted in significant tumor rejection in established MC38 colon tumors. While the combination of anti-4-1BB and anti-CTLA-4 antibodies produced tumor rejection in these two commonly less aggressive tumor types, the same therapy failed to produce tumor growth delay in the highly aggressive B16 melanoma model [25]. Combination immunotherapies have also been tested as a treatment in murine models of glioma: the combination of GVAX followed by CTLA-4 blockade resulted in 50% long-term survival in a murine model of intracranial glioma, whereas CTLA-4 blockade alone did not improve survival in established tumors [26]. Conversely, murine intracranial SMA-560 gliomas treated with anti-CTLA-4 antibodies as a monotherapy elicited long-term survival in 80% of treated animals [27]. Though this particular study found a survival benefit resulting from the administration of one immune modulating agent, the vast majority of immunotherapy studies implicate combination therapy as more efficacious in fighting tumor growth. We found that when both antibodies were combined with radiation, treatment not only resulted in prolonged survival but also produced a durable tumor free long-term survival.

The synergy of immune modulating agents has been well documented, and the specific combination of 4-1BB activation and CTLA-4 blockade offsets any toxicity incurred by using one agent on its own. The addition of 4-1BB activation to CTLA-4 blockade reduced the severe immune related adverse events that result from CTLA-4 blockade in a preclinical study [18]. Treatment with the human monoclonal CTLA-4 blocking antibody ipilimumab resulted in severe immune related adverse events in a clinical trial that made termination of treatment inevitable [14]. It seems that the occurrence of these severe immune related events was related to the mechanism of CTLA-4 blockade. Treatment with nivolumab, a human monoclonal antibody blocking PD-1, resulted in a milder toxicity profile [28]. Furthermore, the addition of nivolumab to ipilimumab reduced the rate of severe immune related events related to CTLA-4 blockade remarkably, which affirms the benefits of combining monoclonal antibodies [29].

The addition of radiation to immunotherapy provides an environment conducive to immune mediated killing of tumor cells in order to activate effective antigen presentation. This strategy prevents cancer cells from escaping immune recognition [19,20,30]. While radiotherapy is part of the standard treatment regimen for malignant glioma, the high number of fractions may actually hinder the ability of the immune system to target and kill cancer cells [31]. We previously published results suggested that focal radiation could augment an immune response [6]. We used a unique small animal irradiator to deliver precise radiation making

our approach an attractive regimen for translation into the clinic [22,23]. Although our results show that treatment with double immunotherapy – without focal RT – resulted in tumor free survival in 17% of treated animals, triple therapy remained superior by consistent tumor rejection in at least 50% in all animals. Interestingly, we found that the treated animals either had a complete objective response to triple therapy that resulted in the formation of a protective memory or failed to respond to treatment. One possible explanation could come from the fact that there is likely variability in the sizes of each animal's tumor (hence some could have margins outside of the treatment field) and perhaps a certain amount of the tumor needed to be exposed to radiation to elicit the protective response. In addition, the addition of focal RT to CTLA-4 blockade resulted in long-term survivors. As a result, our findings suggest that radiation is synergistic when combined with immunotherapy.

In addition, we found that the timing of antibody treatment with regard to RT did not influence treatment efficacy [32]. One point to note was that the timing of the CTLA-4 antibody administration was different due to logistics. In the triple therapy protocol, anti-CTLA-4 antibodies were administered in a six day interval in order to reduce the risk of auto-immunity when combined with anti-4-1BB antibodies. For the CTLA-4 timing experiment, the interval of antibody administration was shortened from six days to two days in order to assess the timing relative to RT delivery. CTLA-4 blockade administered on three separate time schedules relative to RT did not differ in result suggesting that treatment efficacy is independent of a specific therapeutic window. Surprisingly, when CTLA-4 blockade was given in three dosages of 800 μg in a two-day interval – instead of the six day interval employed in our triple therapy protocol – the treatment was able to produce tumor free long-term survival.

We sought to examine the mechanism by which the triple therapy affects T cell infiltration in the brain. It is known that CTLA-4 blockade removes suppressive signals and allows expansion of tumor-specific T cells, in particular of CD4$^+$ effectors [7]. On the other hand, 4-1BB activation is known to co-stimulate CD8$^+$ T cells and increases their proliferation and survival [12]. We hypothesized that triple therapy will result in higher CD4$^+$ and CD8$^+$ tumor infiltrating lymphocytes. When compared to non-tumor bearing mice, our results show that there is indeed an influx of CD4$^+$ and CD8$^+$ T cells into the brains from the groups in which immunotherapy with 4-1BB activation and CTLA-4 blockade is employed. The depletion study provided information about which of these two T cell subsets determines the efficacy of triple therapy. Interestingly, animals treated with triple therapy with CD8$^+$ T cell depletion responded to treatment and resulted in 43% long-term survival whereas depletion of CD4$^+$ T cells completely abolished the effect of triple therapy. This is surprising considering a previously published study stating that the tumor-eradicating effect of 4-1BB activation with CTLA-4 blockade in a MC38 colon cancer model is primarily CD8$^+$ T cell dependent [18]. Furthermore, our recently published study showed that combination therapy with focal RT and PD-1 blockade was primarily CD8$^+$ T cell dependent and that depletion of CD4$^+$ T cells did not interfere with treatment efficacy [6]. We hypothesized that triple therapy would be CD8$^+$ T cell dependent as well, however, our results suggest that triple therapy is CD4$^+$ T cell-dependent and, more surprisingly, CD8$^+$ T cell-independent. The precise mechanism remains unknown.

We have found that our triple therapy regimen has the potential to eliminate tumor cells and confer a survival advantage to over 50% of animals treated with the regimen. One additional desirable outcome of using immunotherapy is to develop a memory response to tumor cells such that highly aggressive tumors such as GBM do not have a chance to recur. To assess the establishment of a protective tumor response, long-term survivors were re-challenged with GL261 cells in both flanks and were capable of rejecting glioma flank tumor formation. In contrast, when long-term survivors were peripherally injected with B16 melanoma cells, flank tumors were formed. It is known that gliomas and melanomas share melanoma-associated antigens like trp2 and gp100 [33,34], however, our results suggest a glioma-specific memory response. This finding is consistent with the concept that the anti-tumor memory response in this model involves glioma-specific antigens. Future work is needed to identify these antigens and evaluate their specificity.

Conclusion

Treatment with focal radiation therapy followed by double immunotherapy with anti-4-1BB and anti-CTLA-4 antibodies significantly extends survival and, more importantly, produces tumor free long-term survival. Triple therapy is dependent on an intact CD4$^+$ T cell compartment, whereas depletion of CD8$^+$ T cells did not abrogate treatment efficacy. Furthermore, triple therapy provides for a durable antigen-specific memory response.

Author Contributions

Conceived and designed the experiments: ZB JAP JZ APS EA CGD ML. Performed the experiments: ZB JAP JZ APS DM CG SN MK JR CJ. Analyzed the data: ZB JAP JZ APS JR XY ML. Contributed reagents/materials/analysis tools: NMD PTT BT JWW HB DMP. Contributed to the writing of the manuscript: ZB JAP JZ APS DM CJ JR ML.

References

1. Stupp R, Hegi ME, Mason WP, van den Bent MJ, Taphoorn MJ, et al. (2009) Effects of radiotherapy with concomitant and adjuvant temozolomide versus radiotherapy alone on survival in glioblastoma in a randomised phase III study: 5-year analysis of the EORTC-NCIC trial. The lancet oncology 10: 459–466.
2. Stupp R, Mason WP, van den Bent MJ, Weller M, Fisher B, et al. (2005) Radiotherapy plus concomitant and adjuvant temozolomide for glioblastoma. The New England journal of medicine 352: 987–996.
3. Pardoll DM (2012) The blockade of immune checkpoints in cancer immunotherapy. Nature reviews Cancer 12: 252–264.
4. Albesiano E, Han JE, Lim M (2010) Mechanisms of local immunoresistance in glioma. Neurosurgery clinics of North America 21: 17–29.
5. Jackson C, Ruzevick J, Phallen J, Belcaid Z, Lim M (2011) Challenges in immunotherapy presented by the glioblastoma multiforme microenvironment. Clinical & developmental immunology 2011: 732413.
6. Zeng J, See AP, Phallen J, Jackson CM, Belcaid Z, et al. (2013) Anti-PD-1 blockade and stereotactic radiation produce long-term survival in mice with intracranial gliomas. International journal of radiation oncology, biology, physics 86: 343–349.
7. Leach DR, Krummel MF, Allison JP (1996) Enhancement of antitumor immunity by CTLA-4 blockade. Science 271: 1734–1736.
8. Callahan MK, Wolchok JD, Allison JP (2010) Anti-CTLA-4 antibody therapy: immune monitoring during clinical development of a novel immunotherapy. Seminars in oncology 37: 473–484.
9. Melero I, Shuford WW, Newby SA, Aruffo A, Ledbetter JA, et al. (1997) Monoclonal antibodies against the 4-1BB T-cell activation molecule eradicate established tumors. Nature medicine 3: 682–685.
10. Melero I, Hervas-Stubbs S, Glennie M, Pardoll DM, Chen L (2007) Immunostimulatory monoclonal antibodies for cancer therapy. Nature reviews Cancer 7: 95–106.
11. Pollok KE, Kim YJ, Zhou Z, Hurtado J, Kim KK, et al. (1993) Inducible T cell antigen 4-1BB. Analysis of expression and function. Journal of immunology 150: 771–781.
12. Shuford WW, Klussman K, Tritchler DD, Loo DT, Chalupny J, et al. (1997) 4-1BB costimulatory signals preferentially induce CD8+ T cell proliferation and lead to the amplification in vivo of cytotoxic T cell responses. The Journal of experimental medicine 186: 47–55.
13. Krummel MF, Allison JP (1996) CTLA-4 engagement inhibits IL-2 accumulation and cell cycle progression upon activation of resting T cells. The Journal of experimental medicine 183: 2533–2540.
14. Hodi FS, O'Day SJ, McDermott DF, Weber RW, Sosman JA, et al. (2010) Improved survival with ipilimumab in patients with metastatic melanoma. The New England journal of medicine 363: 711–723.
15. Robert C, Thomas L, Bondarenko I, O'Day S, Weber J, et al. (2011) Ipilimumab plus dacarbazine for previously untreated metastatic melanoma. The New England journal of medicine 364: 2517–2526.
16. Margolin K, Ernstoff MS, Hamid O, Lawrence D, McDermott D, et al. (2012) Ipilimumab in patients with melanoma and brain metastases: an open-label, phase 2 trial. The lancet oncology 13: 459–465.
17. Silk AW, Bassetti MF, West BT, Tsien CI, Lao CD (2013) Ipilimumab and radiation therapy for melanoma brain metastases. Cancer medicine 2: 899–906.
18. Kocak E, Lute K, Chang X, May KF Jr., Exten KR, et al. (2006) Combination therapy with anti-CTL antigen-4 and anti-4-1BB antibodies enhances cancer immunity and reduces autoimmunity. Cancer research 66: 7276–7284.
19. Ferrara TA, Hodge JW, Gulley JL (2009) Combining radiation and immunotherapy for synergistic antitumor therapy. Current opinion in molecular therapeutics 11: 37–42.
20. Demaria S, Bhardwaj N, McBride WH, Formenti SC (2005) Combining radiotherapy and immunotherapy: a revived partnership. International journal of radiation oncology, biology, physics 63: 655–666.
21. Formenti SC, Demaria S (2009) Systemic effects of local radiotherapy. The Lancet Oncology 10: 718–726.
22. Wong J, Armour E, Kazanzides P, Iordachita I, Tryggestad E, et al. (2008) High-resolution, small animal radiation research platform with x-ray tomographic guidance capabilities. International journal of radiation oncology, biology, physics 71: 1591–1599.
23. Armour M, Ford E, Iordachita I, Wong J (2010) CT guidance is needed to achieve reproducible positioning of the mouse head for repeat precision cranial irradiation. Radiation research 173: 119–123.
24. Youlin K, Li Z, Xiaodong W, Xiuheng L, Hengchen Z (2012) Combination immunotherapy with 4-1BBL and CTLA-4 blockade for the treatment of prostate cancer. Clinical & developmental immunology 2012: 439235.
25. Curran MA, Kim M, Montalvo W, Al-Shamkhani A, Allison JP (2011) Combination CTLA-4 blockade and 4-1BB activation enhances tumor rejection by increasing T-cell infiltration, proliferation, and cytokine production. PloS one 6: e19499.
26. Agarwalla P, Barnard Z, Fecci P, Dranoff G, Curry WT Jr. (2012) Sequential immunotherapy by vaccination with GM-CSF-expressing glioma cells and CTLA-4 blockade effectively treats established murine intracranial tumors. Journal of immunotherapy 35: 385–389.
27. Fecci PE, Ochiai H, Mitchell DA, Grossi PM, Sweeney AE, et al. (2007) Systemic CTLA-4 blockade ameliorates glioma-induced changes to the CD4+ T cell compartment without affecting regulatory T-cell function. Clinical cancer research: an official journal of the American Association for Cancer Research 13: 2158–2167.
28. Topalian SL, Hodi FS, Brahmer JR, Gettinger SN, Smith DC, et al. (2012) Safety, activity, and immune correlates of anti-PD-1 antibody in cancer. The New England journal of medicine 366: 2443–2454.
29. Wolchok JD, Kluger H, Callahan MK, Postow MA, Rizvi NA, et al. (2013) Nivolumab plus ipilimumab in advanced melanoma. The New England journal of medicine 369: 122–133.
30. Hodge JW, Guha C, Neefjes J, Gulley JL (2008) Synergizing radiation therapy and immunotherapy for curing incurable cancers. Opportunities and challenges. Oncology 22: 1064–1070; discussion 1075, 1080–1061, 1084.
31. Grossman SA, Ye X, Lesser G, Sloan A, Carraway H, et al. (2011) Immunosuppression in patients with high-grade gliomas treated with radiation and temozolomide. Clinical cancer research: an official journal of the American Association for Cancer Research 17: 5473–5480.
32. Wada S, Jackson CM, Yoshimura K, Yen HR, Getnet D, et al. (2013) Sequencing CTLA-4 blockade with cell-based immunotherapy for prostate cancer. Journal of translational medicine 11: 89.
33. Chi DD, Merchant RE, Rand R, Conrad AJ, Garrison D, et al. (1997) Molecular detection of tumor-associated antigens shared by human cutaneous melanomas and gliomas. The American journal of pathology 150: 2143–2152.
34. Prins RM, Odesa SK, Liau LM (2003) Immunotherapeutic targeting of shared melanoma-associated antigens in a murine glioma model. Cancer research 63: 8487–8491.

12

Expression and Immune Responses to MAGE Antigens Predict Survival in Epithelial Ovarian Cancer

Sayeema Daudi[1], Kevin H. Eng[2], Paulette Mhawech-Fauceglia[3], Carl Morrison[4], Anthony Miliotto[1,5], Amy Beck[5], Junko Matsuzaki[5,6], Takemasa Tsuji[5,6], Adrienne Groman[2], Sacha Gnjatic[7], Guillo Spagnoli[8], Shashikant Lele[1], Kunle Odunsi[1,5,6]*

1 Department of Gynecologic Oncology, Roswell Park Cancer Institute, Buffalo, New York, United States of America, 2 Department of Biostatisticsm, Roswell Park Cancer Institute, Buffalo, New York, United States of America, 3 Department of Pathology, University Southern California, Los Angeles, California, United States of America, 4 Department of Pathology, Roswell Park Cancer Institute, Buffalo, New York, United States of America, 5 Center for Immunotherapy, Roswell Park Cancer Institute, Buffalo, New York, United States of America, 6 Department of Immunology, Roswell Park Cancer Institute, Buffalo, New York, United States of America, 7 Department of Medicine, Mount Sinai Hospital, New York, New York, United States of America, 8 Department of Biomedicine, University Hospital Basel, Basel, Switzerland

Abstract

The MAGE cancer-testis antigens (CTA) are attractive candidates for immunotherapy. The aim of this study was to determine the frequency of expression, humoral immunity and prognostic significance of MAGE CTA in human epithelial ovarian cancer (EOC). mRNA or protein expression frequencies were determined for MAGE-A1, -A3, -A4, -A10 and -C1 (CT7) in tissue samples obtained from 400 patients with EOC. The presence of autologous antibodies against the MAGE antigens was determined from 285 serum samples. The relationships between MAGE expression, humoral immunity to MAGE antigens, and clinico-pathologic characteristics were studied. The individual frequencies of expression were as follows: A1: 15% (42/281), A3: 36% (131/390), A4: 47% (186/399), A10: 52% (204/395), C1: 16% (42/267). Strong concordant expression was noted with MAGE-A1:-A4, MAGE-A1:-C1 and MAGE-A4:-A10 ($p<0.0005$). Expression of MAGE-A1 or -A10 antigens resulted in poor progression free survival (PFS) (OR 1.44, CI 1.01–2.04, $p=0.044$ and OR 1.3, CI 1.03–1.64, $p=0.03$, respectively); whereas, MAGE-C1 expression was associated with improved PFS (OR 0.62, CI 0.42–0.92, $p=0.016$). The improved PFS observed for MAGE-C1 expression, was diminished by co-expression of MAGE-A1 or -A10. Spontaneous humoral immunity to the MAGE antigens was present in 9% (27/285) of patients, and this predicted poor overall survival (log-rank test $p=0.0137$). These findings indicate that MAGE-A1, MAGE-A4, MAGE-A3, and MAGE-A10 are priority attractive targets for polyvalent immunotherapy in ovarian cancer patients.

Editor: Sophia N. Karagiannis, King's College London, United Kingdom

Funding: This work was supported in part by the Cancer Research Institute Ovarian Cancer Working Group Grant, Cancer Vaccine Collaborative Grant of the Cancer Research Institute and Ludwig Institute for Cancer Research, Anna-Maria Kellen Clinical Investigator Award of the Cancer Research Institute (to Kunle Odunsi), National Institutes of Health 5T32 CA 108456, National Institutes of Health R01CA158318-01A1 and Roswell Park Cancer Institute-University of Pittsburg Cancer Institute Ovarian Cancer Specialized Program of Research Excellence National Institutes of Health P50CA159981-01A1. The funders had no role in study design, data collection and analysis, decision to publish, or preparation of the manuscript.

Competing Interests: The authors have declared that no competing interests exist.

* Email: kunle.odunsi@roswellpark.org

Introduction

Epithelial ovarian cancer (EOC) represents the most lethal gynecologic malignancy in women. Despite considerable efforts directed at early detection and improving response rates, the majority of women present with disseminated disease at initial diagnosis, carry an unacceptable relapse rate of approximately 85% and a 5-year overall survival of 20–30% [1,2]. Consequently, targeted treatment strategies, such as immunotherapy will be required to improve the clinical outcome of ovarian cancer patients.

The development of successful immunotherapy requires the characterization of tumor-associated antigens (TAA) that are commonly expressed in ovarian tumors, with a restricted expression pattern in normal tissues. Moreover, the ideal antigen should exhibit a high frequency of expression in cancer and evidence of immunogenicity. Candidate TAA are often identified in patients with strong cellular and/or humoral immune responses that indicate robust inherent immunogenicity to these antigens [3–5].

The cancer testis antigens (CTA) are a subclass of TAA encoded by approximately 140 genes. Despite their poorly characterized biologic function, expression of these antigens are known to be restricted in immune privileged sites such as the testes, placenta and fetal ovary, but not in other normal tissues. Abnormal expression of these germ-line genes in malignant tumors may reflect the activation of a silenced "gametogenic program", which ultimately leads to tumor progression and broad immunogenicity [6]. The immunogenicity of CTA has led to the widespread development of cancer vaccines targeting these antigens in many solid tumors. Within this large class of TAA, melanoma-associated antigens (MAGE) have emerged as promising candidates for cancer immunotherapy [7–9].

More than 30 cancer testis (CT) genes have been reported as members of multi-gene families that are organized into gene clusters on chromosome X (CT-X antigens). The CT gene clusters are located between Xq24 and Xq28 and include gene families such as MAGE and NY-ESO-1 [10]. Type I MAGE gene clusters are the most extensively characterized and include the MAGE-A, MAGE-B and MAGE-C families. The MAGE-A proteins are encoded by 12 different MAGE-A gene family members (MAGE-A1 to MAGE-A12) and are defined by a conserved 165–171 amino acid base, called the MAGE homology domain (MHD). The MHD corresponds to the only region of shared amino acids by all of the MAGE-A family members. MAGE-C1/CT7 is structurally different from MAGE-A family, with a protein product of 1142 amino acids (vs.<400 residues for the MAGE-A proteins) that contains a tandem repeat sequence that is absent in MAGE-A [11].

In the present study, we have analyzed the expression and immunogenicity of a panel of five MAGE CTA in a large cohort of ovarian cancer patients. In addition, we have examined the relationship between coordinate expression of MAGE genes and clinico-pathologic outcomes.

Materials and Methods

Patients and Specimens

Formalin-fixed paraffin-embedded (FFPE; for immunohisto-chemistry) and snap-frozen tissue specimens (for reverse transcriptase-PCR) were obtained from 400 patients undergoing cytoreductive surgery for ovarian, primary peritoneal and fallopian tube cancer at the Roswell Park Cancer Institute (Buffalo, NY) between 1992 and 2008. We identify, and refer to, these three cancers as EOC due to their common origin in the mullerian epithelium. All tissue specimens were collected under an approved protocol from the institutional review board (IRB) of Roswell Park Cancer Institute. Patients signed an IRB approved written informed consent, and these were filed in the IRB office. All pathology specimens were reviewed in our institution, and the histopatho-logic subtype of the tumors was classified according to the guidelines of the World Health Organization (WHO) [12,13]. The stage and grade of the tumors were assessed according to the International Federation of Gynecology and Obstetrics (FIGO) [14,15]. In a subset of the patients, serum samples were collected at diagnosis. The medical records of these patients were retrospectively reviewed under an approved institutional review board protocol. The review included outpatient and inpatient treatment. Study outcomes included overall survival (OS) and progression free survival (PFS). Both survival criteria were measured from the time of diagnosis. Recurrence was defined via objective criteria as all therapy was given in the adjuvant setting. The duration of OS was the interval between diagnosis and death. PFS represented the interval between diagnosis to disease progression, recurrence or death. The observation time was the interval between diagnosis and last contact (death or last follow-up). Data were censored at the last follow-up for patients with no evidence of recurrence, progression, or death.

Total Tissue RNA Isolation

Total tissue RNA was isolated from frozen tumor tissues by use of the TRI Reagent (Molecular Research Center Inc, Cincinnati, OH, USA) according to the manufacturer's protocol. Potentially contaminating DNA was removed by treating with RNase-free DNase I (Boehringer-Mannheim, Mannheim, Germany), followed

by phenol/chroloform extraction. RNA was dissolved in RNase-free H_2O. The resulting RNA concentration was measured spectrophotometrically (DU500 Spectrophotometer, Beckman Coulter, Fulleron, CA, USA), and the quality of the RNAs was checked by electrophoresis on 1.5% agarose gel.

Table 1. Patient characteristics.

Patients eligible for analysis	400
Age Median (Range) (Years)	63 (21–93)
PFS Median (Range) (Months)	12 (0.1–160)
OS Median (Range) (Months)	40 (0.1–173)
FU Median (Range) (Months)	35 (0.7–176)
Primary Site	
Fallopian Tube	8 (2%)
Ovary	339 (84%)
Primary Peritoneal	53 (14%)
FIGO Stage	
Early Stage	69 (18%)
Advanced Stage	323 (82%)
Histology	
Clear Cell	21 (5%)
Endometrioid	18 (4.5%)
Mucinous	18 (4.5%)
Serous	254 (64%)
Other[a]	89 (22%)
Grade	
1	29 (7%)
2/3	353 (88%)
Debulking Status	
Optimal	301 (75%)
Suboptimal	90 (23%)
Unknown	9 (2%)
Platinum Status	
Sensitive	182 (46%)
Resistant / Refractory	132 (33%)
Unknown	86 (21%)
Recurrences	
No Recurrence	67 (17%)
Recurrence / Persistent Disease	162 (41%)
No Disease Free Interval	98 (25%)
Unknown	65 (17%)
Current Status	
Alive No Evidence of Disease	84 (22%)
Alive with Disease	37 (10%)
Dead	270 (68%)

PFS = Progression Free Survival. OS = Overall Survival. FU = Follow Up.
[a]Other Histology includes Borderline, Carcinosarcoma, Granulosa Cell, Mixed, Sertoli Leydig, Sex Cord Stromal, Signet Ring Cell, Small Cell Type, Transitional, Anaplastic, Undifferentiated and Poorly Differentiated tumors.
[b]Numbers do not add up to 100% due to unknown categories.

Table 2. Serum antibody and co-expression status for MAGE antigens in ovarian cancer.

MAGE Antigen	A1	A3	A4	A10	C1	Any A
Autoantibody (ELISA)	10/285 (4%)	12/285 (4%)	7/115 (6%)	6/86 (7%)	10/93 (11%)	27/285 (9%)
Expression (rt-PCR or IHC)	42/281 (15%)	131/390 (36%)	186/399 (47%)	204/395 (52%)	42/267 (16%)	310/400 (78%)
MAGE Co-expression	**A1**	**A3**	**A4**	**A10**	**C1**	
MAGE-A1		23/281 (8%)	31/281 (11%)	23/277 (8%)	12/258 (5%)	
MAGE-A3			70/289 (18%)	81/386 (21%)	18/267 (7%)	
MAGE-A4				114/394 (29%)	24/267 (9%)	
MAGE-A10					25/264 (10%)	

A total of 400 patients were studied for MAGE expression. A subset of 285 patients were studied for anti-MAGE autoantibody. The numerator represents the number of antigen positive tumors or serology. The denominator represents the total number of successful assays for each antigen. Antigen specific numbers vary due to assay viability. Percentages represent the frequency of MAGE expression or MAGE-specific antibody.

Reverse Transcriptase-PCR Analysis of MAGE-A1, MAGE-A3, MAGE-A4, MAGE-A10 and MAGE-C1 Expression

Two micrograms of each RNA sample were used to generate cDNA with the Ready-To-Go Reverse Transcriptase-PCR (rt-PCR) beads (GE Healthcare, Buckinghamshire, UK). RNA from normal testicular tissue (Clontech, Mountain View, CA) was used as a positive control. PCR was subsequently performed to study the expression of MAGE-A1, -A3, -A4, -A10 and -C1 in 305 patients with EOC. Glyceraldehyde-3-phosphodehydrogenase (GAPDH) primers were used as a test for RNA integrity. **Table S1** lists the primer sequences for each gene and its respective amplicon length. The amplification conditions for all gene

products was 5 min at 95°C, followed by 35 cycles that consisted of 1 min at 95°C, 1 min at 60°C, and 1 min at 72°C. These cycles were followed by a 6-min elongation step at 72°C (BioRad iCycler, BioRad Laboratories, Hercules, CA, USA). The PCR products were separated over a 1.5% agarose gel and visualized with ethidium bromide on an ultraviolet transilluminator (IS-4400 ChemiImager, Alpha Innotech, San Leandro, CA). The intensities of the PCR products were heterogeneous, and some specimens yielded only faint amplicon bands. These were scored positive only if the result could be reproduced by a repeated RNA extraction and specific rt-PCR from the same tumor specimen. Cases with very low transcript levels that were not reproducibly positive were

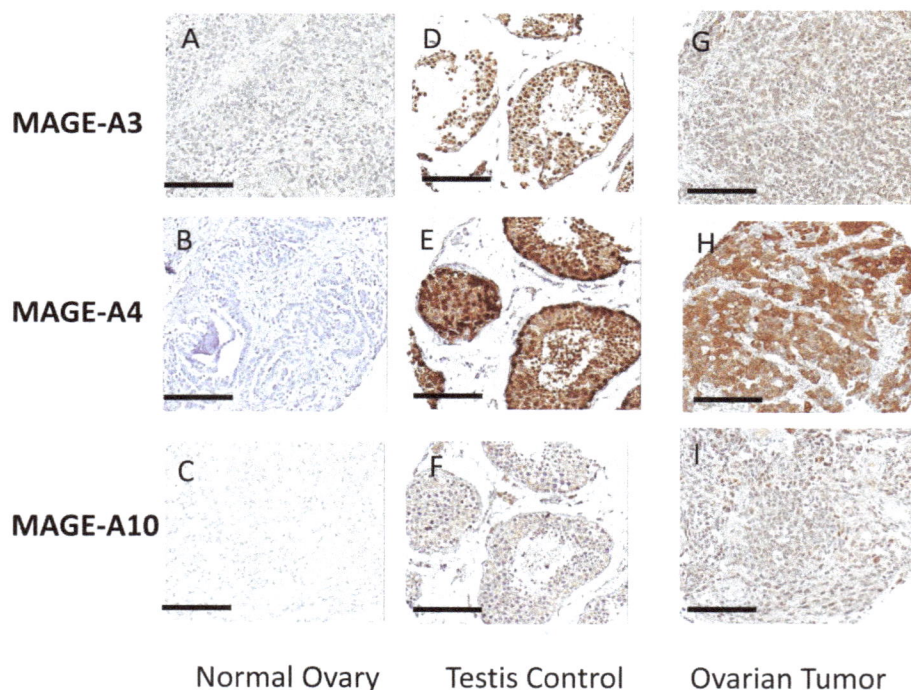

Figure 1. A–I: Immunohistochemical staining for MAGE. Specimens were stained with polyclonal antibody for MAGE-A3 (X20), clones 57b and A3 hybridoma supernatants for MAGE-A4 and MAGE-A10, respectively (x15). Specimens from the normal ovary and testis were used as negative and positive controls, respectively. A–C: Staining of the normal ovary showing no reactivity. D–F: Staining of the testis showing seminiferous tubules with strong intratubular staining, and absent non-specific reactivity. G–I: Staining of ovarian tumor demonstrating strong cytoplasmic and/or nuclear staining patterns.

A

	A3	A4	A10	C1
A1	OR: 2.8 95% CI: [2.2-3.5] $p = 0.0022$	OR: 3.7 95% CI: [3.0-4.4] $p = 0.0003$	OR: 1.2 95% CI: [0.6-1.8] $p = 0.7$	OR: 4.4 95% CI: [3.6-5.2] $p = 0.00015$
A3		OR: 1.5 95% CI: [1.1-2.0] $p = 0.058$	OR: 1.9 95% CI: [1.5-2.4] $p = 0.0028$	OR: 1.6 95% CI: [0.9-2.3] $p = 0.18$
A4			OR: 2.2 95% CI: [1.8-2.6] $p = 0.00013$	OR: 1.6 95% CI: [0.9-2.3] $p = 0.18$
A10				OR: 1.5 95% CI: [0.8-2.1] $p = 0.3$

B

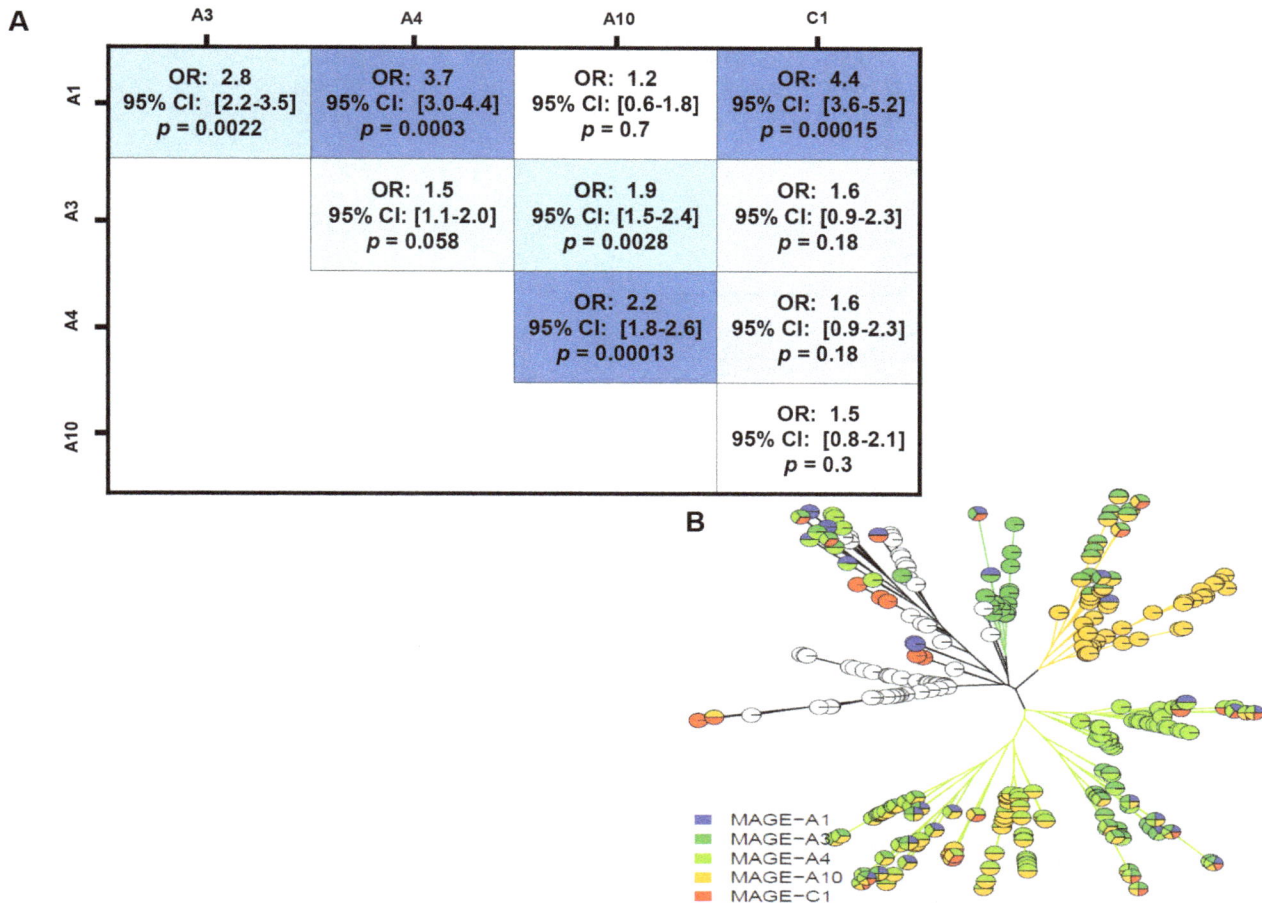

- ■ MAGE-A1
- ■ MAGE-A3
- ■ MAGE-A4
- ■ MAGE-A10
- ■ MAGE-C1

Figure 2. A–B: Co- expression of MAGE antigens in ovarian cancer. (A) MAGE-A1 is co-expressed with –A3 or –A4 or –C1. MAGE-A3 is co-expressed with –A10. MAGE-A4 is co-expressed with MAGE-A10. The darker color intensity represents a stronger significance. The strongest associations are between MAGE-A1 to –A4, MAGE-A1 to –C1 and MAGE-A1 to –A3. Odds ratios (OR) greater than 1 imply the antigens tend to appear together. (B) Phylogenetic tree for MAGE expression. Each leaf ending in a pie chart symbolizes a person.

not regarded as positive. PCR product bands were excised from the agarose gel and the associated DNA was isolated with the QIAquick Gel Extraction Kit (Qiagen, Valencia, CA, USA). DNA samples were submitted for sequencing to verify the PCR product.

Immunohistochemical Analysis of MAGE-A3, MAGE-A4 and MAGE-A10 Expression

Immunohistochemical (IHC) analysis was performed using FFPE tissues from 304 patients on tissue microarrays (TMA). TMA were constructed using 0.6 mm FFPE tissue cores punched from each donor block. To overcome tumor heterogeneity, three representative cores were selected from each tumor. The 4 μm-thick tissue cores were deparaffinized and pretreated with a specific antigen retrieval solution (Dakocytomation, Carpenteria, CA) over 20 minutes. Slides were cooled for 20 minutes and then treated in 3% H_2O_2 to quench endogenous peroxidase activity. The TMA slides were then incubated with a serum-free protein block (Dakocytomation, Carpenteria, CA) for 30 minutes. **Table S2** lists the antibodies and IHC conditions. MAGE-A3 rabbit anti-human polyclonal antibody (LS-B4662, Lifespan Biosciences, Inc.) was commercially acquired. Anti-MAGE-A4 mAb (clone: 57b) and anti-MAGE-A10 (clone: A3) hybridoma supernatants were produced at the University Hospital Basel (Basel, Switzerland) [16,17]. Rabbit IgG or mouse IgG1 (Sigma, St. Louis, MO) was

used as the negative isotype matched control. Labeled streptavidin biotin (LSAB+) reagents (Dakocytomation, Carpenteria, CA) were used according to the manufacturer's instructions followed by a 3,3'-diaminobenzidine (DAB)+ (Dakocytomation, Carpenteria, CA) incubation. Sections were counterstained with hematoxylin. A cut-off of $\geq 5\%$ positive tumor cells was used to define positive expression.

Measurement of serum antibody by ELISA

Serologic analysis of humoral immune responses was performed as previously described [18]. 285 serum samples from a subset of the patients were analyzed by ELISA for seroreactivity to bacterially produced full-length recombinant proteins MAGE-A1, -A3, -A4, -A10 or -C1. As a negative control antigen, recombinant dihydrofolate reductase protein was prepared and used in each assay. Serum was diluted serially from 1:100 – 1:100,000 and added to low-volume 96-well plates (Corning) coated overnight at 4°C with 1 μg/mL antigen in 25 μl and blocked for 2 h at room temperature with PBS containing 5% nonfat milk. After overnight incubation, plates were extensively washed with PBS containing 0.2% Tween 20 and rinsed with PBS (BioTek ELx405 automated washer). Serum IgG bound to antigens was detected with goat anti-human IgG antibodies conjugated to alkaline phosphatase (Southern Biotech). Following

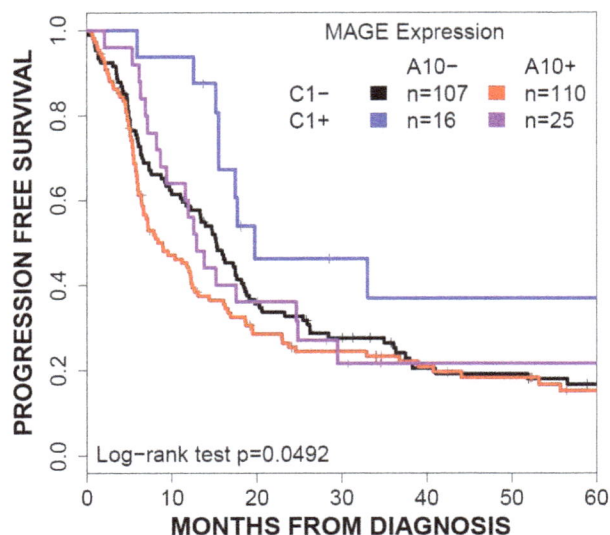

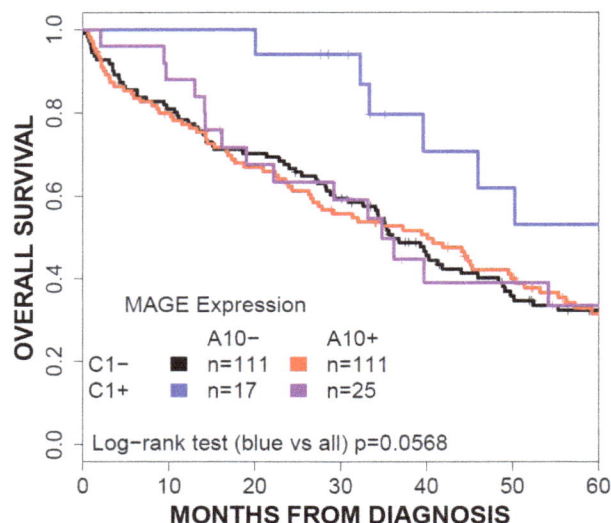

Figure 3. Survival by MAGE expression. Overall survival curves for patient groups based on MAGE-A10 and –C1 expression. MAGE-C1 expression predicts an improved progression free survival and a trend towards improved overall survival. Expression of MAGE-A10 dampens survival outcomes to the degree of patients with negative MAGE expression.

addition of ATTOPHOS substrate (Fisher Scientific), fluorescent signal was measured using a Cytofluor Series 4000 fluorescent reader (PerSeptive Biosystems). A reciprocal titer was calculated for each plasma sample as the maximal dilution still significantly reacting to a specific antigen. Specificity was determined by comparing seroreactivity among the various antigens tested. In each assay, sera of patients with known reactivity were used as controls. A positive result was defined as reciprocal titers >100.

Statistical Analysis

All statistical analyses were generated using SAS software (SAS System Copyright 2002 SAS Institute Inc. v.9.2) and the R 2.15.3 statistical computing language. A nominal significance level of 0.05 was used in all testing. Using a 2×2 contingency table, the level of concordance among the various MAGE gene expression profiles was determined. The distributions of MAGE-A1, -A3, -A4, -A10 and -C1 expression and clinical outcome were analyzed by the Wilcoxon Rank Sum Test or Pearson Chi Square Test. Multivariate analysis for independent predictors of survival were tested using the Cox proportional hazard model [19]. Estimated survival distributions were calculated by the method of Kaplan and Meier [20], and tests of significance with respect to survival distributions were based on the log-rank test. Relative prognosis was summarized using estimates and 95% confidence limits for the hazard ratio (HR). No adjustments were made for multiple comparisons. A phylogenetic tree is constructed by a Manhattan

distance, coding expression as zero (absent) and one (present), and the standard neighbor joining algorithm.

Results

Study Population

A total of 400 tissues from patients with ovarian, primary peritoneal and fallopian tube cancers were investigated by rt-PCR and IHC. The characteristics of the patients in this study are presented in **Table 1**. The median age of the patient sample was 63 (range: 21–93), with a median duration of follow-up of 35 months (range: 1–176 months). As expected, the majority of patients presented with advanced stage disease (82%), poorly differentiated tumors (74%) and with serous histology (64%). Platinum sensitive disease was demonstrated in 182 of the 400 patients (46%), with 116 patients having platinum resistance (29%), and 16 patients with a platinum refractory response (4%). The median OS for all patients was 40 months (range: 0–173), whereas the median PFS was 12 months (range: 0–160).

Expression of MAGE-A1, MAGE-A3, MAGE-A4, MAGE-A10 and MAGE-C1 in Ovarian Cancer

Expression of MAGE antigens was evaluated by both rt-PCR and IHC for the majority of patients from whom appropriate samples were available. The expression of MAGE-A4 and MAGE-A10 was detected concordantly by both methods (r = 0.31,

Table 3. Patient Characteristics by MAGE Expression.

Clinical and Pathologic Features	MAGE-A10(-) MAGE-C1(-)	MAGE-A10(-) MAGE-C1(+)	MAGE-A10(+) MAGE-C1(-)	MAGE-A10(+) MAGE-C1(+)	p value
All tumors (n)	193/258 (75%)	29/258 (11%)	24/258 (9%)	12/258 (5%)	
Age (Years)	63 (21–89)	66 (37–84)	69 (34–91)	62 (35–86)	0.9
PFS (95% CI)	15 (15.7–NA)	20 (15.7–NA)	8 (7–12.2)	13 (10–30)	**0.005**
OS (95% CI)	43 (36–52)	68 (40–NA)	38 (28–45)	35 (23–NA)	0.192
FIGO Stage					0.1373
Early Stage (I–II)	35	6	0	2	
Late Stage (III–)	154	23	24	10	
Tumor Grade					0.4532
1	18	3	1	0	
2/3	171	25	23	12	
Histology					0.737
Clear Cell	12	3	0	0	
Endometrioid	7	1	1	1	
Mucinous	12	0	1	0	
Serous	115	19	17	9	
Other	47	5	4	2	
Primary Site					0.744
Ovarian	159	25	17	11	
Primary Peritoneal	29	3	6	1	
Fallopian Tube	5	1	1	0	
Debulking Status					0.112
Optimal	147	25	16	11	
Suboptimal	38	4	8	1	
Platinum Status					0.008
Sensitive	72	21	7	7	
Resistant / Refractory	70	6	14	4	
Clinical Response					0.018
Complete Response	84	21	8	9	
Persistent Disease	59	6	13	2	

PFS = Months Progression Free Survival. OS = Months Overall Survival. NA = upper limit not estimated.
aOther Histology includes Borderline, Carcinosarcoma, Granulosa Cell, Mixed, Sertoli Leydig, Sex Cord Stromal, Signet Ring Cell, Small Cell Type, Transitional, Anaplastic, Undifferentiated and Poorly Differentiated tumors.
Pvalues are for any difference among the columns.

OR = 3.88, p<0.001; r = 0.14, OR = 2.00, p<.001 respectively) but MAGE-A3 results were not reproducibly concordant (r = − 0.06, OR = 0.86, p = 0.9198) due to a low rate of detection (**Table S3**). Unless otherwise stated, we proceeded by classifying tissues as antigen positive if they were identified by rt-PCR or IHC (**Table 2**). Consequently, when considering all 400 tissues samples analyzed by rt-PCR or IHC in this study, the frequencies for MAGE-A3, -A4 and –A10 expression by either method were 36% (131/390), 47% (186/399) and 52% (204/395) of the tissues, respectively (**Table 2**). MAGE-A1 and -C1 demonstrated the lowest frequency of expression at 15% (42/281) and 16% (42/267), respectively. **Table S3** is a summary of the frequency of MAGE mRNA and protein expression in tumor specimens from the EOC patients.

MAGE-A3, -A4 and -A10 exhibited no immunostaining in normal tissues (**Figs.1A–C**) but intense immunostaining in testis (**Figs.1D–F**). The staining pattern was cytoplasmic and nuclear for MAGE-A3 and A-4, and diffuse cytoplasmic staining for MAGE-A10 (**Figs.1G–I**).

Co-expression of MAGE-A and MAGE-C1 in Ovarian Cancer

The frequencies of co-expression of the MAGE antigens are shown in **Table 2**. The highest frequency of co-expression was observed for -A4:-A10 (29%). While they are both comparatively rare, the MAGE-C family antigen (-C1) tended to be co-expressed with MAGE-A1 [OR 4.4, p = 0.00015, CI 3.6–5.2] and to be expressed independently with the other MAGE-A family antigens (**Figure 2a**). MAGE-A family antigens -A1:-A4 [OR 3.7, p = 0.0003, 3.0-4.4] and –A1:-A3 [OR 2.8 p = 0.0022, CI 2.2–3.5] have the strongest co-expression; nearly every pair is associated except for –A1:-A10 (OR 1.2, p = 0.7 CI 0.6–1.8) which suggests they are expressed independently. To characterize the multivariate pattern of MAGE expression, the phylogenetic tree in **Figure 2b** was created, whereby each leaf ending in a pie

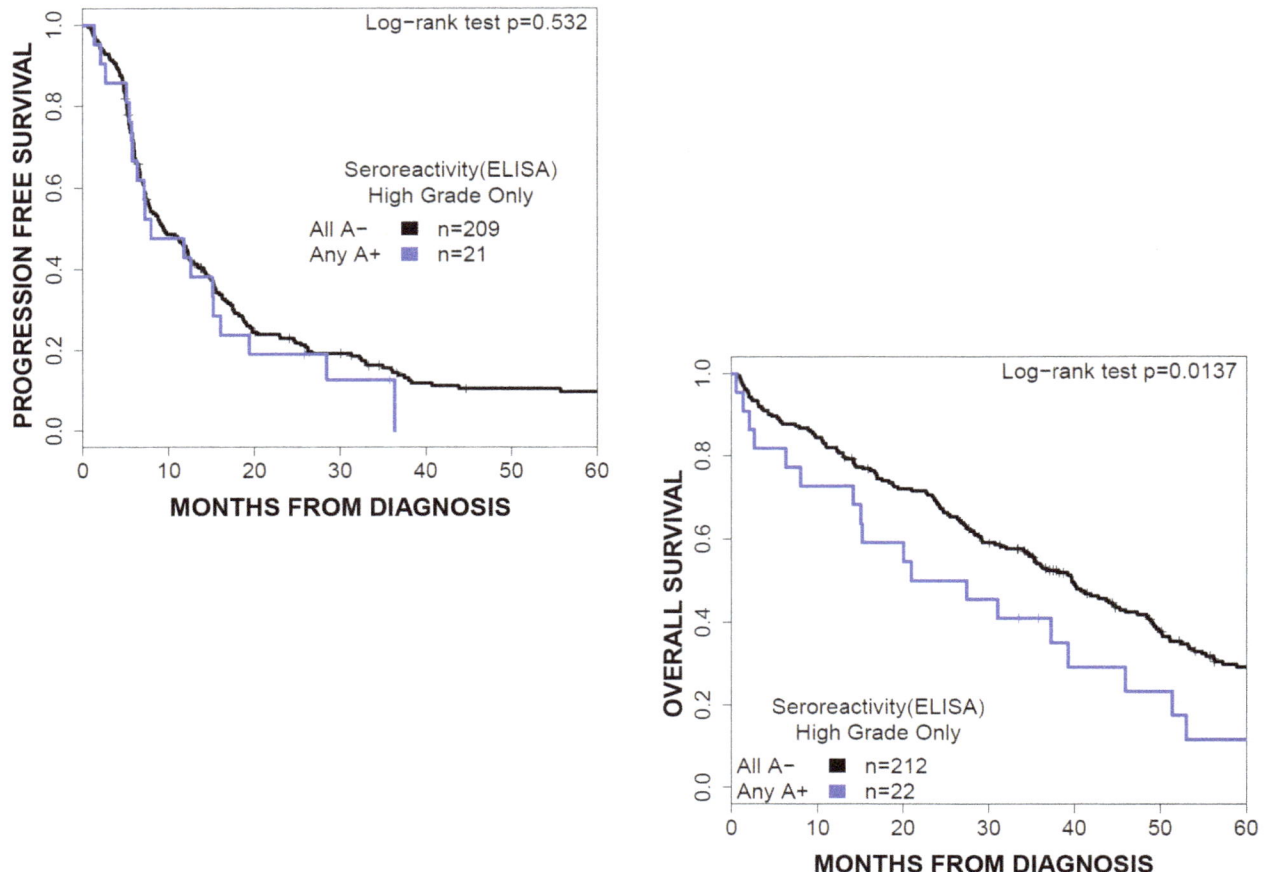

Figure 4. Survival by MAGE serology. Overall survival curves for patients groups based on the presence of anti-MAGE autoantibody. Humoral response to any MAGE antigen predicts poor overall survival, and no significant association with progression free survival.

chart symbolizes a person or set of people. There are two distinct patterns of expression that are observed. The MAGE-A4 gene directs a major pattern of expression (lower right hand clades), and then later develops into MAGE-A3 and -A10 expression in this patient population. The second unique expression pattern consists of an independent expression of MAGE-A3 and -A10, which then develops into -A4 (upper right hand clades). In stark contrast, MAGE-C1 expression rarely appears alone and emerges sporadically throughout the phylogenetic tree. Similarly, MAGE-A1 appears infrequently and rarely in the MAGE-A10 clade. These observations translate into strong clinical implications within this large study cohort.

Correlation of MAGE Antigen Expression with Clinical Outcome

The relationship between MAGE expression and clinic-pathologic parameters was investigated. We found that MAGE-A3 and A4 did not have individual prognostic effects. Consequently, we focused further analysis on MAGE-A1, MAGE-A10, MAGE-C1 and other known clinico-pathologic prognostic factors in ovarian cancer.

Alone, MAGE-A10 expression (204/395, 52%) was associated with worse clinical outcome (median PFS 8.8[7.2–12.3] vs. 15.5[13.6–18.4] months, $p = 0.009$; OS 37.8[28.2–45.0] vs. 45.0[39.8–52.2] months, $p = 0.0781$). Co-expression with MAGE-C1 (25/204, 12%) reversed this trend for PFS but not

OS: A10(+)/C1(−) patients had median PFS of 7.9 months (7.0–12.1) versus A10(+)/C1(+) 13.1 months (CI9.5–29.9). Stratified into four groups based on A10/C1 expression pattern, this pattern holds (log-rank test $p = 0.0133$) and suggests that A10(−)/C1(+) expression may be protective (median PFS 20 [15.7-NA] months) (**Fig. 3**).

Expression patterns were not jointly associated with age ($p = 0.900$), stage ($p = 0.1373$), grade ($p = 0.4532$), histology ($p = 0.737$), primary site ($p = 0744$) or debulking status ($p = 0.112$) (**Table 3**). MAGE-C1 expression was associated with platinum sensitive disease (28/38, 74% vs. 70/142, 49%; $p = 0.009$) and clinical response (30/38, 79% vs. 92/164, 56%, $p = 0.015$).

Although we focused on MAGE-A10, the less prevalent MAGE-A1 (42/281, 15%) was also mildly associated with poorer survival outcomes (median PFS 10.3[6.2–15.0] vs 12.8[10.5–15.7] months $p = 0.043$, OS 38.7[20.3–78.4] vs. 41.3[36.5–46.6] months $p = 0.607$). For PFS, MAGE-A1 co-expression with A10 is redundant (stratified log-rank test $p = 0.57$) however A1(+)/A10(−) patients have slightly poorer prognosis (median PFS 12.7 [5.3–36.6] vs. 16.3 [14.1–19.4] months, $p = 0.0187$). To model all three antigens jointly, we recommend considering the expression of either the A1 or A10 antigen along with the expression of MAGE-C1; the effect is not significantly different from the stratification presented in **Table 3**.

Table 4. Patient Characteristics by MAGE Serology.

Clinical and Pathologic Features	All MAGE-A (−)	Any MAGE-A (+)	p value
All tumors (n)	258/285 (91%)	27/285 (9%)	
Age [Median (range)] (Years)	63 (21–89)	69 (43–89)	0.017
PFS (95% CI)	14 (11–17)	12 (6–20)	**0.231**
OS (95% CI)	45 (40–52)	28 (17–52)	**0.002**
FIGO Stage			0.828
Early Stage (I–II)	43	5	
Late Stage (III–IV)	212	22	
Tumor Grade			0.428
1	20	3	
2/3	233	24	
Histology			0.241
Clear Cell	18	0	
Endometrioid	9	2	
Mucinous	12	2	
Serous	165	13	
Other	54	10	
Primary Site			0.017
Ovarian	215	22	
Primary Peritoneal	38	5	
Fallopian Tube	5	0	
Residual Tumor at Cytoreduction			0.765
Optimal	193	22	
Suboptimal	58	5	
Platinum Status			0.616
Sensitive	110	12	
Resistant / Refractory	104	8	
Clinical Response			0.877
Complete Response	124	12	
Persistent Disease	89	8	

PFS = Progression Free Survival. OS = Overall Survival. FU = Follow Up.
[a]Other Histology includes Borderline, Carcinosarcoma, Granulosa Cell, Mixed, Sertoli Leydig, Sex Cord Stromal, Signet Ring Cell, Small Cell Type, Transitional, Anaplastic, Undifferentiated and Poorly Differentiated tumors.

Correlation of Antibody Response to the MAGE Antigen with Clinical Outcome

ELISA for serum MAGE antigen-specific antibodies was performed on serum samples obtained at diagnosis from 285 of the 400 EOC patients (**Table 2**). Spontaneously induced humoral response to at least one MAGE-A antigen was observed in 9% (27/285) of patients of which 85% (23/27) also expressed a MAGE-A antigen. The serologic response to any MAGE antigen was equally distributed among all clinico-pathologic parameters (**Table 4**). The presence of humoral immune response to any of the MAGE antigens predicted a worse overall survival (median PFS 12.3[6.4–19.7] vs. 13.5[10.9–16.5] months, p = 0.231; median OS 27.8[17.3–52.2] vs 45.4[40.2–51.9] months, p = 0.002) (**Figure 4**).

Discussion

Immunotherapy is a promising approach to improve survival rates and clinical outcomes in ovarian cancer patients [21–23]. Among the possible tumor antigen targets, CTA are considered as

the most promising candidates for the development of anti-cancer vaccines. To assess the utility of the MAGE family CTA as targets for specific immunotherapy in EOC, the present comprehensive analysis was undertaken on a large panel of ovarian tumors. Our results indicate aberrant expression of MAGE-A1, MAGE-A3, MAGE-A4, MAGE-A10 and MAGE-C1 in 15%, 36%, 47%, 52% and 16% of EOC specimens, respectively. In addition, we found that considering any of these MAGE antigens, approximately 78% showed expression of at least one of these five CT antigens. Moreover, MAGE-A1 and MAGE-A10 expression were associated with poor clinical outcome, while MAGE-C1/CT7 was associated with improved survival.

The frequency of MAGE expression in EOC that we report is generally consistent with that reported for the majority of other tumors, except for melanoma and non-small cell lung cancer [16,24]. Expression of MAGE-A3 mRNA has been found in 10–40% of several tumor types, including bladder [25], breast [26] and multiple myeloma [27]. With respect to EOC, the frequency of MAGE-A1 and -A3 expression that we report is similar to that reported in previous studies, with the exception of Zhang *et al* who found a 54% and 37% expression in ovarian cancer tissues, respectively [28–30]. This may reflect differences in the study populations, as there were far more early stage tumors than our study group. In a previous study, the expression of MAGE-A4 adversely correlated with survival or indirectly to established prognostic factors in ovarian cancer [31]. Consistent with these studies, our findings demonstrate a clear association for MAGE expression and prognosis. In this regard, while MAGE-A1 and MAGE-A10 expression were associated with poor clinical outcome, MAGE-C1 was associated with improved survival. These contrasting survival findings among the different MAGE antigen families raise many essential questions regarding the role of the MAGE genes in tumorigenesis, invasion and metastasis in EOC.

In general, MAGE antigens are more often expressed in patients with advanced disease and poor outcome, indicating that their expression might contribute to tumorigenesis [26,32–37]. Several studies have demonstrated that MAGE proteins are critical to cell survival, increasing the tumorigenic properties of cells and therefore, may actively contribute to the development of malignancies [38–40]. Moreover, since CT antigen expression has been associated with tumorigenic transformation of cancer stem cells [41], it is possible that MAGE-A1 and MAGE-A10 expressing ovarian cancer cells represent a population with self-renewing stem cell properties, and therefore more resistant to immune elimination or chemotherapy.

In contrast to MAGE-A1 and MAGE-A10, the possible mechanism(s) by which expression of MAGE-C1/CT7 confers a survival benefit is less clear. In comparing the protein structure of the MAGE family members, while the first and second domains are highly conserved among the MAGE-A and –C family members, the MAGE-C1 protein carries a unique feature. In addition to a 275-amino acid MAGE-homologous segment on its C-terminus, MAGE-C1/CT-7 has an 867-amino acid region composed of three types of tandem repeats in its N-terminus [11]. This region may be of significant importance as the repetitive protein sequence may shape the epitopes presented for immune recognition of MAGEC1/CT-7 and potentially thereby determine the quality of the resulting immune responses.

In addition, our results indicate that patients with anti-MAGE humoral immunity had worse prognosis. These findings do not necessarily imply that anti-MAGE immune responses directly impair treatment outcomes in ovarian cancer patients. Since antigen density presented by antigen-presenting cells *in vivo* differentially affects the generation of anti-tumor humoral and T cell responses [42], we propose that patients who developed spontaneous immune responses are those with high antigen density

because of advanced disease burden, and therefore with worse prognosis. These patients are still likely to benefit from MAGE-directed immunotherapy because their on-going anti-MAGE-A immune responses are not effective. In a previous study of spontaneous humoral immune responses against the NY-ESO-1 CT antigen, the impact of humoral immunity was neutral on patient prognosis [43].

Because the expression of MAGE antigens is regulated by epigenetic mechanisms such as methylation and histone acetylation, we reasoned that MAGE antigen expression in tumors may be the result of the activation of a coordinated gene-expression program, rather than a series of independent events [6]. Using analytical methods, the present study identified significant co-expression among the MAGE antigens. These results support the notion that ovarian cancer acquires a gametogenic transcription profile, in which typically silenced genes are now activated leading to tumor progression. Our results indicate that MAGE-A4 is the central gene that directs the pattern of expression of the other genes, with MAGE-C1 only emerging sporadically in the phylogenetic tree. Taken together, our results suggest that MAGE-A1, -A10 and -C1 are possible prognostic factors in ovarian cancer, with MAGE-A1 and A-10 associated with poor prognosis; and MAGE-C1/CT7 associated with improved prognosis. We propose MAGE-A1 and MAGE-A10 as priority targets for immunotherapy in ovarian cancer. Since MAGE-A4 exhibits a relatively high frequency of expression, and appears to direct a major pattern of co-expression of other MAGE antigens (Fig. 2b), we also propose MAGE-A4 as a priority target for ovarian cancer immunotherapy.

Acknowledgments

The authors would like to thank Erika Ritter and Christina Sedrak, from LICR NY branch, for their excellent technical assistance.

Author Contributions

Conceived and designed the experiments: SD KO. Performed the experiments: SD PMF CM AM AB JM TT AG SG. Analyzed the data: SD KHE PMF AG SG KO. Contributed reagents/materials/analysis tools: GS SG KO. Contributed to the writing of the manuscript: SD KHE TT JM SG SL KO.

References

1. Ozols RF, Bundy BN, Greer BE, Fowler JM, Clarke-Pearson D, et al. (2003) Phase III trial of carboplatin and paclitaxel compared with cisplatin and paclitaxel in patients with optimally resected stage III ovarian cancer: a Gynecologic Oncology Group study. J Clin Oncol 21: 3194–3200.
2. Jemal A, Siegel R, Xu J, Ward E (2010) Cancer statistics, 2010. CA Cancer J Clin 60: 277–300.
3. van der Bruggen P, Traversari C, Chomez P, Lurquin C, De Plaen E, et al. (1991) A gene encoding an antigen recognized by cytolytic T lymphocytes on a human melanoma. Science 254: 1643–1647.
4. Sahin U, Tureci O, Schmitt H, Cochlovius B, Johannes T, et al. (1995) Human neoplasms elicit multiple specific immune responses in the autologous host. Proc Natl Acad Sci U S A 92: 11810–11813.
5. Stockert E, Jager E, Chen YT, Scanlan MJ, Gout I, et al. (1998) A survey of the humoral immune response of cancer patients to a panel of human tumor antigens. J Exp Med 187: 1349–1354.
6. Simpson AJ, Caballero OL, Jungbluth A, Chen YT, Old LJ (2005) Cancer/testis antigens, gametogenesis and cancer. Nat Rev Cancer 5: 615–625.
7. Van den Eynde B, Peeters O, De Backer O, Gaugler B, Lucas S, et al. (1995) A new family of genes coding for an antigen recognized by autologous cytolytic T lymphocytes on a human melanoma. J Exp Med 182: 689–698.
8. Kruit WH, Suciu S, Dreno B, Mortier L, Robert C, et al. (2013) Selection of immunostimulant AS15 for active immunization with MAGE-A3 protein: results of a randomized phase II study of the European Organisation for Research and Treatment of Cancer Melanoma Group in Metastatic Melanoma. J Clin Oncol 31: 2413–2420.
9. Vansteenkiste J, Zielinski M, Linder A, Dahabreh J, Gonzalez EE, et al. (2013) Adjuvant MAGE-A3 immunotherapy in resected non-small-cell lung cancer: phase II randomized study results. J Clin Oncol 31: 2396–2403.
10. Caballero OL, Chen YT (2009) Cancer/testis (CT) antigens: potential targets for immunotherapy. Cancer Sci 100: 2014–2021.

11. Chen YT, Gure AO, Tsang S, Stockert E, Jager E, et al. (1998) Identification of multiple cancer/testis antigens by allogeneic antibody screening of a melanoma cell line library. Proc Natl Acad Sci U S A 95: 6919–6923.

12. Serov S, SCully RE, Sobin LJ. In: Inte (1973) Histological typing of ovarian tumors. International histological classification of tumors No 9 Geneva: World Health Organization: 51–53.

13. Creasman W (1989) Announcements. FIGO stages: 1988 revision. Gynecol Oncol 35: 125–127.

14. (1971) International Federation of Gynecology and Obstetrics. 1–7.

15. Shimizu Y, Kamoi S, Amada S, Akiyama F, Silverberg SG (1998) Toward the development of a universal grading system for ovarian epithelial carcinoma: testing of a proposed system in a series of 461 patients with uniform treatment and follow-up. Cancer 82: 893–901.

16. Schultz-Thater E, Piscuoglio S, Iezzi G, Le Magnen C, Zajac P, et al. (2011) MAGE-A10 is a nuclear protein frequently expressed in high percentages of tumor cells in lung, skin and urothelial malignancies. Int J Cancer 129: 1137–1148.

17. Landry C, Brasseur F, Spagnoli GC, Marbaix E, Boon T, et al. (2000) Monoclonal antibody 57B stains tumor tissues that express gene MAGE-A4. Int J Cancer 86: 835–841.

18. Gnjatic S, Old LJ, Chen YT (2009) Autoantibodies against cancer antigens. Methods Mol Biol 520: 11–19.

19. Cox D (1972) Regression models and life-tables. JR Stat Soc 34: 187–220.

20. Kaplan EaM, P (1958) Nonparametric estimation from incomplete observation. J Am Stat Assoc 53: 457–486.

21. Odunsi K, Qian F, Matsuzaki J, Mhawech-Fauceglia P, Andrews C, et al. (2007) Vaccination with an NY-ESO-1 peptide of HLA class I/II specificities induces integrated humoral and T cell responses in ovarian cancer. Proc Natl Acad Sci U S A 104: 12837–12842.

22. Odunsi K, Matsuzaki J, Karbach J, Neumann A, Mhawech-Fauceglia P, et al. (2012) Efficacy of vaccination with recombinant vaccinia and fowlpox vectors expressing NY-ESO-1 antigen in ovarian cancer and melanoma patients. Proc Natl Acad Sci U S A 109: 5797–5802.

23. Odunsi K, Matsuzaki J, James SR, Mhawech-Fauceglia P, Tsuji T, et al. (2014) Epigenetic potentiation of NY-ESO-1 vaccine therapy in human ovarian cancer. Cancer Immunol Res 2: 37–49.

24. Jang SJ, Soria JC, Wang L, Hassan KA, Morice RC, et al. (2001) Activation of melanoma antigen tumor antigens occurs early in lung carcinogenesis. Cancer Res 61: 7959–7963.

25. Picard V, Bergeron A, Larue H, Fradet Y (2007) MAGE-A9 mRNA and protein expression in bladder cancer. Int J Cancer 120: 2170–2177.

26. Otte M, Zafrakas M, Riethdorf L, Pichlmeier U, Loning T, et al. (2001) MAGE-A gene expression pattern in primary breast cancer. Cancer Res 61: 6682–6687.

27. Andrade VC, Vettore AL, Felix RS, Almeida MS, Carvalho F, et al. (2008) Prognostic impact of cancer/testis antigen expression in advanced stage multiple myeloma patients. Cancer Immun 8: 2.

28. Russo V, Dalerba P, Ricci A, Bonazzi C, Leone BE, et al. (1996) MAGE BAGE and GAGE genes expression in fresh epithelial ovarian carcinomas. Int J Cancer 67: 457–460.

29. Gillespie AM, Rodgers S, Wilson AP, Tidy J, Rees RC, et al. (1998) MAGE, BAGE and GAGE: tumour antigen expression in benign and malignant ovarian tissue. Br J Cancer 78: 816–821.

30. Zhang S, Zhou X, Yu H, Yu Y (2010) Expression of tumor-specific antigen MAGE, GAGE and BAGE in ovarian cancer tissues and cell lines. BMC Cancer 10: 163.

31. Yakirevich E, Sabo E, Lavie O, Mazareb S, Spagnoli GC, et al. (2003) Expression of the MAGE-A4 and NY-ESO-1 cancer-testis antigens in serous ovarian neoplasms. Clin Cancer Res 9: 6453–6460.

32. Brasseur F, Rimoldi D, Lienard D, Lethe B, Carrel S, et al. (1995) Expression of MAGE genes in primary and metastatic cutaneous melanoma. Int J Cancer 63: 375–380.

33. Patard JJ, Brasseur F, Gil-Diez S, Radvanyi F, Marchand M, et al. (1995) Expression of MAGE genes in transitional-cell carcinomas of the urinary bladder. Int J Cancer 64: 60–64.

34. Gure AO, Chua R, Williamson B, Gonen M, Ferrera CA, et al. (2005) Cancer-testis genes are coordinately expressed and are markers of poor outcome in non-small cell lung cancer. Clin Cancer Res 11: 8055–8062.

35. Jungbluth AA, Ely S, DiLiberto M, Niesvizky R, Williamson B, et al. (2005) The cancer-testis antigens CT7 (MAGE-C1) and MAGE-A3/6 are commonly expressed in multiple myeloma and correlate with plasma-cell proliferation. Blood 106: 167–174.

36. Kim J, Reber HA, Hines OJ, Kazanjian KK, Tran A, et al. (2006) The clinical significance of MAGEA3 expression in pancreatic cancer. Int J Cancer 118: 2269–2275.

37. Okabayashi K, Fujita T, Miyazaki J, Okada T, Iwata T, et al. (2012) Cancer-testis antigen BORIS is a novel prognostic marker for patients with esophageal cancer. Cancer Sci 103: 1617–1624.

38. Monte M, Simonatto M, Peche LY, Bublik DR, Gobessi S, et al. (2006) MAGE-A tumor antigens target p53 transactivation function through histone deacetylase recruitment and confer resistance to chemotherapeutic agents. Proc Natl Acad Sci U S A 103: 11160–11165.

39. Kondo T, Zhu X, Asa SL, Ezzat S (2007) The cancer/testis antigen melanoma-associated antigen-A3/A6 is a novel target of fibroblast growth factor receptor 2-IIIb through histone H3 modifications in thyroid cancer. Clin Cancer Res 13: 4713–4720.

40. Liu W, Cheng S, Asa SL, Ezzat S (2008) The melanoma-associated antigen A3 mediates fibronectin-controlled cancer progression and metastasis. Cancer Res 68: 8104–8112.

41. Gjerstorff M, Burns JS, Nielsen O, Kassem M, Ditzel H (2009) Epigenetic modulation of cancer-germline antigen gene expression in tumorigenic human mesenchymal stem cells: implications for cancer therapy. Am J Pathol 175: 314–323.

42. Bullock TN, Mullins DW, Engelhard VH (2003) Antigen density presented by dendritic cells in vivo differentially affects the number and avidity of primary, memory, and recall CD8+ T cells. J Immunol 170: 1822–1829.

43. Odunsi K, Jungbluth AA, Stockert E, Qian F, Gnjatic S, et al. (2003) NY-ESO-1 and LAGE-1 Cancer-Testis Antigens Are Potential Targets for Immunotherapy in Epithelial Ovarian Cancer. Cancer Res 63: 6076–6083.

13

Reciprocal Complementation of the Tumoricidal Effects of Radiation and Natural Killer Cells

Kai-Lin Yang[1,9], Yu-Shan Wang[1,9], Chao-Chun Chang[1], Su-Chen Huang[1], Yi-Chun Huang[1], Mau-Shin Chi[1], Kwan-Hwa Chi[1,2]*

1 Department of Radiation Therapy and Oncology, Shin Kong Wu Ho-Su Memorial Hospital, Taipei, Taiwan, 2 Institute of Radiation Science and School of Medicine, National Yang-Ming University, Taipei, Taiwan

Abstract

The tumor microenvironment is a key determinant for radio-responsiveness. Immune cells play an important role in shaping tumor microenvironments; however, there is limited understanding of how natural killer (NK) cells can enhance radiation effects. This study aimed to assess the mechanism of reciprocal complementation of radiation and NK cells on tumor killing. Various tumor cell lines were co-cultured with human primary NK cells or NK cell line (NK-92) for short periods and then exposed to irradiation. Cell proliferation, apoptosis and transwell assays were performed to assess apoptotic efficacy and cell viability. Western blot analysis and immunoprecipitation methods were used to determine XIAP (X-linked inhibitor of apoptosis protein) and Smac (second mitochondria-derived activator of caspase) expression and interaction in tumor cells. Co-culture did not induce apoptosis in tumor cells, but a time- and dose-dependent enhancing effect was found when co-cultured cells were irradiated. A key role for caspase activation via perforin/granzyme B (Grz B) after cell-cell contact was determined, as the primary radiation enhancing effect. The efficacy of NK cell killing was attenuated by upregulation of XIAP to bind caspase-3 in tumor cells to escape apoptosis. Knockdown of XIAP effectively potentiated NK cell-mediated apoptosis. Radiation induced Smac released from mitochondria and neutralized XIAP and therefore increased the NK killing. Our findings suggest NK cells in tumor microenvironment have direct radiosensitization effect through Grz B injection while radiation enhances NK cytotoxicity through triggering Smac release.

Editor: Gabriele Multhoff, Technische Universitaet Muenchen, Germany

Funding: This study was supported by a grant from the National Science Council, Taiwan (NSC 97-2320-B-341-001-MY2, http://web1.nsc.gov.tw/). The National Science Council had no role in study design, data collection and analysis, decision to publish, or preparation of the manuscript.

Competing Interests: The authors have declared that no competing interests exist.

* E-mail: M006565@ms.skh.org.tw

9 These authors contributed equally to this work.

Introduction

Radiation is a highly effective tumoricidal modality, but its efficacy is modulated by the tumor microenvironment [1,2]. Many clinical studies have shown that the intra-tumoral presence of CD8+ cells, NK cells, CD4+ cells, and dendritic cells (DC) is positively correlated with survival, while the presence of macrophages and regulatory T cells predict poor responsiveness to therapy and survival [3,4,5]. There is increased interest in modulation of immune cells infiltrating the tumor microenvironment to enhance the therapeutic efficacy of radiation [6,7].Patients received vaccine before the standard chemotherapy/radiotherapy to achieve a better result has successfully reported on prostate and head and neck cancer [8,9,10]. There is evidence that immune-mediated microenvironmental change has occurred during tumor progression and after therapy. The specific T cells were present before radiation and a cascade of antigen release after radiation may further enhance polyclonal response [8,10]. The combination of immunotherapy and radiotherapy is theoretically synergistic and complementary to each other. Nevertheless, it is not clearly understood why an improved immunological environment is critical for the efficacy of subsequent radiotherapy nor why an irradiated tumor improves the subsequent immunotherapy effect.

The creation of a favorable host anti-tumor immune microenvironment by in situ delivery of interleukin-2 (IL-2) and granulocyte macrophage colony growth factor (GM-CSF) genes into the peri-tumoral site resulted in improved radio-responsiveness and systemic anticancer immunity [11]. Timar et al. reported that peri-tumoral injection of neoadjuvant leukocyte interleukin augmented the tumor sensitivity to subsequent radiation therapy and chemotherapy in oral cancer [12]. We found that neoadjuvant immunotherapy given before radiotherapy improved the radiosensitization effect over immunotherapy given after radiotherapy, through activation of NK cells [13].

We hypothesized that NK cells sensitized target cells to radiotherapy. The most important apoptotic machinery activated by effector-target cell contact is likely caspase, which is initiated by granzyme B (Grz B)/perforin [14]. Various mechanisms contribute to resistance of tumor cells to immune cell killing [15,16,17]. In general, the XIAP/Smac pathway is important for full activation of autoprocessing of caspases [18,19]. The XIAP protein can directly inhibit caspase activity and regulate death receptor-mediated apoptosis induced by immune cells [20]. The inhibitory action of XIAP is counteracted by Smac, a mitochondrial protein that is released into the cytosol during apoptosis, binds to XIAP, and disrupts its activity [21]. Breaking tumor resistance to immune

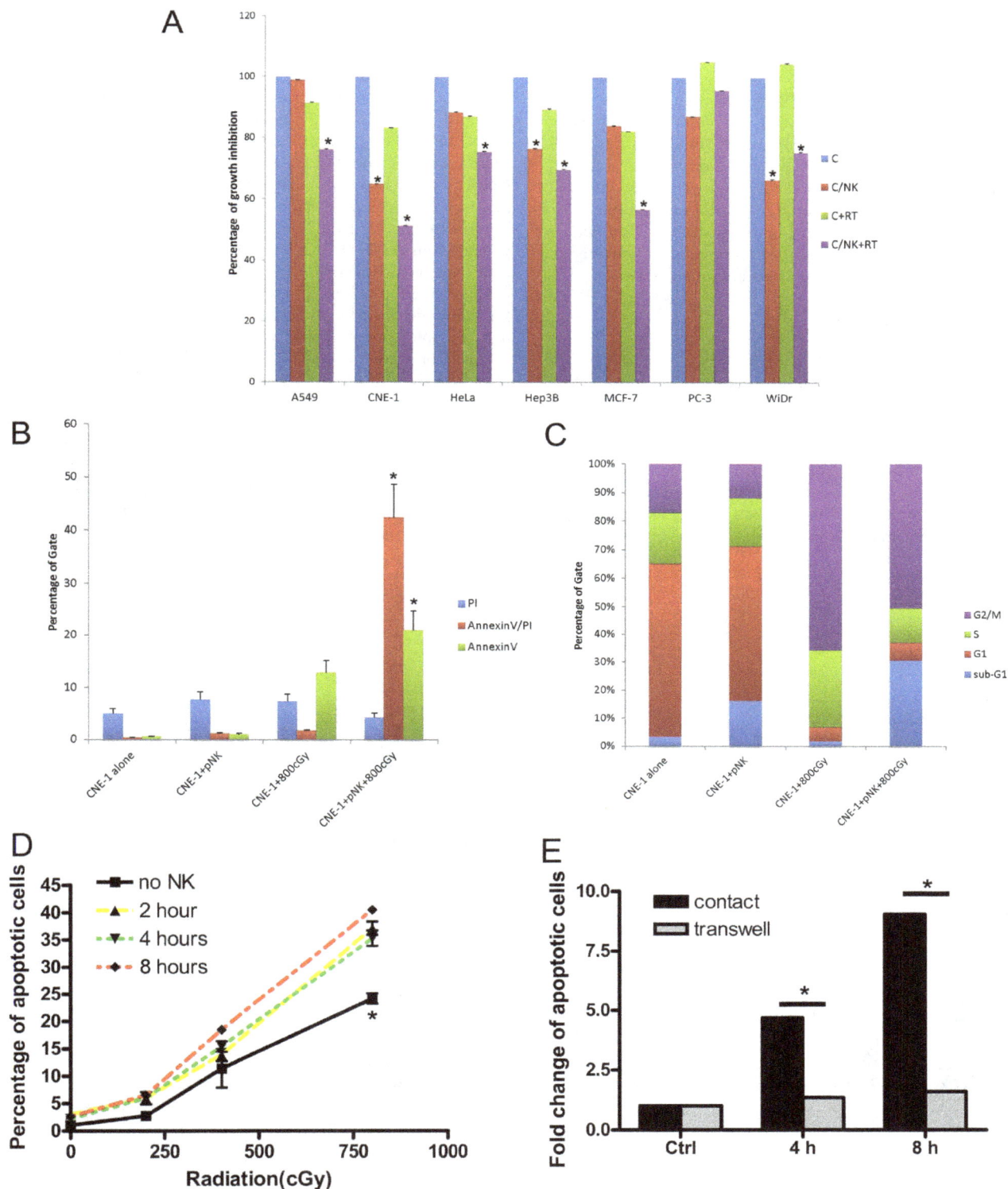

Figure 1. pNK and NK-92 cells sensitized tumor cells. 1×10^5 of various tumor cells were seeded in 96-well tissue-culture plates, co-cultured with 2.5×10^5 pNK cells for 4 h, washed and then exposed to 800 cGy of irradiation and evaluated 48 h late for cell proliferation by the MTS (A). C, cancer cell alone; C/NK, cancer cell and NK coculture; C+RT, cancer cell treated with 800 cGy radiation; C/NK+RT, cancer cell and pNK coculture followed by radiation. The apoptosis of CNE-1 cells after irradiation 48 h under various co-culture conditions that described previously was analyzed by (B) Annexin-V assay and (C) cell cycle analysis. (D) CNE-1 cells were incubated with NK-92 cells in 1:2.5 ratios for 2, 4, and 8 h and irradiated at indicated doses. (E) 1×10^5 CNE-1 cells were cultured in the lower chambers of transwells, and 2.5×10^5 NK-92 cells were cultured in the upper chambers for 4 and 8 h. Both of (D) and (E) were assayed using Annexin-V to detect apoptotic cells (AnnexinV+). (*, $p < 0.05$).

cells by concomitant low-dose radiation has been reported, but the underlying mechanism is poorly understood [22].

We show here that NK cells significantly enhance the radiation effect on target cells without killing them. Caspase activation after radiation was induced in target cells after co-culture with NK cells but not in target cells without co-culture. Immunotherapy alone (co-cultured only) resulted in increased XIAP binding of caspase-3 in the cytosol, thus escaping apoptosis, whereas irradiating co-cultured cells resulted in a re-localization of XIAP into the mitochondria and induced a release of Smac from the mitochondria to inhibit cytosolic XIAP to enhance apoptosis. This finding provides new evidence of reciprocal complementation between the tumoricidal effects of radiotherapy and immunotherapy.

Materials and Methods

Cells and Culture Conditions

The effector cells including primary human NK cells (pNK) isolated from Human peripheral mononuclear cells (PBMC) and human NK-92 cell line. The PBMC was provided by the Taipei Blood Center (TBC) following the guidelines of the Institutional Review Board of TBC. The TBC provide the donor bloods who have already signed the consent of donation to research use and our proposal has to be passed their IRB. The target cells including human lung adenocarcinoma cells (A549), nasopharyngeal cancer

cell line (CNE-1), cervical cancer cells (HeLa), hepatoma cells (Hep3B) and breast cancer cells (MCF-7) were purchased from American Type Culture Collection (ATCC), and maintained in DMEM (Invitrogen, Verviers, Belgium) containing 10% heat-inactivated fetal bovine serum (FBS), 2 mM L-glutamine, 100 units/mL penicillin, and 100 μg/mL streptomycin (Sigma, St. Louis, MO). The prostate carcinoma cell line PC-3 and colon carcinoma cell line WiDr were purchased from the Culture Collection and Research Center (Hsinchu, Taiwan), and cultured respectively in complete Ham's F-12 and α-medium (Invitrogen) supplemented with 10% FBS, glutamine, penicillin, and streptomycin. Human NK-92 cell line was purchased from the Culture Collection and Research Center (Hsinchu, Taiwan), and fresh batches were thawed every year. NK-92 cells were propagated in α-medium supplemented with 12.5% heat-inactivated FBS, 12.5% horse serum, 1.5 g/L sodium bicarbonate, 0.2 mM myo-inositol, 0.1 mM 2-mercaptoethanol, 0.02 mM folic acid (Sigma) and 100 units/mL IL-2 (Proleukin, Chiron, Emeryville, CA). Unconjugated anti-FasL (clone 100419; R&D systems) antibody was used for neutralization experiments.

Primary Human NK Cell Isolation

pNK cells were isolated from PBMC by negative selection using pNK cell Isolation Kit II and MACS columns (Miltenyi Biotech) following the manufacturer's protocol. Experiments were per-

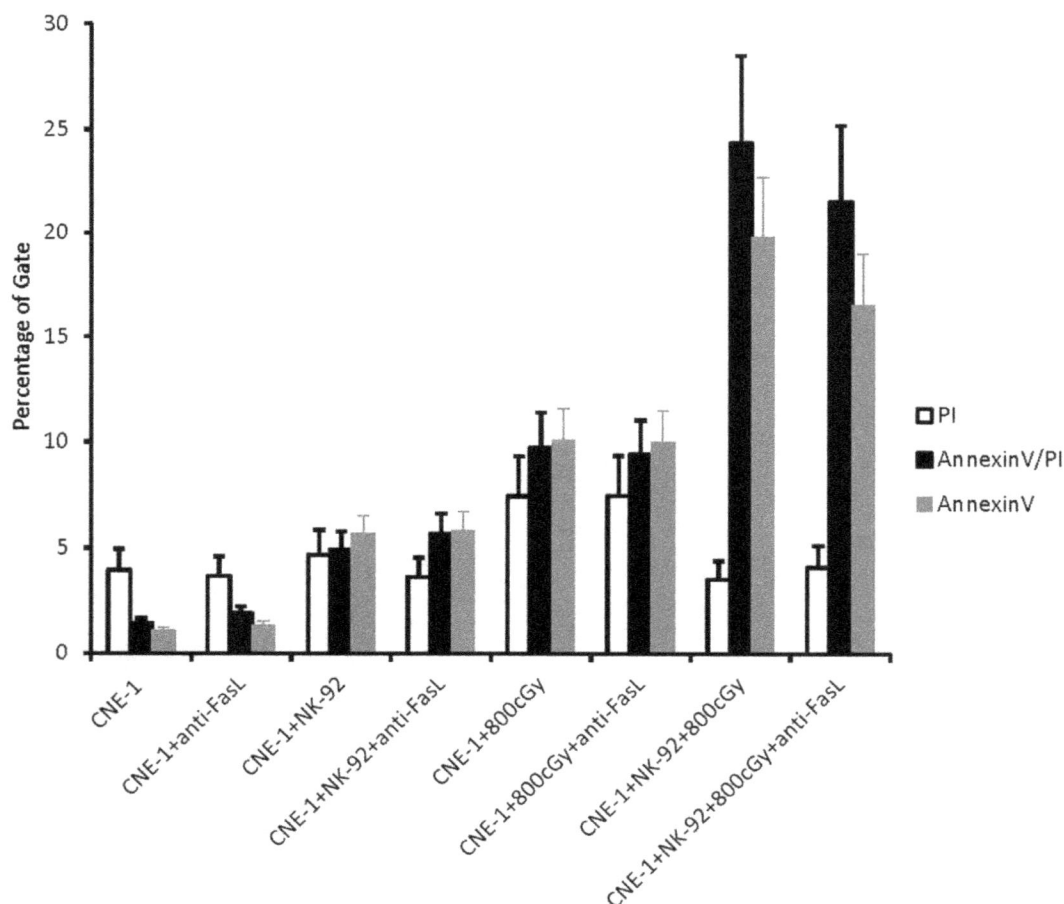

Figure 2. Effect of NK-92-treated CNE-1 cells on Fas blockage. CNE-1 cells were co-cultured with 2.5 fold NK-92 cells for 4 h in presence of anti-FasL blocking antibody (10 μg/ml). The percentage of apoptotic cells after irradiation 48 h under various co-culture conditions was analyzed by Annexin-V assay (AnnexinV+, D). Results from 3 independent experiments are shown; bars indicate mean ± SD.

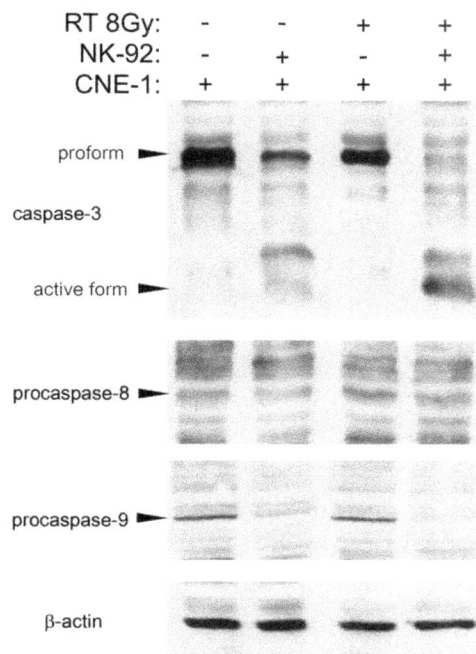

Figure 3. The caspase signaling pathway was induced after co-culture. CNE-1 cells were co-cultured with 2.5 fold of NK-92 cells for 4 h, then NK-92 cells were washed away, and CNE-1 cells were exposed to 800 cGy of radiation. Control cells of CNE-1 alone or CNE-1 cells that had been co-cultured were not irradiated. After 24 h of incubation, cells were harvested for western blot analysis of procaspase/caspase-3, procaspase-8, and procaspase-9 protein in lysates of CNE-1 alone (lane C), CNE-1 cells cultures with NK-92 cells (lane C/N). The arrows indicate cleaved (activated) caspase 3 at about 17 kDa and its precursor, pro-caspase 3, at about 43 kDa; precaspase 8, at about 55kDa; procaspase 9, at about 45kDa. β-actin was used as the internal control.

formed when purity of pNK cells was more than 95% as determined by flow cytometry.

MTS Cell Proliferation Assay

Various tumor cell lines were cultured at a density of 1.0×10^5 cells/well in 96-well round-bottom plates (Falcon) containing 200 µl of medium. Tumor cells (1×10^6) were cultured with or without NK cells (2.5×10^6) in different combinations for 4 h. After 4 h, the non-adherent NK cells were washed away and tumor cells were exposed to 800 cGy of irradiation. Tumor cells were maintained for 2 days at 37°C in a 5% CO_2 humidified atmosphere. The proliferation rate of the cells was measured using an MTS assay (CellTiter 96 aqueous one-solution cell proliferation assay; Promega). Forty microliters of CellTiter 96 aqueous one-solution were added to each well. After 4 h of incubation, the UV absorbance of the solution was measured at a wavelength of 490 nm. All MTS assays were done in triplicate.

Apoptosis Assay

CNE-1 cells and pNK or NK-92 cells were cultured, trypsinized as described above, and washed twice with PBS. Apoptosis was confirmed using an Annexin V Apoptosis Kit (BD Pharmingen) according to the manufacturer's instructions. Briefly, tumor cells were washed 3 times with PBS; then, some cells were analyzed immediately for apoptosis using Annexin V/PI staining. Washed cells were supplemented with 1% BSA and then stained directly

with 10 µL of PI and 2.5 µL Annexin V-FITC, after the addition of 222.5 µL of binding buffer. Immediately after 10 min incubation in the dark on ice, the cells were analyzed by flow cytometry. The percentage of positive cells was determined by using a FACSCalibur cytometer and Cell Quest Pro software (Becton Dickinson, Mountain View, CA).

Transwell Assay

CNE-1 cells (0.5×10^6) were placed in the lower Transwell chamber (Corning Glass Works, Corning, NY) and a filter with a 0.8-µm pore size was placed on top of the chamber. Aliquots of NK-92 cells (1.25×10^6 cells) were applied to the upper chamber, and the chambers were incubated at 37°C in 5% CO_2 for 4 h. CNE-1 cells were analyzed by Annexin V/PI apoptosis detection kit as described above.

Western Blot Analysis

For protein analysis, cells were lysed for 5 min at room temperature in a buffer of 150 mM NaCl, 50 mM Tris (pH 8.0), 5 mM EDTA, 1% (v/v) Nonidet p-40, 1 mM phenylmethylsulfonyl fluoride, 20 µg/mL aprotinin, and 25 µg/mL leupeptin (Sigma). Total protein concentration of lysates was measured using the Bio-Rad protein assay reagent. Cell lysates (100 µg) were electrophoresed on a 12% polyacrylamide gel, transferred onto Immobilon-P PVDF membrane (Millipore, Bedford, MA), and blocked in PBS-Tween 20 and 10% nonfat milk for 2 h at room temperature. The filter was incubated with specific antibodies to anti-Fas, anti-caspase-3, -8, or -9 (Santa Cruz Biotechnology, Santa Cruz, CA), anti-XIAP, or anti-Smac antibody (Cell Signaling Technology, Beverly, CA) for 2 h at room temperature in PBS-0.05% Tween 20 containing 5% nonfat milk, followed by 1 h incubation at room temperature with horseradish peroxidase-conjugated secondary antibodies (Jackson ImmunoResearch Laboratories, West Grove, PA) in the same buffer. Blots were developed on X-ray film by using a chemiluminescent detection system (ECL; GE Life Science, Buckinghamshire, UK). The protein bands of caspase 3 and pro-caspase 3 on X-ray film were scanned and densitometrically analysed with ImageJ software (US National Institutes of Health). Results are expressed as the ratio pro-caspase/caspase 3 (a low ratio is indicative of apoptosis) [23].

RNA Preparation and Real-time PCR

RNA was extracted with Trizol (Invitrogen, Carlsbad, CA) and chloroform, then precipitated with isopropanol, according to the manufacturer's recommendations. Further purification was obtained with the RNeasy Mini Kit (Qiagen, Valencia, CA). Integrity and purity were verified by spectrophotometry, and the quality was assessed by electrophoresis on agarose gels. Double-stranded cDNA was synthesized from total RNA. Real-time PCR was performed using a LightCycler rapid thermal cycler system (Roche Diagnostics Ltd, Lewes, UK) according to the manufacturer's instructions. Reactions were performed in a 20-µL volume with 0.5 µM primers and $MgCl_2$ concentration optimized between 2–5 mM. Nucleotides, Taq DNA polymerase, and buffer were included in the LightCycler-DNA Master SYBR Green I mix (Roche Diagnostics). A typical protocol took approximately 15 min to complete and included a 30-s denaturation step followed by 45 cycles with denaturation at 95°C for 10 s, annealing at 55°C for 5 s, and extension at 72°C for 10 s. To confirm amplification specificity, the PCR products from each primer pair were subjected to melting curve analysis and subsequent agarose gel electrophoresis. The baseline of each reaction was equalized by calculating the mean value of the 5

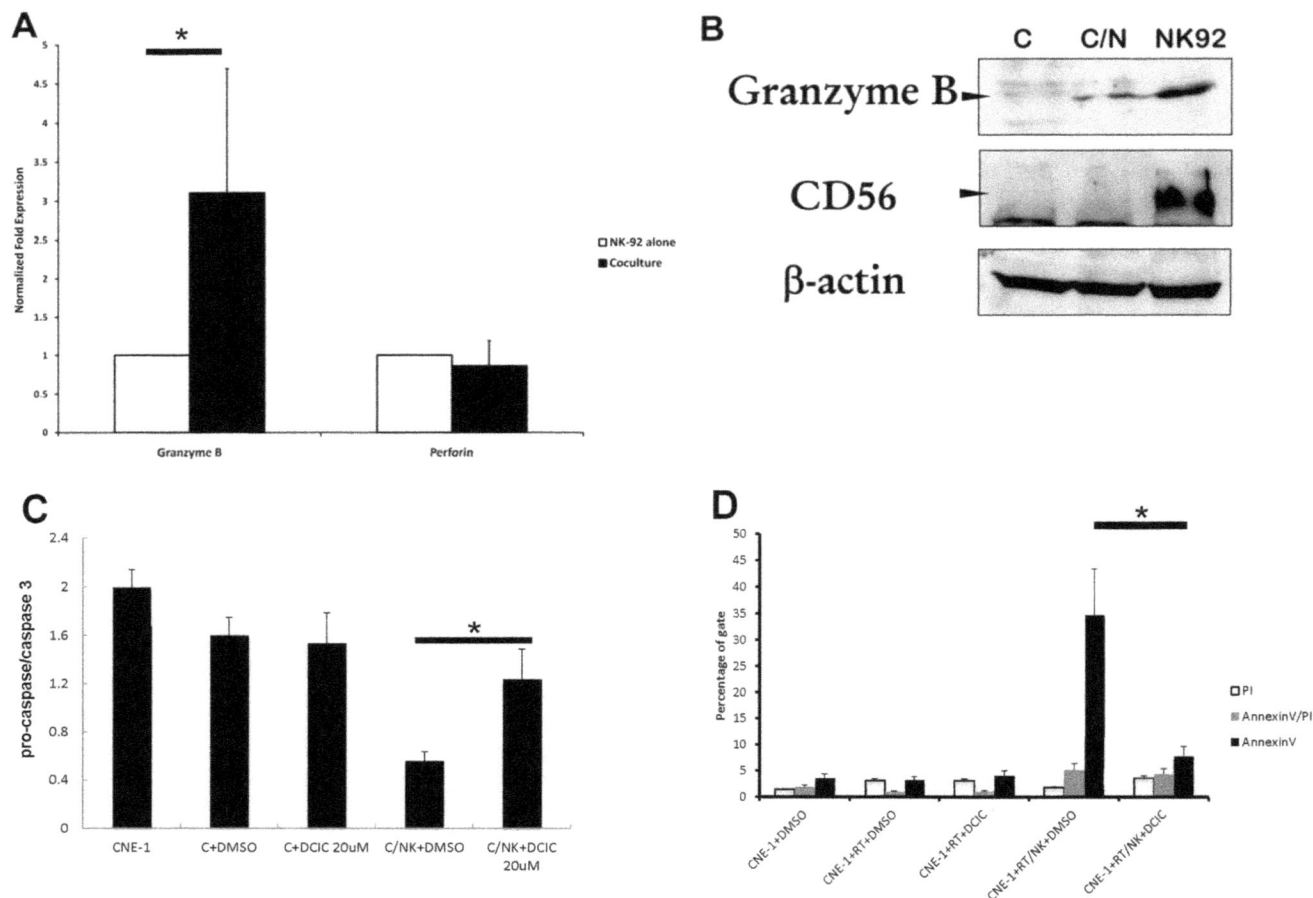

Figure 4. Granzyme B was secreted by NK-92 cells and penetrated into CNE-1 cells during co-culture. (A) Levels of Granzyme B and perforin mRNA expression in NK-92 cells co-cultured with or without CNE-1 cells for 4 h were measured by real-time RT-PCR. The amounts of mRNA are expressed relative to the amount of MBD-4 in each sample and are shown as the mean ± SD of 3 separate experiments. Significant differences in the expression in the presence or absence of the stimulators are indicated as * ($p < 0.05$). (B) Quantitative analysis of Granzyme B protein in lysates of CNE-1 alone by western blotting (lane C); CNE-1 treated with NK-92 cells for 4 h then NK-92 cells removed (lane C/N); NK-92 cells that had been washed from CNE-1 cell co-culture (lane NK92). CD56 was used to demonstrate exclusion of contamination with NK-92 cells, and β-actin was used as the internal control. (C) DCIC pretreated with CNE-1 cells for 1 h, then co-cultured with 2.5 fold of NK92 cells for 4 h. After washing NK92 cells away, and CNE-1 cells were exposed to 800 cGy of radiation and analyzed for the ratio procaspase/caspase-3 by ImageJ (a decreased ratio is indicative of apoptosis). The bar chart was average of three independent experiments. (D) Annexin-V assay. (*, $p < 0.05$).

lowest measured data points for each sample and subtracting this from each reading point. Background fluorescence was removed by setting a noise band. The number of cycles at which the best-fit line through the log-linear portion of each amplification curve intersects the noise band is inversely proportional to the log of copy number.

Immunoprecipitation Assay

Cell extracts were incubated with 1 μg of anti-XIAP or -Smac antibody for 24 h at 4°C. The precipitates were further reacted with protein A-Sepharose beads (GE Healthcare/Amersham Biotech, Piscataway, NJ) and eluted by boiling for 5 min in Laemmli sample buffer. Electrophoretic separation of the immuno-precipitated proteins or cell lysates was done in 10% acrylamide gels, and bands were transferred onto Immobilon NC membranes (Millipore, Bedford, MA). For immuno-blotting, the membranes were probed with anti-XIAP, Smac, or caspase-3 antibody at 1/200 dilution. The blots were incubated with species-specific conjugated HRP secondary Abs (Jackson ImmunoRe-

search Laboratories) and signals revealed by ECL (GE Healthcare).

Data Analysis

Each experiment was performed in duplicate and its average was used for quantification. Data are expressed as the mean ± SEM of averages from at least 3 experiments. ANOVA was used to assess the statistical significance of the differences, and a value of $p < 0.05$ was considered statistically significant.

Results

NK Cells Enhance Radiosensitivity

The ability of pNK cells to enhance radiation in cancer cell lines was examined by irradiating cells after a 4-h co-incubation with pNK. As shown in Fig. 1A, pNK cells were found to enhance radiation cytotoxicity in most cell lines in compared with medium alone control or radiation alone except PC-3 cell line. It seems to be a general phenomenon in rest cell lines. Since CNE-1 showed the most significant radiosensitization effect on pNK cells

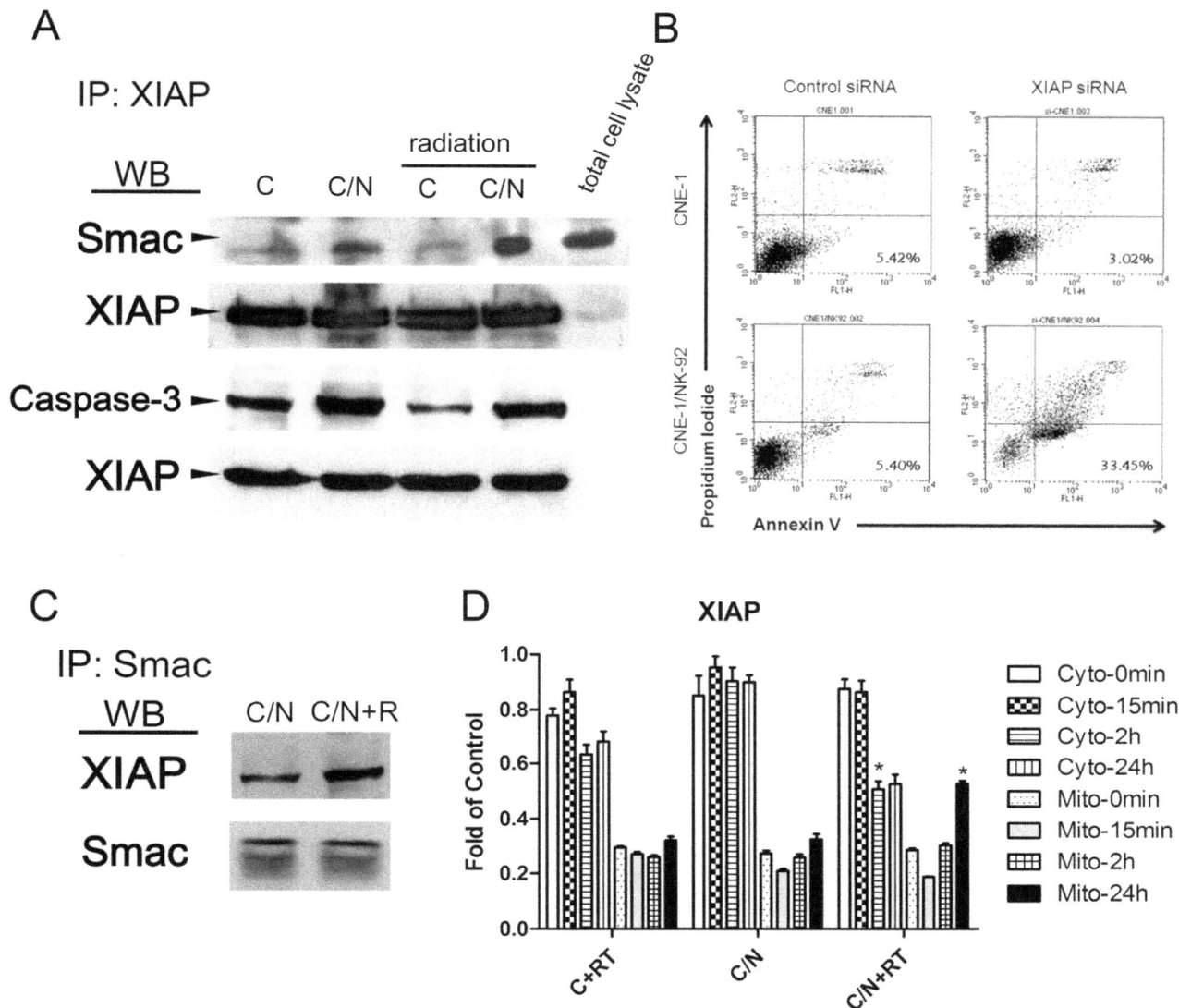

Figure 5. Caspase-3 was inhibited by XIAP and XIAP was downregulated by binding of Smac after radiation. CNE-1 cells (lane C) were treated with NK-92 cells for 4 h (lane C/N) before combined treatment with 800 cGy of radiation. (A) Cell lysates were immunoprecipitated with anti-XIAP antibody and immunoblotted with anti-Smac, anti-caspase-3 or anti-XIAP antibody. (B) CNE-1 cells were transfected with 80 nM of XIAP siRNA for 16 h and co-cultured with NK-92 cells for 4 h before NK-92 cells were washed away. The cells were assayed using Annexin-V to determine the percentage of apoptotic cells (AnnexinV+). (C) Cell lysates were immunoprecipitated by anti-Smac antibody and detected with anti-XIAP antibody by Western blot. (D) CNE-1 cells were treated with NK-92 cells for 4 h (C/N) before combined treatment with 800 cGy of radiation (C/N+RT) or CNE-1 treated with 800 cGy of radiation alone (C+RT). After treatment, cells were further incubated for 0 min, 15 min, 2 h, or 24 h, then harvested and fractionated into cytosolic (Cyto) and mitochondrial (Mito) fractions for assay by western blot. β-actin was used as the loading control for each fraction. Density of the XIAP normalized with β-actin was assayed by Image J. The bar chart was average of three independent experiments.

treatment (P<0.001), we choose CNE-1 cell for the following mechanistic study. Apoptotic efficacy of CNE-1 cells co-cultured with pNK cells was assessed by apoptosis assay and cell cycle analysis. Both of the percentage of late apoptotic cells (AnnexinV/ PI) and early apoptotic cells (AnnexinV) were significantly increased as compared to the pNK control or the radiation treatment control (p<0.05) (Figure 1B) as well as sub-G1 ratio in cell cycle analysis (Figure 1C). Although CNE-1, Hep3B and WiDr showed significant growth inhibition by MTS assay after 4 h co-culture with NK cells (Figure 1A), the apoptosis assay did not reveal cell death (CNE-1, Figure 1 C and D; Hep3B and WiDr, Figure S1). The representative data for annexin-V and cell cycle analysis were showed in Figure S2A and B. Longer exposure to

pNK before irradiation resulted in a greater effect of cytotoxicity significantly (p<0.05, Figure 1D). The decline in the radiation enhancing effect observed in cells co-cultured in transwells indicated a cell-cell contact-dependent mechanism (Figure 1E). These data suggest that a short, sublethal contact with NK cells increases the susceptibility of CNE-1 cells to radiation. Similar results for tumor cells cocultured with NK cell line (NK-92) was showed in Figure S2C and D. A dose response relationship that below 2.5:1 of NK/tumor cells coculture resulted in less effect was found (Figure S3). Thus, we used NK-92 cell line to surrogate pNK cells and 2.5:1 of NK/tumor cells ratio for the following experiments.

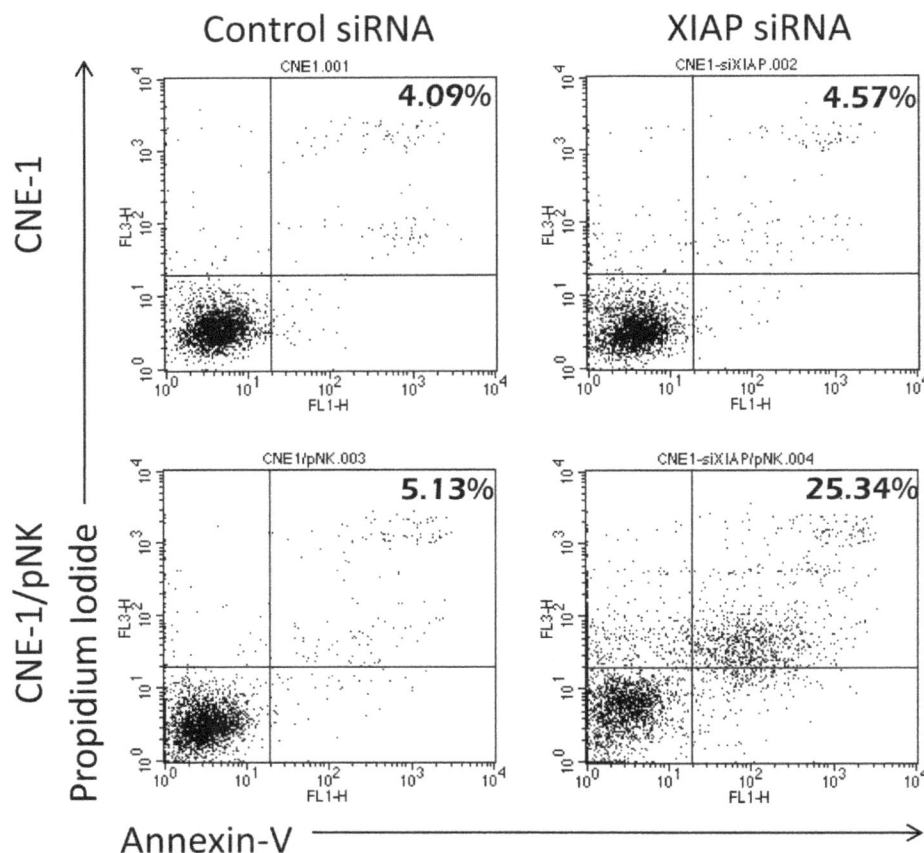

Figure 6. Primary NK cells sensitized tumor cells with same pathway. CNE-1 cells were transfected with 80 nM of XIAP siRNA for 16 h and co-cultured with pNK cells for 4 h before pNK cells were washed away. The cells were assayed using Annexin-V to determine the percentage of apoptotic cells.

NK-92 Contact Induced Extrinsic Pathway on CNE-1 Cells only Partially Related to NK-induced Radiation Enhancing Effect

NK-92 cell is known to trigger apoptotic signals via death receptor on target cells [24], whether death receptor activation plays the major role in NK cells radiosensitization effect is basically unknown. We found that Fas protein was significantly increased in CNE-1 cells after co-culture with NK-92 cells in a time and dose-dependent manner (Figure S4). Nevertheless, the radiation-enhancing effect was not significantly abolished by anti-FasL (Figure 2). A similar result was found in the TRAIL/DR5 system (data not shown). Both indicated death receptors were only partially involved in the radiosensitization effect of NK cells.

Intrinsic Pathway of Apoptotic Protein Caspase-9 Involved in the NK-induced Radiation Enhancing Effect

The effect of NK co-culture on caspase activation in CNE-1 cells with or without radiation was investigated next. Western blot analysis confirmed that procaspase-9 was cleavaged after NK cell co-culture (Figure 3). The cleavage of procaspase-9 indicated the activation of caspase-9 [25]. Caspase-3 activity was only slightly increased in the absence of radiation. On the other hand, caspase-8 was not activated in all treatments. Since caspase-9 is the primary caspase involved in the intrinsic mitochondrial pathway and caspase-8 is involved in the death receptor pathway, our

results suggest that NK-92 may sensitize CNE-1 cells to radiation chiefly by activation of the intrinsic mitochondrial apoptosis pathway.

Grz B Plays A Key Role in NK-92-induced Radiation Enhancing Effect

Cytosolic Grz B is a major effector molecule of NK cells that initiates the proteolytic cascade inducing target cell death. The gene expression of Grz B, but not perforin, was increased in NK-92 cells after co-culture (Figure 4A). The release of Grz B into CNE-1 cells is evident in Figure 4B. As shown in Figure 4B, the level of Grz B in CNE-1 is very low (first line, top plant and Figure S5). After co-culture with NK cells, the level of Grz B was significantly increased (second line, middle plant) while radiation alone did not increase the Grz B level (Figure S5). The NK cell marker, CD56, was used to demonstrate the lack of contamination of NK-92 cells in the harvested CNE-1 cells after co-culture. Since Grz B play a role in the NK-92-induced radiation enhancing effect, DCIC, a Grz B inhibitor, was used to block the NK-92-induced signaling pathway. We found that 20 mM DCIC was the maximal dose that did not affect cell survival. This dose was used to inhibit the NK/radiation induced apoptosis by both procaspase/caspase 3 ratio and annexin-V assay (Figure 4C and D, $p < 0.05$). These data further confirmed that Grz B was involved in the NK-92-induced radiation-enhancing effect.

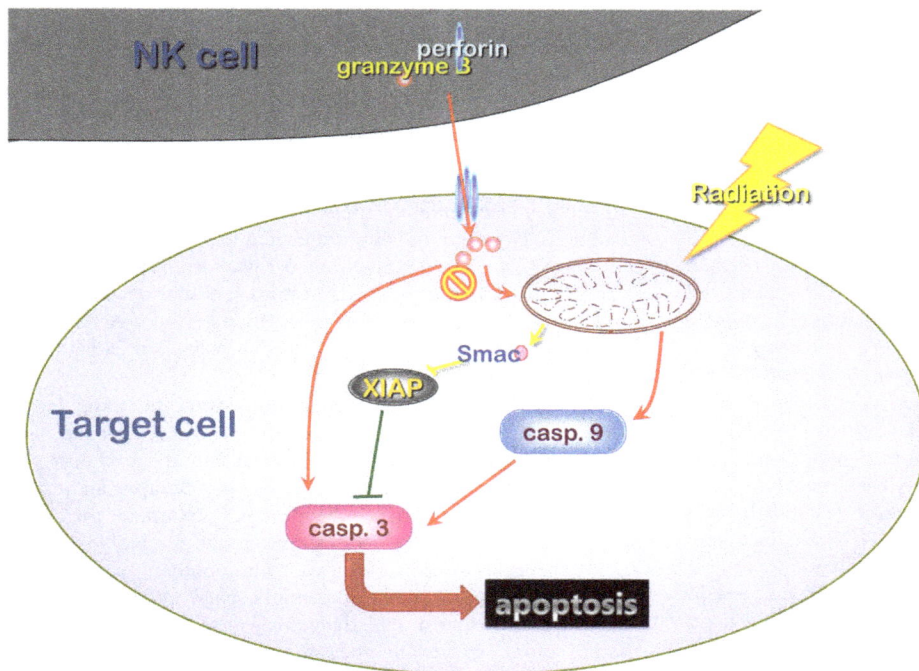

Figure 7. Mechanism of reciprocal interaction between NK cells and radiation in target cells. NK cells damage target cell through perforin/granzyme B and death receptor/caspase mediated pathway. The radiosensitisation effect through NK cell depends more on the perforin/granzyme B pathway. Without radiation, the suboptimal activation of NK cells cause up-regulation of XIAP. With radiation, the mitochondria releases Smac to neutralize XIAP and enhances NK cell-mediated cytotoxicity.

Radiation INDUCED SMAC to Counteract XIAP Binding of Caspase-3

To address the question of how NK-92 cells activated the caspase pathway without completing the apoptotic process, we further investigated the changes of XIAP, an important anti-apoptotic molecule. Immunoprecipitated XIAP was exposed to caspase-3 and Smac (a proapoptotic protein); then, the binding efficiency was assessed by western blot. We tested whether radiation treatment facilitates the activation of the Smac to bind XIAP. Immunoprecipitation analysis showed that Smac binding to XIAP was markedly increased as compared with C/N without radiation (Figure 5A). After co-culture with NK-92 cells (C/N), XIAP binding of activated caspase-3 in CNE-1 cells increased without a change in the total amount of XIAP (Figure 5A). To confirm the key role of XIAP in resistance to NK-92-mediated killing, we specifically down-regulated XIAP by transfecting siRNA into CNE-1 cells. As shown in Figure 5B, knockdown of XIAP significantly enhanced NK-92-induced apoptosis. The finding was further confirmed by immunoprecipitation of Smac, and then incubating the precipitate with XIAP. XIAP/Smac complexes was increased in C/N plus radiation, as predicted (Figure 5C). A detailed time-dependent translocation of XIAP from the cytosol to mitochondria was investigated by analyzing mitochondrial and cytosolic fractions from 15 min to 24 h after radiation. A migration of XIAP from the cytosol to mitochondria was observed between 2 h and 24 h after RT (Figure 5D). The decreasing of XIAP in cytosol was significantly revealed at 2 h after RT, whereas increasing of XIAP in mitochondria was significantly shown at 24 h after RT. NK-92 cell treatment alone did not promote XIAP translocation (Figure 5D). The transloca-tion of XIAP into mitochondria may initiate the release of Smac inside the mitochondria [26]. These data indicated that NK-92 co-

culture with CNE-1 cells was insufficient to achieve apoptosis due to the induction of XIAP binding with caspase, while subsequent radiation released Smac into the cytosol to bind cytosolic XIAP, thus enabling apoptosis to proceed.

pNK Cells Induced Radiation-enhancing Effect through XIAP

To further investigate whether the pNK cells could also sensitize CNE-1 cells to radiotherapy as well, we further knock-out XIAP by transfecting siRNA into CNE-1 cells. As shown in Figure 6, knockdown of XIAP also significantly enhanced pNK-induced apoptosis. These data indicated that both pNK and NK-92 shared similar mechanisms to induce radiosensitization effect. NK cells released granzyme B/perforin into target cells, triggered activation of the caspase pathway, and directly increased radiation-induced cell damage. The radiosensitising effect was significantly reduced when granzyme B was inhibited. If radiation was not adminis-tered, "the suboptimal activated" NK cells up-regulated of XIAP in target cells and thereby inhibited apoptosis. The adding of radiation significantly increased apoptosis by stimulating the release of mitochondrial Smac to neutralize the inhibitory effects of XIAP. Therefore, radiation is, in a broad sense, a Smac-inducing agent that may significantly increase the killing effect of NK cells. This model of reciprocal interaction between NK cells and radiation in target cells is illustrated in Figure 7.

Discussion

Although the clinical benefits of combined immunotherapy and conventional therapy are well acknowledged, the underlying mechanisms involved in cell-cell contact level have not been well defined. Here, we show that NK cells and radiation could reciprocally help each other to induce tumor cell death. NK cells sensitize target cells to radiation by injection with Grz B upon cell-cell contact. Radiation induces the release of mitochondrial Smac to counteract the cytosolic XIAP self-protection mechanism and to enhance NK cell-mediated lysis.

Evidence in the literature suggests that combining vaccines and monoclonal antibody treatments with chemotherapy or radiotherapy has higher clinical response rates than individual treatment modalities [27,28,29]. Phase III clinical trials have shown the survival benefit [30]. Chemotherapy-treated tumor cells became sensitive to lysis by low-avidity cytotoxic T lymphocytes induced by specific immunotherapy [29]. Immune and tumor cell crosstalk must occur in the tumor microenvironment. We have tested seven tumor cell lines in NK/tumor coculture system, only PC-3 did not express significant radiosensitization effect after pre-incubation with NK cells. The reason for PC-3 did not respond to what we expect may due to PC-3 was more resistant to radiation according to previous publication [31]. Rudner et al. has found that PC-3 could be reversed to high levels of apoptotic cell death after radiation when Akt inhibitor was combined [31]. The induction of proapoptotic signals to certain cancer cells by NK/tumor cells coculture may depend on different experimental conditions in order to show optimal result. However, it should be a general phenomenon. In our study, we chose 2.5:1 of NK/tumor cells ratio, this ratio is relatively high as compared to the in vivo tumor microenvironment. However, clinical results have long suggested the importance of healthy immune microenvironment but the mechanism remains unclear. Our result on NK cells just a small brick of whole picture of immune microenvironment.

NK cells are known to initiate tumor cell death, either by binding the death receptor CD95/Fas or by the release of granules containing perforin and the enzymatic molecule Grz B [32]. In spite of optimal cell engaging mechanisms, NK cell-mediated Grz B or death receptor signaling appears insufficient to induce the level of caspase-3 activity required to achieve target cell death without the help of radiation. Grz B fails to induce mitochondrial release of cytochrome c, and as a result, tumor cells escape from immune destruction.

A number of mechanisms were proposed to explain the failure of natural defense immunity [33,34]. After serial analysis of the molecular mechanisms, we found that XIAP machinery is likely the most important defense mechanism. XIAP is the first well-characterized member of the inhibition of apoptosis protein family [35]. Knockdown of XIAP significantly enhanced the cytotoxic effect of NK92 cells. While a similar finding has been reported in cytotoxic T cells [36], we are the first group to propose that radiation may be regarded as a Smac-mediated agent to overcome immune resistance.

Radiation targets mitochondria and potentiates the effects of intermembrane space proteins, such as Smac. Both Smac and cytochrome c are co-released from mitochondria during UV-induced apoptosis, and this process is caspase-independent [37]. This release was believed to be triggered by the aggregation of Bax in the outer mitochondrial membrane to form a lipid-protein complex [37]. The release of additional apoptotic factors from the mitochondria, such as Smac, to inhibit XIAP activity, and to further activate caspase-9 to promote the cascade of activation events is necessary to complete the apoptotic pathway [36]. Our data provides evidence that Smac is a downstream effector molecule of radiation. Interestingly, Streceli et al. has reported that endogenous XIAP translocates from the cytosol to mitochondria to induce permeabilization of the outer membrane of mitochondria, leading to Smac release, which occurs early in the apoptosis process [26]. We agree with their observation that XIAP may

switch the mitochondrial function from the anti- to pro-apoptotic form when radiation provides additional suicide signal to NK-contacted cells.

Apoptosis activation by NK-92 cells by the extrinsic pathway, which increased death receptor-mediated caspase 8, and the intrinsic pathway from Grz B, which induced caspase 9, is not sufficient to induce CNE-1 cell death. This phenomenon may present in most tumor microenvironment. Under such sublethal conditions, NK immunity is not sufficient to control tumor growth. The extrinsic or intrinsic apoptotic pathway from NK cell contact is not lethal without a concomitant mitochondrial release of Smac modality such as radiation proposed in this study. A reciprocal complementary relationship between NK cells and radiation on tumoricide is evident.

The concept of combined immunotherapy and radiotherapy has advanced recently [38]. Several studies have revealed that the quantitative measurement of tumor infiltrating lymphocytes in biopsy samples before chemotherapy or radiotherapy can be used as a predictor of the clinical effectiveness of treatment for cancer [39,40]. Our findings provide a conceptual acceptable link for clinical implications on neoadjuvant immunotherapy. We found that NK cells that infiltrate tumors have potent radiation-enhancing effects in a sublethal dosage. Neoadjuvant immuno-therapy aims to create a microenvironment favorable to cells of the innate immune system before radiotherapy is given. Theoretically, this is more effective than providing specific immunotherapy after radiotherapy, while ignoring the tumor microenvironment before radiation. We also found that radiation greatly enhanced the tumor susceptibility to immunologically mediated cell death, through the release of Smac. The dead cells, along with the danger signals delivered by irradiated tumor tissue, serve as links between the local response and the subsequent specific immune response [41]. Innate effector cells, including NK cells and dendritic cells in the tumor microenvironment, orchestrate the entire scenario [42].

In conclusion, we found that NK cells sensitize tumor cells to radiation and radiation sensitizes tumor cells to NK cell attack. Grz B transfer into tumor cells results in a radiation enhancing effect. Resistance of tumor cells to NK cell-mediated death is associated with endogenous XIAP inhibiting the caspase-3 triggered by immune cell attack. Radiation induced mitochondrial release of Smac to neutralize cytosolic XIAP. Therefore, the reciprocal complementation between NK cells and radiation to effect tumoricide is intriguing and important. A strategy of neoadjuvant immunotherapy to alter the immune milieu before radiotherapy is suggested.

Supporting Information

Figure S1   Apoptosis assay. 1×10^5 of (A) Hep3B cells and (B) WiDr cells were seeded in 96-well tissue-culture plates, co-cultured with 2.5×10^5 pNK cells for 4 h, washed and then exposed to 800 cGy of irradiation and evaluated 48 h late for Annexin-V.

Figure S2   The representative data for annexin-V and cell cycle analysis. 1×10^5 of CNE-1 cells were seeded in 96-well tissue-culture plates, co-cultured with 2.5×10^5 pNK (A, B) or NK-92 (C, D) cells for 4 h, washed and then exposed to 800 cGy of irradiation and evaluated 48 h late for Annexin-V assay (A, C) and cell cycle analysis (B, D).

Figure S3   Dosage analysis on NK/tumor cells ratio. CNE-1 cells were seeded into 6-well plates and co-cultured with

NK-92 cells at the indicated ratios for 4 h. The apoptotic cells were measured by Annexin-V assay.

Figure S4 CNE-1 expressed Fas after co-culture with NK-92 cells. The expression of Fas was measured by flow cytometry. CNE-1 cells were seeded into 6-well plates and co-cultured with 2.5 fold NK-92 cells at the indicated times (A). CNE-1 cells were co-cultured with NK-92 cells at the indicated ratios for 4 h (B).

Figure S5 Granzyme B expression assay. Granzyme B protein in lysates of CNE-1 alone by western blotting (lane C); CNE-1 treated with 800 cGy of irradiation (lane C/RT); lysates of NK-92 cells (lane NK92). β-actin was used as the internal control.

Author Contributions

Conceived and designed the experiments: KLY YSW KHC. Performed the experiments: CCC YCH MSC. Analyzed the data: SCH. Contributed reagents/materials/analysis tools: KLY YSW KHC. Wrote the paper: KLY YSW KHC.

References

1. Chi KH, Wang YS, Kao SJ (2012) Improving radioresponse through modification of the tumor immunological microenvironment. Cancer Biother Radiopharm 27: 6–11.
2. Ahn GO, Brown JM (2009) Influence of bone marrow-derived hematopoietic cells on the tumor response to radiotherapy: experimental models and clinical perspectives. Cell Cycle 8: 970–976.
3. Fuertes MB, Kacha AK, Kline J, Woo S-R, Kranz DM, et al. (2011) Host type I IFN signals are required for antitumor CD8+ T cell responses through CD8+ dendritic cells. The Journal of Experimental Medicine 208: 2005–2016.
4. Grabenbauer GG, Lahmer G, Distel L, Niedobitek G (2006) Tumor-infiltrating cytotoxic T cells but not regulatory T cells predict outcome in anal squamous cell carcinoma. Clin Cancer Res 12: 3355–3360.
5. Cortez-Retamozo V, Etzrodt M, Newton A, Rauch PJ, Chudnovskiy A, et al. (2012) Origins of tumor-associated macrophages and neutrophils. Proc Natl Acad Sci U S A 109: 2491–2496.
6. Shiao SL, Ganesan AP, Rugo HS, Coussens LM (2011) Immune microenvironments in solid tumors: new targets for therapy. Genes & Development 25: 2559–2572.
7. Sommariva M, De Cecco L, De Cesare M, Sfondrini L, Menard S, et al. (2011) TLR9 agonists oppositely modulate DNA repair genes in tumor versus immune cells and enhance chemotherapy effects. Cancer Res 71: 6382–6390.
8. Cha E, Fong L (2011) Immunotherapy for Prostate Cancer: Biology and Therapeutic Approaches. Journal of Clinical Oncology 29: 3677–3685.
9. Tímár J, Forster-Horváth C, Lukits J, Döme B, Ladányi A, et al. (2003) The Effect of Leukocyte Interleukin Injection (Multikine®) Treatment on the Peritumoral and Intratumoral Subpopulation of Mononuclear Cells and on Tumor Epithelia: A Possible New Approach to Augmenting Sensitivity to Radiation Therapy and Chemotherapy in Oral Cancer–A Multicenter Phase I/II Clinical Trial. The Laryngoscope 113: 2206–2217.
10. Gulley JL, Arlen PM, Bastian A, Morin S, Marte J, et al. (2005) Combining a recombinant cancer vaccine with standard definitive radiotherapy in patients with localized prostate cancer. Clin Cancer Res 11: 3353–3362.
11. Wang YS, Tsang YW, Chi CH, Chang CC, Chu RM, et al. (2008) Synergistic anti-tumor effect of combination radio- and immunotherapy by electro-gene therapy plus intra-tumor injection of dendritic cells. Cancer Lett 266: 275–285.
12. Timar J, Ladanyi A, Forster-Horvath C, Lukits J, Dome B, et al. (2005) Neoadjuvant immunotherapy of Oral Squamous Cell Carcinoma Modulates Intratumoral CD4/CD8 Ratio and Tumor Microenvironment: A Multicenter Phase II Clinical Trial. J Clin Oncol 23: 3421–3432.
13. Chi CH, Wang YS, Yang CH, Chi KH (2010) Neoadjuvant immunotherapy enhances radiosensitivity through natural killer cell activation. Cancer Biother Radiopharm 25: 39–45.
14. Metkar SS, Wang B, Aguilar-Santelises M, Raja SM, Uhlin-Hansen L, et al. (2002) Cytotoxic cell granule-mediated apoptosis: perforin delivers granzyme B-serglycin complexes into target cells without plasma membrane pore formation. Immunity 16: 417–428.
15. Campoli M, Ferrone S (2008) Tumor escape mechanisms: potential role of soluble HLA antigens and NK cells activating ligands. Tissue Antigens 72: 321–334.
16. Hersey P, Zhang XD (2001) How melanoma cells evade trail-induced apoptosis. Nat Rev Cancer 1: 142–150.
17. Thomas DA, Massague J (2005) TGF-beta directly targets cytotoxic T cell functions during tumor evasion of immune surveillance. Cancer Cell 8: 369–380.
18. Wang C-Y, Mayo MW, Korneluk RG, Goeddel DV, Baldwin AS Jr (1998) NF-kB Antiapoptosis: Induction of TRAF1 and TRAF2 and c-IAP1 and c-IAP2 to Suppress Caspase-8 Activation. Science 281: 1680–1683.
19. Du C, Fang M, Li Y, Li L, Wang X (2000) Smac, a mitochondrial protein that promotes cytochrome c-dependent caspase activation by eliminating IAP inhibition. Cell 102: 33–42.
20. Dubrez-Daloz L, Dupoux A, Cartier J (2008) IAPs: more than just inhibitors of apoptosis proteins. Cell Cycle 7: 1036–1046.
21. Wu H, Tschopp J, Lin SC (2007) Smac mimetics and TNFalpha: a dangerous liaison? Cell 131: 655–658.
22. Farooque A, Mathur R, Verma A, Kaul V, Bhatt AN, et al. (2011) Low-dose radiation therapy of cancer: role of immune enhancement. Expert Review of Anticancer Therapy 11: 791–802.
23. Iuvone T, Esposito G, Esposito R, Santamaria R, Di Rosa M, et al. (2004) Neuroprotective effect of cannabidiol, a non-psychoactive component from Cannabis sativa, on β-amyloid-induced toxicity in PC12 cells. Journal of Neurochemistry 89: 134–141.
24. Ames E, Hallett WHD, Murphy WJ (2009) Sensitization of human breast cancer cells to natural killer cell-mediated cytotoxicity by proteasome inhibition. Clinical & Experimental Immunology 155: 504–513.
25. Liu Q, Hilsenbeck S, Gazitt Y (2003) Arsenic trioxide-induced apoptosis in myeloma cells: p53-dependent G1 or G2/M cell cycle arrest, activation of caspase-8 or caspase-9, and synergy with APO2/TRAIL. Blood 101: 4078–4087.
26. Owens TW, Foster FM, Valentijn A, Gilmore AP, Streuli CH (2010) Role for X-linked Inhibitor of Apoptosis Protein Upstream of Mitochondrial Permeabilization. Journal of Biological Chemistry 285: 1081–1088.
27. Weiner LM, Surana R, Wang S (2010) Monoclonal antibodies: versatile platforms for cancer immunotherapy. Nat Rev Immunol 10: 317–327.
28. Dietrich P-Y, Dutoit V, Tran Thang NN, Walker PR (2010) T-cell immunotherapy for malignant glioma: toward a combined approach. Current Opinion in Oncology 22: 604–610.
29. Ramakrishnan R, Assudani D, Nagaraj S, Hunter T, Cho H-I, et al. (2010) Chemotherapy enhances tumor cell susceptibility to CTL-mediated killing during cancer immunotherapy in mice. The Journal of Clinical Investigation 120: 1111–1124.
30. Drake CG (2011) Prostate cancer as a model for tumour immunotherapy. Nat Rev Immunol 10: 580–593.
31. Rudner J, Ruiner CE, Handrick R, Eibl HJ, Belka C, et al. (2010) The Akt-inhibitor Erufosine induces apoptotic cell death in prostate cancer cells and increases the short term effects of ionizing radiation. Radiat Oncol 5: 108.
32. Shresta S, Pham CTN, Thomas DA, Graubert TA, Ley TJ (1998) How do cytotoxic lymphocytes kill their targets? Current Opinion in Immunology 10: 581–587.
33. Wahl SM, Wen J, Moutsopoulos N (2006) TGF-β: a mobile purveyor of immune privilege. Immunological Reviews 213: 213–227.
34. Wilczynski JR, Radwan M, Kalinka J (2008) The characterization and role of regulatory T cells in immune reactions. Front Biosci 13: 2266–2274.
35. Deveraux Q, Reed J (1999) IAP family proteins - suppressors of apoptosis. Genes Dev 13: 239–252.
36. Seeger JM, Schmidt P, Brinkmann K, Hombach AA, Coutelle O, et al. (2010) The proteasome inhibitor bortezomib sensitizes melanoma cells toward adoptive CTL attack. Cancer Res 70: 1825–1834.
37. Zhou LL, Zhou LY, Luo KQ, Chang DC (2005) Smac/DIABLO and cytochrome c are released from mitochondria through a similar mechanism during UV-induced apoptosis. Apoptosis 10: 289–299.
38. Westwood JA, Berry LJ, Wang LX, Duong CP, Pegram HJ, et al. (2010) Enhancing adoptive immunotherapy of cancer. Expert Opin Biol Ther 10: 531–545.
39. Yasuda K, Nirei T, Sunami E, Nagawa H, Kitayama J (2011) Density of CD4(+) and CD8(+) T lymphocytes in biopsy samples can be a predictor of pathological response to chemoradiotherapy (CRT) for rectal cancer. Radiation Oncology 6: 49.
40. Dahlin AM, Henriksson ML, Van Guelpen B, Stenling R, Oberg A, et al. (2011) Colorectal cancer prognosis depends on T-cell infiltration and molecular characteristics of the tumor. Mod Pathol 24: 671–682.
41. Zitvogel L, Casares N, Peuignot MO, Chaput N, Albert ML, et al. (2004) Immune Response Against Dying Tumor Cells. Advances in Immunology: Academic Press. 131–179.
42. Croci D, Zacarías Fluck M, Rico M, Matar P, Rabinovich G, et al. (2007) Dynamic cross-talk between tumor and immune cells in orchestrating the immunosuppressive network at the tumor microenvironment. Cancer Immunology, Immunotherapy 56: 1687–1700.

14

Engineered Drug Resistant γδ T Cells Kill Glioblastoma Cell Lines during a Chemotherapy Challenge: A Strategy for Combining Chemo- and Immunotherapy

Lawrence S. Lamb Jr[1,2]*, Joscelyn Bowersock[1], Anindya Dasgupta[3], G. Yancey Gillespie[2], Yun Su[1], Austin Johnson[1], H. Trent Spencer[3]*

1 Department of Medicine, University of Alabama at Birmingham, Birmingham, Alabama, United States of America, **2** Department of Surgery, University of Alabama at Birmingham, Birmingham, Alabama, United States of America, **3** Emory University School of Medicine, Department of Pediatrics, Aflac Cancer Center and Blood Disorders Service, Atlanta, Georgia, United States of America

Abstract

Classical approaches to immunotherapy that show promise in some malignancies have generally been disappointing when applied to high-grade brain tumors such as glioblastoma multiforme (GBM). We recently showed that *ex vivo* expanded/activated γδ T cells recognize NKG2D ligands expressed on malignant glioma and are cytotoxic to glioma cell lines and primary GBM explants. In addition, γδ T cells extend survival and slow tumor progression when administered to immunodeficient mice with intracranial human glioma xenografts. We now show that temozolomide (TMZ), a principal chemotherapeutic agent used to treat GBM, increases the expression of stress-associated NKG2D ligands on TMZ-resistant glioma cells, potentially rendering them vulnerable to γδ T cell recognition and lysis. TMZ is also highly toxic to γδ T cells, however, and to overcome this cytotoxic effect γδ T cells were genetically modified using a lentiviral vector encoding the DNA repair enzyme O(6)-alkylguanine DNA alkyltransferase (AGT) from the O(6)-methylguanine methyltransferase (MGMT) cDNA, which confers resistance to TMZ. Genetic modification of γδ T cells did not alter their phenotype or their cytotoxicity against GBM target cells. Importantly, gene modified γδ T cells showed greater cytotoxicity to two TMZ resistant GBM cell lines, U373[TMZ-R] and SNB-19[TMZ-R] cells, in the presence of TMZ than unmodified cells, suggesting that TMZ exposed more receptors for γδ T cell-targeted lysis. Therefore, TMZ resistant γδ T cells can be generated without impairing their anti-tumor functions in the presence of high concentrations of TMZ. These results provide a mechanistic basis for combining chemotherapy and γδ T cell-based drug resistant cellular immunotherapy to treat GBM.

Editor: Maria G. Castro, University of Michigan School of Medicine, United States of America

Funding: This work was supported by grants from CURE Childhood Cancer to HTS. The funders had no role in study design, data collection and analysis, decision to publish, or preparation of the manuscript.

Competing Interests: The authors have declared that no competing interests exist.

* E-mail: Lawrence.Lamb@ccc.uab.edu (LSL); hspence@emory.edu (HTS)

Introduction

Treatment strategies for high-grade primary brain tumors such as glioblastoma multiforme (GBM) have failed to significantly and consistently extended survival despite 50 years of advances in radiotherapy, chemotherapy, and surgical techniques [1]. Immunotherapy remains an attractive option, although classical approaches that have shown some promise in other malignancies have generally been disappointing when applied to GBM [2–7]. A variety of immune cell therapy approaches to GBM have been attempted over the past several years. *Ex vivo* culture of cytotoxic T lymphocytes (CTL) from tumor-draining lymph nodes [8,9], tumor-infiltrating lymphocytes (TIL), and HLA-mismatched T cells from healthy donors with systemic and intracranial infusion have all met with limited success. The most predominant cell therapy consisted of autologous lymphokine-activated killer (LAK) cells, a combination of NK and T lymphocytes cultured in high doses of IL-2. Although promising in early studies, these therapies fall short for several reasons. CTL therapies are based on adaptive immunity (i.e. MHC-restricted, antigen-specific responses) and are therefore dependent upon the dose of T cell clones that specifically recognize various tumor-associated peptide antigens dispersed among various subsets of glioma cells. Infusion or intracranial placement of HLA-mismatched CTL relies on allogeneic recognition of transplantation antigens and is highly dependent on glioma cell MHC Class I expression [10,11]. LAK cell preparations are difficult to consistently manufacture, are short-lived *in vivo* [12], and are complicated by IL-2 related toxicity once infused or placed in the tumor resection cavity [2,13–16].

To overcome these issues, during the past six years, we developed a robust method for generating anti-glioma immunocompetent γδ T cells. We have shown that *ex vivo* expanded/activated γδ T cells from healthy volunteers are cytotoxic to high-grade gliomas in both *in vitro* and in specific *in vivo* models designed to replicate therapeutic conditions [17–19]. The anti-tumor cytotoxicity of γδ T cells is at least partially due to innate recognition of stress-induced NKG2D ligands such as MICA/B and UL-16 binding proteins (ULBP) that are expressed on GBM but not on adjacent normal brain tissue [17,20,21].

One of the most formidable obstacles in the treatment of cancer has been chemotherapy-induced hematopoietic cell toxicity and the associated loss of an effective and robust immune response [22]. To circumvent these consequences, concurrent with the development of immunocompetent cell expansion methods, we developed a gene therapy-based strategy whereby anti-cancer immune cells are genetically engineered to resist the toxic effects of chemotherapy drugs, which allows for the combined administration of chemotherapy and immunotherapy. This drug resistant immunotherapy (or DRI) approach has been shown to be effective in animal models of sarcoma and neuroblastoma. [23–25].

Temozolomide (TMZ) - induced DNA damage induces transient expression of NKG2D ligands on cells that are generally resistant to the drug, rendering them vulnerable to recognition and lysis by γδ T cells [26]. Strategies that protect cellular therapy products from chemotherapy induced toxicity could likely improve the effectiveness of combined immune and chemotherapy regimens. In this report, an *in vitro* proof of concept evaluation of a DRI-based strategy using lentiviral genetic modification of γδ T cells for enforced expression of P140KMGMT, which confers resistance to TMZ, is presented as a previously unexplored avenue for treatment of high-grade gliomas.

Methods

Blood samples were obtained from consenting volunteers, in writing, in accordance with the principles expressed in the Declaration of Helsinki and was approved by the University of Alabama at Birmingham's Institutional Review Board.

Glioblastoma cell lines and cloning of TMZ-resistant cells

Human glioma cell lines U87, U373, and SNB-19 were used in this study. The U87 is a grade IV glioma that originated from a 44-year-old Caucasian woman [27]. The genetic characteristics of the cell line have been well-described [28]. The cell line was obtained from the ATCC by the UAB Brain Tumor Tissue Core, a unit of the UAB NCI SPORE in Brain Cancer. Its origin has been verified by STR PCR and has been found to agree with the original cell source. U373MG is a grade III astrocytoma that was cultured from a 61 year old male [27] and was obtained directly from Darell D. Bigner (Duke University) who obtained them from Jan Ponten of Uppsala University. The cell line has been verified as authentic (Rb-deleted, p15/p16 wildtype) and has the same STR pattern as the original line. SNB-19 is a grade IV glioma cell line derived from the resection of a glioblastoma multiforme from a 47 year old male [29] and was obtained directly from Richard Morrison who extensively characterized the cell line [30]. The cells have been verified as authentic by STR PCR.U87 cells, known to be resistant to TMZ, were not modified. SNB-19 and U373 glioma cells, normally sensitive to TMZ, were cultured in incremental concentrations of TMZ up to 400 μM over several weeks in our laboratory with stepwise selection and subculture of resistant clones as described by Zhang [31].

Expansion and activation of human γδ T Cells

Peripheral blood (50 ml) was obtained from healthy volunteers. Mononuclear cells were isolated by density gradient centrifugation and resuspended at 1.0×10^6/ml in RPMI 1640+10% autologous serum +1 μM Zoledronic Acid (Novartis Oncology; East Hanover, NJ) with 50 U/ml IL-2 (Chiron; Emeryville, CA). Cells were transduced with lentivirus on culture day +6 and +7 as described below, and the culture was maintained at the original density for 14 days with addition of 50 U/ml IL-2 on post-culture days 2, 6, and 10 and addition of complete media as determined by pH and cell density. Composition, purity, and viability were determined by flow cytometry at day 0, +7 and +14 following initiation of the culture. A final viability determination was obtained by flow cytometric analysis of ToPro Iodide (Molecular Probes; Eugene, OR) incorporation. Our final product routinely contains ≥80% γδ T cells, ≤5% αβ T cells, and ≤15% NK cells to be acceptable for further studies.

Lentivirus vector production and titer

The SIV vector used in the proposed studies is based on the SIVmac viral system obtained from Dr. Arthur Nienhius (St. Jude Children's Hospital, Memphis, TN) and has been described previously [24,32,33]. Transgenes that confer drug resistance were cloned into the SIV transfer vector, pCL20cSLFR MSCVGFP, between the BstEII and Not1 restriction sites. A CMV promoter was then cloned in place of the MSCV promoter to generate pCL20-CMV-P140KMGMT. The control vector, pCL20-CMV-GFP, contains GFP driven by the CMV promoter. All recombinant viral-based vectors were prepared by transient co-transfection of 293T cells with the following plasmids: pSIV:2.06 μg, PCAG4:1.25 μg, pVSVG:1.25 μg, pCL20 expression vector:1.67 μg using 40 μl of Lipofectamine 2000 per 10 cm plate. One day post-transfection, the media was replaced with fresh DMEM-F12, 10% FBS, 1% penicillin/streptomycin and viral supernatant was collected every 24 hours for three days. Pooled viral supernatant was filtered through a 0.45 μM filter and concentrated overnight by sedimentation at $10,000 \times g$. The pellet was resuspended in StemPro 34 media at $1/100^{th}$ the initial volume and frozen in 1 ml aliquots. The concentrated vector was titered by transducing HEK-293T cells with increasing vector volumes. Seventy two hours post-transduction genomic DNA was isolated and DNA copy number was estimated by quantitative PCR. Titers were determined using primers designed specifically to amplify the transgene. Typically, virus titers of 10^8 TU/ml were obtained.

Lentiviral transduction of γδ T cells

On the previously described days of expansion culture, 1×10^6 γδ T cells were added to 1 ml of pre-warmed culture medium and plated in a 6 well culture dish. To each well varying amounts of virus were added to achieve an MOI of 5, 10, 20, and 50, with 2 control wells, as well as 50 U of IL-2. For 3 consecutive days, beginning on day 6, viable cell counts were performed and virus was added to the media to obtain the desired MOI. Additional media was added to each well to bring the total volume to 1 mL if needed. On day 9, 11, 13 and 15 a viable cell count was performed and media added to bring the concentration of viable cells to 1×10^6 cells/mL; with additional IL-2 added to a concentration of 50 U/mL On day 15 the cells were incubated in media containing 400 μM TMZ for 24 hours. Following incubation viable cell counts were measured using an automated Trypan-blue dye exclusion and counting system(Vi-Cell: Beckman-Coulter; Miami, FL).

To prepare a bulk γδ T cell culture, lentivirus was added to the cell culture medium at an MOI of 20 and supplemented with 6 μg/ml polybrene. The transduction was repeated the following day with additional lentivirus particles, also at an MOI of 20. Twenty four hours after the second transduction, fresh medium was added to the virus containing medium and the transduced cells were used within a week of preparation.

Flow cytometry and NKG2DL assays

Cultured peripheral lymphocytes were labeled with fluoro-chrome-conjugated antibodies to CD3 (SK7) and TCR-γδ (11F2)

(BD Biosciences: San Jose, CA). For NKG2DL assays, SNB-19, U373, and U87MG human glioma cells were cultured as described below in equal volumes of DMEM-F12 and HAM's media with 10%FCS supplemented with 2 mM l-glutamine until confluent. Cells were removed, washed in PBS, and resuspended in PBS containing 5% FBS and 100 μM aqueous TMZ (control cells received PBS only) and labeled with NKG2D ligands MIC-A/B conjugated with Phychoerythrin (PE), ULBP-1 PE, ULBP-2 conjugated wit Allophycocyanin (APC), ULBP-3 PE, ULBP-4 PE, and appropriately matched isotype controls (R&D Systems; Minneapolis, MN) for 20 min at 4°C. Following a second wash, the cells were acquired on a BD FACS Canto Flow Cytometer at intervals of 1,2,4,8, and 24 hours. Minimums of 10,000 events were acquired and analyzed using FACS DiVa and CellQuest Pro software (BD Biosciences; San Jose, CA). Median Fluorescence Intensity (MFI) was calculated from individual histograms and expressed as MFI ± SD of each curve. Single tubes were acquired for each experiment and separate duplicate experiments were performed to verify trends.

Cloning of TMZ Resistant Cell Lines

TMZ-resistant cells were cloned as described by Zhang [31]. SNB19 and U373 cell lines were cultured in six-well polypropylene plates in equal volumes of DMEM-F12 and HAM's media. Starting with 1 μM, cells were cultured in incrementally increasing TMZ concentrations of 1, 2, 5, 10, 20, 50 and finally 100 μM until cells could be passaged in 100 μM TMZ. The procedure required approximately six months to achieve small numbers of replicating TMZ-resistant cells that are highly resistant to TMZ and show strong expression of NKG2DL ULBP-2 and ULBP-3.

Cytotoxicity assays

Potency of the cell product was determined using *in vitro* cytotoxicity assays against the unmodified and TMZ-resistant clones of the SNB-19 and U373 cell lines and normal astrocyte cultures (control for toxicity). Targets were labeled with the membrane dye PKH26 (Sigma; St. Louis, MO). Expanded/activated γδ T cells were then added to the tubes at ratios of 0:1 (Background), 5:1, 10:1, 20:1 and 40:1 effectors/GBM targets, incubated for four hours at 37°C and 5% CO_2, washed once and resuspended in 1 ml HBSS. ToPro Iodide solution (20 μl) (Molecular Probes; Eugene, OR) was added prior to acquisition on the flow cytometer. Cytotoxicity was calculated as: (Toprolo-dide$^+$PKH26$^+$ events/total PKH26$^+$ events) ×100. Single tubes were acquired for each experiment and duplicate experiments were performed as quality control.

Statistical analysis

Descriptive statistics were used to characterize mean, standard deviation, and standard error of populations. For comparison of antigen expression, median fluorescence intensity (MFI) was obtained from single parameter histograms. Comparisons between groups was accomplished by single parameter t-test for differences between means and the Wilcoxon Signed-Rank test for differences in medians. A result was considered significant at a *p* value of 0.05.

Results

NKG2D Ligands are transiently upregulated on TMZ-resistant U87MG glioma cells after exposure to TMZ

In this experiment, we sought to determine if TMZ exposure stresses a TMZ-resistant U87 culture that had not previously been exposed to TMZ, NKG2D ligand expression was examined at incremental time intervals following TMZ exposure. Chemother-

apy-induced stress was observed as demonstrated by transient up-regulation of the NKG2D ligands ULBP-1, -2, -4, and MIC A/B over the first several hours following exposure (**Figure 1**). In most cases, upregulated surface expression of NKG2DL began to normalize within 24 hours. These results indicate that the increase in NKG2D ligand expression in response to TMZ could increase the vulnerability of glioma cells to recognition and lysis by γδ T cells within the first 4 to 6 hours following TMZ-based chemotherapy.

Generation of TMZ-resistant γδ T cells

To produce expanded/activated γδ T cells that retain function when exposed to high concentrations of TMZ chemotherapy, vectors were generated that confer TMZ-resistance based on enforced expression of AGT. SIV- and HIV- based lentiviral vectors were initially compared to optimize the transduction efficiency of γδ T cells. Using the 14 day expansion culture described above, γδ T cells were transduced at an initial MOI of 15 with HIV-GFP or SIV-GFP vectors on days 6, 7, and 8. Transgene expression was assessed using flow cytometry. As shown in *Figure 2*, the SIV-based vector transduced γδ T cells with a higher efficiency (Q2 = 65%) compared to an HIV-based vector (Q2 = 42%) (n = 3, p = 0.04).

An SIV-based vector expressing the MGMT transgene was then tested from an MOI of 5 to 50 at cell concentrations of approximately 3.5×10^3 cells/μL (range 2.9–4.2 × 10^3) to determine the ability of SIV-based vectors to modify and protect γδ T cells from TMZ-induced cytotoxicity. Following a three day transduction protocol and 14 days of culture, expanded/activated γδ T cells were incubated in media containing 400 μM TMZ for 24 h. Control γδ T cells not transduced with vector were virtually 100% non-viable when TMZ was added, but MGMT transduced cells were TMZ resistant as demonstrated by cell viability at each MOI tested (**Figure 3A**). The γδ T cells were then transduced at an MOI of 15 and cultured in 0, 200 or 400 μM TMZ. Copy number determined by quantitative PCR increased with increasing TMZ concentrations, likely due to the selection of cells expressing greater amounts of MGMT (*Figure 3B*).

Genetic engineering of γδ T cells does not alter their response to Zoledronic acid/IL-2 expansion or cytotoxic function

We then tested whether genetic modification with the MGMT vector had an effect on the the proliferative or cytotoxic function of γδ T cells (TMZ-transduced/resistant T cells - γδ^{TMZ-R}) in response to the Zoledronic acid and IL-2 expansion protocol. Two representative experiments using expanded/activated γδ T cells from separate donors are shown. When comparing genetically-modified γδ T cells to unmodified cells we found no difference in the proliferative response, as all populations routinely yielded an expansion of γδ T cells comprising 65% - 90% of the total lymphocyte population (*Figure 4a and 4b*). The cytotoxicity of unmodified to modified γδ T cells to the U87 glioma cell line was nearly equivalent at all E:T ratios (*Figure 4c and 4d*), verifying that γδ^{TMZ-R} genetically-modified T cell function is equivalent to that of unmodified γδ T cells.

For three separate donors, the expanded cells comprised approximately $2.0–12.0 \times 10^8$ cells with transduced cell number yields generally less than unmodified cells due to cell loss during lentivirus transduction (*Table 1*). However, a 50 ml blood draw routinely yielded ≥2 × 10^8 transduced γδ T cells, which is sufficient for a therapeutic intracranial cell dose.

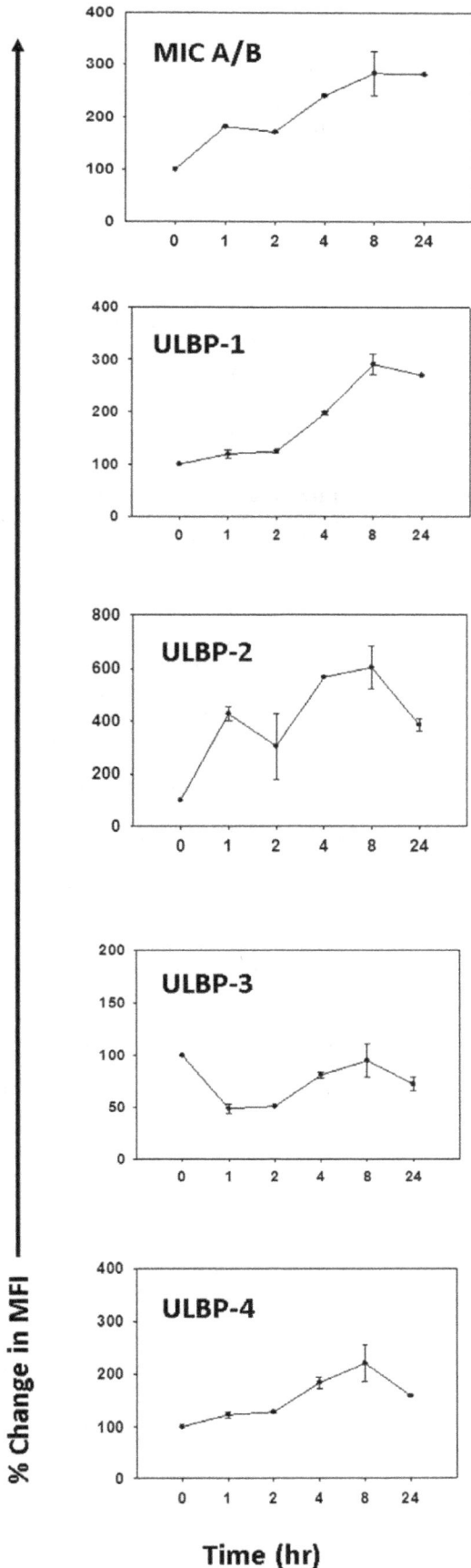

Figure 1. Transitory increase in stress-associated antigens on TMZ-resistant cell line U87 after exposure to TMZ. U87 cells were cultured to confluence and incubated in media containing 100 μM TMZ. Stress antigens were assessed at the time intervals noted on the x axis by flow cytometry and the increase in median fluorescence intensity over isotype control were calculated. Data are shown as percentage increase over unmanipulated U87 cells. SD of 3 experiments are shown.

Gene-modified γδ T cells function in the presence of TMZ

Cytolytic function of MGMT-modified γδ T cells was evaluated against TMZ-resistant clones of SNB-19 and U373 in the presence of TMZ using the cytotoxicity assay procedure described above but modified to include 100 μM TMZ during the four-hour incubation. TMZ-resistant clones from both cell lines propagated slowly in TMZ-supplemented media but were highly resistant to the drug. As proof-of-concept, cytotoxicity against SNB-19^{TMZ-R} cells was assessed in separate experiments from U373^{TMZ-R} cells using different donors in order to conserve available cells while conducting the experiment in such a manner as to determine if expanded/activated γδ^{TMZ-R} function was consistent across donors and cell lines. TMZ-resistant clones remained viable in the absence of TMZ for the length of the assay as shown in the upper panels of Figure 5a and 5b. When both cell lines were incubated in the presence of TMZ and expanded/activated γδ^{TMZ-R}, viability as measured by the uptake of the dye ToPro Iodide was noticeably increased after four hours in culture, as shown in the lower panels of Figure 5a and 5b. Dose-dependent cytotoxicity of WT γδ was significantly less when assayed against SNB-19^{TMZ-R} (c) with no TMZ in the media vs. γδ^{TMZ-R} against SNB-19^{TMZ-R} in the presence of TMZ (p = 0.0085). Cytotoxicity was also trended greater against TMZ-resistant U373 with γδ^{TMZ-R} as effectors as well when the assay was conducted in the presence of TMZ (p = .0875) but did not achieve significance at the p = 0.05 level. These assays were conducted as separate experiments from different donors.

Discussion

No treatment options are currently available to control the progression of rapidly proliferating invasive high-grade gliomas. Intensive chemotherapeutic strategies, such as high dose temozolomide can lead to lymphodepletion, impaired T cell function, and consequent suppression of anti-tumor immune responses [34]. We have previously shown that local placement of allogeneic γδ T cells can slow progression of small established intracranial tumors and significantly extend survival in a human GBM xenograft model [35]. The characteristically rapid growth of high-grade gliomas as well as both systemic and local immunosuppression, however, remain formidable barriers to cellular therapy.

Several recent studies on solid extra-cranial neoplasms have shown that strategic timing of chemotherapy and immunotherapy, taking advantage of innate response to chemotherapy-induced expression of stress-associated antigens on tumor cells and depletion of regulatory T cells in the local microenvironment, can achieve synergies that are significantly greater than either individual approach [36–42]. It is envisioned that novel approaches to combine either traditional or new chemo- and immunotherapies can potentially improve upon the conventional treatment modalities for GBM.

Our DRI strategy presents an attractive avenue to effectively partner both immuno- and chemo- therapies by genetically engineering anti-cancer immune cells to confer anti-tumor immunity during aggressive dosing of chemotherapy. We recently showed that cultured leukemia cells can be eliminated by the

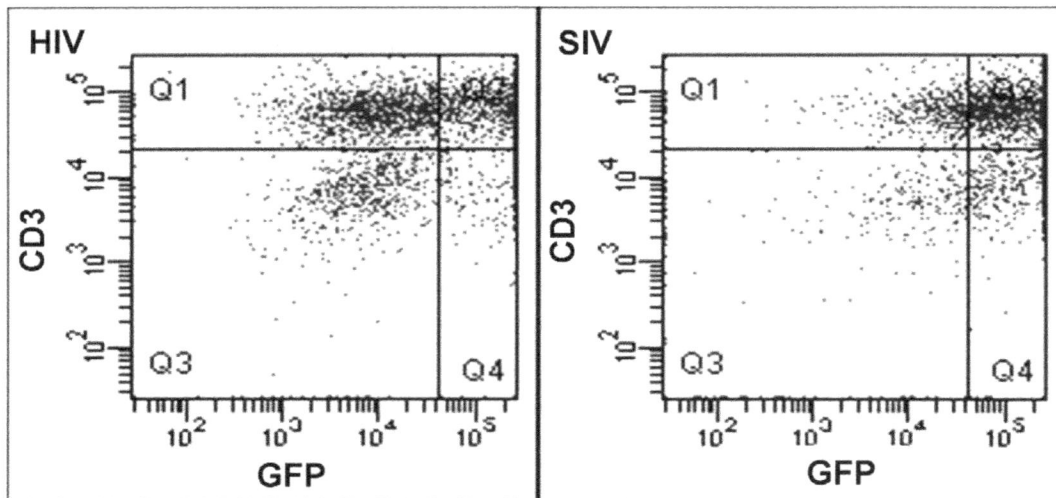

Figure 2. Genetic modification of expanded/activated γδ T cells by HIV (a) and SIV-GFP (b) lentiviral vectors 6 days following transduction with an MOI of 15. Mean fluorescence intensity (MFI) is approximately the same for both vectors, but transduction efficiency and expression from the SIV-derived vector is higher when measured on day+6. Quadrant values are noted to the right of each plot.

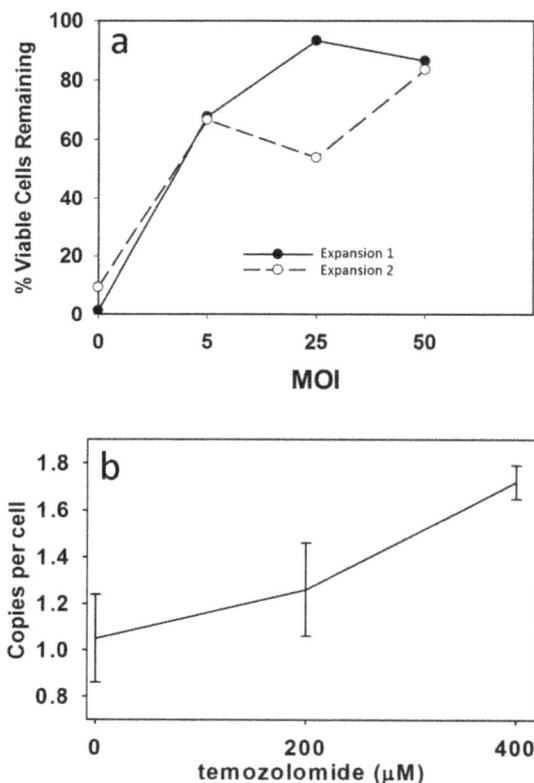

Figure 3. Transduction of γδ T cells with lentivirus vector was performed on day 6, 7 and 8 of expansion culture (see text) with increasing MOI. (a) On day +14 cells were incubated in media supplemented with 400 μM TMZ and viable cell counts were obtained for each MOI. Two separate experiments are shown. (b) Quantitative PCR analysis to measure P140KMGMT copy numbers of the bioengineered γδ T cells in the presence of increasing concentrations of TMZ, which are indicated in the figure.

combined additions of chemotherapy and genetically engineered immune effector cells [24]. We also showed that systemic administration of bioengineered chemotherapy-resistant hematopoietic cells has shown promise in animal models [23]. However, in the context of GBM therapy, systemic cell therapy will likely be an ineffective DRI strategy for established tumors due to their highly immunosuppressive nature of the tumor and the difficulty of the immune cells to cross the blood-brain barrier. However, systemic therapies incorporating DRI may be useful when directed at microscopic post-resection GBM. In the present study, we evaluated the effectiveness of a DRI strategy to enhance GBM cell clearance by the combined additions of genetically engineered γδ T cells with temozolomide to tumor cells that are refractory to high concentrations of the drug. Our choice to test a γδ T cell mediated DRI strategy is based upon our previous finding that γδ T cells, injected stereotactically either during intracranial transplantation or a few days after the transplantation of GBM cells in mice can extend the survival of the treated animals when compared to the survival of the tumor bearing animals that were not treated [35]. The exploitation of a γδ T cell based DRI strategy to target GBM is a practical approach since the tumor is partially shielded from the immune system, thereby preventing the elucidation of an immune response against locally infused cells.

A γδ T cell based DRI strategy against GBM cells can provide several benefits compared to chemotherapy alone, as cytotoxic drugs can potentially augment the cytolytic properties of the expanded γδ T cells. These cells express activating receptors for NKG2D family of ligands, such as ULBPs and MIC A/B, which are generally upregulated on stressed tumor cells. It has been established that tumors that express NKG2D ligands can readily be killed by immune effector cells that contain recognition receptors for these ligands [43,44]. Such tumors are also often rejected during transplantation [45], while tumorigenesis is favored in mice that lack the expression of NKG2D receptors [46]. Surprisingly, in GBM cells, the efficacy of NKG2D mediated tumor destruction may be decreased in part due to elevated expression of MHC class I molecules on their surface [47]. However, tumor cell killing can be enhanced by forced expression of NKG2D ligands in GBM tumors [48]. We showed that the

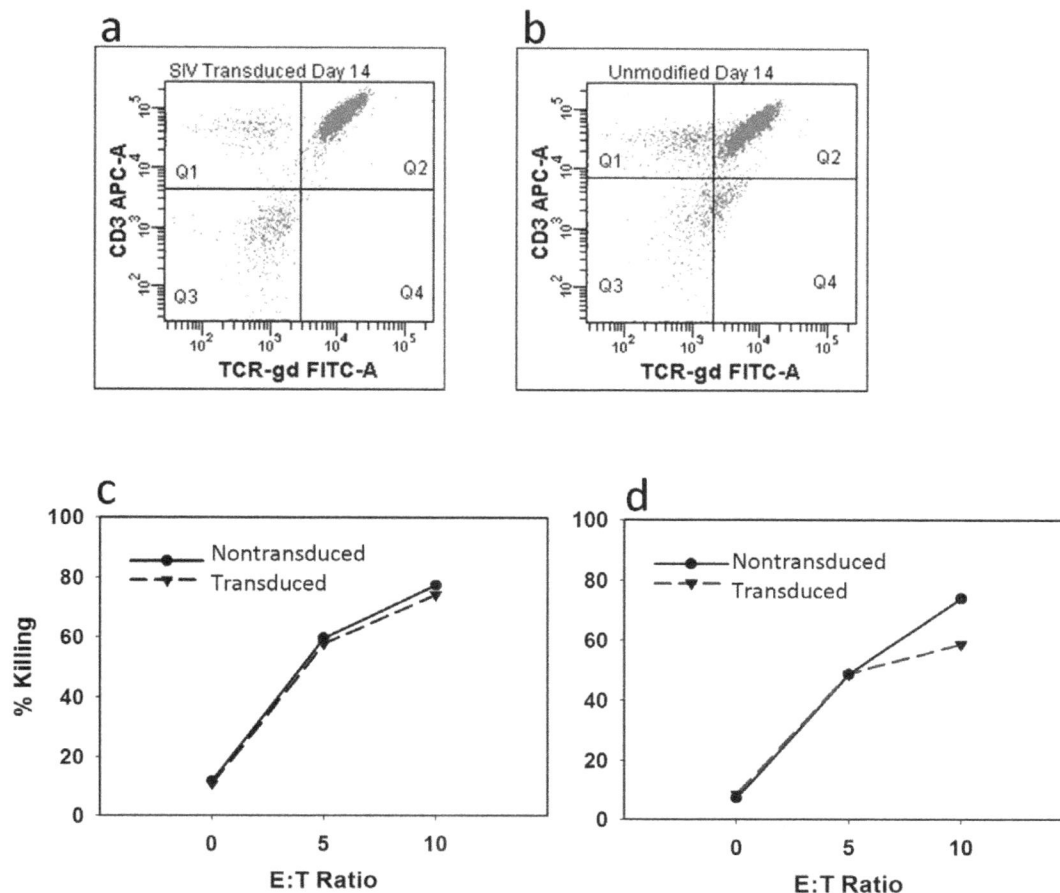

Figure 4. Expanded/activated γδ T cells were manufactured as described in the text. Flow cytometry from two separate donors shown from (*a*) unmanipulated and (*b*) P140KMGMT-transduced γδ T cells. For both panels (a) and (b) quadrant 2 (Q2) represents γδ T cells. As discussed in the text, the yield of γδ T cells was slightly lower than control due to loss of cells during the transduction procedure; however, purity of the final product was not affected as both products from a single donor show >90% purity of γδ T cells. (c and d) Cytotoxicity assays from two separate expansions (panel c and d, respectively) of unmodified γδ T cells (solid line) versus TMZ P140KMGMT transduced γδ T cells (dashed line) against the TMZ-resistant glioma cell line U87 were conducted to determine if genetic modification impairs γδ T cell function. Cytolytic activity of γδ T cells against U87 cells was nearly equivalent at all E:T ratios, verifying that P140KMGMT transduced γδ T cells function is equivalent to that of unmodified γδ T cells.

addition of temozolomide to drug resistant GBM cells induces transient but consistent upregulation of several NKG2D ligands on the U87 GBM cell line that displays partial resistance to TMZ. In this scenario, the addition of genetically engineered variants of the parental γδ T cells, that possess MHC unrestricted cytolytic properties, can potentially enhance tumor cell killing. The strategy of up-regulation of the stress/danger response of malignant cells following chemotherapy as a means of increasing their vulnerability to immune recognition and attack has been recently reviewed by others [26,49,50]. Consequently, up-regulation of stress-induced expression of NKG2D ligands on gliomas during chemotherapy can potentiate a DRI based anti-tumor strategy provided that immunocompetent cell therapies maintain efficacy during cytoreductive therapy.

We have also shown that in the presence of high concentrations of temozolomide the genetically engineered γδ T cells mediate significant killing of GBM cells that have been rendered resistant to temozolomide, whereas non-modified cells are ineffective. SNB-

Table 1. Proliferation of Modified vs. Transduced γδ T cells in Culture.

Specimen	Initial γδ T cell number	Final* (unmodified)	Fold Expansion	Final* (transduced)	Fold Expansion
20100504	5.1×10^6	2.3×10^8	46.3	2.0×10^8	39.9
20100812	3.4×10^6	1.6×10^8	73.1	2.5×10^8	46.1
20110308	2.8×10^6	1.2×10^9	438.5	5.4×10^8	191.4

*Cell dose is extrapolated to final volume of unmodified cells based on starting volume removed for transfection.

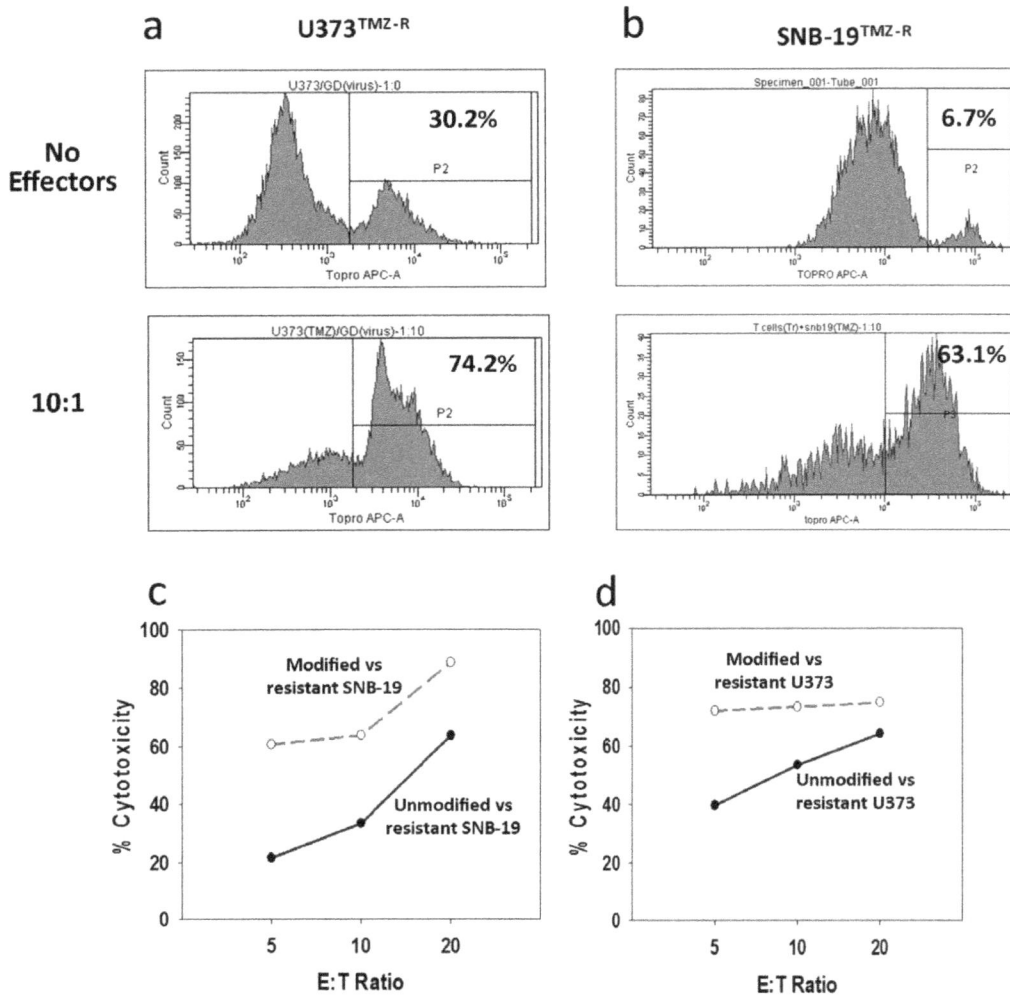

Figure 5. TMZ-resistant clones of the GBM cell line (a) U373^{TMZ-R} and (b) SNB-19^{TMZ-R} were selected by incubation in increasing concentrations of TMZ over 60 days. The cell lines were labeled with PKH-26 and incubated for 4 hours in the presence of 100 μM TMZ alone (upper panel) and with P140KMGMT transduced γδ T cells (γδ^{TMZ-R}) at a 10:1 effector:target ratio. The culture was then labeled with ToPro Iodide and acquired for flow cytometric phenotyping. A minimum of 5000 PKH26+ events was acquired to insure statistical validity of the data. All plots gated on PKH-26+ target cells. Note that the cloned cell lines are resistant to killing in media supplemented with TMZ with SNB-19^{TMZ-R} showing less cell loss than U373^{TMZ-R}. Addition of γδ^{TMZ-R} results in much greater incorporation of ToPro Iodide after 4 h incubation suggesting that the increased cytotoxicity is overwhelmingly due to genetically modified γδ T cells. Dose-dependent cytotoxicity of γδ^{TMZ-R} is significantly less when assayed against SNB-19^{TMZ-R} (c) with no TMZ in the media vs. γδ^{TMZ-R} against SNB-19^{TMZ-R} in the presence of TMZ (p = 0.0085). Cytotoxicity was also trended greater against TMZ-resistant U373 with γδ^{TMZ-R} as effectors as well when the assay was conducted in the presence of TMZ (p = .0875). These assays were conducted as separate experiments from different donors.

19 and U373 cell lines constitutively express high levels of surface NKD2D ligands ULBP-2 and ULBP-3 (data not shown) as well as MIC-A for U373, suggesting that the additive effect of TMZ on γδ T cell-based cytotoxicity may be partially mediated by nonpeptide ligands [51]. Besides inducing tumor associated stress molecules, chemotherapy can also augment immunotherapy in several ways, such as by enhancing the persistence of tumor reactive T lymphocytes and by increasing tumor trafficking of tumor responsive T cells, and by modulating immunosuppressive factors [52]. Thus administration of chemotherapy prior to cellular immunotherapy can modulate an immune environment that can be beneficial to the infused immune effector cells, such as γδ T cells. It has been shown that chemotherapy treatments can facilitate the rapid infiltration of large numbers of γδ T cells into tumors and prior to invasion of Tc1 cells [53]. Furthermore,

temozolomide based chemotherapy has been shown to decrease the population of Fox-P3+ regulatory T cells, which provides an environment to further enhance the immune response [54].

Therefore, rapidly emerging evidence supports the crucial contribution of the innate immune system to the anti-tumorigenicity of conventional chemotherapy-based cancer treatments [22,26,49]. In the context of GBM therapy, in order to access the chemotherapy derived window of opportunity of tumor vulnerability it may be beneficial to place a high concentration of γδ T cells at the tumor site and to protect these effector cells, by gene transfer of MGMT, from the cytotoxic effects of TMZ chemotherapy, which would otherwise reduce or abrogate their function. In the present study, we successfully demonstrated two key aspects that are essential to the success of such a localized and a passive immunotherapy approach to target GBM: i) the genetic engineering of γδ T cells and their expansion to concentrations sufficient for a therapeutic dose based on previous studies of γδ T cell therapy of human xenografts in immunodeficient mice [35], and ii) the retention of anti-tumor cytotoxicity of the genetically engineered cells at concentrations of temozolomide that up-regulate tumor associated stress molecules that activate effector cell functions. Intra-cavity post-resection administration of glioma-reactive genetically engineered γδ T cells presents one of the few opportunities to deliver concentrated cellular immunotherapy directly to the site of residual malignancy at the time of maximal tumor vulnerability during high dose chemotherapy. The in vitro effectiveness of our γδ T cell-based DRI strategy provides the necessary foundation to pursue such an innovative approach to the treatment of high-grade gliomas.

Acknowledgments

We would like to thank Arthur Nienhuis (St. Jude University, Memphis, TN) for the SIV vector system.

Author Contributions

Conceived and designed the experiments: LSL GYG HTS. Performed the experiments: JB AD YS AJ. Analyzed the data: LSL AD HTS. Contributed reagents/materials/analysis tools: LSL GYG HTS. Wrote the paper: LSL AD HTS.

References

1. Castro MG, Cowen R, Williamson IK, David A, Jimenez-Dalmaroni MJ, et al. (2003) Current and future strategies for the treatment of malignant brain tumors. Pharmacol Ther 98: 71–108.
2. Merchant RE, Ellison MD, Young HF (1990) Immunotherapy for malignant glioma using human recombinant interleukin-2 and activated autologous lymphocytes. A review of pre-clinical and clinical investigations. J Neurooncol 8: 173–188.
3. Farkkila M, Jaaskelainen J, Kallio M, Blomstedt G, Raininko R, et al. (1994) Randomised, controlled study of intratumoral recombinant gamma-interferon treatment in newly diagnosed glioblastoma. Br J Cancer 70: 138–141.
4. Mahaley MS Jr, Bertsch L, Cush S, Gillespie GY (1988) Systemic gamma-interferon therapy for recurrent gliomas. J Neurosurg 69: 826–829.
5. Boiardi A, Silvani A, Ruffini PA, Rivoltini L, Parmiani G, et al. (1994) Loco-regional immunotherapy with recombinant interleukin-2 and adherent lympho-kine-activated killer cells (A-LAK) in recurrent glioblastoma patients. Cancer Immunol Immunother 39: 193–197.
6. Rainov NG, Kramm CM, Banning U, Riemann D, Holzhausen HJ, et al. (2000) Immune response induced by retrovirus-mediated HSV-tk/GCV pharmacogene therapy in patients with glioblastoma multiforme. Gene Ther 7: 1853–1858.
7. Yu JS, Liu G, Ying H, Yong WH, Black KL, et al. (2004) Vaccination with tumor lysate-pulsed dendritic cells elicits antigen-specific, cytotoxic T-cells in patients with malignant glioma. Cancer Res 64: 4973–4979.
8. Merchant RE, Baldwin NG, Rice CD, Bear HD (1997) Adoptive immunother-apy of malignant glioma using tumor-sensitized T lymphocytes. Neurol Res 19: 145–152.
9. Plautz GE, Barnett GH, Miller DW, Cohen BH, Prayson RA, et al. (1998) Systemic T cell adoptive immunotherapy of malignant gliomas. J Neurosurg 89: 42–51.
10. Kruse CA, Cepeda L, Owens B, Johnson SD, Stears J, et al. (1997) Treatment of recurrent glioma with intracavitary alloreactive cytotoxic T lymphocytes and interleukin-2. Cancer Immunol Immunother 45: 77–87.
11. Read SB, Kulprathipanja NV, Gomez GG, Paul DB, Winston KR, et al. (2003) Human alloreactive CTL interactions with gliomas and with those having upregulated HLA expression from exogenous IFN-gamma or IFN-gamma gene modification. J Interferon Cytokine Res 23: 379–393.
12. Komatsu F, Kajiwara M (2000) CD18/CD54(+CD102), CD2/CD58 pathway-independent killing of lymphokine-activated killer (LAK) cells against glioblas-toma cell lines T98G and U373MG. Oncol Res 12: 17–24.
13. Barba D, Saris SC, Holder C, Rosenberg SA, Oldfield EH (1989) Intratumoral LAK cell and interleukin-2 therapy of human gliomas. J Neurosurg 70: 175–182.
14. Saris SC, Patronas NJ, Rosenberg SA, Alexander JT, Frank J, et al. (1989) The effect of intravenous interleukin-2 on brain water content. J Neurosurg 71: 169–174.
15. Hayes RL, Koslow M, Hiesiger EM, Hymes KB, Hochster HS, et al. (1995) Improved long term survival after intracavitary interleukin-2 and lymphokine-activated killer cells for adults with recurrent malignant glioma. Cancer 76: 840–852.
16. Dillman RO, Duma CM, Schiltz PM, DePriest C, Ellis RA, et al. (2004) Intracavitary placement of autologous lymphokine-activated killer (LAK) cells after resection of recurrent glioblastoma. J Immunother 27: 398–404.
17. Bryant NA, Rash AS, Woodward AL, Medcalf E, Helwegen M, et al. (2010) Isolation and characterisation of equine influenza viruses (H3N8) from Europe and North America from 2008 to 2009. Vet Microbiol.
18. Bryant NL, Suarez-Cuervo C, Gillespie GY, Markert JM, Nabors LB, et al. (2009) Characterization and immunotherapeutic potential of gammadelta T-cells in patients with glioblastoma. Neuro Oncol 11: 357–367.
19. Lamb LS Jr (2009) gammadelta T cells as immune effectors against high-grade gliomas. Immunol Res 45: 85–95.
20. Wu J, Groh V, Spies T (2002) T cell antigen receptor engagement and specificity in the recognition of stress-inducible MHC class I-related chains by human epithelial gamma delta T cells. J Immunol 169: 1236–1240.
21. Poggi A, Carosio R, Fenoglio D, Brenci S, Murdaca G, et al. (2004) Migration of V delta 1 and V delta 2 T cells in response to CXCR3 and CXCR4 ligands in healthy donors and HIV-1-infected patients: competition by HIV-1 Tat. Blood 103: 2205–2213.
22. van der Most RG, Robinson BW, Lake RA (2005) Combining immunotherapy with chemotherapy to treat cancer. Discov Med 5: 265–270.
23. McMillin DW, Hewes B, Gangadharan B, Archer DR, Mittler RS, et al. (2006) Complete regression of large solid tumors using engineered drug-resistant hematopoietic cells and anti-CD137 immunotherapy. Hum Gene Ther 17: 798–806.
24. Dasgupta A, McCarty D, Spencer HT (2010) Engineered drug-resistant immunocompetent cells enhance tumor cell killing during a chemotherapy challenge. Biochem Biophys Res Commun 391: 170–175.
25. Dasgupta A, Shields J, Spencer HT (2012) Treatment of a solid tumor using engineered drug resistant immunocompetent cells and cytotoxic chemotherapy. Hum Gene Ther.
26. Zitvogel L, Apetoh L, Ghiringhelli F, Kroemer G (2008) Immunological aspects of cancer chemotherapy. Nat Rev Immunol 8: 59–73.
27. Ponten J, Macintyre EH (1968) Long term culture of normal and neoplastic human glia. Acta pathologica et microbiologica Scandinavica 74: 465–486.
28. Clark MJ, Homer N, O'Connor BD, Chen Z, Eskin A, et al. (2010) U87MG decoded: the genomic sequence of a cytogenetically aberrant human cancer cell line. PLoS genetics 6: e1000832.
29. Gross JL, Behrens DL, Mullins DE, Kornblith PL, Dexter DL (1988) Plasminogen activator and inhibitor activity in human glioma cells and modulation by sodium butyrate. Cancer Research 48: 291–296.
30. Welch WC, Morrison RS, Gross JL, Gollin SM, Kitson RB, et al. (1995) Morphologic, immunologic, biochemical, and cytogenetic characteristics of the human glioblastoma-derived cell line, SNB-19. In Vitro Cellular & Develop-mental Biology Animal 31: 610–616.
31. Zhang J, Stevens MF, Laughton CA, Madhusudan S, Bradshaw TD (2010) Acquired resistance to temozolomide in glioma cell lines: molecular mechanisms and potential translational applications. Oncology 78: 103–114.
32. Hanawa H, Hematti P, Keyvanfar K, Metzger ME, Krouse A, et al. (2004) Efficient gene transfer into rhesus repopulating hematopoietic stem cells using a simian immunodeficiency virus-based lentiviral vector system. Blood 103: 4062–4069.
33. Doering CB, Denning G, Dooriss K, Gangadharan B, Johnston JM, et al. (2009) Directed engineering of a high-expression chimeric transgene as a strategy for gene therapy of hemophilia A. Mol Ther 17: 1145–1154.
34. Liseth K, Ersvaer E, Hervig T, Bruserud O (2010) Combination of intensive chemotherapy and anticancer vaccines in the treatment of human malignancies: the hematological experience. J Biomed Biotechnol 2010: 692097.
35. Bryant NL, Gillespie GY, Lopez RD, Markert JM, Cloud GA, et al. (2011) Preclinical evaluation of ex vivo expanded/activated gammadelta T cells for immunotherapy of glioblastoma multiforme. J Neurooncol 101: 179–188.
36. Ramakrishnan R, Assudani D, Nagaraj S, Hunter T, Cho HI, et al. (2010) Chemotherapy enhances tumor cell susceptibility to CTL-mediated killing during cancer immunotherapy in mice. J Clin Invest 120: 1111–1124.
37. Gulley JL, Madan RA, Arlen PM (2007) Enhancing efficacy of therapeutic vaccinations by combination with other modalities. Vaccine 25 Suppl 2: B89–96.
38. Fridlender ZG, Sun J, Singhal S, Kapoor V, Cheng G, et al. (2010) Chemotherapy delivered after viral immunogene therapy augments antitumor efficacy via multiple immune-mediated mechanisms. Mol Ther 18: 1947–1959.
39. Arlen PM, Gulley JL, Parker C, Skarupa L, Pazdur M, et al. (2006) A randomized phase II study of concurrent docetaxel plus vaccine versus vaccine alone in metastatic androgen-independent prostate cancer. Clin Cancer Res 12: 1260–1269.
40. Ramakrishnan R, Antonia S, Gabrilovich DI (2008) Combined modality immunotherapy and chemotherapy: a new perspective. Cancer Immunol Immunother 57: 1523–1529.
41. Mitchell MS (2003) Combinations of anticancer drugs and immunotherapy. Cancer Immunol Immunother 52: 686–692.
42. Antonia SJ, Mirza N, Fricke I, Chiappori A, Thompson P, et al. (2006) Combination of p53 cancer vaccine with chemotherapy in patients with extensive stage small cell lung cancer. Clin Cancer Res 12: 878–887.

43. Bauer S, Groh V, Wu J, Steinle A, Phillips JH, et al. (1999) Activation of NK cells and T cells by NKG2D, a receptor for stress-inducible MICA. Science 285: 727–729.

44. Gonzalez S, Lopez-Soto A, Suarez-Alvarez B, Lopez-Vazquez A, Lopez-Larrea C (2008) NKG2D ligands: key targets of the immune response. Trends Immunol 29: 397–403.

45. Diefenbach A, Jensen ER, Jamieson AM, Raulet DH (2001) Rae1 and H60 ligands of the NKG2D receptor stimulate tumour immunity. Nature 413: 165–171.

46. Guerra N, Tan YX, Joncker NT, Choy A, Gallardo F, et al. (2008) NKG2D-deficient mice are defective in tumor surveillance in models of spontaneous malignancy. Immunity 28: 571–580.

47. Wischhusen J, Friese MA, Mittelbronn M, Meyermann R, Weller M (2005) HLA-E protects glioma cells from NKG2D-mediated immune responses in vitro: implications for immune escape in vivo. J Neuropathol Exp Neurol 64: 523–528.

48. Friese MA, Platten M, Lutz SZ, Naumann U, Aulwurm S, et al. (2003) MICA/NKG2D-mediated immunogene therapy of experimental gliomas. Cancer Res 63: 8996–9006.

49. Lake RA, Robinson BW (2005) Immunotherapy and chemotherapy-a practical partnership. Nat Rev Cancer 5: 397–405.

50. van der Most RG, Currie AJ, Robinson BW, Lake RA (2008) Decoding dangerous death: how cytotoxic chemotherapy invokes inflammation, immunity or nothing at all. Cell death and differentiation 15: 13–20.

51. Kato Y, Tanaka Y, Miyagawa F, Yamashita S, Minato N (2001) Targeting of tumor cells for human gammadelta T cells by nonpeptide antigens. J Immunol 167: 5092–5098.

52. Dudley ME, Wunderlich JR, Robbins PF, Yang JC, Hwu P, et al. (2002) Cancer regression and autoimmunity in patients after clonal repopulation with antitumor lymphocytes. Science 298: 850–854.

53. Ma Y, Aymeric L, Locher C, Mattarollo SR, Delahaye NF, et al. (2011) Contribution of IL-17-producing gamma delta T cells to the efficacy of anticancer chemotherapy. The Journal of experimental medicine 208: 491–503.

54. Banissi C, Ghiringhelli F, Chen L, Carpentier AF (2009) Treg depletion with a low-dose metronomic temozolomide regimen in a rat glioma model. Cancer immunology, immunotherapy : CII 58: 1627–1634.

15

Autologous Tumor Lysate-Pulsed Dendritic Cell Immunotherapy with Cytokine-Induced Killer Cells Improves Survival in Gastric and Colorectal Cancer Patients

Daiqing Gao[1]*, Changyou Li[1], Xihe Xie[1], Peng Zhao[1], Xiaofang Wei[1], Weihong Sun[1], Hsin-Chen Liu[2], Aris T. Alexandrou[2], Jennifer Jones[3], Ronghua Zhao[3], Jian Jian Li[2]*

1 Biotherapy Center, Qingdao Center Hospital, The Second Affiliated Hospital, Qingdao University Medical College, Qingdao, China, 2 Department of Radiation Oncology, NCI-Designated Comprehensive Cancer Center, University of California at Davis Sacramento, Sacramento, California, United States of America, 3 Department of Medicine, University of Saskatchewan, Saskatoon, Canada

Abstract

Gastric and colorectal cancers (GC and CRC) have poor prognosis and are resistant to chemo- and/or radiotherapy. In the present study, the prophylactic effects of dendritic cell (DC) vaccination are evaluated on disease progression and clinical benefits in a group of 54 GC and CRC patients treated with DC immunotherapy combined with cytokine-induced killer (CIK) cells after surgery with or without chemo-radiotherapy. DCs were prepared from the mononuclear cells isolated from patients using IL-2/GM-CSF and loaded with tumor antigens; CIK cells were prepared by incubating peripheral blood lymphocytes with IL-2, IFN-γ, and CD3 antibodies. The DC/CIK therapy started 3 days after low-dose chemotherapy and was repeated 3–5 times in 2 weeks as one cycle with a total of $188.3\pm79.8\times10^6$ DCs and $58.8\pm22.3\times10^8$ CIK cells. Cytokine levels in patients' sera before and after treatments were measured and the follow-up was conducted for 98 months to determine disease-free survival (DFS) and overall survival (OS). The results demonstrate that all cytokines tested were elevated with significantly higher levels of IFN-γ and IL-12 in both GC and CRC cohorts of DC/CIK treated patients. By Cox regression analysis, DC/CIK therapy reduced the risk of post-operative disease progression (p<0.01) with an increased OS (<0.01). These results demonstrate that in addition to chemo- and/or radiotherapy, DC/CIK immunotherapy is a potential effective approach in the control of tumor growth for post-operative GC and CRC patients.

Editor: Michael Lim, Johns Hopkins Hospital, United States of America

Funding: The authors have no support or funding to report.

* E-mail: gaodaiqing@126.com (DG); jian-jian.li@ucdmc.ucdavis.edu (JJL)

Introduction

Gastric cancer (GC) and colorectal cancer (CRC) are major malignant diseases of alimentary tract. While GC is the most common cancer in the Asian-Pacific region, CRC is ranked as the fourth most common malignancy world-wide, with about 1.2 million new cases and 609,051 deaths annually [1]. Surgical resection with or without adjuvant chemo- and/or radiation therapy remains the key modality for GC and CRC, but unfortunately shows limited clinical benefits due to high rate of tumor metastasis. Although current adjuvant chemo-radiation therapy has been shown to extend patient survival in the presence of recurrent lesions [2,3], severe side effects usually limit the efficacy of this anti-cancer modality [2–4]. To further improve the overall survival for GC and CRC patients, it is critical to explore novel approaches to control tumor metastasis with or without the use of traditional chemo-and/or radiotherapy.

The dendritic cells (DCs) play a crucial role in the induction of antigen-specific T-cell responses to provide active immunotherapy [5–7]. Clinical studies using specifically designed DC-targeted cancer cell vaccines demonstrated different clinical benefits. Patients with lymphoma [8,9], metastatic melanoma [10,11], colon cancer, and non-small cell lung cancer [12] showed that vaccination with tumor antigen-pulsed DCs, either isolated directly from blood or generated *ex vivo* from blood precursors, elicited antigen specific immune reaction and, in some cases, significant tumor responses. In fact, application of an active immunotherapy regimen, Sipuleucel-T (APC8015) used by activating peripheral blood mononuclear cells (PBMCs) with a prostatic acid phosphatase (PAP), a fusion protein of prostate cancer antigen, with GM-CSF, resulted in approximately 4 month-prolonged median survival in prostate cancer patients [13–15], and was approved by FDA for the treatment of metastatic prostate cancers [14,16,17]. CIK cells are a subset of natural killer T lymphocytes (NKT) that are predominantly CD3+CD56+ type II NKT cells [18], and such cells can be generated *ex vivo* by incubating peripheral blood lymphocytes with an agonistic anti-CD3 monoclonal antibody, interleukin (IL)-2, IL1-β and interferon (IFN)-γ. CIK cells, supported by encouraging clinical trial results in both autologous and allogeneic contexts, are known to cytolytically eliminate tumor cells [19]. In contrast to lymphokine-activated killer (LAK) cells, which are cytotoxic effector T-cells stimulated predominantly in response to high concentration of interleukin-2 (IL-2), CIK cells exhibit enhanced tumor cell lytic activity [20,21], higher proliferation rate [22], and relatively lower toxicity [23]. Although passive immunotherapy by adoptive transfer of T cells is believed to be effective in the control of primary tumors, it is unclear whether passive immunotherapy is effective in the long-term control of tumor relapse [24]. On the other hand, the active immunotherapy using tumor-specific vaccines, such as DC vaccine, has the potential benefit to significantly enhance tumor-specific effector and memory T cells. The anti-tumor responses triggered by DC/CIK therapy have been reported in a number of *ex vivo* [25–29] and *in vivo* [30] studies as well as in preliminary clinical trials in patients with non-Hodgkin's and Hodgkin's lymphoma [31,32] and non-small cell lung cancer with few side effects [33]. In the present study, clinical benefits are evaluated in a group of 54 GC and CRC patients treated with DC immunotherapy combined with cytokine-induced killer (CIK) cells after surgery with or without chemo-radiotherapy. The results demonstrate improved rates of DFS and OS with elevated levels of IFN-γ and IL-12 in both GC and CRC cohorts of DC/CIK treated patients.

Patients and Methods

Study design, patient recruitment, and data collection

We conducted the study with patients treated in the Department of Surgery and Center of Biological Therapy, Qingdao Central Hospital, Qingdao, China from 2005 to 2010 (Table 1). Patients were recruited with the following criteria: 1) 18 years and older, 2) pathologically confirmed GC or CRC, 3) underwent surgical resection of primary tumors, 4) no evidence of tumor metastasis or recurrence before receiving cell-based immunotherapy, 5) having completed chemo-and/or radiotherapy for at least 1 month, and 6) signing the consent form. Patients in the control group were recruited with demographic and clinical pathological characteristics. A total of 27 patients were randomly assigned to cell-based immunotherapy and 27 patients were included in the control group. Tumors were staged according to the International Union Against Cancer's (UICC) classification based on pTNM subsets. All patients' informed consents were obtained and the

Table 1. Demographic and pathological data of patients recruited for treatment and control groups*

	Treatment	Control	P
Age	61.56±12.82	64.48±12.77	0.41
Sex (male/female)	16/11	16/11	1.00
Diagnosis (gastric/colorectal)	14/13	14/13	1.00
Differentiation (well/moderate/poor)	13/14	14/13	0.76
Tumor (T1-2/T3-4)	6/21	4/23	0.73
Lymph nodes (N negative/N positive)	7/20	15/12	0.03
TNM stage (I II/III IV)	5/22	16/11	<0.01
Radiotherapy	0	0	1.00
Chemotherapy	13	22	0.04
Radiotherapy and Chemotherapy	1	5	0.02
Metastasis/recurrence(gastric/colorectal)	2/5	7/12	<0.05

*All patients were recruited as control and treatment groups following the protocol approved by Ethics Committee at Qingdao Central Hospital Informed Consent).

procedures of the study were reviewed and approved by the Ethic Review Board of Qingdao Central Hospital. After cell-based immunotherapy, all patients obtained follow-up by hospital visits and/or telephone interviews in at least every 6 months. Local tumor recurrence and distant metastasis were examined by imaging analyses. DFS (disease-free survival, the time interval between surgery and tumor recurrence) and OS (overall survival, the time between surgery and last follow-up) were collected in the project research database. DFS and OS rates were calculated in both treatment and control groups from the dates of surgery and the follow-ups were completed for all patients by August 2011, including the patients with 12 month or longer period after immunotherapy.

DC vaccine and CIK cellular therapy

A dosage of 1×10^6 units IL-2 (Quangang Pharma Co. Shandong, China) in 250 ml physiological saline was prepared

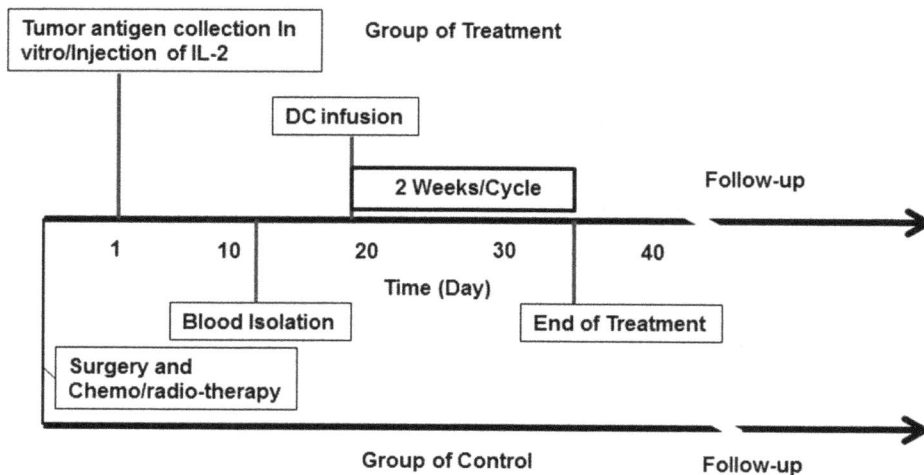

Figure 1. Following up of DC/CIK therapy and control patients. The prognoses of patients were recorded up to 98 months after the dates of surgery in both treatment and control groups.

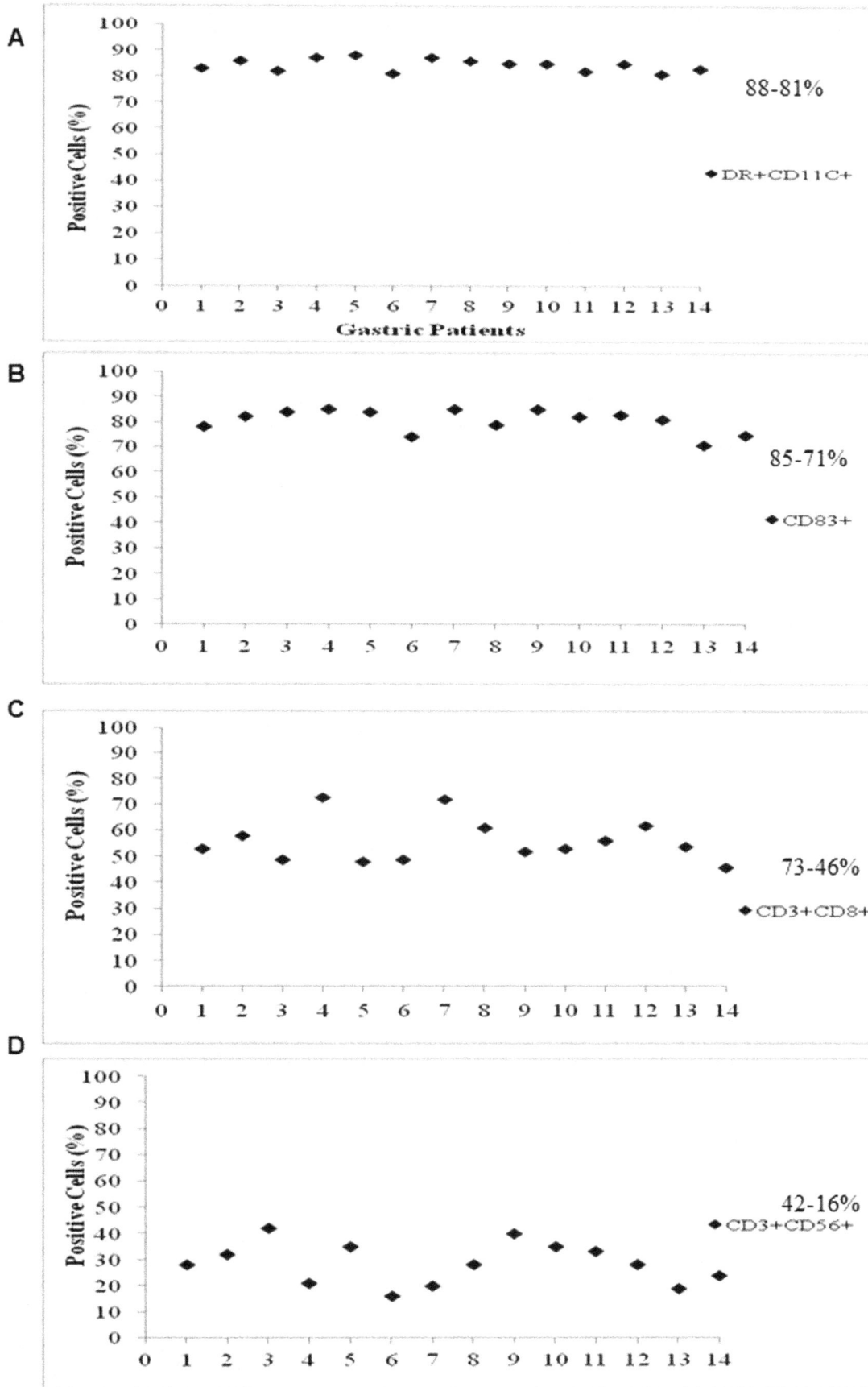

Figure 2. The maturity of dendritic cells (A,C) and CIK cells (B, D) was determined by measuring the percentage of cells expressing DR and CD11c, CD83 (DC markers), and CD3/CD8, CD3/CD56 (CIK cell markers) in blood samples collected from treated gastric cancer patients.

and intravenously administered to patients in the treatment group, once a day for 5 consecutive days. Three to six days post-IL-2 injection, mononuclear cells (4–6×10^9) were collected from total 6–9 liters of circulating blood by COBE Spectra Apheresis System (Gambro BCT, Inc., Colorado, USA) and stored in 120–150 ml plasma. If the mononuclear cells were less than 4×10^8/Liter, GM-CSF (150 μg) were subcutaneously applied to the patients—once a day for 1–3 days before further collection of mononuclear cells was processed.

Antigen preparation

Tumor antigen was prepared by following the established protocol [34,35] from human AGS gastric cancer or LS-174T colon cancer cells. Tumor cells were cultured for 2–3 passages (1–2×10^8), and collected, and washed with normal saline for 3 times, and lysed by freezing-thawing three times, and analyzed with ultrasonic cell disruption. Lysates from tumor cells were then fractionated by centrifugation (1200 rpm $\times$ 5 min), and the supernatant was collected and filtered with a 0.22 filter (Carrighwohill, Co. Cork, Ireland), and protein concentration in the supernatant was measured before storage at $-80°C$.

Preparation of DC and CIK cells

Mononuclear cells were isolated from the collected cells from peripheral blood of GC and CRC patient by following an established method [36,37] using Ficoll (GE Healthcare life Science, Shanghai, China). Isolated cells were suspended in RPMI 1640 medium at a concentration of 1×10^7 mL^{-1} and cultured in 175 cm^2 cell culture flasks at 37°C, 5% CO_2 for 2 hrs. Adherent cells were cultured in serum free DC culture medium (CellGenix, Freiburg, Germany) containing 20 ng/mL interleukin 4 (IL-4) and 50 ng/mL GM-CSF at 37°C, 5% CO_2 for 6 days. DC culture medium containing prepared tumor antigen was then added in cultured cells to a final concentration of 50 μg/ml, and cultured for another 2 days. Matured DCs were examined by flow cytometry for DC markers CD83 and HLA-DR. Preparations were tested as bacteria and pyrogen free. A portion of the prepared DC was infused into the patients and the remaining DCs were stored at $-80°C$. Suspension cells were cultured in RPMI 1640 medium (2×10^6/mL) containing 10% BFS, 100 U/mL IL-2, 300 U/mL IFN-γ, 20 ng/mL CD3 monoclonal antibody (R&D Systems, Minneapolis, MN, USA), and 40 U/mL gentamycin. On day 8, a portion of the cells were examined by flow cytometry for CIK cell markers with antibodies against CD3, CD8, and CD56. Cells were then kept in normal saline with 1% albumin, and the rest of suspensions cells were kept in culture for another 7 days.

DC vaccine and CIK cell administration

Patients in the treatment group received one cycle of low dose chemotherapy starting on the day after mononuclear cells collection with Carmofure (100 mg, po., bid) for 5~6 days. The infusion of DCs and CIK cells was started on day 2 or day 3 after chemotherapy. Prepared DC cells were divided into two parts: one part was mixed with CIK cells in 250 ml normal saline containing 1500 U/mL IL-2 and 1% albumin, and infused into the patients intravenously. The other part was suspended in 1.5 ml normal saline and injected subcutaneously into the area of draining lymph nodes adjacent to the tumor sites. The treatment was repeated 3–5 times in 2 weeks as one cycle. Patients with advanced stage

diseases received 2 cycles of the treatment, while early stage patients were treated with one cycle. The immune responses of patients were monitored before and after the treatment by measuring serum levels of IFN-γ, IL-2, IL-6, IL-10, and IL-12 determined by ELISA (R&D systems, Minneapolis, MN, USA). The time schedules of DC and CIK preparation and infusion were shown in Figure 1.

Statistical analysis

Data was presented as percentages, means with standard deviation (mean $\pm$ SD), or median with 95% confidence intervals (95% CI). Chi square test, Student's t-test or Mann–Whitney test, Pearson's linear or Spearman rank tests were used for analysis as appropriate. Treatment outcome was analyzed by Kaplan–Meier survival curves with log rank test, and multivariate Cox proportional hazards regression tests. Statistical significance was set at $p < 0.05$. All statistical analyses were performed using SPSS 16.0 for Windows (SPSS, Chicago, IL, USA).

Results

Baseline information

A total of 54 patients with histological confirmed gastric or colorectal adenocarcinoma were randomly recruited into this study consisting of 27 patients in each group. The demographic and clinical pathological data of patients in the treatment and control groups were presented in Table 1. Half of the patients in the treatment group and all patients in control group had received at least one cycle of chemo-radiation before enrollment. Immunotherapy was initiated at least one month after the termination of chemo- and/or radiation therapy and follow-up time was 98 months for all patients in treatment and control groups.

Characteristics of DC/CIK cells for cell infusion

The average number of cells infused into patients in one cycle was $188.3 \pm 79 \times 10^6$ for DCs and $58.8 \pm 22.3 \times 10^8$ for CIK cells. Cells expressing DR/CD11C and CD83 (DC markers) or CD3/CD8 and CD3/CD56 (CIK markers) were analyzed. DCs prepared from GC patients were 88%-81% positive for DR/CD11C and 85%-71% positive for CD83 (Fig. 2A, B). CIK cells prepared from GC patients showed 73%-46% positive for CD3/CD8 and 42%-16% positive for CD3/CD56 (Fig. 2C, D). In addition, DC prepared from CRC patients were 87%-80% positive for DR/CD11C and 84%-71% positive for CD83 (Fig. 3A, B), and CIK cells from CRC patients were 75%-48% positive for CD3/CD8 and 41%-11% positive for CD3/CD56 respectively (Fig. 3C, D). The overall cytolytic efficacy of CIK cells from all patients was enhanced ~2.5 fold. These results indicate that the majority of the DCs and CIK cells prepared from patients were mature and functional.

Serum cytokine levels after DC/CIK therapy

We examined serum levels of a group of cytokine for each patient before and after DC/CIK treatments (Figure 4 for GC (A) and CRC (B)). The levels of IL-2, IL-6 and IL-10 slightly enhanced, with no statistical significance in the sera of GC and CRC patients (Fig. 4A, B). However, serum IL-12 and IFN-γ levels were significantly increased in both GC and CRC patients, indicating that DC/CIK therapy may specifically promote a Th1

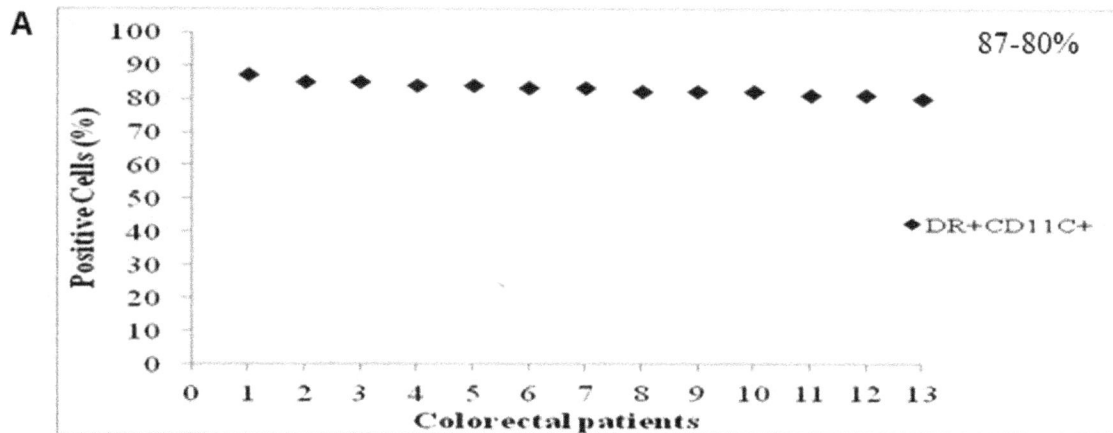

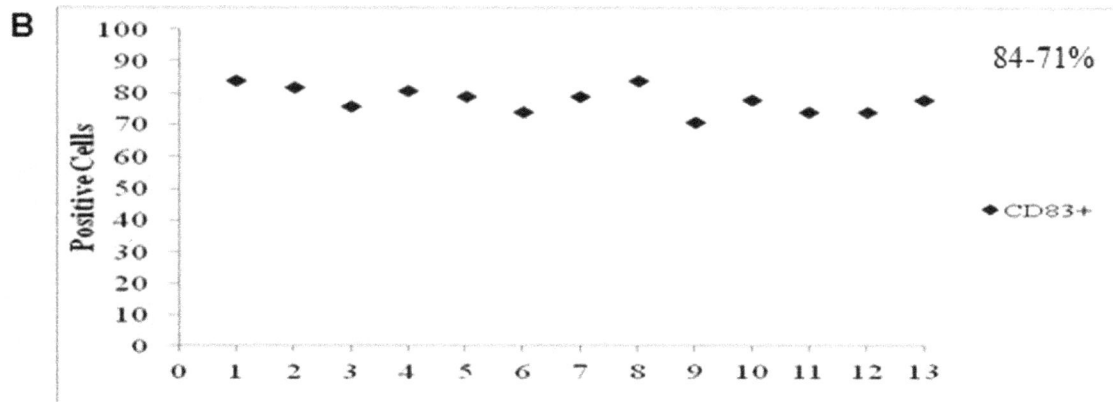

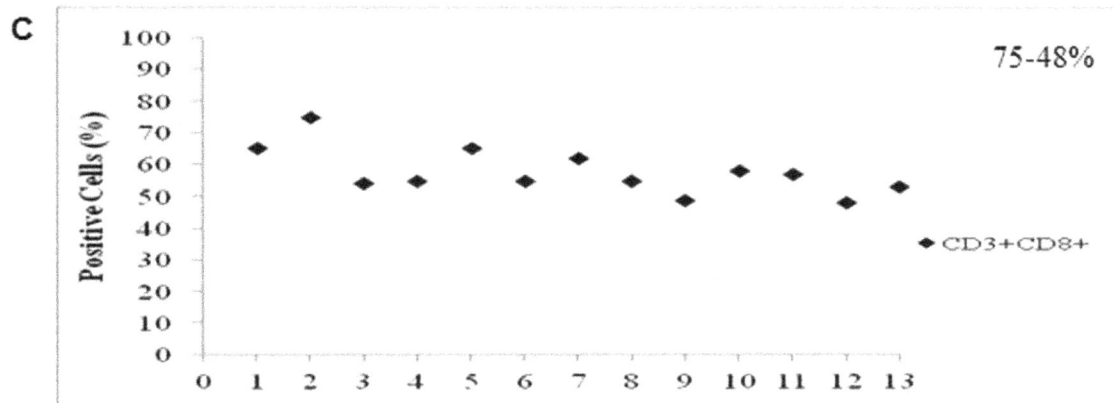

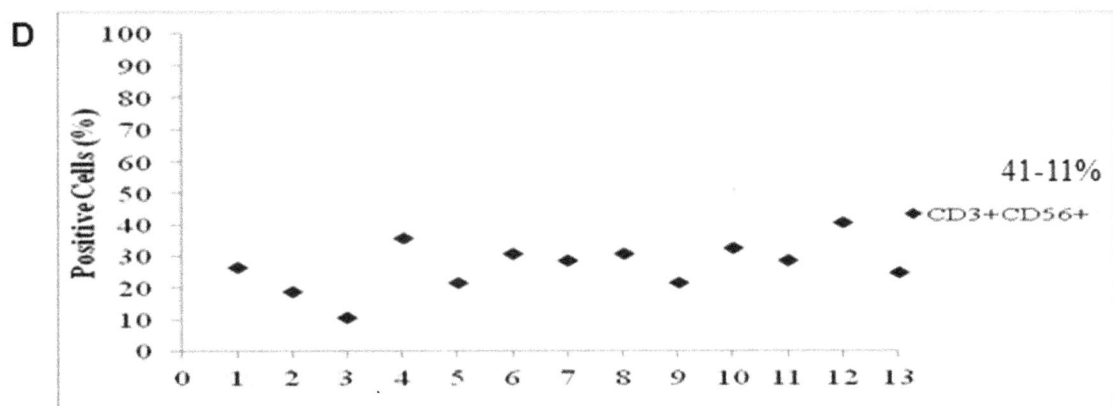

Figure 3. The maturity of dendritic cells (A,C) and CIK cells (B, D) was determined by measuring the percentage of cells expressing DR and CD11c, CD83 (DC markers), and CD3/CD8, CD3/CD56 (CIK cell markers) in blood samples collected from treated colorectal cancer patients.

immune response to mediate tumor killing effect of DC/CIK therapy.

Disease-free survival (DFS) and overall survival (OS) of patients after cell-based immunotherapy

As shown in Figures 5 and 6, DFS and OS were both significantly prolonged in patients in DC/CIK treatment groups (GC: 5-year DFS rate: 66%, OS rate: 66%; CRC: 5-year DFS rate: 66%, OS rate: 75%) compared with the patients in control groups (GC: 5-year DFS rate: 34%, OS rate: 34%; CRC: 5-year DFS rate: 8%, OS rate: 15%; $p<0.01$). To examine the differential response of GC and CRC, we analyzed two cohorts (GC: $p<0.05$; CRC: $p<0.01$) and found that CRC are more sensitive to DC/CIK therapy than GC. In addition, analysis with multivariate Cox proportional regression confirmed that DC/CIK therapy significantly and independently reduced the risk of post-operative disease progression (Odd ratio: 0.09, 95% CI: 0.02–0.42; $p<0.01$) or patient deceases (Odd ratio: 0.05, 95% CI: 0.01–0.37; $p<0.01$) after adjusting for age, sex, tumor grade, TNM stages, and previous chemo- and/or radiation treatments.

Potential adverse effects of cell-based immunotherapy

The most common adverse effect observed in all patients receiving DC/CIK therapy was fever, which occurred in 9 of 27 treated patients (33%) in the range of 37.5–40°C. All patients recovered spontaneously or after antipyretic treatment with non-steroid medicine. No other significant complications accompanying cell-based immunotherapy were observed.

Discussion

Cancer immunotherapy had shown a potential efficacy in tumor growth control and patient survival [14,38,39] as the news released that "Instead of using surgery, chemotherapy, or radiotherapy, researchers from the National Institutes of Health are finding so-far limited but inspiring success in a new approach for fighting cancer, using the immune system to attack the tumors the way it would be a cold or flu. -CNN.com (August 2006)". Although extensively studied in cells and animal models, the clinical data regarding the exact benefit of immunotherapy in patient survival and disease progression remain to be further investigated [17,40]. Despite limited size of cohorts, this study demonstrates a remarkable enhancement in the post-surgical control of tumor recurrence and survival rates in GC and CRC patients treated with combined DC/CIK therapy. It has been well established that

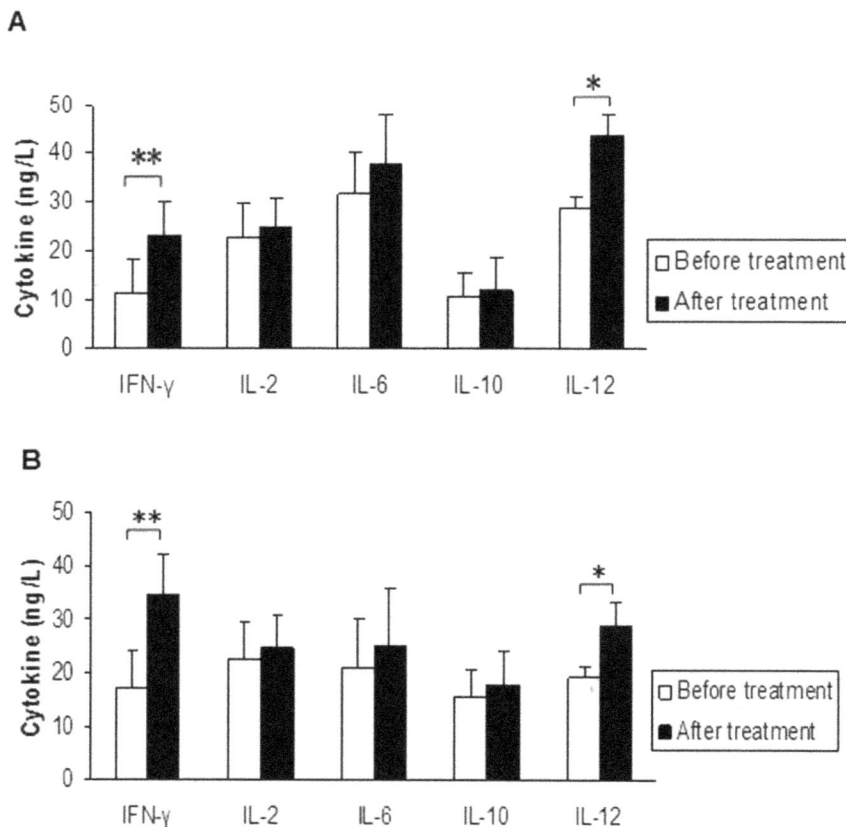

Figure 4. Serum levels of INF-γ, IL-2, IL-6, IL-10 and IL-12 measured from gastric (A) and colorectal (B) cancer patients before and after a 2-week cycle of treatment with DC/CIK cells (A, n = 14, B, n = 13, *p<0.05, **p<0.01).

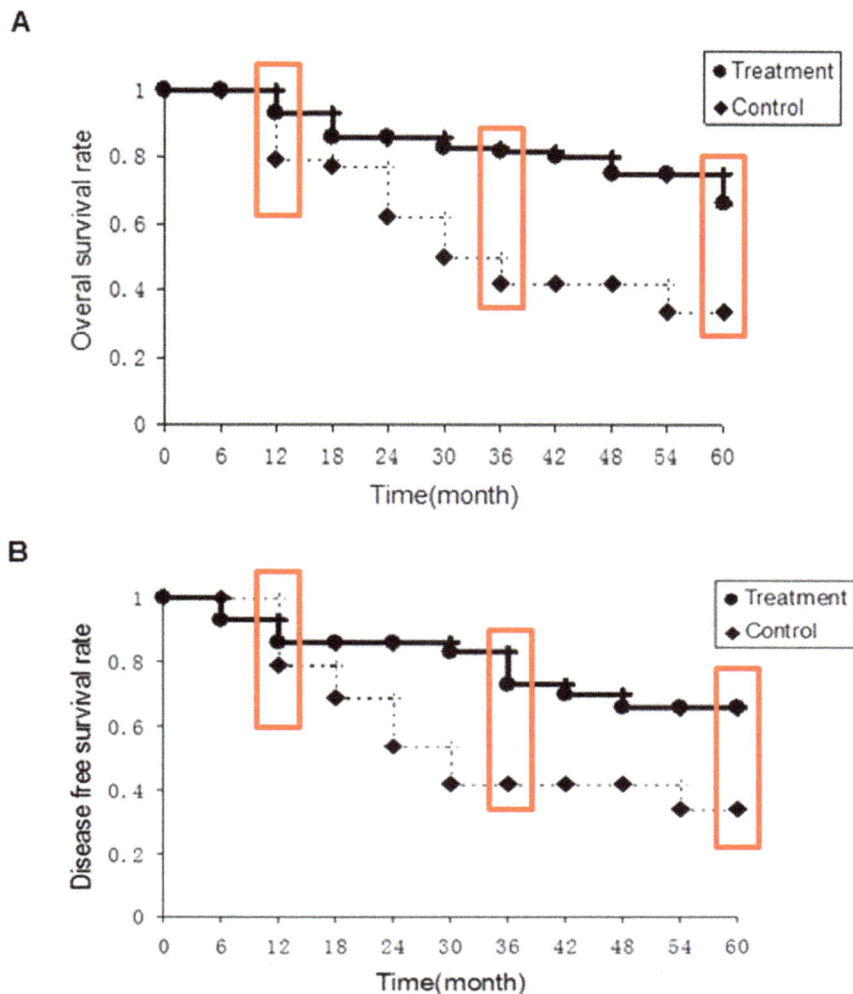

Figure 5. (A) The overall survival rate of the gastric cancer patients. The 1-, 3-, and 5-year survival rates in the treatment group was 93%, 82%, and 66%, compared with the control 79%, 42%, and 34% respectively. B) Disease free survival rate of the gastric cancer patients. The 1-, 3-, and 5-year survival rates in the treatment groups (red box marked) were 86%, 73%, and 66%, compared with the control 79%, 42%, and 34% respectively. The cumulative survival curves in A and B were analyzed by the Kaplan-Meier method.

the DCs prime naïve T-cells and DC vaccine combined with CIK cell therapy has achieved encouraging promise as a novel therapeutic approach for disease control in specific cancers [41]. DCs [6,7,42] have the capability to present tumor antigens to T lymphocytes and induce the specific cytotoxic T cells against tumor antigens [43]. Sipuleucel-T, the first DC vaccine, was approved for clinical application by FDA in USA to treat asymptomatic metastatic castrate-resistant prostate cancer, improving patients' OS in phase III trial [14]. Additional promising results were reported in recent phase III trials using tumor vaccine to treat various late stage cancers [44], including melanoma, follicular lymphoma, CRC, and NSCLC. Studies in the clinics have established that DCs capture and process tumor-associated antigens and secrete cytokines to initiate an immune response [45].

In addition to DC vaccine, CIKs are induced by cytokines and possess nonspecific cytotoxicity against tumors [24]. CIK cells can kill tumor cells directly, but have significantly short term anti-cancer efficacy and they are less likely to control tumor outgrowth in the long-term [24]. In contrast, DC vaccine is shown to induce tumor-specific effector and memory T cells [24]. Therefore, the

combination of DC vaccine with CIK treatment may have a potential higher cytotoxic activity and specificity in the effector T cells, which shows both short and long term anti-tumor efficacy. In agreement with the clinical benefits observed in other clinical trials[44], our study suggests that DC/CIK treatment can significantly enhance patient survival, prompting its future clinical investigation.

Although a number of pro-inflammatory cytokines were elevated in the DC/CIK treated patients, only two Th1 cytokines, IL-12 and IFN-γ, showed a significant increase in patients' sera in our study. Studies demonstrated that IFN-γ and IL-12 play critical roles in immunotherapy using DC and CIK [28,33]. Tumor cells are highly heterogeneous [46] and a specific tumor may contain cells with both high and low MHC-I populations [47,48]. Interestingly, MHC-I expression shows heterogeneous among tumor cells and radiation promotes the immunological recognition of the tumor cells by immune cells via MHC-I [49]. However, probably due to the heterogeneity in a given tumor, a single type of immune therapy may only be effective in a subpopulation of cancer patients. Similarly, tumor cells with higher MHC-I

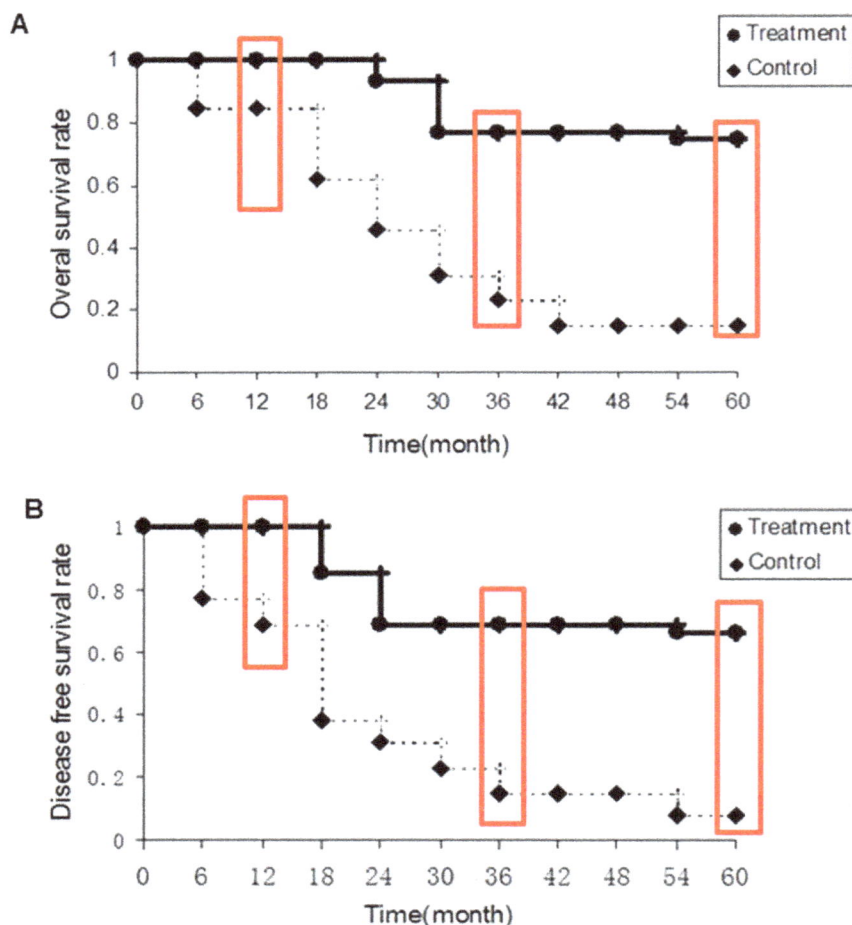

Figure 6. (A) The overall survival rate of the colorectal cancer patients. The 1-, 3-, and 5-year survival rates in the treatment group were 100%, 77%, and 75%, compared with the control 85%, 23%, and 15% respectively. (B) Disease free survival of the gastric cancer patients. The 1-, 3-, and 5-year survival rates in the treatment group were 100%, 69%, and 66%, compared with the control 69%, 15%, and 8% respectively. The cumulative survival curves in A and B were analyzed by the Kaplan-Meier method.

expression may be more sensitive to DC vaccine therapy while cells with lower MHC-I expression may be killed by CIK. Our results support that combined DC/CIK therapy may promote tumor cell cytotoxicity by targeting different populations of tumor cells, such as those with various levels of MHC-I.

The doses of DC and CIK to the patients in this study were determined based on previous dose escalating test, and found to be safe in all patients. It should be noted that in the current study, data were derived from patients treated with a modified regimen, i.e., before lymphocyte collection by intravenously administration of IL-2 to improve function and number of lymphocytes, which may contribute a significant role in DC/CIK therapy. In addition, patients also received 1 cycle of low dose chemotherapy prior to the DC and CIK infusion, which may also affect the overall effectiveness of DC/CIK therapy. We hypothesized that a 3-day gap is critical for sufficient "washout" of chemotherapeutic agent, so as not to affect the effectiveness of infused DC and CIK. Patients in the control group had been previously treated with at least 1 cycle of chemotherapy, comparable to patients enrolled in the immunotherapy group (Table 1 and Figures, 5, 6). The potential effects of low dose chemotherapy before cell infusion [28]

may also induce tumor cell killing, up-regulate the expression of tumor antigen and contribute to the composition of host immune cells. Therefore, further studies will be conducted with larger patient cohorts. In conclusion, this clinical study indicates that the combination of DC vaccine and CIK therapy may significantly improve the disease-free survival in gastric and colorectal cancer patients.

Acknowledgments

We thank Dr. William Murphy and Dr. Cheikh Menaa at the NCI-designed comprehensive cancer center of University of California at Davis for helpful discussions, and the prodigious support of doctors and nurses in the biotherapy center, Qingdao Central Hospital.

Author Contributions

Conceived and designed the experiments: DG CL JJ RZ JL. Performed the experiments: DG CL XX PZ XW WS HL JJ RZ JL. Analyzed the data: DG CL RZ JL. Contributed reagents/materials/analysis tools: DG JL. Wrote the paper: DG AA JL.

References

1. Jemal A, Bray F, Center MM, Ferlay J, Ward E, et al (2011) Global cancer statistics. CA Cancer J Clin 61: 69–90.

2. Ottoman RE, Langdon EA, Rochlin DB, Smart CR (1963) Side-Effects of Combined Radiation and Chemotherapy in the Treatment of Malignant Tumors. Radiology 81: 1014–1017.

3. Palesty JA, Wang W, Javle MM, Yang GY (2004) Side effects of therapy: case 3. Gastric cancer after radiotherapy of pediatric Hodgkin's disease. J Clin Oncol 22: 2507–2509.

4. Boulikas T, Vougiouka M (2004) Recent clinical trials using cisplatin, carboplatin and their combination chemotherapy drugs (review). Oncol Rep 11: 559–595.

5. Frankenberger B, Schendel DJ (2012) Third generation dendritic cell vaccines for tumor immunotherapy. Eur J Cell Biol 91: 53–58.

6. Steinman RM, Banchereau J (2007) Taking dendritic cells into medicine. Nature 449: 419–426.

7. Melief CJ (2007) Cancer: immune pact with the enemy. Nature 450: 803–804.

8. Hsu FJ, Benike C, Fagnoni F, Liles TM, Czerwinski D, et al. (1996) Vaccination of patients with B-cell lymphoma using autologous antigen-pulsed dendritic cells. Nat Med 2: 52–58.

9. Timmerman JM, Czerwinski DK, Davis TA, Hsu FJ, Benike C, et al. (2002) Idiotype-pulsed dendritic cell vaccination for B-cell lymphoma: clinical and immune responses in 35 patients. Blood 99: 1517–1526.

10. Nestle FO, Alijagic S, Gilliet M, Sun Y, Grabbe S, et al. (1998) Vaccination of melanoma patients with peptide- or tumor lysate-pulsed dendritic cells. Nat Med 4: 328–332.

11. Thurner B, Haendle I, Roder C, Dieckmann D, Keikavoussi P, et al. (1999) Vaccination with mage-3A1 peptide-pulsed mature, monocyte-derived dendritic cells expands specific cytotoxic T cells and induces regression of some metastases in advanced stage IV melanoma. J Exp Med 190: 1669–1678.

12. Fong L, Hou Y, Rivas A, Benike C, Yuen A, et al. (2001) Altered peptide ligand vaccination with Flt3 ligand expanded dendritic cells for tumor immunotherapy. Proc Natl Acad Sci U S A 98: 8809–8814.

13. Higano CS, Schellhammer PF, Small EJ, Burch PA, Nemunaitis J, et al. (2009) Integrated data from 2 randomized, double-blind, placebo-controlled, phase 3 trials of active cellular immunotherapy with sipuleucel-T in advanced prostate cancer. Cancer 115: 3670–3679.

14. Kantoff PW, Higano CS, Shore ND, Berger ER, Small EJ, et al. (2010) Sipuleucel-T immunotherapy for castration-resistant prostate cancer. N Engl J Med 363: 411–422.

15. Higano CS, Small EJ, Schellhammer P, Yasothan U, Gubernick S, et al. (2010) Sipuleucel-T. Nat Rev Drug Discov 9: 513–514.

16. Huber ML, Haynes L, Parker C, Iversen P (2012) Interdisciplinary critique of sipuleucel-T as immunotherapy in castration-resistant prostate cancer. J Natl Cancer Inst 104: 273–279.

17. Frohlich MW (2012) Sipuleucel-T for the treatment of advanced prostate cancer. Semin Oncol 39: 245–252.

18. Gutgemann S, Frank S, Strehl J, Schmidt-Wolf IG (2007) Cytokine-induced killer cells are type II natural killer T cells. Ger Med Sci 5: Doc07.

19. Mesiano G, Todorovic M, Gammaitoni L, Leuci V, Giraudo Diego L, et al. (2012) Cytokine-induced killer (CIK) cells as feasible and effective adoptive immunotherapy for the treatment of solid tumors. Expert Opin Biol Ther 12: 673–684.

20. Lu PH, Negrin RS (1994) A novel population of expanded human CD3+CD56+ cells derived from T cells with potent in vivo antitumor activity in mice with severe combined immunodeficiency. J Immunol 153: 1687–1696.

21. Margolin KA, Negrin RS, Wong KK, Chatterjee S, Wright C, et al. (1997) Cellular immunotherapy and autologous transplantation for hematologic malignancy. Immunol Rev 157: 231–240.

22. Linn YC, Hui KM (2003) Cytokine-induced killer cells: NK-like T cells with cytolytic specificity against leukemia. Leuk Lymphoma 44: 1457–1462.

23. Hontscha C, Borck Y, Zhou H, Messmer D, Schmidt-Wolf IG (2011) Clinical trials on CIK cells: first report of the international registry on CIK cells (IRCC). J Cancer Res Clin Oncol 137: 305–310.

24. Thanendrarajan S, Nowak M, Abken H, Schmidt-Wolf IG (2011) Combining cytokine-induced killer cells with vaccination in cancer immunotherapy: more than one plus one? Leuk Res 35: 1136–1142.

25. Gonzalez-Carmona MA, Marten A, Hoffmann P, Schneider C, Sievers E, et al. (2006) Patient-derived dendritic cells transduced with an a-fetoprotein-encoding adenovirus and co-cultured with autologous cytokine-induced lymphocytes induce a specific and strong immune response against hepatocellular carcinoma cells. Liver Int 26: 369–379.

26. Wongkajornsilp A, Sangsuriyong S, Hongeng S, Waikakul S, Asavamongkolkul A, et al. (2005) Effective osteosarcoma cytolysis using cytokine-induced killer cells pre-inoculated with tumor RNA-pulsed dendritic cells. J Orthop Res 23: 1460–1466.

27. Marten A, Greten T, Ziske C, Renoth S, Schottker B, et al. (2002) Generation of activated and antigen-specific T cells with cytotoxic activity after co-culture with dendritic cells. Cancer Immunol Immunother 51: 25–32.

28. Marten A, Ziske C, Schottker B, Weineck S, Renoth S, et al. (2001) Transfection of dendritic cells (DCs) with the CIITA gene: increase in immunostimulatory activity of DCs. Cancer Gene Ther 8: 211–219.

29. Su X, Zhang L, Jin L, Ye J, Guan Z, et al. (2010) Coculturing dendritic cells with zoledronate acid efficiently enhance the anti-tumor effects of cytokine-induced killer cells. J Clin Immunol 30: 766–774.

30. Chan JK, Hamilton CA, Cheung MK, Karimi M, Baker J, et al. (2006) Enhanced killing of primary ovarian cancer by retargeting autologous cytokine-induced killer cells with bispecific antibodies: a preclinical study. Clin Cancer Res 12: 1859–1867.

31. Sun Y, Chen J, Cai P, Hu YH, Zhong GC, et al. (2010) [Therapy of relapsed or refractory non-Hodgkin's lymphoma by antigen specific dendritic cells-activated lymphocytes]. Zhongguo Shi Yan Xue Ye Xue Za Zhi 18: 219–223.

32. Leemhuis T, Wells S, Scheffold C, Edinger M, Negrin RS (2005) A phase I trial of autologous cytokine-induced killer cells for the treatment of relapsed Hodgkin disease and non-Hodgkin lymphoma. Biol Blood Marrow Transplant 11: 181–187.

33. Li H, Wang C, Yu J, Cao S, Wei F, et al. (2009) Dendritic cell-activated cytokine-induced killer cells enhance the anti-tumor effect of chemotherapy on non-small cell lung cancer in patients after surgery. Cytotherapy 11: 1076–1083.

34. Pan Y, Zhang J, Zhou L, Zuo J, Zeng Y (2006) In vitro anti-tumor immune response induced by dendritic cells transfected with EBV-LMP2 recombinant adenovirus. Biochem Biophys Res Commun 347: 551–557.

35. Pan Y, Chefalo P, Nagy N, Harding C, Guo Z (2005) Synthesis and immunological properties of N-modified GM3 antigens as therapeutic cancer vaccines. J Med Chem 48: 875–883.

36. Moiseyenko V, Imyanitov E, Danilova A, Danilov A, Baldueva I (2007) Cell technologies in immunotherapy of cancer. Adv Exp Med Biol 601: 387–393.

37. Schadendorf D, Algarra SM, Bastholt L, Cinat G, Dreno B, et al. (2009) Immunotherapy of distant metastatic disease. Ann Oncol 20 Suppl 6: vi41–50.

38. Morse MA, Deng Y, Coleman D, Hull S, Kitrell-Fisher E, et al. (1999) A Phase I study of active immunotherapy with carcinoembryonic antigen peptide (CAP-1)-pulsed, autologous human cultured dendritic cells in patients with metastatic malignancies expressing carcinoembryonic antigen. Clin Cancer Res 5: 1331–1338.

39. O'Neill D, Bhardwaj N (2005) Exploiting dendritic cells for active immunotherapy of cancer and chronic infection. Methods Mol Med 109: 1–18.

40. Madan RA, Schwaab T, Gulley JL (2012) Strategies for optimizing the clinical impact of immunotherapeutic agents such as sipuleucel-T in prostate cancer. J Natl Compr Canc Netw 10: 1505–1512.

41. O'Neill DW, Bhardwaj N (2007) Exploiting dendritic cells for active immunotherapy of cancer and chronic infections. Mol Biotechnol 36: 131–141.

42. Banchereau J, Steinman RM (1998) Dendritic cells and the control of immunity. Nature 392: 245–252.

43. van Broekhoven CL, Parish CR, Demangel C, Britton WJ, Altin JG (2004) Targeting dendritic cells with antigen-containing liposomes: a highly effective procedure for induction of antitumor immunity and for tumor immunotherapy. Cancer Res 64: 4357–4365.

44. Schlom J (2012) Recent advances in therapeutic cancer vaccines. Cancer Biother Radiopharm 27: 2–5.

45. Marten A, Ziske C, Schottker B, Renoth S, Weineck S, et al. (2001) Interactions between dendritic cells and cytokine-induced killer cells lead to an activation of both populations. J Immunother 24: 502–510.

46. Duru N, Fan M, Candas D, Menaa C, Liu HC, et al. (2012) HER2-associated radioresistance of breast cancer stem cells isolated from HER2-negative breast cancer cells. Clin Cancer Res 18: 6634–6647.

47. Li CD, Zhang WY, Li HL, Jiang XX, Zhang Y, et al. (2005) Mesenchymal stem cells derived from human placenta suppress allogeneic umbilical cord blood lymphocyte proliferation. Cell Res 15: 539–547.

48. Beutler N, Hauka S, Niepel A, Kowalewski DJ, Uhlmann J, et al. (2013) A natural tapasin isoform lacking exon 3 modifies peptide loading complex function. Eur J Immunol 43: 1459–1469.

49. Sharma A, Bode B, Wenger RH, Lehmann K, Sartori AA, et al. (2011) gamma-Radiation promotes immunological recognition of cancer cells through increased expression of cancer-testis antigens in vitro and in vivo. PLoS One 6: e28217.

16

Interleukin-15-Induced CD56$^+$ Myeloid Dendritic Cells Combine Potent Tumor Antigen Presentation with Direct Tumoricidal Potential

Sébastien Anguille[1,2]*, Eva Lion[1], Jurjen Tel[3], I. Jolanda M de Vries[3], Karen Couderé[1], Phillip D. Fromm[4], Viggo F. Van Tendeloo[1], Evelien L. Smits[1,2❥], Zwi N. Berneman[1,2❥]

1 University of Antwerp, Faculty of Medicine and Health Sciences, Vaccine and Infectious Disease Institute (VAXINFECTIO), Laboratory of Experimental Hematology, Antwerp, Belgium, 2 Antwerp University Hospital, Center for Cell Therapy and Regenerative Medicine, Antwerp, Belgium, 3 Radboud University Nijmegen Medical Centre and Nijmegen Centre for Molecular Life Sciences, Department of Tumor Immunology, Nijmegen, The Netherlands, 4 ANZAC Research Institute, Dendritic Cell Biology and Therapeutics Group, Sydney, Australia

Abstract

Dendritic cells (DCs) are the quintessential antigen-presenting cells of the human immune system and play a prime role in coordinating innate and adaptive immune responses, explaining the strong and still growing interest in their application for cancer immunotherapy. Much current research in the field of DC-based immunotherapy focuses on optimizing the culture conditions for *in vitro* DC generation in order to assure that DCs with the best possible immunogenic qualities are being used for immunotherapy. In this context, monocyte-derived DCs that are alternatively induced by interleukin-15 (IL-15 DCs) have attracted recent attention due to their superior immunostimulatory characteristics. In this study, we show that IL-15 DCs, in addition to potent tumor antigen-presenting function, possess tumoricidal potential and thus qualify for the designation of killer DCs. Notwithstanding marked expression of the natural killer (NK) cell marker CD56 on a subset of IL-15 DCs, we found no evidence of a further phenotypic overlap between IL-15 DCs and NK cells. Allostimulation and antigen presentation assays confirmed that IL-15 DCs should be regarded as *bona fide* myeloid DCs not only from the phenotypic but also from the functional point of view. Concerning their cytotoxic activity, we demonstrate that IL-15 DCs are able to induce apoptotic cell death of the human K562 tumor cell line, while sparing tumor antigen-specific T cells. The cytotoxicity of IL-15 DCs is predominantly mediated by granzyme B and, to a small extent, by tumor necrosis factor-α (TNF-α)-related apoptosis-inducing ligand (TRAIL) but is independent of perforin, Fas ligand and TNF-α. In conclusion, our data provide evidence of a previously unappreciated role for IL-15 in the differentiation of human monocytes towards killer DCs. The observation that IL-15 DCs have killer DC capacity lends further support to their implementation in DC-based immunotherapy protocols.

Editor: Jacques Zimmer, Centre de Recherche Public de la Santé (CRP-Santé), Luxembourg

Funding: This work was supported in part by research grants of the Research Foundation Flanders (FWO Vlaanderen, www.fwo.be), the Belgian Foundation against Cancer (Stichting tegen Kanker, www.kanker.be), the Methusalem program of the Flemish Government attributed to Prof Herman Goossens (University of Antwerp, Belgium), the Interuniversity Attraction Pole program (IAP #P6/41) of the Belgian Government and the Belgian Hercules Foundation (www.herculesstichting.be). SA is a PhD fellow of the Research Foundation Flanders and received financial support from the Belgian Foundation against Cancer and the Belgian public utility foundation VOCATIO (www.vocatio.be). EL holds an Emmanuel van der Schueren Fellowship of the Flemish League against Cancer (Vlaamse Liga tegen Kanker, www.tegenkanker.be). JT was supported by a grant from The Netherlands Organization for Scientific Research (NWO ZonMW, www.zonmw.nl). YW is funded by a PhD grant of the Institute for the Promotion of Innovation through Science and Technology (IWT, www.iwt.be). NC and ELS are post-doctoral fellows of the Research Foundation Flanders. The funders had no role in study design, data collection and analysis, decision to publish, or preparation of the manuscript.

Competing Interests: The authors have declared that no competing interests exist.

* E-mail: sebastien.anguille@uza.be

❥ These authors are joint senior authors on this work.

Introduction

Over the past years, the phenotypic and functional boundaries distinguishing the main cell subsets of the human immune system have become increasingly blurred. While it has already been well established that T cells may share some phenotypic and functional features with natural killer (NK) cells [1], more recent evidence also points to the existence of such overlap between NK cells and dendritic cells (DCs) [2]. NK cells have been shown capable of antigen presentation, a classical function of DCs [3]. In mice, specialized NK cell subsets, collectively designated as 'natural killer dendritic cells' (NKDCs), have been identified that display a hybrid NK cell/DC phenotype and combine functional properties of NK cells (cytotoxicity) and DCs (antigen presentation) [4–9]. Conversely, evidence from both rodent and human studies is emerging that DCs may exhibit NK-like activity and play a direct role in innate immunity as killer cells; in the literature, these cells are designated as 'killer DCs' [10–13]. Such killer DCs that can combine both tumor antigen presentation function with direct tumoricidal activity are garnering increasing attention as potential new, multifunctional tools for cancer immunotherapy [10–12,14].

Hitherto, monocyte-derived DCs represent the DC type most widely used in human immunotherapy trial protocols [15,16]. They are classically obtained through *in vitro* differentiation of peripheral blood monocytes in the presence of granulocyte macrophage colony-stimulating factor (GM-CSF) and interleukin (IL)-4 [17], followed by induction of DC maturation using a pro-inflammatory cytokine cocktail composed of tumor necrosis factor (TNF)-α, IL-1β, IL-6 and prostaglandin E_2 (PGE$_2$) [18]. Over the years, it has become apparent that these "gold-standard" DCs, commonly referred to as 'IL-4 DCs', are suboptimal in terms of antigen presentation function and T cell stimulatory capacity [17]. This explains the impetus behind the many efforts that are currently being made to optimize the culture conditions for *ex vivo* monocyte-derived DC generation [19,20].

Within this context, we and others have shown that the immunostimulatory properties of monocyte-derived DCs can be significantly enhanced by replacing IL-4 with IL-15 for DC differentiation and by using Toll-like receptor (TLR) stimuli to trigger DC maturation [17,21–23]. In addition, we have found that these so-called 'IL-15 DCs' display a rather unconventional DC phenotype, with a subset of these cells being positive for the cell surface marker CD56 [17]. Since CD56 is the archetypal phenotypic marker of NK cells, we here aimed to investigate whether IL-15 DCs also bear functional resemblance with NK cells in terms of cytotoxic activity. In this study, IL-15 DCs are shown to possess potent tumor antigen presentation function in combination with lytic potential against the classical NK cell target cell line K562, thus confirming the hypothesis that IL-15 DCs qualify for the designation of killer DCs.

Methods

Ethics statement

This study was approved by the Ethics Committee of the University of Antwerp (Antwerp, Belgium) under the reference number 11/47/366. All experiments were performed using blood samples from anonymous volunteer donors, provided through the Antwerp Blood Transfusion Center of the Red Cross (Edegem, Belgium).

Human cell lines

The human myeloid leukemia cell lines K562 and U937 were obtained from American Type Culture Collection (Rockville, MD, USA) and maintained in Iscove's modified Dulbecco's medium (IMDM; Invitrogen, Merelbeke, Belgium) supplemented with 10% fetal bovine serum (FBS; Invitrogen). The human cytotoxic T lymphocyte (CTL) clone specific for the HLA-A*0201-restricted epitope 126–134 of the Wilms' tumor 1 protein (WT1) [24] was kindly provided by Dr C. Bonini (San Raffaele Scientific Institute, Milan, Italy) and maintained in IMDM/10% FBS and 60 IU/mL IL-2 (Immunotools, Friesoythe, Germany).

DC culture

Mature IL-15 DCs were generated according to our previously described protocol [17]. Briefly, peripheral blood mononuclear cells (PBMCs) were prepared from buffy coats by standard Ficoll density gradient centrifugation (Ficoll-Paque^{TM} PLUS; GE Healthcare, Diegem, Belgium). CD14$^+$ monocytes were purified using a positive immunomagnetic cell selection kit (Miltenyi, Amsterdam, The Netherlands) and seeded into 6-well culture plates (Corning Life Sciences, Schiphol-Rijk, The Netherlands) at a density of $1–1.2 \times 10^6$/mL in DC differentiation medium containing Roswell Park Memorial Institute medium (RPMI-1640; Invitrogen), 2.5% heat-inactivated human AB serum

(Invitrogen), 800 IU/mL GM-CSF (Invitrogen) and 200 ng/mL IL-15 (Immunotools). After 24–36 hr of *in vitro* culture, CD56$^+$ and CD56$^-$ IL-15 DC populations were separated using anti-CD56 magnetic microbeads according to the manufacturer''s instructions (Miltenyi). Both fractions were resuspended in DC differentiation medium and cultured for an additional 16–20 hr in the presence of a DC maturation cocktail containing 3 μg/mL of the TLR7/8 ligand R-848 (Enzo Life Sciences, Antwerp, Belgium), 2.5 ng/mL TNF-α (Gentaur, Brussels, Belgium), 5000 IU/mL interferon-γ (IFN-γ; Immunotools) and 1 μg/mL PGE$_2$ (Pfizer, Puurs, Belgium). In some experiments, IL-15 DC function was compared to that of conventional 7-day GM-CSF/IL-4 monocyte-derived DCs (IL-4 DCs), which were generated as described previously [17].

Flow cytometric immunophenotyping

Purity of IL-15 DC cultures was checked on a routine basis by multiparameter flow cytometry using a combination of FITC-, PE-, PB-/V450- and APC-conjugated monoclonal antibodies (mAbs) specific for CD3, CD7, CD11c, CD19 and CD56. All mAbs were from Becton Dickinson (BD; Erembodegem, Belgium) unless specified otherwise. Cell surface staining of mature IL-15 DCs was performed using FITC-, PE-, PB-/V450-, or APC-conjugated mAbs against various NK cell markers (CD7, CD16, CD56, CD69, NKG2D [Miltenyi], NKp46), NKDC-associated surface antigens (CD11c, B220 [eBioscience, Halle-Zoersel, Belgium], NKR-P1A/CD161 [Miltenyi]) and monocyte/DC markers (BDCA-1/CD1c [Miltenyi], CD14, CD40, CD80, CD83 [Invitrogen], CD86, CD209/DC-SIGN, CCR7 [R&D Systems, Minneapolis, MN, USA], HLA-DR). For detection of membrane-bound cytolytic effector molecules, DCs were stained with PE-labeled mAbs against TNF-α, Fas ligand/CD178 (eBioscience) and TNF-α-related apoptosis-inducing ligand (TRAIL). Dead cells were excluded by 7-amino actinomycin D (7-AAD; 5 μL/sample; BD) staining 10 min prior to acquisition on a FACSAria II (BD) flow cytometer. In each experiment, isotype-matched control mAbs were included to determine non-specific background staining. Results were expressed as delta mean fluorescence intensity (ΔMFI) (calculated by subtracting MFI values of isotype controls from sample MFI values) and as percentages of marker-positive cells (determined by Overton subtraction of isotype control histograms from sample histograms).

CD56 expression kinetics

In a separate experiment designed to study the kinetics of CD56 expression during IL-15 DC differentiation, ultra-purified FACS-sorted monocytes were used as precursor cells for IL-15 DC differentiation. For this specific experiment, CD14 magnetic bead-selected monocytes were stained with CD14-PerCP-Cy5.5/CD16-V500 (both from BD) and then flow-sorted using an Influx cytometer (BD). Sorting gates were set conservatively on CD14^{++}CD16$^-$ cells to ensure high-purity isolation (>99.9%) of the "classical" monocyte subset. Sorted monocytes were then subjected to IL-15 DC differentiation as described above. Flow cytometric analysis of CD56 expression on IL-15 DCs was performed at different time points following start of culture (4 hr, 16 hr, 24 hr, 40 hr, 48 hr, 64 hr, 72 hr, 96 hr and 7 days) by double surface staining with CD11c-APC (BD) and CD56-PB (BioLegend, San Diego, CA, USA). At each time point, samples were stained in parallel with CD11c-APC (BD) and a PB-labeled isotype-matched control mAb (mouse IgG2a, κ; BioLegend) to determine non-specific background labeling. Samples were acquired on an Influx cytometer (BD).

Combined cell surface and intracellular staining

Brefeldin A (1 μL/10^6 cells; Invitrogen) was added to the DC cultures 180 min prior to harvesting the cells. After harvest, cells were surface-stained with CD11c-V450 and CD56-APC (both from BD). The LIVE/DEAD® fixable violet stain with 405 nm excitation (1 μL/10^6 cells; Invitrogen) was concomitantly added to allow discrimination between viable and non-viable cells. After 30 min incubation at room temperature, cells were treated sequentially with FACS lysing solution and FACS permeabilizing solution 2 (BD). Intracellular expression of cytolytic effector molecules was assessed after 4–6 hr incubation at 4°C with one of the following mAbs or their corresponding isotype controls: perforin-FITC, granzyme B-PE or TRAIL-PE (all from BD). Samples were acquired using a FACSAria II cytometer (BD). Results were expressed as ΔMFI values, as specified above.

Granzyme B secretion

CD56$^+$ and CD56$^-$ IL-15 DCs were harvested 16–20 hours following addition of the maturation cocktail, washed, and resuspended in IMDM/10% FBS at a density of 2×10^6 viable cells/mL. Cell-free culture supernatants were collected after overnight incubation and cryopreserved at -20°C for later analysis. Thawed supernatants were diluted 5-fold to allow quantification of granzyme B using a commercially available ELISA kit according to the manufacturer's instructions (Diaclone, Besançon, France).

Allogeneic mixed lymphocyte reaction (allo-MLR)

To prepare the responder cells for the MLR, frozen CD14$^+$ monocyte-depleted PBMCs of an allogeneic blood donor were thawed and further depleted of NK cells and NKT cells using anti-CD56 magnetic microbeads (Miltenyi). The resultant lymphocyte fraction was then labeled with 5,6-carboxyfluorescein diacetate succinimyl ester (CFSE; 5 μM; Invitrogen), and co-cultured with mature CD56$^+$ and CD56$^-$ IL-15 DCs in a 96-well round-bottom plate (Corning) at a stimulator:responder ratio of 1:10. Unstimulated CFSE-labeled cells served as negative control, while CFSE-labeled responders cells stimulated by either IL-4 DCs or a combination of phytohemagglutinin (PHA; 1 μg/mL; Sigma-Aldrich, Bornem, Belgium) and IL-2 (20 IU/mL; Immunotools) served as positive controls. After 5 days, cells were stained with CD11c-V450, CD3-APC and CD4-APC-H7 (all from BD) and analyzed using a FACSAria II cytometer (BD). T cell proliferation was assessed by quantifying the percent of CFSE-diluted (CFSE^{low}) cells within the CD11c$^-$CD3$^+$CD4$^+$ gate after background subtraction.

Antigen presentation assay

To evaluate their capacity for tumor antigen processing and presentation, IL-15 DCs were loaded by electroporation with *in vitro* transcribed *WT1*-encoding RNA. *WT1* RNA was produced by eTheRNA (Prof K. Thielemans, Free University of Brussels, Brussels, Belgium) starting from a T7 promotor-driven plasmid containing the codon-optimized (GeneArt, Regensburg, Germany) human *WT1* gene, lacking its 5'-,3'-untranslated regions as well as the aa292–348 nuclear localization sequence and flanked at its 5'- and 3'-sides, respectively, by the signal sequence and the HLA class II-targeting sequence of DC-lysosome-associated membrane protein [20]. IL-15 DCs from HLA-A*0201$^+$ individuals were prepared and electroporated as previously described [17], with minor modifications. Briefly, 5×10^6 cells were transferred to a 4-mm electroporation cuvette (Bio-Rad, Hercules, CA, USA) and electrotransfected with 20 μg RNA by an exponential decay pulse

of 300 V/300 μF using the Gene Pulser Xcell device (Bio-Rad). Four hours post-electroporation, cells were transferred to 96-well round-bottom plates (Corning) and co-cultured in triplicate with the WT1$_{126-134}$-specific CTL clone at a DC-to-T cell ratio of 1:1. The next day, supernatants were collected and analyzed for IFN-γ production by ELISA as per the manufacturer's instructions (Peprotech, Rocky Hill, NJ, USA). In parallel experiments, *WT1* RNA-electroporated IL-15 DCs were co-cultured with the CTL clone at a DC-to-T cell ratio of 40:1 in triplicate wells of anti-IFN-γ-antibody-coated 96-well PVDF-bottom ELISpot plates (Millipore, Bedford, MA, USA). After overnight co-culture at 37°C, plates were developed using a commercially available IFN-γ ELISpot kit (Diaclone). IFN-γ spot-forming cells (SFCs) were counted with a computerized ELISpot plate reader (Autoimmun Diagnostika, Strassberg, Germany). In each assay, the following controls were included to determine the levels of non-antigen-specific IFN-γ production: T cells cultured alone, DCs cultured alone and T cells cultured with non-antigen-loaded DCs.

Cytotoxicity assays

A flow cytometry-based lysis assay [25] was used to determine the cytotoxic activity of IL-15 DCs against the following potential targets: the K562 human myeloid leukemia cell line (major histocompatibility complex [MHC] class I-negative), the U937 human myeloid leukemia cell line (MHC class I-positive) and the WT1$_{126-134}$-specific CTL clone. Briefly, target cells were labeled with the PKH67 green fluorescent cell linker (Sigma-Aldrich). DCs were harvested following maturation, rigorously washed, and co-cultured overnight with PKH67-labeled target cells in fresh IMDM/10% FBS medium at different effector-to-target (E:T) ratios (50:1, 25:1, 12:1, 6:1 and 1:1). Prior to flow cytometric measurement, the cell surface was stained with CD11c-V450 (BD) to allow further discrimination between effector cells (PKH67$^-$CD11c$^+$) and targets cells (PKH67$^+$CD11c$^-$). The cells were then washed and resuspended in Annexin-V-binding buffer (BD) containing Annexin-V-APC (1 μL/100 μL buffer; BD). After 15 min incubation at room temperature, samples were stained with propidium iodide (PI; Sigma-Aldrich) and immediately acquired on a Partec CyFlow ML (Partec, Münster, Germany) or a FACSAria II (BD) multiparameter flow cytometer. PKH67-labeled target cells cultured without DCs served as controls to determine spontaneous cell death. Percentages of viable target cells (i.e. percentages of PI$^-$/Annexin-V$^-$ cells within the PKH67$^+$/CD11c$^-$ target cell gate) were used to quantify the cytotoxic responses according to the following formula: % of specific lysis = 100– [(% viable target cells in the presence of DCs/% viable target cells without DCs) ×100].

Cytotoxicity blocking studies

Cytotoxicity blocking experiments were performed as described above, except that effector cells (CD56$^+$ IL-15 DCs) were pre-incubated at 37°C with either neutralizing TRAIL mAbs (40 μg/10^6 cells; R&D Systems) or concanamycin A (200 nM/10^6 DCs; Tocris Bioscience, Bristol, UK) before addition of PKH67-labeled K562 target cells at a 50:1 E:T ratio. Control experiments were run in parallel using TRAIL isotype control mAbs (mouse IgG1; R&D Systems) or concanamycin A control medium, respectively.

Data mining and statistical analysis

Flow cytometry data were analyzed using FlowJo software (v9.3; Treestar, Ashland, OR, USA). GraphPad Prism software (v5.0; San Diego, CA, USA) was used for statistical analysis and graphing. Statistical comparisons were performed using Wilcoxon's matched-pairs signed rank test or paired Student's *t*-test, where appropriate. *P*-values <0.05 were considered statistically significant. All data were expressed as means ± standard error of the mean (SEM).

Results

IL-15 DCs are CD56$^{+/-}$ myeloid DCs that are phenotypically unrelated to NK cells

Exposure of human peripheral blood CD14$^+$ monocytes to GM-CSF and IL-15 resulted in their rapid differentiation into CD11c$^+$ DCs with subset expression of CD56 (Figure 1A, left panel). Acquisition of CD56 was also demonstrable on IL-15 DCs differentiated from ultra-purified, FACS-sorted CD14$^+$ monocytes, with CD56 being detectable already within the first 24 hr of culture. Maximal CD56 surface expression was observed between 24–48 hr after start of IL-15 DC culture, after which expression gradually declined toward the non-specific background level at day 7 (Figure S1).

Further phenotypic analysis of the CD56$^+$ IL-15 DC fraction revealed that this subset displayed the characteristic forward scatter (FSC)/sideward scatter (SSC) profile of DCs (data not shown) and that it co-expressed CD11c and BDCA-1, indicating a myeloid DC phenotype (Figure 1A, middle panel). In addition, CD56$^+$ IL-15 DCs were found to lack co-expression of CD7, which confirmed that these cells are unrelated to NK cells (Figure 1A, right panel) [26]. Natural cytotoxicity receptors (NCRs), such as the NK cell-specific marker NKp46 [27], and other typical NK cell-associated markers, such as CD16, CD69 or NKG2D, were not expressed on the cell surface of CD56$^+$ IL-15 DCs (Figure 1B, 'NK panel').

The co-expression of CD11c with the prototypical NK cell marker CD56 led us to further investigate whether the phenotype of CD56$^+$ IL-15 DCs might correspond to that of the so-called NKDCs in mice [5–7]. Notwithstanding expression of CD11c, we were unable to classify CD56$^+$ IL-15 DCs as their human counterpart due to the lack of NKDC-associated surface hallmarks such as NKR-P1A/CD161, which is the human homologue of murine NK1.1 [28], and B220 (Figure 1B, 'NKDC panel').

After 2–3 days of culture, including a maturation step during the final 16–20 hr, both CD56$^+$ and CD56$^-$ IL-15 DC populations developed a mature DC phenotype characterized by a marked down-regulation of CD14, up-regulation of DC-SIGN, high-level expression of co-stimulatory molecules (CD40, CD80 and CD86) and of HLA-DR as well as of the maturation markers CD83 and CCR7 (Table 1 and Figure 1B, 'DC panel'). Compared to their CD56$^-$ counterparts, CD56$^+$ IL-15 DCs showed more prominent down-regulation of CD14 along with significantly higher expression levels of CD40, CD80, CD86, CD83 and CCR7, indicative of a more differentiated and/or activated DC phenotype (Table 1).

IL-15 DCs possess allo-stimulatory capacity

Next, CD56$^+$ and CD56$^-$ IL-15 DC subpopulations were subjected to an allo-MLR in order to examine their ability to stimulate allogeneic T cell proliferation, one of the defining functional characteristics of DCs [29]. While NK cells were unable to stimulate allogeneic T cell proliferation (data not shown), IL-15 DCs were found to possess potent allostimulatory capacity, as determined by CFSE dilution analysis (Figure 2). There was no statistically significant difference between the percent of CFSE^{low} CD4$^+$ T cells in CD56$^+$ as compared to CD56$^-$ IL-15 DC-stimulated cultures (background-subtracted % CFSE^{low} CD4$^+$ T cells following stimulation with CD56$^+$ *vs.* CD56$^-$ DCs: 24.1±3.9% vs. 19.7±2.6%; *P*>0.05).

IL-15 DCs are functional DCs with potent tumor antigen-presenting capacity

To determine their capacity for tumor antigen presentation, IL-15 DCs were loaded by RNA electroporation with the WT1 tumor antigen [30] and examined for their ability to trigger IFN-γ production by a WT1$_{126-134}$-specific CTL clone. *WT1* RNA-electroporated IL-15 DCs elicited a marked increase in IFN-γ secretion, as determined by ELISA, indicating that RNA translation and processing for MHC class I presentation had occurred in these cells. Production of IFN-γ in response to non-antigen-loaded IL-15 DCs was approximately 3.3-fold lower as compared to *WT1* RNA-electroporated IL-15 DCs, confirming the antigen specificity of the responses observed (Figure 3A; *WT1* RNA EP *vs.* non/mock EP: *P*<0.001 and *P* = 0.01 for CD56$^+$ and CD56$^-$ IL-15 DCs, respectively). *WT1* RNA-electroporated CD56$^+$ IL-15 DCs were significantly more efficient at antigen presentation than their CD56$^-$ counterparts, as was demonstrated by their superior capacity to stimulate the CTL clone to secrete IFN-γ (Figure 3A, *WT1* RNA EP CD56$^+$ *vs.* CD56$^-$ IL-15 DCs: *P* = 0.003).

Results of the IFN-γ ELISpot assay were similar to those obtained by ELISA. As shown in Figure 3B, both CD56$^+$ and CD56$^-$ *WT1* RNA-electroporated IL-15 DCs were able to induce robust IFN-γ ELISpot responses. Numbers of IFN-γ SFCs/well in non-antigen-stimulated cultures (i.e. CTL clone cultured with non-antigen-loaded DCs) did not differ significantly between CD56$^+$ and CD56$^-$ IL-15 DCs and were found to be consistently lower than those in corresponding cultures stimulated with *WT1* RNA-electroporated IL-15 DCs (Figure 3B; *WT1* RNA EP *vs.* non/mock EP: *P*<0.001 for both CD56$^+$ and CD56$^-$ IL-15 DCs). Although *WT1* RNA-electroporated CD56$^-$ IL-15 DCs induced a potent IFN-γ ELISpot response (SFCs/well: 141.4±3.3), significantly higher numbers of IFN-γ SFCs/well (184.4±8.0) were observed when *WT1* RNA-electroporated CD56$^+$ IL-15 DCs were used as effectors (*P*<0.001), confirming the superiority of CD56$^+$ over CD56$^-$ IL-15 DCs in terms of antigen-presenting capacity (Figure 3B).

IL-15 DCs are killer DCs capable of tumor lysis while sparing antigen-specific T cells

The observation that a subset of IL-15 DCs expressed the classical NK cell marker CD56 prompted us to examine whether these DCs have cytolytic effector function. Therefore, both CD56$^+$ and CD56$^-$ IL-15 DC fractions were co-cultured with the K562 tumor cell line and examined for lytic activity using a PI/Annexin-V-based flow cytometric lysis assay. After 16–18 hr of co-culture, CD56$^+$ IL-15 DCs were found to have reduced K562 cell viability by 22.7±1.0% at an E:T ratio of 50:1 (Figure 4). This decrease in K562 cell viability was due to an increase in apoptotic cell death, as indicated by the higher frequency of PI$^+$Annexin-V$^+$ K562 target cells after co-culture with CD56$^+$ IL-15 DCs (Figure 4A). As shown in Figure 4B, the cytotoxic action of CD56$^+$ IL-15 DCs was titratable and most apparent at high E:T ratios, where levels of cytotoxicity between CD56$^+$ and CD56$^-$ IL-15 DCs were found to differ significantly (Figure 4B; *P*<0.001 and *P* = 0.006 for E:T ratios of 50:1 and 25:1, respectively). At these E:T ratios, lytic activity of CD56$^-$ IL-15 DCs was markedly lower as compared to that of CD56$^+$ DCs, but still higher than that of conventional IL-4 DCs which failed to induce any significant cytotoxicity (Figure 4B).

We next sought to determine whether IL-15 DCs display any non-specific cytotoxic activity against tumor antigen-specific T cells, which would be unwanted in the context of immunotherapy. To this end, mature CD56$^+$ and CD56$^-$ IL-15 DCs derived from HLA-A*0201$^+$ donors were added to the WT1$_{126-134}$-specific

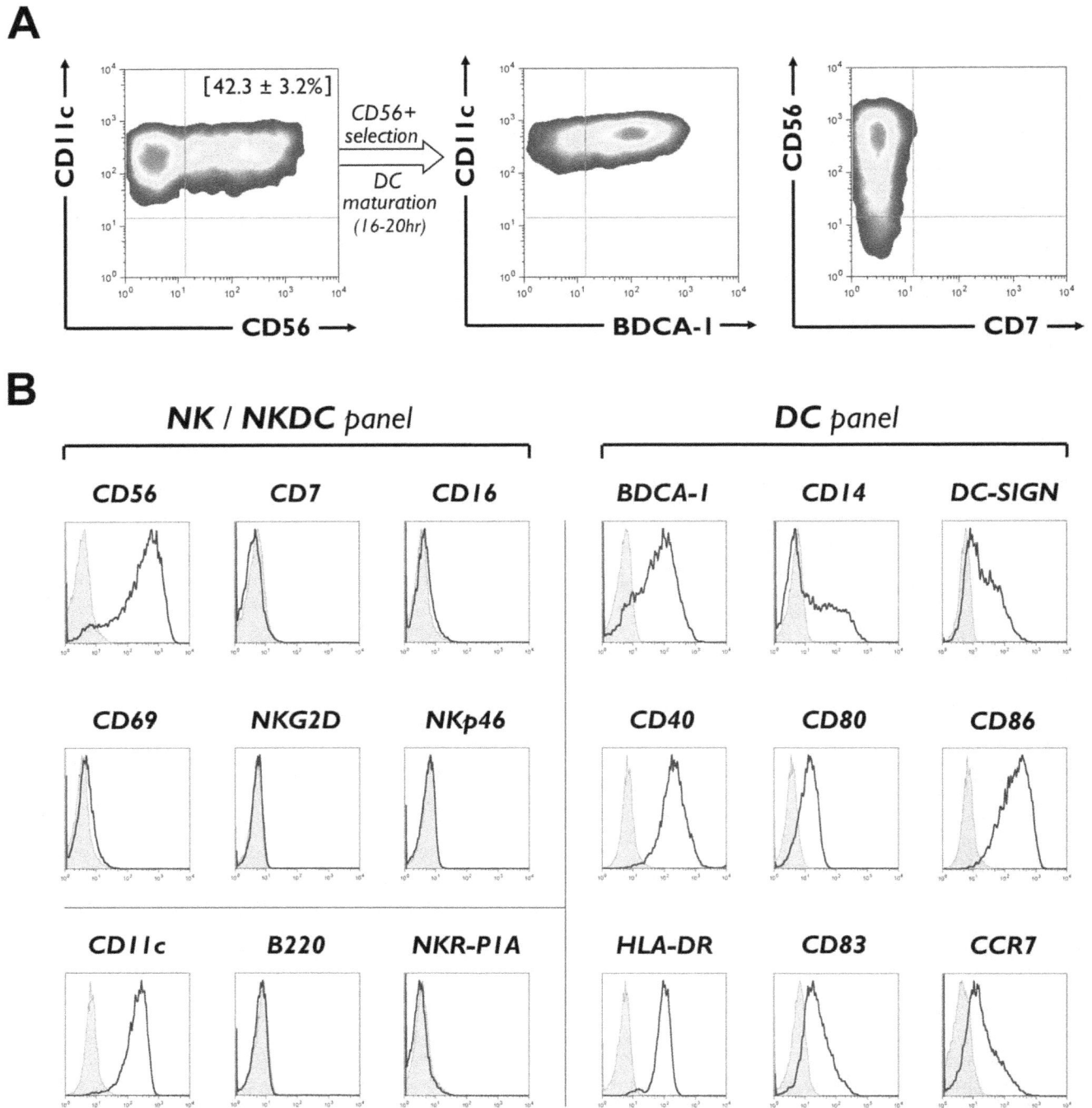

Figure 1. Phenotypic characteristics of CD56⁺ IL-15 DCs. (A) CD14⁺ monocytes were cultured for 24–36 hr in the presence of GM-CSF and IL-15 (IL-15 DCs) and analyzed by flow cytometry for expression of CD11c/CD56 (left). The percentage between parentheses indicates the mean (± SEM) percentage of CD56⁺ cells among the total IL-15 DC population ($n = 17$). These CD56⁺ cells were then immunomagnetically separated, cultured for another 16–20 hr in the presence of DC maturation cocktail and analyzed for co-expression of CD11c/BDCA-1 (middle) and CD56/CD7 (right). Quadrant gates were set using corresponding isotype controls. (B) Matured CD56⁺ IL-15 DCs were further analyzed by flow cytometry for expression of the indicated NK cell-associated (CD56, CD7, CD16, CD69, NKG2D, NKp46), NKDC-associated (CD11c, B220, NKR-P1A) and DC-related surface antigens. Histogram overlays show expression of the indicated markers (solid line histograms) compared to their respective isotype controls (filled grey histograms). All plots are representative of at least 4 independent experiments.

CTL clone at a 50:1 E:T ratio. Residual cell viability was determined after overnight incubation by PI/Annexin-V staining. Figure 4C shows that there was no significant difference in T cell clone viability regardless of the presence or absence of IL-15 DCs,

confirming that IL-15 DCs lack lytic activity against WT1-specific T cells (Figure 4C; T cells *vs.* T cells + DCs: $P > 0.05$ for both CD56⁺ and CD56⁻ IL-15 DCs).

Table 1. Phenotypic difference between matured CD56$^+$ and CD56$^-$ IL-15 DCs.

	ΔMFI		% positive cells	
	CD56$^-$ IL-15 DCs	CD56$^+$ IL-15 DCs	CD56$^-$ IL-15 DCs	CD56$^+$ IL-15 DCs
CD11c	262.6±40.1	364.0±51.5*	98.5±0.6	99.0±0.6*
BDCA-1/CD1c (n=4)	19.1±5.3	39.7±9.3	60.0±4.4	74.5±4.0
CD14 (n=6)	16.3±4.2	10.9±3.5*	51.5±5.8	40.5±5.4*
DC-SIGN/CD209	4.7±1.1	6.0±1.6	40.9±4.4	44.0±5.4
CD40	169.7±21.8	227.6±23.6*	97.9±0.9	98.9±0.5*
CD80	6.8±1.3	9.3±1.8*	59.7±4.8	65.0±4.8
CD86	168.4±21.3	223.5±28.9*	97.1±0.6	98.1±0.5*
HLA-DR	106.3±12.9	107.0±13.9	96.5±0.8	96.0±1.1
CCR7	7.2±3.1	11.1±3.7*	35.8±8.7	46.4±8.8*
CD83	13.8±3.6	19.1±5.4*	62.3±6.4	68.1±5.7*

Pairwise comparison of CD56$^-$ and CD56$^+$ IL-15 DC surface phenotypes. Results are presented as mean (± SEM) ΔMFI values and as mean (± SEM) percentage of cells staining positive for the indicated cell surface marker. Data are from 7 independent experiments, except if specified otherwise. Asterisks indicate a statistically significant difference in cell surface marker expression between CD56$^+$ and CD56$^-$ IL-15 DC populations ($P<0.05$).

Lysis by IL-15 DCs is not due to contamination by cytotoxic lymphocytes

IL-15 DC cultures were routinely checked for purity by multiparameter flow cytometry in order to exclude the possibility that cytotoxicity results were confounded by culture contamination with cytotoxic lymphocytes. As mentioned above, IL-15 DCs could be clearly distinguished from residual lymphocyte subsets on the basis of their distinct FSC/SSC profile, their intense uniform expression of CD11c and lack of CD7 expression. Both CD56$^+$ and CD56$^-$ IL-15 DC preparations were found to contain minute numbers of contaminating lymphocytes. The percentage of CD7$^+$ cells within the contaminating lymphocyte cluster, which includes NK cells and other cytotoxic lymphocytes [26], was 0.9±0.2% for CD56$^+$ IL-15 DC cultures and 1.1±0.3% for CD56$^-$ IL-15 DC cultures (n = 12).

To further address the possibility that the observed lytic activity against K562 cells might have resulted from this low-level contamination with NK cells, we additionally performed a cytotoxicity assay against the U937 cell line, another known NK cell-sensitive target cell line [25,31]. As shown in Figure S2, both CD56$^+$ and CD56$^-$ IL-15 DC preparations failed to affect the viability of U937 cells, even at the high 50:1 E:T ratio used, indicating that the presence of these few NK cell contaminants was not a major concern in our experimental design.

IL-15 DCs contain TRAIL, express and secrete granzyme B but lack perforin

The logical next step was to determine the mechanisms that underlie the killing activity of IL-15 DCs. In view of the above observation that the cytotoxic action of these cells relies primarily

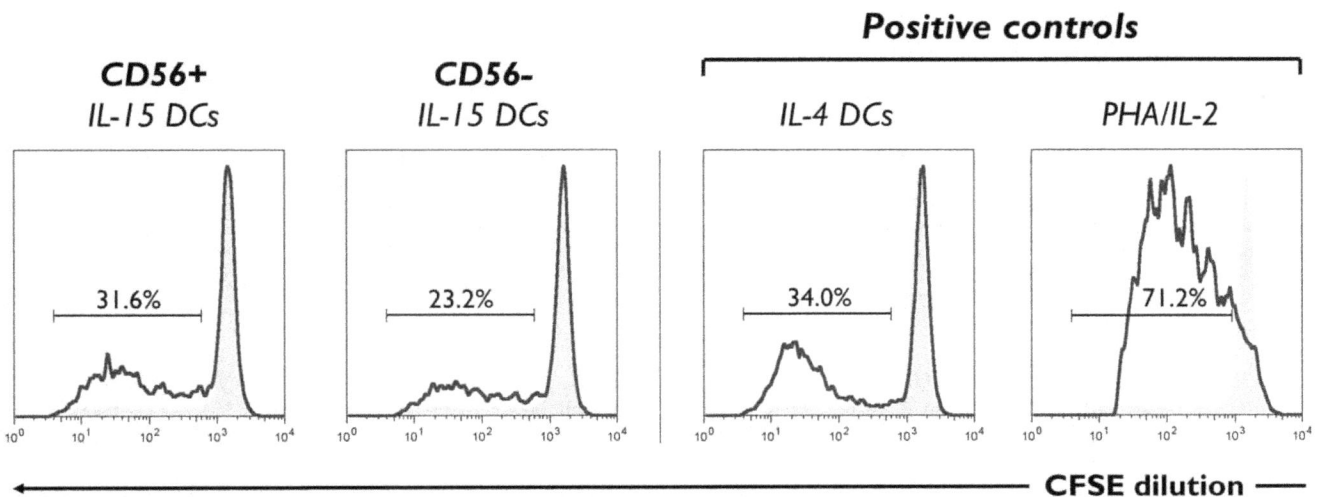

Positive controls

CD56+ IL-15 DCs — 31.6%
CD56- IL-15 DCs — 23.2%
IL-4 DCs — 34.0%
PHA/IL-2 — 71.2%

CFSE dilution →

Figure 2. Allostimulatory capacity of CD56$^+$ and CD56$^-$ IL-15 DCs in a MLR. CD56$^+$ and CD56$^-$ IL-15 DCs were co-cultured with allogeneic, CFSE-labeled lymphocytes at a 1:10 ratio for 5 days. CFSE-labeled cells stimulated with IL-4 DCs (1:10 stimulator/responder ratio) or PHA/IL-2 were used as positive controls. Histograms show the degree of CFSE dilution, indicative of T cell proliferation, among gated CD3$^+$CD4$^+$ T cells in the absence (filled grey histograms) and presence (solid line histograms) of the indicated stimulators. Numbers above the bracketed lines indicate the background-subtracted percentages of proliferated (i.e. CFSE^{low}) T cells within the CD3$^+$CD4$^+$ gate. Data shown are representative of three donors.

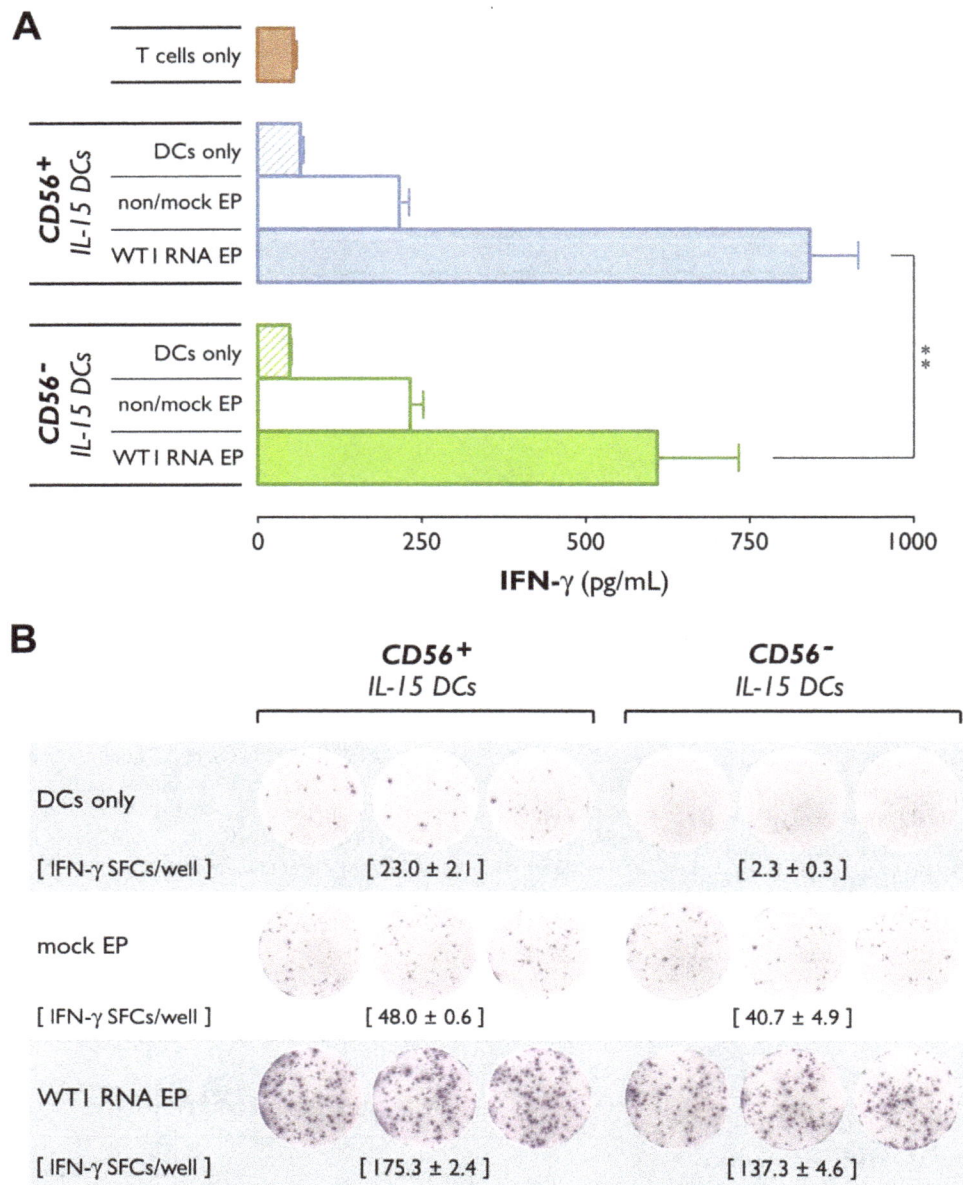

Figure 3. Differential ability of CD56$^+$ and CD56$^-$ IL-15 DCs to stimulate a WT1-specific CTL clone. Mature CD56$^+$ and CD56$^-$ IL-15 DCs were electroporated (EP) with *WT1* RNA and co-cultured with an HLA-A*0201-restricted WT1$_{126-134}$-specific CTL clone. Negative controls included: T cells cultured without DCs (T cells only), *WT1* RNA-electroporated DCs cultured without T cells (DCs only), and T cells cultured with non-antigen-loaded DCs (non/mock EP). (A) After overnight incubation, IFN-γ concentrations (pg/mL) in the culture supernatants were measured by ELISA. Bars represent mean ($\pm$ SEM) IFN-γ concentrations of triplicate wells of three independent experiments (**, $P = 0.003$). (B) Antigenic responses were quantified in parallel by IFN-γ ELISpot. Illustrative single-well images from an IFN-γ ELISpot plate of one representative experiment are shown. Values in parentheses indicate the mean ($\pm$ SEM) number of IFN-γ spot-forming cells (SFCs) of triplicate ELISpot wells.

on the induction of apoptosis, we focused on the most common apoptotic cell death pathways. As shown in Figure 5A, we found no evidence for cell surface expression of the apoptotic death receptor ligands TNF-α, FasL or TRAIL. We next performed intracellular staining experiments to examine the possible involvement of intracellular lytic molecules. In these experiments, DCs were identified on the basis of their characteristic FSC/SSC profile and CD11c positivity. Interestingly, both CD56$^+$ and CD56$^-$ IL-15 DCs contained intracellular TRAIL protein, which was found to be expressed at a significantly higher level in the CD56$^+$ IL-15 DC subset (Figure 5B; ΔMFI for intracellular

TRAIL in CD56$^+$ *vs.* CD56$^-$ IL-15 DCs: $P = 0.03$). Furthermore, intracellular cytokine staining revealed that both CD56$^+$ and CD56$^-$ IL-15 DCs expressed considerable levels of granzyme B, albeit that the CD56$^+$ fraction expressed significantly more granzyme B than the CD56$^-$ DC subset (Figure 5B; ΔMFI for intracellular granzyme B in CD56$^+$ *vs.* CD56$^-$ IL-15 DCs: 33.0 ± 10.7 *vs.* 23.3 ± 7.8; $P = 0.004$). In line with this, we observed a superior granzyme B secretory capacity of CD56$^+$ IL-15 DCs (1121.0 ± 353.3 pg/mL) over their CD56$^-$ counterparts (452.3 ± 117.0 pg/mL) (Figure 5C; $P = 0.047$). Strikingly, whereas

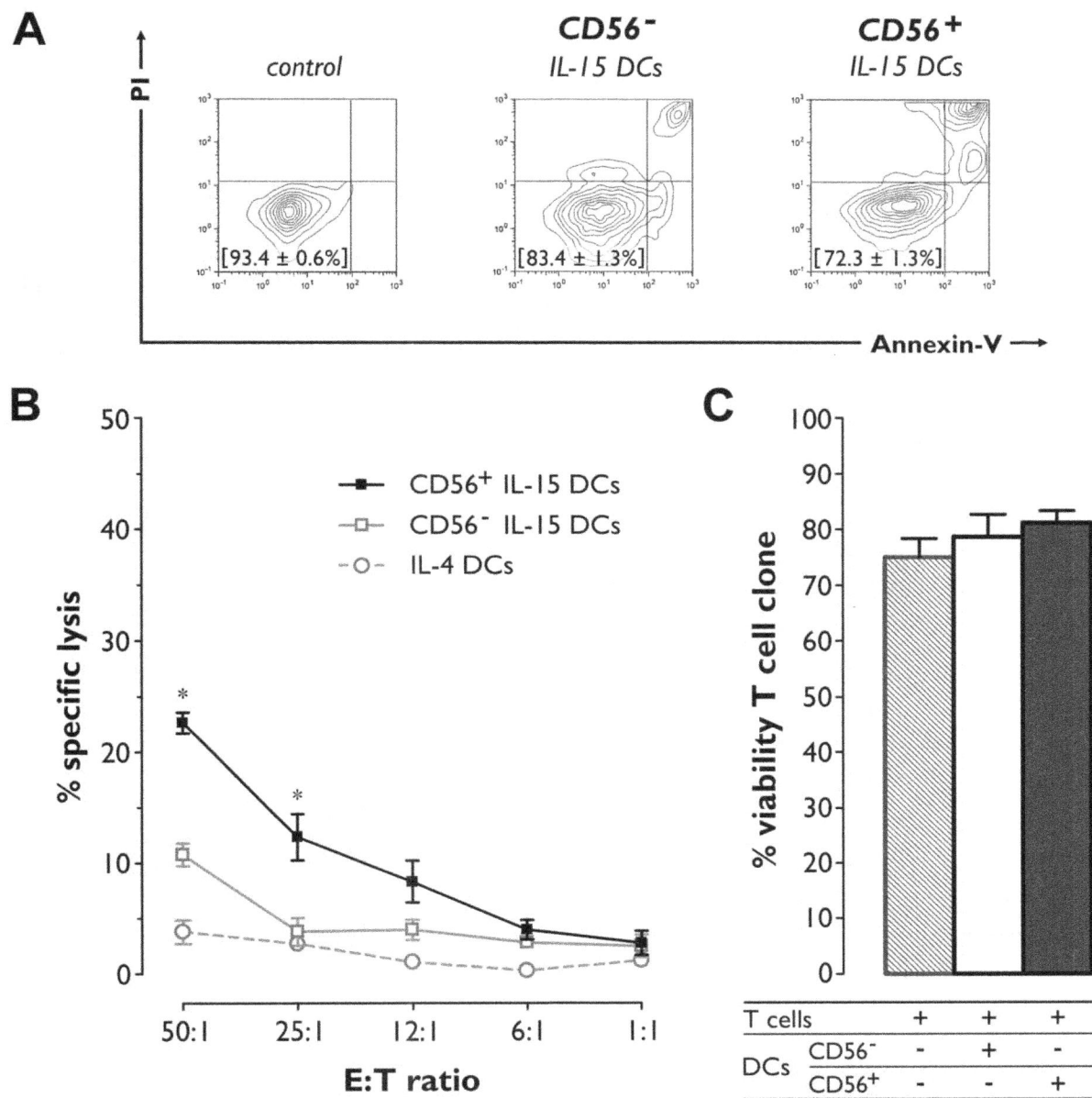

Figure 4. Lysis of K562 cells but not of a WT1-specific CTL clone by IL-15 DCs. PKH67-labeled target cells were mixed at varying E:T ratios with mature CD56+ and CD56− IL-15 DCs or, where indicated, with conventionally generated IL-4 DCs and then subjected to PI/Annexin-V staining after overnight incubation. Target cell viability was defined as the percentage of PI−/Annexin-V− cells within the PKH67+CD11c− gate. (A) Viability profiles of gated K562 tumor cells cultured alone (control) or with either CD56− or CD56+ IL-15 DCs at an E:T ratio of 50:1. One representative experiment out of five is shown. Percentages of viable K562 cells are displayed in the lower left quadrants and expressed as mean (± SEM) of 5 independent experiments. (B) Graph depicting the specific lysis of K562 tumor cells by CD56+ IL-15 DCs (solid black line, ■; $n = 5$), CD56− IL-15 DCs (solid grey line, □; $n = 5$) and IL-4 DCs (dashed grey line, ○; $n = 3$) at the indicated E:T ratios. Results are expressed as mean (± SEM) percentages of specific lysis. Asterisks refer to a statistically significant difference in cytotoxic activity at the indicated E:T ratio between CD56+ and CD56− IL-15 DCs. (C) Bar graphs showing the viability of a WT1$_{126-134}$-specific CTL clone after overnight culture in the absence or presence of either CD56− (□) or CD56+ (■) IL-15 DCs at an E:T ratio of 50:1. Data are presented as mean (± SEM) percentages of viable T cells from three experiments.

intracellular levels of TRAIL and granzyme B were increased, perforin expression was found to be absent (Figure 5B).

The cytotoxic activity of IL-15 DCs predominantly relies on granzyme B

Based on the data above, we envisaged two putative mechanisms underlying the cytotoxic action of CD56+ IL-15 DCs: TRAIL- and/or granzyme B-dependent apoptosis. To further dissect the relative contributions of these pathways to the pro-apoptotic effect of CD56+ IL-15 DCs on K562 cells, we performed cytotoxicity blocking experiments using anti-TRAIL neutralizing antibodies and concanamycin A, a selective inhibitor of vacuolar-type H+-ATPase that prevents acidification and degranulation of perforin/granzyme-containing cytotoxic granules. Since cytotoxicity of CD56+ IL-15 DCs against K562 cells was most prominent at high E:T ratios, we chose the E:T ratio of 50:1 for all further

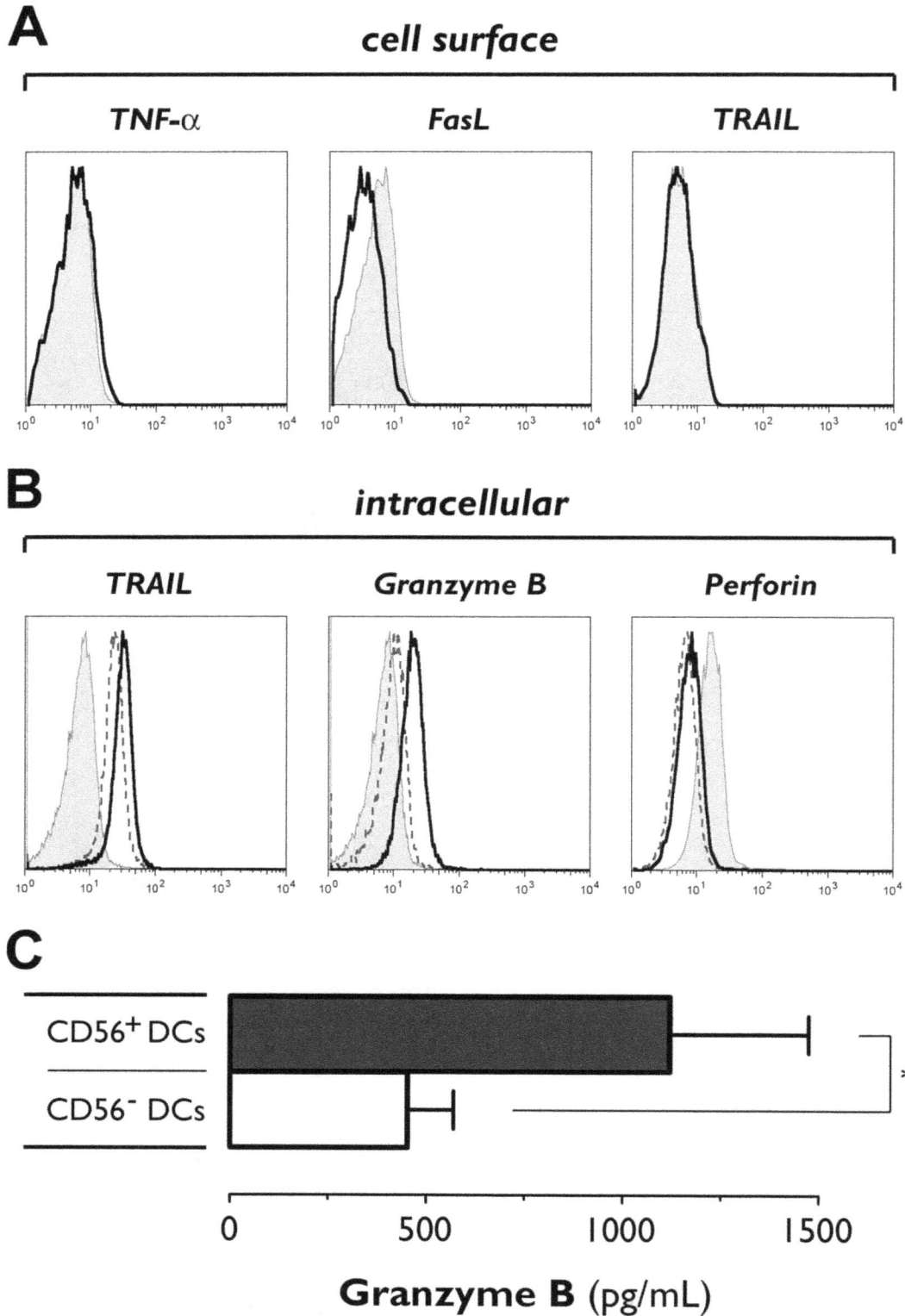

Figure 5. Expression of lytic molecules by IL-15 DCs. (A) Matured CD56[+] IL-15 DCs were analyzed by flow cytometry for cell surface expression of TNF-α, FasL and TRAIL (solid line histograms). Filled grey histograms represent isotype controls. Data are from one experiment representative of three. (B) Both CD56[+] (solid line) and CD56[−] (dashed line) IL-15 DCs were stained for intracellular expression of TRAIL, granzyme B and perforin. Filled grey histograms represent isotype controls. One representative experiment out of 6 (for TRAIL) and 9 (for granzyme B and perforin) is shown. (C) Supernatants from overnight washout cultures of CD56[+] (■) and CD56[−] (□) IL-15 DCs were analyzed for granzyme B release by ELISA. Bars represent mean (± SEM) granzyme B concentrations (pg/mL) from 7 experiments.*, $P<0.05$.

blocking experiments. As shown in Figure 6, neutralization of TRAIL activity resulted in a net decrease in cytotoxicity by $4.6\pm0.7\%$ as compared to isotype control, corresponding to a $22.5\pm2.8\%$ inhibition (Figure 6; $P=0.03$). Upon incubation with concanamycin A, cytotoxicity of CD56$^+$ IL-15 DCs against K562 was reduced from $24.2\pm6.3\%$ (control medium) to $6.4\pm1.1\%$, corresponding to a $62.9\pm6.1\%$ inhibition (Figure 6, $P=0.001$). Taken together, these results confirmed that granzyme B and, to a small extent, TRAIL participated in the observed cytotoxicity of IL-15 DCs.

Discussion

Dendritic cells, the quintessential antigen-presenting cells of the human immune system, have attracted much interest for active, specific immunotherapy of cancer over the years [32]. Despite some clinical successes, there is a general consensus that DC-based anti-tumor immunotherapy has not yet fulfilled its full therapeutic potential and that there remains considerable room for improvement, especially when it comes to optimizing the immunostimulatory activity of the DCs used for clinical application [32,33]. Due to their potent immunostimulatory properties, monocyte-derived DCs generated in the presence of GM-CSF and IL-15 (IL-15 DCs) have been advocated as promising new vehicles for DC-based immunotherapy [17,21–23]. In this study, we reveal for the first

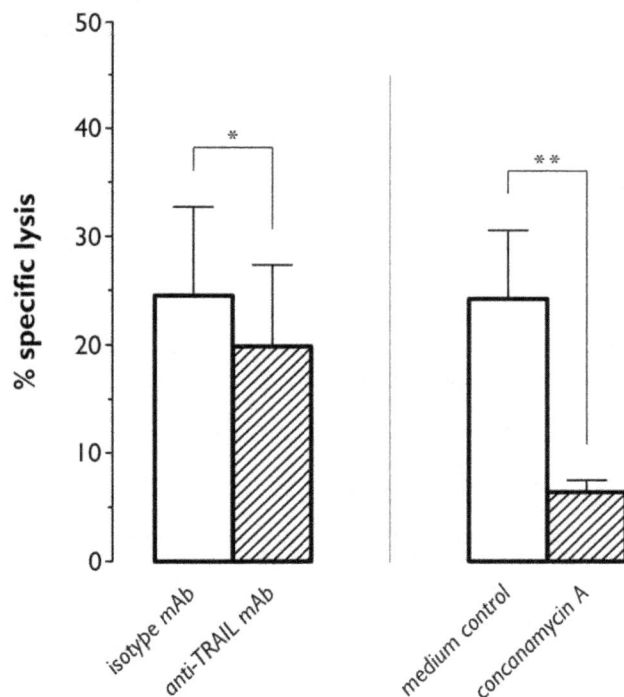

Figure 6. Inhibition of CD56$^+$ IL-15 DC-mediated cytotoxicity by neutralizing anti-TRAIL mAbs and concanamycin A. Matured CD56$^+$ IL-15 DCs were co-cultured with PKH67-labeled K562 target cells at an E:T ratio of 50:1 in the presence of either anti-TRAIL blocking mAb (left) or the granule exocytosis inhibitor concanamycin A (right). Parallel experiments were performed using TRAIL isotype-matched control mAb and medium control devoid of concanamycin A, respectively. Lysis of target cells was determined after overnight incubation using a flow cytometry-based cytotoxicity assay, as described above. Results are expressed as mean ($\pm$ SEM) percentages of specific target cell lysis. Data are from 5 (for TRAIL) and 10 (for concanamycin) independent experiments. *, $P<0.05$; **, $P<0.01$.

time that IL-15 DCs, in addition to a robust capacity for tumor antigen presentation, possess tumor cell killing potential. Our findings thus establish a previously unrecognized 'killer DC' function for IL-15 DCs, providing further support to their application in DC-based cancer immunotherapy protocols.

Although a subset of IL-15 DCs expresses the archetypal NK cell marker CD56 [34], we found no evidence for a further phenotypic overlap between IL-15 DCs and NK cells, nor could these cells be identified as the human homologue of murine NKDCs [4–9]. Our phenotypic data unequivocally establish that IL-15 DCs are genuine monocyte-derived DCs despite the rather unconventional expression of CD56. Perhaps the most compelling evidence for this comes from our cell sorting experiment in which CD14$^+$ monocytes were flow sorted to ultra-high purity and then subjected to IL-15 DC differentiation. In this experiment, we showed that CD56$^+$ IL-15 DCs can also be differentiated from a virtually pure, FACS-sorted CD14^{++}CD16$^-$ monocyte starting population, thus confirming that these cells are truly monocyte-derived and not related to NK cells. In addition, CD56$^+$ IL-15 DCs fall within the flow cytometric scatter gate of DCs, but not of lymphocytes. The co-expression of the myeloid DC lineage markers BDCA-1 and CD11c along with the absence of CD7 expression, which allows their accurate discrimination from NK cells [26,35], lends further support to the notion that IL-15 DCs are unrelated to NK cells in spite of their partial positivity for CD56.

To corroborate these phenotypic data and to confirm that IL-15 DCs also functionally qualify as DCs, we performed an allo-MLR as well as an antigen presentation assay. Both CD56$^+$ and CD56$^-$ IL-15 DCs are able to stimulate allogeneic T cell proliferation, thereby fulfilling one of the basic functional criteria for being qualified as DCs [29]. Furthermore, in this study, we also show that IL-15 DCs, as would be expected from DCs, are capable of processing and presenting the WT1 tumor antigen [30] to CD8$^+$ T cells. Together with previous observations from our group and others [17,21,22], these data confirm that IL-15 DCs are "authentic" myeloid DCs not only from the phenotypic but also from the functional point of view. Strikingly, in the WT1 antigen presentation assay, CD56$^+$ IL-15 DCs were found to have a superior antigen-presenting capacity over their CD56$^-$ counterparts. Both fractions had comparable expression of the WT1 protein following electroporation (data not shown), suggesting that CD56$^+$ DCs have a higher intrinsic ability to process and present endogenously synthesized antigen to T cells. Although the precise functional role of CD56 on DCs remains to be elucidated, the above data suggest that the expression of CD56 on DCs is linked with superior immunostimulatory activity. This mirrors the situation in NK cells and CD56-expressing T cells where CD56 expression and antigen density correlate with activation status and enhanced immune function [1,36–43]. Further support for this statement comes from the phenotypic data presented in Table 1, which show that CD56$^+$ IL-15 DCs are in a more differentiated and activated modus as compared to their CD56$^-$ counterparts.

The observation that CD56$^+$ IL-15 DCs, in addition to being potent allostimulatory and antigen-presenting cells, are endowed with a cytotoxic capacity is a novel finding that adds to the growing body of evidence that DCs can adopt an "unconventional" cytotoxic effector function and act as killer cells (reviewed in [10–12,14]). Among the stimuli capable of triggering such 'killer DC' function are type I and II IFNs [44–49], TLR ligands [13,48,50–53] and, as shown here and in another recent study, IL-15 [54]. The fact that IL-15, a known growth factor for NK cells [34], was used in this study for DC differentiation as well as the fact that IL-15 DCs were found to be cytotoxic against the NK prototype target K562 [25], prompted us to perform rigorous culture purity assessments in order to exclude the possibility that the observed cytotoxic effects were due to the presence of contaminating NK cells. Based on the model proposed by Stary *et al.* [53], at least 10% of NK cell contaminants would have been needed to account for the cytotoxic activity reported in the present study. The trace contamination (<1%) of IL-15 DC cultures by lymphocytes was thus far too low to account for the observed cytotoxic effects and was therefore considered negligible [53]. This was also further supported by the finding that neither CD56⁻ nor CD56⁺ IL-15 DC preparations had cytotoxic activity against the U937 cell line, another well-recognized NK-sensitive target [25,31].

The lack of cytotoxicity against U937 identifies a second point of difference between IL-15 DCs and NK cells, in addition to the finding that these cells do not share any phenotypic resemblance except for CD56 surface expression. Indeed, as discussed above, IL-15 DCs do not bear any other NK cell-associated surface markers, such as NKG2D or NCRs. The mechanism underlying the ability of NK cells to induce U937 cell death has been recently identified as being NCR-mediated [31], likely explaining the absent cytotoxic activity of IL-15 DCs against U937 cells. Another striking dissimilarity between IL-15 DCs and NK cells that merits further discussion is their differential pattern of cytotoxicity against the K562 cell line. While NK cells are strong and rapid inducers of K562 cell death, the anti-K562 cytotoxic activity of IL-15 DCs occurs only in the higher E:T range and with much slower dynamics. Interestingly, this intrinsically lower lytic potential has also been reported in other 'killer DC' studies and thus appears to be a common feature that distinguishes killer DCs from "classical" cytotoxic effector cells such as NK cells [46,52,53,55–57]. The observation that IL-15 DCs display a distinct lytic profile further supports our view that these cells, despite the non-conforming expression of CD56, should be regarded as *bona fide* DCs endowed will killing potential and not as NK cells with antigen-presenting function [2].

An important finding from this study is that IL-15 killer DCs do not induce cell death of tumor antigen-specific T cells, suggesting that their cytotoxic action is tumor-selective. This is especially noteworthy in view of recent data from Luckey *et al.*, who showed that murine killer DCs are capable of eliminating allergen-specific T cells through a TNF-α-dependent mechanism and, as such, of preventing mice from developing allergic contact dermatitis [58]. In line with this, murine CD8⁺ DCs have been previously shown to be capable of inducing T cell apoptosis through the Fas/FasL pathway [59]. DC-mediated killing of T cells has also been demonstrated in the context of HIV infection [11,60]. Evidently, the possibility of T cell killing would represent a major obstacle to the exploitation of killer DCs for cancer immunotherapy. Our data, however, indicate that T cell-directed cytotoxicity is not a general feature of killer DCs. This is consistent with the emerging view that killer DCs are a heterogeneous population, containing subsets that are preferentially tumoricidal as well as others that appear to be more biased toward a tolerogenic profile (e.g. through their ability for T cell killing) [10].

This heterogeneity also applies to the different cytotoxic effector mechanisms that can be used by killer DCs. FasL and TNF-α, previously described as key components of the lytic armamentarium of killer DCs [10,11,45,59], are not found to be expressed on the IL-15 DC surface, thus arguing against their possible involvement in IL-15 DC-mediated killing. Although they lack membrane expression of TRAIL, IL-15 DCs – in particular the CD56⁺ fraction – harbor an internal pool of TRAIL molecules. Nevertheless, TRAIL neutralization resulted only in a marginal reduction of the lytic activity of CD56⁺ IL-15 DCs against K562 cells, indicating that TRAIL is not a major contributor to the cytotoxic action of these DCs. This is in contrast to several other studies that implied an important role for this death receptor ligand in DC-mediated cytotoxicity [44,46,48,53]. Our results point to granzyme B-induced apoptosis as the main cell death pathway used by IL-15 DCs. The presence of intracellular granzyme B deposits in IL-15 DCs was ascertained by direct gating on the DC population on the basis of a combination of scatter profile and CD11c positivity. The functional importance of this expression was further supported by the capacity of IL-15 DCs to release granzyme B extracellularly and ultimately confirmed by the profound reduction of their cytotoxic activity using concanamycin A, which is commonly used to inhibit the perforin/granzyme B cytotoxic pathway [13,53]. Intriguingly, we were unable to reveal expression of perforin in IL-15 DCs. This observation is in contrast to the study of Stary *et al.* in which TLR7/8-stimulated blood myeloid DCs were found to express both perforin and granzyme B [53], but is congruent with a recent report showing that mouse plasmacytoid DCs can kill in a granzyme B-dependent, perforin-independent fashion [13]. Although puzzling at first sight, the discordant expression of perforin and granzyme B apparently does not preclude IL-15 DCs from inducing K562 cell death. This complements the notion that granzyme B-induced apoptosis can still occur in the absence of perforin, although not with the same efficiency or rapidity [61–63]. The lack of perforin expression in IL-15 DCs may thus provide a plausible explanation for their differential lytic profile as compared to "classical" cytotoxic effector cells such as NK cells, which typically contain high levels of both perforin and granzyme B enabling them to induce rapid target cell death [63,64].

In conclusion, we show here that IL-15 can drive the functional repertoire of human monocyte-derived DCs toward a killer DC profile. This study showcases the considerable potential for phenotypic and functional flexibility of human DCs and provides new converging evidence of the possibility that DCs can adopt a cytotoxic effector function. The observation that IL-15 DCs, in addition to being potent tumor antigen-presenting cells, are endowed with tumoricidal potential provides further strong support to the implementation of IL-15 DCs in DC-based anti-tumor immunotherapy strategies and to the use of IL-15 as an immunostimulatory adjunct in cancer therapy.

Supporting Information

Figure S1 Kinetics of CD56 expression on IL-15 DCs. FACS-purified (>99.9% purity) CD14⁺ monocytes were cultured for 7 days with GM-CSF and IL-15 and analyzed by flow cytometry at the time points indicated for co-expression of CD11c/CD56 (right panels). Samples were stained in parallel with CD11c and an isotype-matched control mAb for CD56 to allow proper gate setting (left panels). Data shown are from a single donor and are representative of two separate experiments.

Figure S2 Lack of cytotoxicity by CD56⁺ and CD56⁻ IL-15 DCs against the U937 target cell line. Residual viability of PKH67-labeled U937 cells after overnight incubation in the absence or presence of either CD56⁻ (□) or CD56⁺ (■) mature IL-15 DCs at an E:T ratio of 50:1. Viability was determined by flow cytometric quantitation of the percentage of PI⁻/Annexin-V⁻ – cells within the PKH67⁺CD11c⁻ gate. Bars represent mean (± SEM) percentages of viable cells from three independent experiments.

Acknowledgments

The authors would like to thank Dr Nathalie Cools for assistance with flow cytometry.

Author Contributions

Conceived and designed the experiments: SA EL IJMdV PDF VFVT ELS ZNB. Performed the experiments: SA EL JT KC PDF. Analyzed the data: SA ZNB. Wrote the paper: SA EL PDF VFVT ELS ZNB.

References

1. Lanier LL, Testi R, Bindl J, Phillips JH (1989) Identity of Leu-19 (CD56) leukocyte differentiation antigen and neural cell adhesion molecule. J Exp Med 169: 2233–2238.
2. Spits H, Lanier LL (2007) Natural killer or dendritic: what's in a name? Immunity 26: 11–16.
3. Hanna J, Gonen-Gross T, Fitchett J, Rowe T, Daniels M, et al. (2004) Novel APC-like properties of human NK cells directly regulate T cell activation. J Clin Invest 114: 1612–1623.
4. Pillarisetty VG, Katz SC, Bleier JI, Shah AB, Dematteo RP (2005) Natural killer dendritic cells have both antigen presenting and lytic function and in response to CpG produce IFN-gamma via autocrine IL-12. J Immunol 174: 2612–2618.
5. Chan CW, Crafton E, Fan HN, Flook J, Yoshimura K, et al. (2006) Interferon-producing killer dendritic cells provide a link between innate and adaptive immunity. Nat Med 12: 207–213.
6. Taieb J, Chaput N, Menard C, Apetoh L, Ullrich E, et al. (2006) A novel dendritic cell subset involved in tumor immunosurveillance. Nat Med 12: 214–219.
7. Blasius AL, Barchet W, Cella M, Colonna M (2007) Development and function of murine B220+CD11c+NK1.1+ cells identify them as a subset of NK cells. J Exp Med 204: 2561–2568.
8. Vosshenrich CA, Lesjean-Pottier S, Hasan M, Richard-Le Goff O, Corcuff E, et al. (2007) CD11cloB220+ interferon-producing killer dendritic cells are activated natural killer cells. J Exp Med 204: 2569–2578.
9. Caminschi I, Ahmet F, Heger K, Brady J, Nutt SL, et al. (2007) Putative IKDCs are functionally and developmentally similar to natural killer cells, but not to dendritic cells. J Exp Med 204: 2579–2590.
10. Wesa AK, Storkus WJ (2008) Killer dendritic cells: mechanisms of action and therapeutic implications for cancer. Cell Death Differ 15: 51–57.
11. Chauvin C, Josien R (2008) Dendritic cells as killers: Mechanistic aspects and potential roles. J Immunol 181: 11–16.
12. Larmonier N, Fraszczak J, Lakomy D, Bonnotte B, Katsanis E (2010) Killer dendritic cells and their potential for cancer immunotherapy. Cancer Immunol Immunother 59: 1–11.
13. Drobits B, Holcmann M, Amberg N, Swiecki M, Grundtner R, et al. (2012) Imiquimod clears tumors in mice independent of adaptive immunity by converting pDCs into tumor-killing effector cells. J Clin Invest 122: 575–585.
14. Chan CW, Housseau F (2008) The 'kiss of death' by dendritic cells to cancer cells. Cell Death Differ 15: 58–69.
15. Anguille S, Van Tendeloo V, Berneman Z (2012) Dendritic cell-based therapeutic vaccination for acute myeloid leukemia. Bull Cancer 99: 635–642.
16. Anguille S, Willemen Y, Lion E, Smits EL, Berneman ZN (2012) Dendritic cell vaccination in acute myeloid leukemia. Cytotherapy 14: 647–656.
17. Anguille S, Smits ELJM, Cools N, Goossens H, Berneman ZN, et al. (2009) Short-term cultured, interleukin-15 differentiated dendritic cells have potent immunostimulatory properties. J Transl Med 7: 109.
18. Jonuleit H, Kuhn U, Muller G, Steinbrink K, Paragnik L, et al. (1997) Pro-inflammatory cytokines and prostaglandins induce maturation of potent immunostimulatory dendritic cells under fetal calf serum-free conditions. Eur J Immunol 27: 3135–3142.
19. Anguille S, Lion E, Smits E, Berneman ZN, van Tendeloo VF (2011) Dendritic cell vaccine therapy for acute myeloid leukemia: questions and answers. Hum Vaccin 7: 579–584.
20. Smits EL, Anguille S, Cools N, Berneman ZN, Van Tendeloo VF (2009) Dendritic cell-based cancer gene therapy. Hum Gene Ther 20: 1106–1118.
21. Mohamadzadeh M, Berard F, Essert G, Chalouni C, Pulendran B, et al. (2001) Interleukin 15 skews monocyte differentiation into dendritic cells with features of Langerhans cells. J Exp Med 194: 1013–1020.
22. Dubsky P, Saito H, Leogier M, Dantin C, Connolly JE, et al. (2007) IL-15-induced human DC efficiently prime melanoma-specific naive CD8+ T cells to differentiate into CTL. Eur J Immunol 37: 1678–1690.
23. Harris KM (2011) Monocytes differentiated with GM-CSF and IL-15 initiate Th17 and Th1 responses that are contact-dependent and mediated by IL-15. J Leukoc Biol 90: 727–734.
24. Provasi E, Genovese P, Lombardo A, Magnani Z, Liu PQ, et al. (2012) Editing T cell specificity towards leukemia by zinc finger nucleases and lentiviral gene transfer. Nat Med 18: 807–815.
25. Lion E, Anguille S, Berneman ZN, Smits EL, Van Tendeloo VF (2011) Poly(I:C) enhances the susceptibility of leukemic cells to NK cell cytotoxicity and phagocytosis by DC. PLoS One 6: e20952.
26. Milush JM, Long BR, Snyder-Cappione JE, Cappione AJ, York VA, et al. (2009) Functionally distinct subsets of human NK cells and monocyte/DC-like cells identified by coexpression of CD56, CD7, and CD4. Blood 114: 4823–4831.
27. Walzer T, Jaeger S, Chaix J, Vivier E (2007) Natural killer cells: from CD3(−)NKp46(+) to post-genomics meta-analyses. Curr Opin Immunol 19: 365–372.
28. Lanier LL, Chang C, Phillips JH (1994) Human NKR-P1A. A disulfide-linked homodimer of the C-type lectin superfamily expressed by a subset of NK and T lymphocytes. J Immunol 153: 2417–2428.
29. Steinman RM, Nussenzweig MC (1980) Dendritic cells: features and functions. Immunol Rev 53: 127–147.
30. Anguille S, Van Tendeloo VF, Berneman ZN (2012) Leukemia-associated antigens and their relevance to the immunotherapy of acute myeloid leukemia. Leukemia 26: 2186–2196.
31. Welte S, Kuttruff S, Waldhauer I, Steinle A (2006) Mutual activation of natural killer cells and monocytes mediated by NKp80-AICL interaction. Nat Immunol 7: 1334–1342.
32. Palucka K, Banchereau J (2012) Cancer immunotherapy via dendritic cells. Nat Rev Cancer 12: 265–277.
33. Figdor CG, de Vries IJ, Lesterhuis WJ, Melief CJ (2004) Dendritic cell immunotherapy: mapping the way. Nat Med 10: 475–480.
34. Farag SS, Caligiuri MA (2006) Human natural killer cell development and biology. Blood Rev 20: 123–137.
35. Bigley V, Spence LE, Collin M (2010) Connecting the dots: monocyte/DC and NK subsets in human peripheral blood. Blood 116: 2859–2860.
36. Robertson MJ, Caligiuri MA, Manley TJ, Levine H, Ritz J (1990) Human natural killer cell adhesion molecules. Differential expression after activation and participation in cytolysis. J Immunol 145: 3194–3201.
37. Pittet MJ, Speiser DE, Valmori D, Cerottini JC, Romero P (2000) Cutting edge: cytolytic effector function in human circulating CD8+ T cells closely correlates with CD56 surface expression. J Immunol 164: 1148–1152.
38. Santin AD, Hermonat PL, Ravaggi A, Bellone S, Roman JJ, et al. (2001) Expression of CD56 by human papillomavirus E7-specific CD8+ cytotoxic T lymphocytes correlates with increased intracellular perforin expression and enhanced cytotoxicity against HLA-A2-matched cervical tumor cells. Clin Cancer Res 7: 804s–810s.
39. Cookson S, Reen D (2003) IL-15 drives neonatal T cells to acquire CD56 and become activated effector cells. Blood 102: 2195–2197.
40. Kelly-Rogers J, Madrigal-Estebas L, O'Connor T, Doherty DG (2006) Activation-induced expression of CD56 by T cells is associated with a reprogramming of cytolytic activity and cytokine secretion profile in vitro. Hum Immunol 67: 863–873.
41. Alexander AA, Maniar A, Cummings JS, Hebbeler AM, Schulze DH, et al. (2008) Isopentenyl pyrophosphate-activated CD56+ {gamma}{delta} T lymphocytes display potent antitumor activity toward human squamous cell carcinoma. Clin Cancer Res 14: 4232–4240.
42. Urban EM, Li H, Armstrong C, Focaccetti C, Cairo C, et al. (2009) Control of CD56 expression and tumor cell cytotoxicity in human Vgamma2Vdelta2 T cells. BMC Immunol 10: 50.
43. Correia MP, Costa AV, Uhrberg M, Cardoso EM, Arosa FA (2011) IL-15 induces CD8+ T cells to acquire functional NK receptors capable of modulating cytotoxicity and cytokine secretion. Immunobiology 216: 604–612.
44. Fanger NA, Maliszewski CR, Schooley K, Griffith TS (1999) Human dendritic cells mediate cellular apoptosis via tumor necrosis factor-related apoptosis-inducing ligand (TRAIL). J Exp Med 190: 1155–1164.
45. Schmitz M, Zhao S, Deuse Y, Schakel K, Wehner R, et al. (2005) Tumoricidal potential of native blood dendritic cells: direct tumor cell killing and activation of NK cell-mediated cytotoxicity. J Immunol 174: 4127–4134.
46. Papewalis C, Jacobs B, Wuttke M, Ullrich E, Baehring T, et al. (2008) IFN-alpha skews monocytes into CD56(+)-expressing dendritic cells with potent functional activities in vitro and in vivo. J Immunol 180: 1462–1470.
47. Anguille S, Lion E, Willemen Y, Van Tendeloo VF, Berneman ZN, et al. (2011) Interferon-alpha in acute myeloid leukemia: an old drug revisited. Leukemia 25: 739–748.
48. Kalb ML, Glaser A, Stary G, Koszik F, Stingl G (2012) TRAIL+ human plasmacytoid dendritic cells kill tumor cells in vitro: mechanisms of imiquimod- and IFN-alpha-mediated antitumor reactivity. J Immunol 188: 1583–1591.
49. Lacasse CJ, Janikashvili N, Larmonier CB, Alizadeh D, Hanke N, et al. (2011) Th-1 lymphocytes induce dendritic cell tumor killing activity by an IFN-gamma-dependent mechanism. J Immunol 187: 6310–6317.
50. Chapoval AI, Tamada K, Chen L (2000) In vitro growth inhibition of a broad spectrum of tumor cell lines by activated human dendritic cells. Blood 95: 2346–2351.
51. Vidalain PO, Azocar O, Yagita H, Rabourdin-Combe C, Servet-Delprat C (2001) Cytotoxic activity of human dendritic cells is differentially regulated by double-stranded RNA and CD40 ligand. J Immunol 167: 3765–3772.
52. Manna PP, Mohanakumar T (2002) Human dendritic cell mediated cytotoxicity against breast carcinoma cells in vitro. J Leukoc Biol 72: 312–320.
53. Stary G, Bangert C, Tauber M, Strohal R, Kopp T, et al. (2007) Tumoricidal activity of TLR7/8-activated inflammatory dendritic cells. J Exp Med 204: 1441–1451.

54. Manna PP, Hira SK, Das AA, Bandyopadhyay S, Gupta KK (2012) IL-15 activated human peripheral blood dendritic cell kill allogeneic and xenogeneic endothelial cells via apoptosis. Cytokine 61: 118–126.

55. Matsui T, Connolly JE, Michnevitz M, Chaussabel D, Yu CI, et al. (2009) CD2 distinguishes two subsets of human plasmacytoid dendritic cells with distinct phenotype and functions. J Immunol 182: 6815–6823.

56. Koski GK, Koldovsky U, Xu S, Mick R, Sharma A, et al. (2012) A novel dendritic cell-based immunization approach for the induction of durable Th1-polarized anti-HER-2/neu responses in women with early breast cancer. J Immunother 35: 54–65.

57. Tel J, Smits EL, Anguille S, Joshi RN, Figdor CG, et al. (2012) Human plasmacytoid dendritic cells are equipped with antigen presenting- and tumoricidal-capacities. Blood 120: 3936–3944.

58. Luckey U, Maurer M, Schmidt T, Lorenz N, Seebach B, et al. (2011) T cell killing by tolerogenic dendritic cells protects mice from allergy. J Clin Invest 121: 3860–3871.

59. Suss G, Shortman K (1996) A subclass of dendritic cells kills CD4 T cells via Fas/Fas-ligand-induced apoptosis. J Exp Med 183: 1789–1796.

60. Barblu L, Machmach K, Gras C, Delfraissy JF, Boufassa F, et al. (2012) Plasmacytoid dendritic cells from HIV controllers produce IFN-alpha and differentiate into functional killer pDC under HIV activation. J Infect Dis 206: 790–801.

61. Choy JC, Hung VH, Hunter AL, Cheung PK, Motyka B, et al. (2004) Granzyme B induces smooth muscle cell apoptosis in the absence of perforin: involvement of extracellular matrix degradation. Arterioscler Thromb Vasc Biol 24: 2245–2250.

62. Pardo J, Wallich R, Ebnet K, Iden S, Zentgraf H, et al. (2007) Granzyme B is expressed in mouse mast cells in vivo and in vitro and causes delayed cell death independent of perforin. Cell Death Differ 14: 1768–1779.

63. Pipkin ME, Lieberman J (2007) Delivering the kiss of death: progress on understanding how perforin works. Curr Opin Immunol 19: 301–308.

64. Thiery J, Keefe D, Boulant S, Boucrot E, Walch M, et al. (2011) Perforin pores in the endosomal membrane trigger the release of endocytosed granzyme B into the cytosol of target cells. Nat Immunol 12: 770–777.

17

Clinical Efficacy of Tumor Antigen-Pulsed DC Treatment for High-Grade Glioma Patients

Jun-Xia Cao[1,2]*, **Xiao-Yan Zhang**[1], **Jin-Long Liu**[1], **Duo Li**[1], **Jun-Li Li**[1], **Yi-Shan Liu**[1], **Min Wang**[1], **Bei-Lei Xu**[1], **Hai-Bo Wang**[1], **Zheng-Xu Wang**[1]*

1 Biotherapy Center, the General Hospital of Beijing Military Command, Beijing, People's Republic of China, **2** Tsinghua-Peking Center for Life Sciences, Laboratory of Dynamic Immunobiology, School of Medicine, School of Life Sciences, Tsinghua University, Beijing, People's Republic of China

Abstract

Background: The effectiveness of immunotherapy for high-grade glioma (HGG) patients remains controversial. To evaluate the therapeutic efficacy of dendritic cells (DCs) alone in the treatment of HGG, we performed a systematic review and meta-analysis in terms of patient survival with relevant published clinical studies.

Materials and methods: A total of 409 patients, including historical cohorts, nonrandomized and randomized controls with HGG, were selected for the meta-analysis.

Results: The treatment of HGG with DCs was associated with a significantly improved one-year survival (OS) ($p < 0.001$) and 1.5-, 2-, 3-, 4-, and 5-year OS ($p < 0.001$) compared with the non-DC group. A meta-analysis of the patient outcome data revealed that DC immunotherapy has a significant influence on progression-free survival (PFS) in HGG patients, who showed significantly improved 1-,1.5-, 2-, 3- and 4-year PFS ($p < 0.001$). The analysis of Karnofsky performance status (KPS) demonstrated no favorable results for DC cell therapy arm ($p = 0.23$). The percentages of $CD3^+CD8^+$ and $CD3^+CD4^+$ T cells and $CD16^+$ lymphocyte subset were not significantly increased in the DC group compared with the baseline levels observed before treatment ($p > 0.05$), whereas $CD56^+$ lymphocyte subset were significantly increased after DC treatment ($p = 0.0001$). Furthermore, the levels of IFN-γ in the peripheral blood of HGG patients, which reflect the immune function of the patients, were significantly increased after DC immunotherapy ($p < 0.001$).

Conclusions: Thus, our meta-analysis showed that DC immunotherapy markedly prolongs survival rates and progression-free time, enhances immune function, and improves the efficacy of the treatment of HGG patients.

Editor: Christopher Wheeler, Cedars-Sinai Medical Center, United States of America

Funding: This research work was supported by the National Natural Science Foundation of China (No. 31171427 and 30971651 to Zheng-Xu Wang); Beijing Municipal Science & Technology Project; Clinical characteristics and Application Research of Capital (No. Z121107001012136 to Zheng-Xu Wang); the National Natural Science Foundation of China (No. 30700974 to Jun-Xia Cao); and the Postdoctoral Foundation of China (No. 20060400775 to Jun-Xia Cao). The funders had no role in study design, data collection and analysis, decision to publish, or preparation of the manuscript.

Competing Interests: The authors have declared that no competing interests exist.

* Email: zhxwang18@hotmail.com (ZXW); 13716111318@139.com (JXC)

Introduction

High-grade gliomas (HGGs) have an incidence currently estimated at 14,000 new diagnoses per year, according to the 2007 World Health Organization (WHO) classification, which includes patients with anaplastic astrocytomas (WHO grade III) and with glioblastoma multiforme (GBM, WHO grade IV) [1]. GBM is the most common and most malignant glioma in adults and represents approximately 75% of all newly diagnosed glioma cases; moreover, the prognosis of these patients remains poor, with a median survival of less than 15 months, despite the use of trimodal therapy [2]. Indeed, there is no conventional treatment that specifically targets tumor cells and spares normal brain parenchyma. Immunologic approaches are theoretically able to

trace, identify, and kill dispersed tumor cells with great accuracy and are being tested to enhance the response of these tumors to existing therapy and/or to stimulate innate immune responses [3].

Based on previous studies, it was assumed that immune reactions do not occur in the brain because of the blood-brain barrier (BBB); however, we now have an in-depth understanding that the central nervous system maintains a two-way communication network with the immune system, with each having a profound influence on the other [4]. Several studies have clarified that lymphocytes and antigen-presenting cells (APCs), including macrophages and dendritic cells (DCs), are able to cross the blood-brain barrier and migrate to a tumor within the brain parenchyma [5]. Thus, in phase I and phase II trials, adoptive immunotherapy including lymphokine-activated killer cells (LAK), cytotoxic T lymphocytes (CTLs) and tumor-infiltrating T lymphocytes (TILs) and active immunotherapy using autologous tumor cells (ATCs) and DCs have demonstrated clinical efficacy, suggesting that immunotherapy may be a useful strategy to combat HGGs [6].

DCs are the most potent APCs in the human body. Importantly, DCs can cross the BBB and traffic into perivascular and parenchymal spaces in the glioma [5,7]. An important milestone has been reached with the recent approval in 2010 of sipuleucel-T (Provenge), the first DC vaccine for hormone-resistant metastatic prostate cancer. This vaccine is primarily an active immunologic agent with proven activity against solid tumors [8]. In HGG, a cohort comparison trial involving 45 children, HGG-IMMUNO-2003, has been conducted since 2001 to implement and improve immunotherapeutic approaches [9]. Additionally, another clinical trial of 77 newly diagnosed glioblastoma patients was performed [10]. In addition, a Phase I/II single-arm clinical trial, HGG-2006, was designed and conducted using 117 patients [11]. In brief, all of the data showed a remarkable overall survival (OS) compared with the generally expected progression of this disease. Thus, both hope and challenges exist for DC-based immunotherapy. These data compelled the design of the current prospective placebo-controlled, double-blind Phase IIb stratified randomized clinical trial (EudraCT number 2009-018228-14) and the Phase III study of DCVax in GBM, which has been registered at ClinicalTrials.gov (NCT00045968).

Unfortunately, due to profound tumor-associated mechanisms of immunosuppression and evasion, immunotherapeutic strategies have thus far not translated into clinical success [12]. There are several reviews that summarize more than 21 DC clinical trials that were performed in HGG in which up to 500 patients were involved, excluding controls. These studies always used historical or nonrandomized cohorts due to the disease's malignancy [13–15]. However, evidence from the meta-analysis through logistic regression regarding the OS, PFS, and other outcomes of the therapy remains scarce. Here, we addressed the effect of the autologous tumor antigen-pulsed DCs on the treatment of glioma patients in terms of survival compared with historical cohorts or nonrandomized and randomized control groups.

Materials and Methods

2.1 Literature search and inclusion and exclusion criteria

The trials analyzed in this study were identified through an electronic search of the PubMed database, the Cochrane Central Registry of Controlled Trials, the Wanfang Database, the China Science and Technology Periodical Database, China Journal Net, reference lists of published trials, and relevant review articles. The search strategy included the medical subject headings "glioma", "immunotherapy", "dendritic cells", and free text search. No language limits were applied. The initial search was performed on Nov 2013 and was updated in Jan 2014. Furthermore, manual searches were performed in reference lists and conference proceedings of the American Society of Clinical Oncology (ASCO) Annual Meetings and the European Cancer Conference (ECCO). We excluded abstracts that were never subsequently published as full papers and studies on animals and cell lines.

2.2 Study selection and data extraction

We collected various sets of information, including the authors' names, journal and year of publication, sample size per arm, newly or recurrent, regimen used, median or mean age of the patients, Karnofsky performance status (KPS), DC antigen, delivery route and dose, and characteristics of the study design (i.e., whether the

trial reported the mode of randomization, allocation concealment, description of withdrawals per arm, and blinding) for all of the trials included in the study. The data were independently screened by two reviewers.

2.3 Definition of outcome measures

Overall survival (OS) was defined as the time from the initiation of treatment until death from any cause. The secondary endpoint was progression-free survival (PFS), which was documented and extracted for analysis. Quality of Life (QoL) was assessed by the KPS. The immune response was assessed by evaluating and comparing the data of surface phenotype of the patients' peripheral blood lymphocytes by FACScan from the recruited papers, including $CD3^+$, $CD4^+$, $CD8^+$, $CD16^+$ and $CD56^+$ of each study. Furthermore, we approximately collected the data of $CD3^+CD8^+$ and $CD3^+CD4^+$ as the T cell subpopulation and $CD16^+$ and $CD56^+$ as other cell subset. In addition we also extracted the data of the cytokine IFN-γ tested by ELISA kit from the included papers.

2.4 Statistical analysis

The analysis was performed using Review Manager Version 5.0 (Nordic Cochran Centre, Copenhagen, Denmark). In our meta-analysis, we compared the immunotherapy-containing arms of the selected trials to the respective non-immunotherapy arms. The treatment effects are reflected by the odds ratios (OR) for OS and PFS. The OS and PFS data in each arm were extracted from each included study, and the pooled odds ratio (OR) was calculated through the Mantel and Haenszel method. A pooled OR<1 indicated a lower recurrence or lower survival in the immunotherapy arm. We used Cochran's Q test, a chi-squared test with a df equal to the number of studies minus one that tests the null hypothesis and demonstrates whether the difference among the studies based on the OR is due to chance, to evaluate whether the studies' results were homogeneous. Also calculated in the analysis was the quantity I^2, which describes the percentage of variation across studies that is due to heterogeneity rather than chance. Generally speaking, I^2 values of 25% represent low heterogeneity, and subsequently, I^2 values of 50% and 75% were used as evidence of moderate and high heterogeneity, respectively. When no statistically significant heterogeneity existed, the OR was calculated with a fixed-effect model; otherwise, a random-effect model was employed. P-values of <0.05 were considered to be statistically significant. All reported P-values resulted from two-sided versions of the respective tests [16].

Results

3.1 Selection of the trials

The electronic search yielded 189 references. After a title and abstract review, 158 publications were excluded for different reasons (nine for being review articles, 11 for using *in vitro* experiments, 26 for being animal models, 91 for being case reports, and 21 for being DC protocol studies or comments) (Tables S1–S5 in File S1). A total of 31 clinical trials were selected as potentially relevant, and their full texts were retrieved for a more detailed assessment. We then excluded 22 of these 31 studies for not having a control arm or not providing detailed patient clinical data and details on the therapeutic response (Table S6 in File S1). The procedure used to select the clinical trials is shown in Figure 1. As a result, 9 articles reporting clinical trials of DC-based therapy were selected for the meta-analysis [17–25] (Table S7 in File S1).

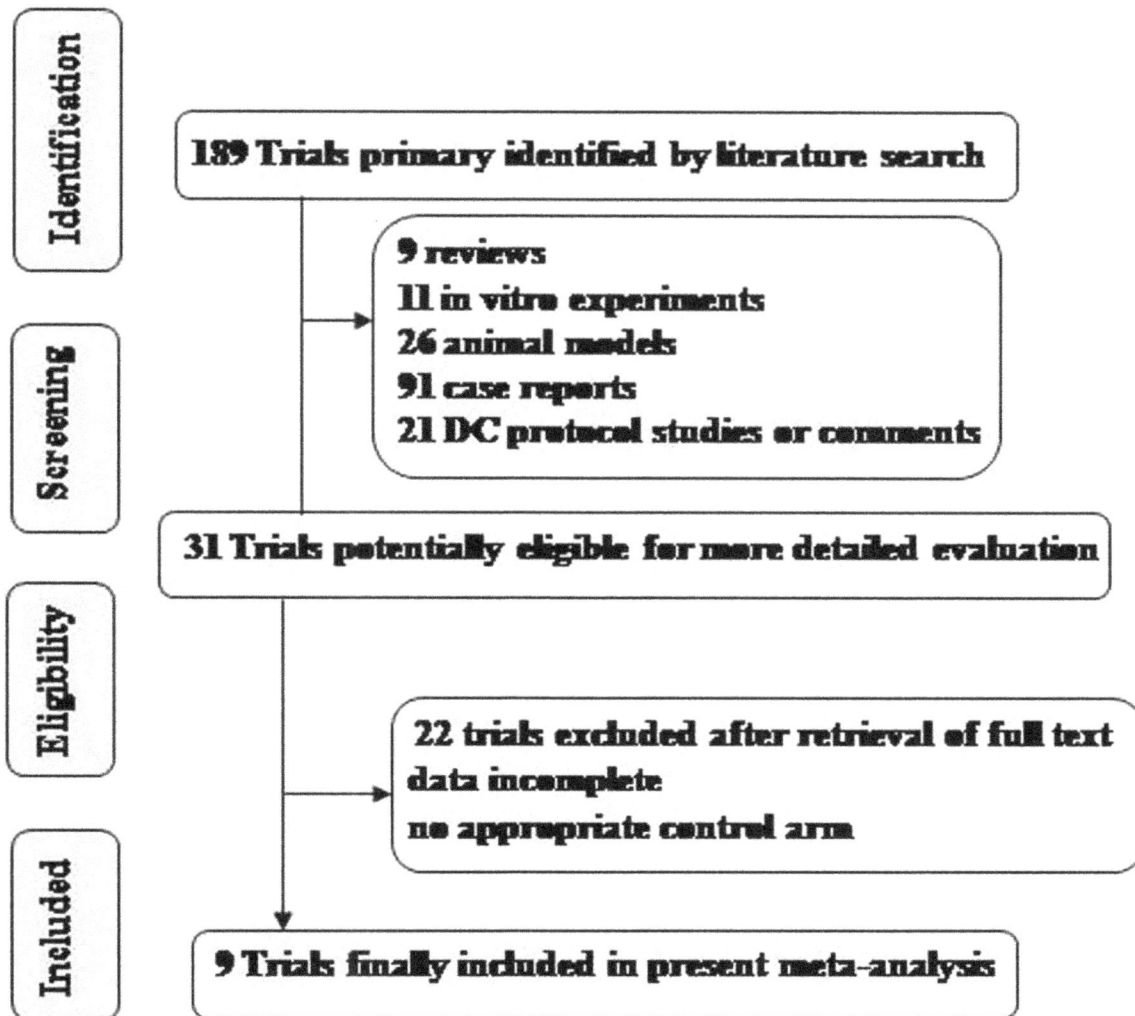

Figure 1. Flow diagram showing record identification, screening and study inclusion process.

3.2 Characteristics of DC cell-based therapy

After the selection process, 9 eligible trials with a total of 409 patients to date were included in the present analysis. All of the trials were fully published: three phase I trials [20,21,23], five phase I/II trials [17,18,19,22,24] and one phase II trials [25]. The clinical data of the trials are shown in Table 1. The median age of the included patients was <50 years. The WHO grade was mainly IV for the included HGG patients. All of the patients had experienced surgery (ST, surgical resection), chemotherapy (CT, chemical therapy), radiotherapy (RT, radiation therapy), and intra-cellular hyperthermia (ICH). The included patients were mainly recurrent containing some of new ones, and also only one trial recruited the new patients [25], which have been listed on Table 1. The patients' KPS have all been reported before immunotherapy and the value was mainly more than 60, but after the treatment only two of them reported [17,25]. Additionally, most of the included patients received the DC therapy without any other simultaneous treatment, and the controls were four historical cohorts [17,18,20,23], three nonrandomized cohorts [19,21,22] and two randomized cohorts [24,25].

The method for the preparation of DCs is now well established, and a sufficient number of DCs can be generated for injection into patients. In Table 1, we summarized the patient information about the DC treatment. DCs were matured using cocktails containing GM-CSF, IL-4, TNF-α, IL-1β, or PGE2. The number of DCs injected ranged from 1×10^6 to 5×10^8. The frequency of the injections was highly variable in different trials. The sources of antigen were also different, but most that were included in our meta-analysis were derived from tumor cells: autologous irradiated tumor cells (AIT), autologous tumor lysate (ATL), HLA-1-eluted peptides (HLP), autologous acid-eluted tumor peptides (ATP), and autologous heat-shock tumor cells (AHT). One trial reported DC treatment with fusions of glioma cells [21]. The routes of DC injection used were mainly intradermal (i.d.), intratumoral (i.t.), and subcutaneous (s.c.).

3.3 Survival

0.5-year overall survival. Information on the 0.5-year survival was available for six trials [17–19,20,23,24]. These six trials contained 320 patients in total (80 patients received DC therapy, and 240 patients not receiving DC therapy were used as a control). Although the 0.5-year OS rates were 96% (77/80) for glioma patients receiving the DC treatment and 88% (211/240) for the historical or nonrandomized and randomized control

Table 1. Clinical information of the eligible trials for the meta-analysis.

Trial reference	Tumor characteristics WHO grade	Clinical trial phase	Patients (male) and control	Median age	Pre-Therapy KPS	Previous treatment	DC Arm Injection	DC regimens	Culture of DC cells
Chen-Nen Chang2011[17]	New or Recurrent III/IV	I/II	17(8); 63(UK); historical	44.7; UK	Median; 90	CT/RT	DCs loaded with AIT (s.c)	1.0–6.1×10^7/course	GM-CSF, IL-4
Ryuya Yamanaka 2005[18]	RecurrentIII/IV	I/II	24(16); 27(UK); historical	48.9; 55.9	Median; 62.5	SR/RT, CT	DCs loaded with ATL (i.d or i.t)	3.9–240.9×10^6/course	GM-CSF, IL-4, KLH
Christopher J Wheeler 2004[19]	De novo IV	I/II	25(11); 25(13); randomized	55; 50	>60	SR/CT, RT	DCs loaded with ATL or HLP	10–40×10^6/course	UK
Linda M.Liau 2005[20]	New or Recurrent IV	I	12(5); 99(UK); historical	40.4; <50	≥60	CT/ICH	DCs loaded with ATP	1–10×10^6/course	GM-CSF, IL-4
Tetsuro Kikuchi 2001[21]	Recurrent UK	I	8(7)	38	Median 70	SR/CT, RT	DCs fused with AIT (i.d)	2.4–8.7×10^6/course	GM-CSF, IL-4, TNF-α
R Yamanaka 2003[22]	Recurrent UK	I/II	10(4)	46	Median 54	SR/RT	DCs loaded with ATL (i.d)	10–137.2×10^6/course	GM-CSF, IL-4, KLH
John S. Yu 2004[23]	New or Recurrent UK	I	14(10); 26(UK); historical	45; 53	≥60	SR/CT	DCs loaded with ATL (i.d)	10^7–10^8/course	GM-CSF, IL-4
X.Jie 2012[24]	Recurrent IV	I/II	13(10); 12(9); randomized	40.2; 43.1	≥60	SR/RT, CT	DCs loaded with AHT and GM-CSF(s.c)	6×10^6/course	GM-CSF, IL-4, IL-1β, PGE2, TNF-α
Der-Yang Cho 2011[25]	New IV	II	18(8); 16(8); randomized	58.6; 55.8	>70	SR/CT, RT	DCs loaded with ATL(s.c)	2–5×10^7/course	GM-CSF, IL-4

The table summarizes the patients' basic information about the tumor stage, newly or recurrent, cases, age, KPS, operative method before the immunotherapy and details of the immunotherapy including the DC, tumor antigen, and loading route. The last row is the culture conditions used for the cells. KPS: Karnofsky performance status; AIT: Autologous irradiated tumor cells; ATL: Autologous tumor lysate; HLP: HLA-1-eluted peptides; ATP: Autologous acid-eluted tumor peptides; AHT: Autologous heat-shock tumor cells; CT: Chemical therapy; SR: Surgical resection; RT: Radiation therapy; KLH: Keyhole limpet hemocyanin; PGE2: Prostaglandin E2; TNF-α: Tumor necrosis factor-α; IL-4: Interleukin-4; i.d: intradermalvaccination; i.t.: intratumoral vaccination; s.c.:subcutaneous injection; ICH: intra-cellular hyperthermia; UK: Unknown.

cohorts, the estimated pooled OR for these six trials did not show a significantly improved 0.5-year OS for patients who received DC therapy compared with the non-DC therapy group (OR 2.49, 95% CI 0.85 – 7.26, $P = 0.09$). Cochran's Q test yielded a P value of 0.45, and the corresponding I^2 quantity was 0%, indicating that the degree of variability between the trials was consistent with what would be expected to occur by chance alone (Figure 2A).

1-year overall survival. Information on the 1-year survival was available for seven trials [17–20,23–25]. These seven trials contained 354 patients in total (98 patients received DC therapy, and 256 control patients did not receive DC therapy). The 1-year overall survival rate was 82% (80/98) for glioma patients receiving the DC treatment, whereas it was 63% (160/256) for the controls. The meta-analysis showed a significantly improved 1-year OS for the patients who received DC therapy compared with those who did not (OR 2.89, 95% CI 1.58–5.27, $P = 0.0006$). Cochran's Q test yielded a P value of 0.09, and the corresponding I^2 quantity was 45% (Figure 2A).

1.5-year overall survival. Information on the 1.5-year survival was available for six trials [17–20,23,24]. These six trials contained 320 patients in total (80 patients received DC therapy, and 240 patients who did not receive DC therapy served as a control). The 1.5-year overall survival rates were 59% (47/80) for glioma patients receiving DC treatment and 28% (66/240) for controls. The meta-analysis showed a significant benefit for the 1.5-year OS in the HGG patients who received DC therapy compared with non-DC therapy (OR 5.13, 95% CI 2.80–9.41, $P<0.00001$). Cochran's Q test yielded a P value of 0.35, and the corresponding I2 quantity was 10% ($<50\%$), indicating that the degree of variability between the trials was consistent with what would be expected to occur by chance alone (Figure 2A).

2-year overall survival. Information on the 2-year survival was available for seven trials [17–20,23–25]. These seven trials contained 354 patients in total (98 patients received DC therapy, and 256 patients who did not receive DC therapy served as a control). The 2-year OS rates were 34% (33/98) for glioma patients receiving DC treatment and 14% (35/256) for the controls. The estimated pooled OR for these seven trials showed a significantly increased 2-year OS for the patients who received DC therapy compared with those who did not (OR 4.69, 95% CI 2.48–8.85, $P<0.00001$). Cochran's Q test had a P value of 0.50, and the corresponding I^2 quantity was 0% (Figure 2A).

3-year overall survival. Information on the 3-year survival was available for six trials [17–20,23,25]. These six trials included 354 patients in total (98 patients received DC therapy, and 256 patients who did not receive DC therapy were used as controls). The 3-year OS rate was 24% (24/98) for glioma patients receiving DC treatment, whereas it was 4% (10/256) for the controls. The meta-analysis showed a significantly longer 3-year OS for the patients who received DC therapy compared with those who did not (OR 11.52, 95% CI 4.66–28.45, $P<0.00001$). Cochran's Q test had a P value of 0.82, and the corresponding I^2 quantity was 0% (Figure 2B).

4-year overall survival. Information on the 4-year survival was available for five trials [17–20,23]. These five trials contained 320 patients in total (80 patients received DC therapy, and 240 patients who did not receive DC therapy were used as a control). The 4-year OS rates were 20% (16/80) for glioma patients receiving DC treatment and 1% (3/240) for the controls. The meta-analysis showed a significant improvement of the 4-year OS in the HGG patients who received DC therapy compared with those who did not (OR 16.61, 95% CI 5.06–54.52, $P<0.00001$). Cochran's Q test had a P value of 0.97, and the corresponding I^2 quantity was 0% (Figure 2B).

5-year overall survival. Information on the 5-year survival was available for two trials [17,20]. These two trials contained 216 patients in total (42 patients received DC therapy, and 174 control patients did not). The 5-year OS rate was 14% (6/42) for glioma patients receiving the DC treatment, whereas it was ultimately 0% (0/174) for the controls. The meta-analysis showed a significantly greater 5-year OS for the patients who received DC therapy compared with those who did not (OR 44.40, 95% CI 5.00–394.16, $P = 0.0007$). Cochran's Q test had a P value of 0.69, and the corresponding I^2 quantity was 0% (Figure 2B), indicating that the degree of variability between the trials was consistent with what would be expected to occur by chance alone.

0.5-year progression-free survival. Information on the 0.5-year PFS was available for two trials [20,25] and contained 145 patients (30 patients received DC immunotherapy) (Figure 3A). DC immunotherapy led to a 0.5-year PFS in 77% (23/30) of glioma patients. In contrast, the 0.5-year PFS was only 68% (78/115) in patients without DC immunotherapy. However, the results showed that there was no significant improvement of the 0.5-year PFS for the patients who received DC therapy compared with the non-DC therapy group (OR 1.89, 95% CI 0.66–5.42, $P = 0.24$). Cochran's Q test had a P value of 0.73, and the corresponding I^2 quantity was 0%.

1-, 1.5-, and 2-year progression-free survival. Information on the 1-, 1.5-, and 2-year PFS was available for two trials [20,25], which contained 145 patients (30 patients received DC immunotherapy) (Figure 3A). DC immunotherapy led to a 1-, 1.5-, and 2-year PFS of 70%, 50%, and 37% (21/30, 15/30 and 11/30), respectively, in HGG patients who received DC treatment, whereas the 1-, 1.5-, and 2-year PFS in the controls was only 32%, 15%, and 3% (37/115, 17/115, and 4/115), respectively. Both of the trials showed a longer disease-free survival for patients who received DC immunotherapy in comparison to the historical or randomized cohorts at one, one and a half and two years. The estimated pooled OR for the two trials showed a highly significantly improved one, one and a half, and two-year PFS for patients receiving DC immunotherapy (OR 5.33, 95% CI 1.98–14.36, $P = 0.0009$; OR 7.49, 95% CI 2.58–21.75, $P = 0.0002$; OR 17.04, 95% CI 3.76–77.17, $P = 0.0002$) (Figure 3A). The overall Cochran's Q test yielded a P value of 0.36, and the corresponding I^2 quantity was 9% ($<50\%$).

3- and 4-year progression-free survival. Information on the 3- and 4-year PFS was available for two trials [20,25] and contained 145 patients (30 patients received DC immunotherapy) (Figure 3B). DC immunotherapy led to a 3- and 4-year PFS of 27% (8/30) in glioma patients. In contrast, the 3- and 4-year PFS was only 1% (1/115) in patients who did not receive DC immunotherapy. Both trials showed a longer PFS for DC immunotherapy in comparison to the controls at three and four years. The estimated pooled OR for the two trials showed a highly significantly improved three- and four-year PFS for patients receiving DC immunotherapy (OR 17.99, 95% CI 2.16–149.80, $P = 0.008$). The overall Cochran's Q test had a P value of 1.00, and the corresponding I^2 quantity was 0%.

3.4 Function response rate

The analysis of KPS demonstrated no favorable results for the DC cell therapy arm, with the OR being 26.58 (95% CI −16.71–69.86, $P = 0.23$). The overall Cochran's Q test yielded $P<0.00001$, and the corresponding I^2 quantity was 95% ($>50\%$) (Figure 4).Thus the random effects model was used in this analysis and it showed that the significant heterogeneity exist between the extracted data of KPS.

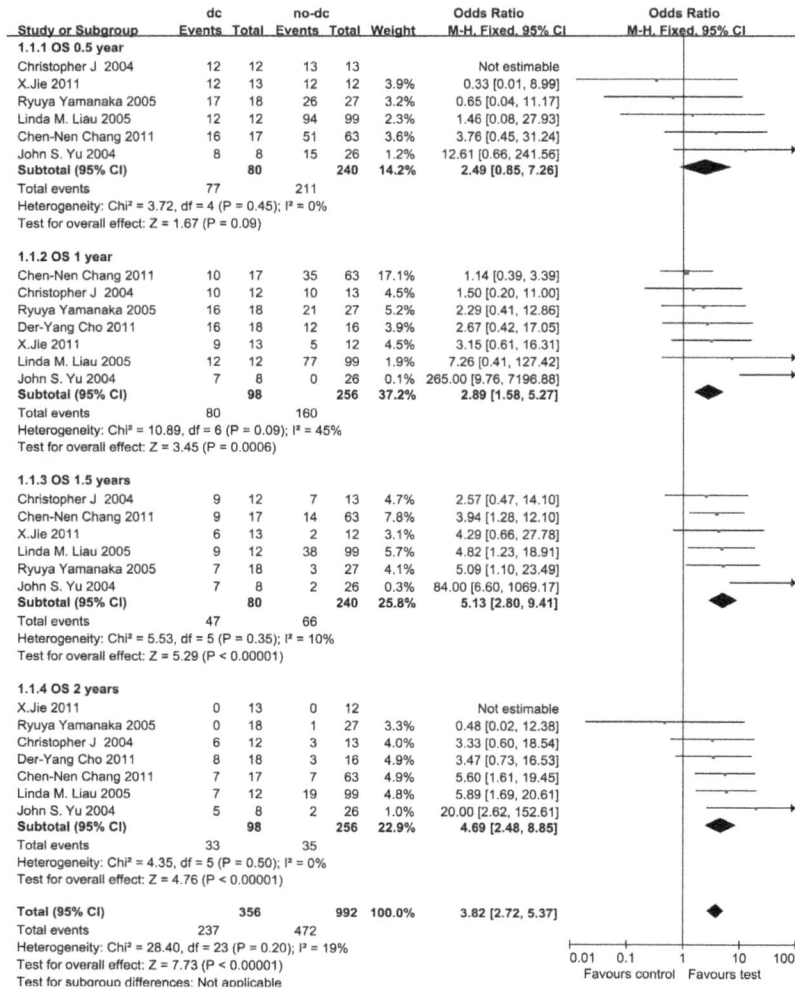

A

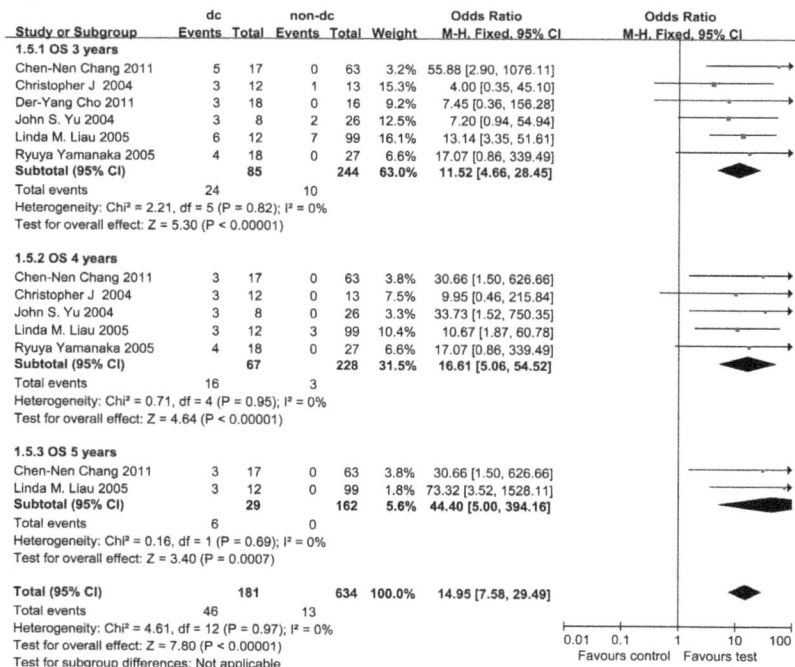

B

Figure 2. Comparison of 0.5-, 1-, 1.5- and 2-year overall survival (OS) between the non-DC and DC groups (A); Forest plot for 3-, 4-, and 5-year OS between the non-DC and DC groups in HGG patients (B). The fixed-effects meta-analysis model (Mantel-Haenszel method) was used. OR, odds ratio. DC, DC-containing therapy; non-DC, non-DC-containing therapy. Each trial is represented by a square, the center of which gives the odds ratio for that trial. The size of the square is proportional to the information in that trial. The ends of the horizontal bars denote a 95% CI. The black diamond gives the overall odds ratio for the combined results of all trials.

3.5 Immune response

Lymphocyte/monocyte subsets in patients. The analysis showed that the proportions of $CD3^+CD8^+$ and $CD3^+CD4^+$ cells were not significantly increased in the DC group compared with the baseline levels observed before treatment, as reflected by pooled MD values of -1.21 (95% CI $= -7.89$–5.48, $p = 0.72$) and -0.46 (95% CI $= -8.31$–7.39, $p = 0.91$) [21,22,24]. Cochran's Q test had P values of 0.14 and 0.02, while the corresponding I^2 quantities were 49% and 73%. $CD16^+$ cells were also not significantly increased in the DC group compared with the baseline levels observed before treatment, as reflected by pooled MD values of -0.79 (95% CI $= -4.62$–3.05, $p = 0.69$), cochran's Q test had a P value of 0.86, while the corresponding I^2 quantity was 0%. Whereas $CD56^+$ lymphocyte subset was significantly increased after DC treatment with pooled MD values of -5.26 (95% CI $= -7.96$–-2.55, $p = 0.0001$) (Figure 5A). Cochran's Q test had a P value of 0.93, while the corresponding I^2 quantity was 0%.

Immune cytokine levels of patients. As a consequence of stimulation by DCs, the $CD4^+$ cells release cytokines, such as IL-2, IL-6, IFN-γ, TNF, and lymphotoxin (LT), which assist in the expansion of the $CD8^+$ cytotoxic T lymphocytes (CTLs). In our analysis, the levels of IFN-γ (OR = -53.16, 95% CI $= -59.72$–-46.59, $p < 0.00001$) were significantly increased after DC treatment (Figure 5B) [21,24]. Cochran's Q test had a P value of 0.41, while the corresponding I^2 quantity was 0%, indicating that there was no evidence of heterogeneity among the individual studies. This finding indicated that the degree of variability among the trials was consistent with what would occur by chance.

Discussion

DC therapy is based on the concept that GBM cells are poor APCs because of the down regulation of costimulatory molecules and the release of immunoinhibitory cytokines [6]. DCs are professional APCs that phagocytose foreign antigens and present them in the context of MHC to activate innate and adaptive immune cells [8]. Thus, DC immunotherapy is widely considered as the fourth treatment modality for patients with cancer [26].

Our systematic meta-analysis yielded several major findings. First, we demonstrated that DC immunotherapy can significantly improve the 1-, 1.5-, 2-, 3-, 4-, and 5-year OS ($p < 0.001$) of HGG patients compared with the non-treatment group. Then, a meta-analysis of the outcome of the patient data revealed that DC immunotherapy has a significant influence on the 1-, 1.5-, 2-, 3-, and 4-year PFS ($p < 0.001$). But, the results of the analysis of KPS demonstrated no favorable outcome for DC cell therapy arm ($p = 0.23$). Furthermore, the percentages of $CD3^+CD8^+$ and $CD3^+CD4^+$ T cells and $CD16^+$ lymphocyte cells were not significantly increased in the DC group compared with the baseline levels observed before treatment ($p > 0.05$), but $CD56^+$ lymphocyte cells were significantly increased after DC treatment ($p < 0.001$). In addition, after DC immunotherapy, the levels of IFN-γ in the peripheral blood of HGG patients, which reflect the immune function of the patients, were significantly increased ($p < 0.001$). Overall, according to our analysis, DC therapy can prolong OS, improve the disease recurrence time, and would involve in the immunity function. Hence, our meta-analysis

demonstrated that DC immunotherapy is a promising therapy method for HGG patients.

To date, most recent phase I and II trials have exhibited the median overall survival is increased by 20% after administration of an autologous DC vaccine for patients with GBM [17,27]. Thus, in a meta-analysis of the collected data, our comprehensive results showed that the 1-, 1.5-, 2-, 3-, 4-, and 5-year OS rates were 82%, 59%, 34%, 24%, 20%, and 14%, respectively, which is slightly different from the results observed with the independent trials and the median overall survival was about 29%. Yet, the positive trend held consistent compared with the historical or the randomized and nonrandomized controls, which maintained 63%, 28%, 14%, 4%, 1%, and 0 OS rates, respectively and the median overall survival was about 9%. So through logistic regression, our data analysis also showed that DC immunotherapy can significantly prolong the OS in HGG patients ($p < 0.001$) by increasing median OS 20%.

Regarding PFS, the data were described in only two studies of 145 patients with historical cohorts or randomized controls. The summarized results showed that the 1-, 1.5-, 2-, 3-, and 4-year PFS rates were 70%, 50%, 37%, and 27%, respectively, compared with the controls, which maintained 32%, 15%, 3%, and 1% PFS rates. Our meta-analysis showed that DC immunotherapy benefits the PFS, which could be up to 50% at the 1.5-year mark. It was previously reported that independent clinical trials of Phase II studies with other immunotherapy methods in recurrent GBM showed that the median PFS is 20 weeks [28], and in another Phase II trial with newly diagnosed GBM, the time for the median PFS is 14.2 months [29]. Although there are quite a few differences among the trials, the positive trend of the meta-analysis was fully confirmed, and the advantage of logistic regression for the data analysis was obvious, revealing that DC immunotherapy has a significant influence on the 1-, 1.5-, 2-, 3-, and 4-year PFS ($p < 0.001$). As a matter of fact, immunotherapy would ameliorate some of the symptoms: patients had increased appetite, improved sleep, gained body weight, and pain relief. But in our meta-analysis, DC immunotherapy may not improve the life quality of postoperative patients ($p = 0.23$) by comparing KPS before and after treatment on the Figure 4.

Immunologic evidence of the response to DC therapy was assessed by comparing the levels of immunologic cell types ($CD3^+CD8^+$, $CD4^+CD8^+$, $CD16^+$ and $CD56^+$ cells) and certain cytokines (IFN-γ) before and after DC treatment. Our meta-analysis showed that following DC therapy, there was a significant increase in the IFN-γ ($p < 0.001$) levels compared with those in non-DC patients, suggesting the induction of an immune response in these patients with DC treatment. The concept of immune-editing is to use immunotherapy as a treatment strategy in response to a major challenge presented to the immune system [30]. Immune-editing consists of 3 phases: elimination, equilibrium, and escape. Elimination refers to the antitumor function of both the adaptive and innate immune system and is driven by the production of IFN-γ. It was demonstrated that IFN-γ production levels from post-vaccine peripheral blood mononucleated cell (PBMC) correlated significantly with patient survival and time to progression [31]. Here, our meta-analysis demonstrated that IFN-γ was significantly increased after DC treatment and thus would

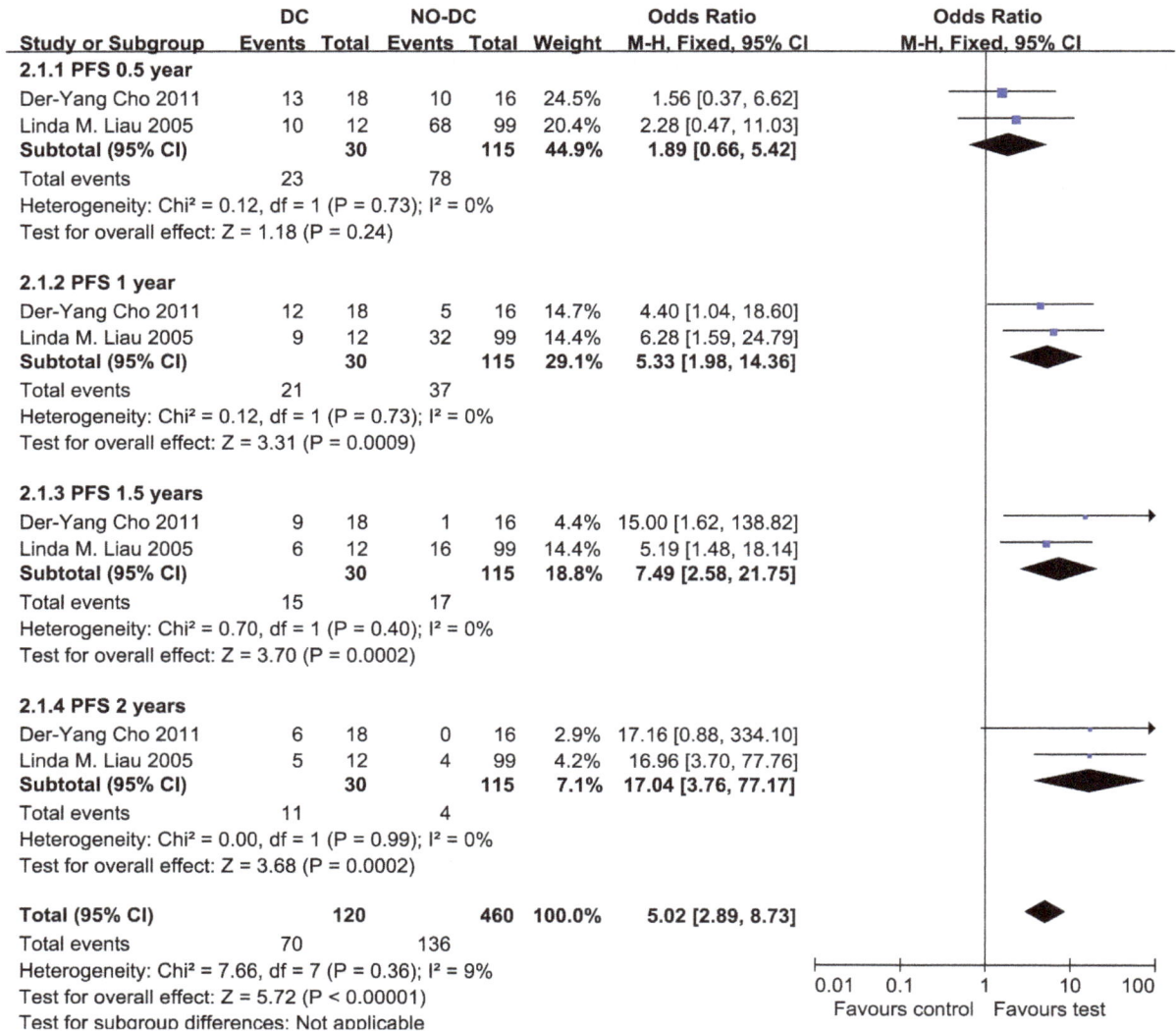

A

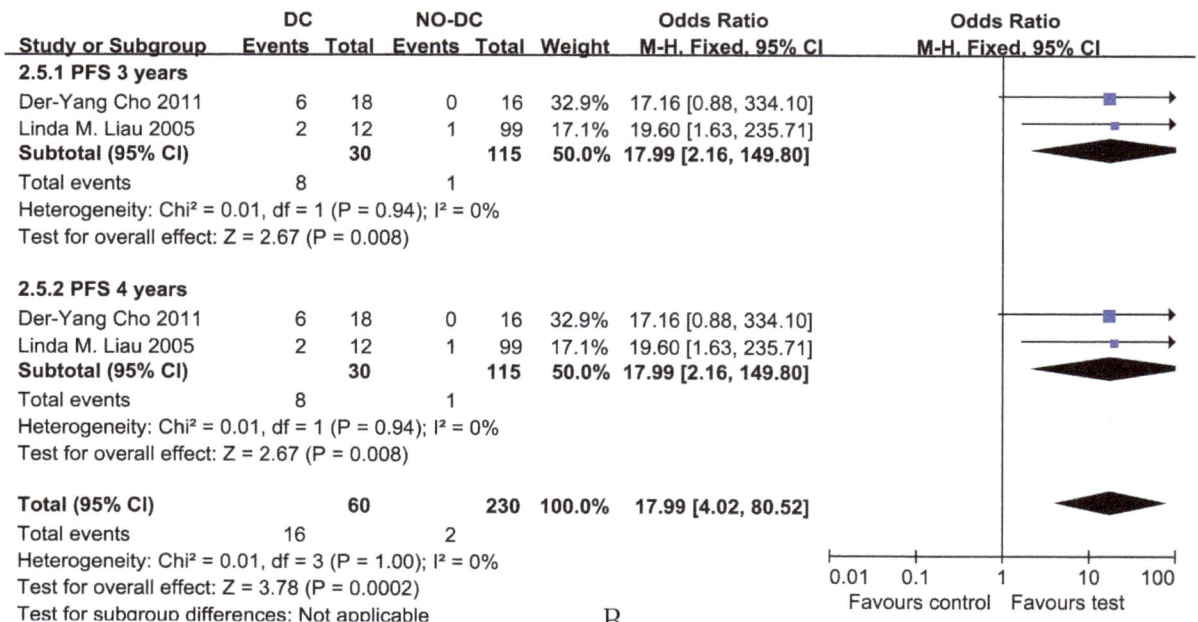

B

Figure 3. Comparison of 0.5-, 1-, 1.5-, and 2-year progression-free survival (PFS) between the non-DC and DC groups (A); Forest plot for 3-, 4-, and 5-year PFS between the non-DC and DC groups in HGG patients (B). The fixed effects meta-analysis model (Mantel-Haenszel method) was used in this analysis.

be helpful in immune-editing to compensate for the elimination. But it should be noted that only two trials were included, and the method for measure IFN-γ was not used ELISPOT and/or ICS. Furthermore, in the included studies, there were some trials in which they detected the IFN-γ with ELISPOT only reported the individual response of the patients [18,22] or qPCR to calculate the multiples or the percentage of the response after the immunotherapy [19,23], but could not be analyzed in our meta-analysis. Thus the quantification of IFN-γ in sera was not consistent in all the studies, that could induce the big heterogeneity among these studies.

Another notable challenge is the presence of an immunosuppressive tumor microenvironment, which causes decreased antigen recognition and depressed immune cell activation. Although increased CD8+ infiltrating lymphocytes have been shown in some studies to be associated with increased patient survival, Hussain et al. reported that most tumor-infiltrating CD8+ cells are not activated [2,32]. In our meta-analysis, the results showed that the CD3+CD8+ and CD4+CD8+ levels were not significantly changed after DC treatment. In addition, our meta-analysis that included only three trials showed CD16+ and CD56+ lymphocyte cells which would denote some of the NK cells, could combat the tumor cells and play an immunomodulatory function, inducing a Th1 immune response and improving antitumor immunoreactivity in the body [33]. Among them CD16+ was not significantly increased after DC treatment, but CD56+ was significantly increased after DC immunotherapy according to our meta-analysis with the included papers.

Equilibrium is the period in which immune cells become latent to a partially eradicated tumor. Escape occurs when the tumor escapes from immunosurveillance and becomes resistant to antitumor immune function, usually via genomic instability or downregulation of key antigens [34]. Thus, to induce a tumor-specific immune reaction via DCs, which is the basis of DC immunotherapy, DCs are loaded with various antigens and then activate both helper T cells and B cells. So far, the different tumor-associated antigens (TAAs) used include specific tumor-associated peptides, tumor-derived RNA and cDNA, tumor cell lysate, apoptotic tumor cells, and gene transfer methods using retroviral vectors, recombinant adenoviruses or lentiviruses encoding tumor antigens, and electroporation of tumor RNA into DCs to increase the target accuracy and overcome the tumor immunosuppression [35]. In our meta-analysis, the selected

clinical trials with DC only used the following tumor antigens: autologous irradiated tumor cells, tumor lysate and acid-eluted tumor peptides or heat-shock tumor cells that compensate for tumor antigen exposure. Other antigens were not included in our meta-analysis, especially EGFRvIII, IL-13Rα, EphA2, survivin, Wilms' tumor 1 (WT1), Sry-related high mobility group box (SOX), and cytomegalovirus (CMV), but have been tested in some clinical trials [36]. Furthermore, cancer stem cells (CSCs) or cancer-initiating cells can also be a potentially useful source of tumor antigens in DC-based immunotherapy, and some of the preclinical data are potentially encouraging [37]. Thus, multiple questions need to be clarified regarding the identification of suitable antigens and improvement of the tumor cell targeting accuracy precluding the eventually successful translation of DC immunotherapy into clinical applications.

More recent transcriptional profiling has classified GBM molecularly into four subtypes with distinct clinical features. Prins et al. showed the difference of sensitivity to a whole-cell lysate DC vaccination between two of the GBM subtypes with MGMT promoter methylation and IDH1 mutation [38]. Interestingly, it was also demonstrated that the mesenchymal gene expression profile may represent a population of patients with favorable responses to their DC vaccine, so the GBM microenvironment is also a double-edged sword concerning DC immunotherapy [39]. Despite these challenges, DC immunotherapy still showed an appealing benefit in terms of extending the survival of patients with HGG. The heterogeneous methods use and the complexity of designing and reporting on the immunotherapy trials will be overcome in the near future, providing stronger evidence to establish DC treatment as the standard for HGG patients.

In brief, DC immunotherapy has yielded encouraging results with immunological and clinical benefits for HGG patients and needs to be further tested to demonstrate significant therapeutic efficacy in phase III clinical trials.

Limitations of the study

Although several early-phase clinical trials have demonstrated promising therapeutic outcomes to date, clinical immunotherapy trials for gliomas have not yet demonstrated objective proof of clinical trials for lacking the randomized studies, so limitations in our analyses should be considered in interpreting the results. Many intrinsic and extrinsic factors might influence the systemic review's reliability. First, no one trial has more than 100 patients per arm.

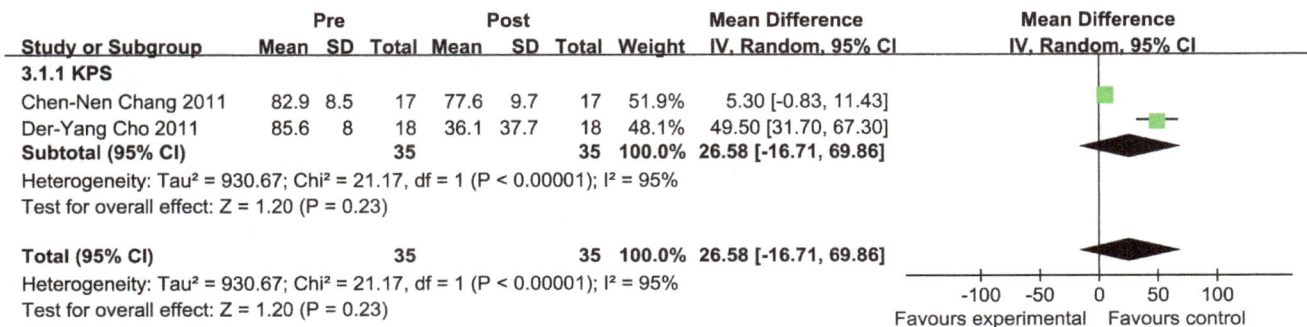

Figure 4. Forest plot for KPS before and after DC treatment. The random effects model (Mantel-Haenszel method) was used in this analysis.

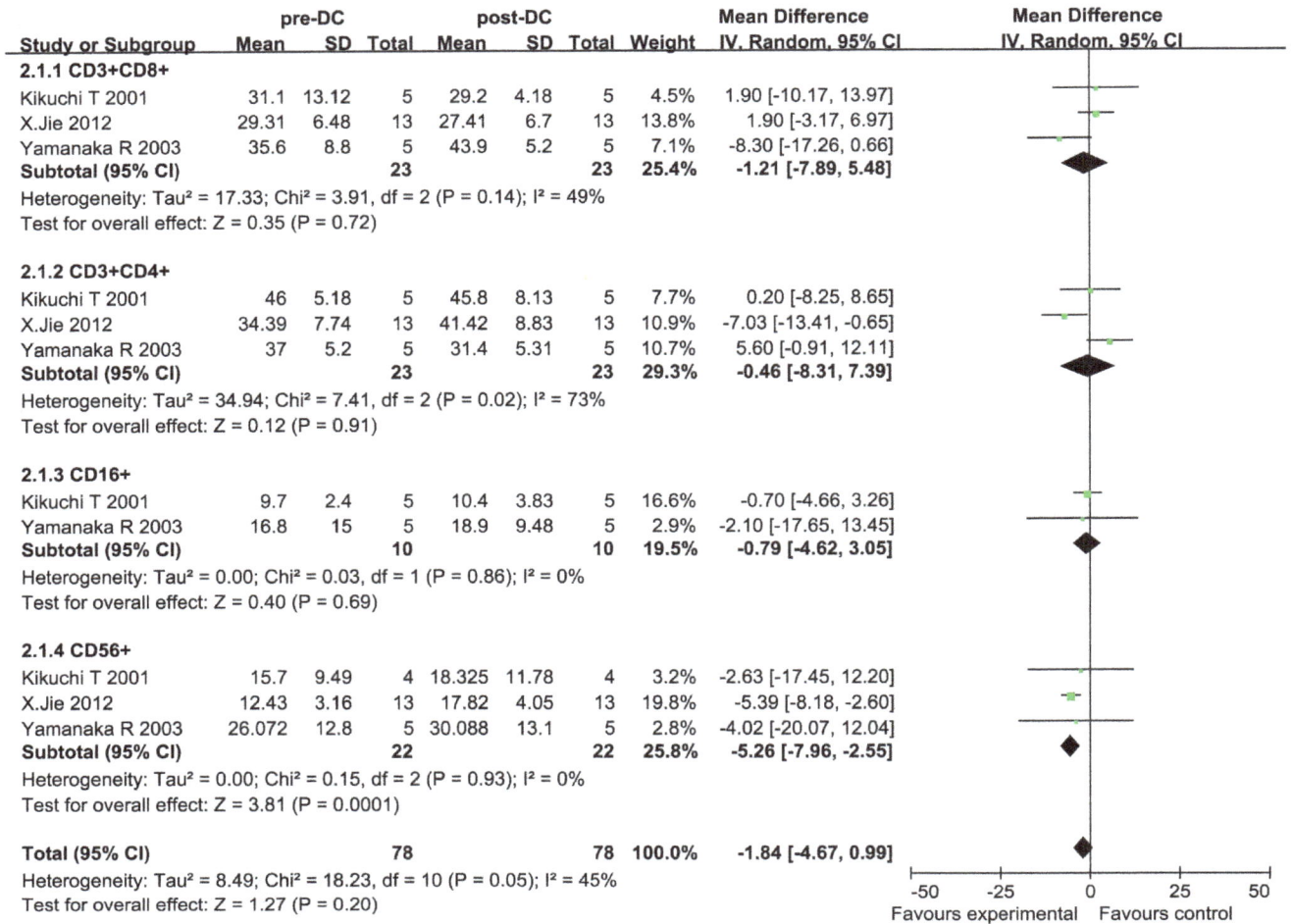

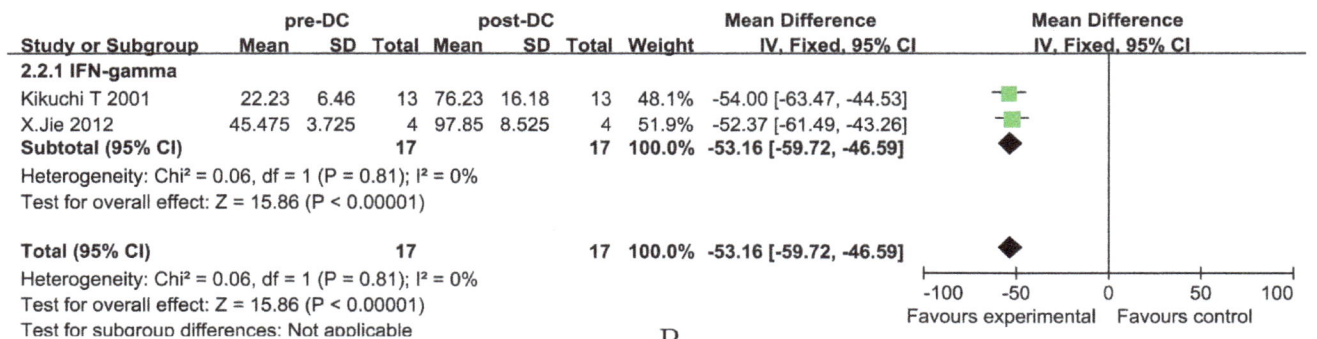

Figure 5. Forest plot for the immunophenotype (A) and immune cytokine (B) assessment. The data were collected from the patients before and after DC treatment. The random and fixed effects meta-analysis model (Mantel-Haenszel method) was used in this analysis.

Therefore, there is a lack of multinational, large-samples, multicenter clinical trials regarding DC cell therapy for HGG. Second, not all of the included studies reported clinical random allocation concealment, and in most cases, we collected data from the nonrandomized and randomized control or historical cohorts; thus, distribution and implementation biases may exist in our meta-analysis. Moreover, the analysis performed in this study was not based on individual patient data and was not subjected to an open external evaluation procedure. Maybe here one should refer

to the proposed HGG-IMMUNO RPA model for use in future reports for relapsed patients treated with immunotherapy [11]. In addition, to maintain consistency during our systematic review, we selected only assessable patients for our analysis. These sampling factors may also introduce bias into our conclusions, for example considering the age-, degree of resection and therapy, gender- and disease-matched controls, and thus our analysis may have led to an overestimation of the treatment effects. However, we expect that our study will be valuable for the design of more comprehensive, larger, controlled clinical trials.

Furthermore, the blood sample sources, injection modes, cell numbers, cell purity, tumor antigen, and cell phenotype may also affect the outcome of individual trials. All of these variables may introduce some level of bias; for instance, there is significant heterogeneity in the extracted data shown in Figure 4 and 5. It is important to standardize not only the DC cell preparation but also the criteria of the immune phenotyping system and the clinical response assessment. Our analysis may be valuable for the standardization of DC immune therapy as an adjuvant treatment for patients with HGG.

Conclusions

Taken together, our data suggest that DC cells have great potential to be a clinically efficacious therapy in the treatment of patients suffering from advanced-stage HGG malignancies who exhibit poor tolerance of chemotherapy or radiotherapy. These early results from clinical trials are very promising and must be verified more stringently before DC immunotherapy can be applied at the bedside.

Supporting Information

Checklist S1 PRISMA Checklist.

File S1 Contains Tables S1–S7. **Table S1**. List 9 excluding papers for reviews. **Table S2**. List 11 excluding papers for being in vitro experiments. **Table S3**. List 26 excluding papers for being animal models experiments. **Table S4**. List 91 case reports for being no enough data. **Table S5**. List 21 DC protocol studies and comments for being no clinical data. **Table S6**. List 22 clinical trials for no appropriate control arm. Specify the reasons of excluded clinical trial study's PICOS characteristics and report characteristics. P: participants; I: interventions; C: comparison; O: outcomes; S: setting (study design). **Table S7**. List 9 including clinical trials. Separately specify all the selected information sources in the included 9 clinical trials for our meta-analysis with PICOS, report characteristics, and clinical data source which denoted every data extracted from the paper's Title, Abstract, Introduction, Material and methods, Results, Figure, Table, Discussion, or Supplementary material.

Author Contributions

Conceived and designed the experiments: ZXW JXC. Performed the experiments: ZXW JXC XYZ JL-Liu YSL MW DL JL-Li BLX HBW. Analyzed the data: JXC XYZ JL-Liu YSL DL MW JL-Li BLX HBW. Contributed reagents/materials/analysis tools: JXC DL MW. Contributed to the writing of the manuscript: ZXW JXC XYZ JL-Liu.

References

1. Louis DN, Ohgaki H, Wiestler OD, Cavenee WK, Burger PC, et al. (2007) The 2007 WHO classification of tumours of the central nervous system. Acta Neuropathol. 114(2):97–109. Epub 2007 Jul 6.
2. Ruzevick J, Jackson C, Phallen J, Lim M (2012) Clinical trials with immunotherapy for high-grade glioma. Neurosurg Clin N Am. 23(3):459-470. doi: 10.1016/j.nec.2012.04.003. Epub 2012 Jun 8.
3. Badhiwala J, Decker WK, Berens ME, Bhardwaj RD (2013) Clinical trials in cellular immunotherapy for brain/CNS tumors. Expert Rev Neurother. 13(4):405–424. doi: 10.1586/ern.13.23.
4. Wilson EH, Weninger W, Hunter CA (2010) Trafficking of immune cells in the central nervous system. J Clin Invest. 120(5):1368–1379. doi: 10.1172/JCI41911. Epub 2010 May 3.
5. Sagar D, Foss C, Baz ER, Pomper MG, Khan ZK, et al. (2012) Mechanisms of dendritic cell trafficking across the blood-brain barrier. J Neuroimmune Pharmacol. 7(1):74–94. doi: 10.1007/s11481-011-9302-7. Epub 2011 Aug 6.
6. Xu X, Stockhammer F, Schmitt M (2012) Cellular-based immunotherapies for patients with glioblastoma multiforme. Clin Dev Immunol. 2012:764213. doi: 10.1155/2012/764213. Epub 2012 Feb 28.
7. Fabry Z, Raine CS, Hart MN (1994) Nervous tissue as an immune compartment: the dialect of the immune response in the CNS. Immunol Today. 15(5):218–224.
8. Palucka K, Bancheraud J (2012) Cancer immunotherapy via dendritic cells. Nat Rev Cancer. 22;12(4):265–277. doi: 10.1038/nrc3258. Review.
9. Ardon H, De Vleeschouwer S, Van Calenbergh F, Claes L, Kramm CM, et al. (2010) Adjuvant dendritic cell-based tumour vaccination for children with malignant brain tumours. Pediatr Blood Cancer. 54(4):519–525. doi: 10.1002/pbc.22319.
10. Ardon H, Van Gool SW, Verschuere T, Maes W, Fieuws S, et al. (2012) Integration of autologous dendritic cell-based immunotherapy in the standard of care treatment for patients with newly diagnosed glioblastoma: results of the HGG-2006 phase I/II trial. Cancer Immunol Immunother. 61(11):2033–2044. doi: 10.1007/s00262-012-1261-1. Epub 2012 Apr 22.
11. De Vleeschouwer S, Ardon H, Van Calenbergh F, Sciot R, Wilms G, et al. (2012) Stratification according to HGG-IMMUNO RPA model predicts outcome in a large group of patients with relapsed malignant glioma treated by adjuvant postoperative dendritic cell vaccination. Cancer Immunol Immunother. 61(11):2105–2112. doi: 10.1007/s00262-012-1271-z. Epub 2012 May 8.
12. Van Gool S, De Vleeschouwer S (2012) Should dendritic cell-based tumor vaccination be incorporated into standard therapy for newly diagnosed glioblastoma patients? Expert Rev Neurother. 12(10):1173–1176. doi: 10.1586/ern.12.107.
13. Bregy A, Wong TM, Shah AH, Goldberg JM, Komotar RJ (2013) Active immunotherapy using dendritic cells in the treatment of glioblastoma multi-forme. Cancer Treat Rev. 39(8):891–907. doi: 10.1016/j.ctrv.2013.05.007. Epub 2013 Jun 21.
14. Van Gool S, Maes W, Ardon H, Verschuere T, Van Cauter S, et al. (2009) Dendritic cell therapy of high-grade gliomas. Brain Pathol. 19(4):694–712. doi: 10.1111/j.1750-3639.2009.00316.x.
15. Mineharu Y, Castro MG, Lowenstein PR, Sakai N, Miyamoto S. (2013) Dendritic Cell-Based Immunotherapy for Glioma: Multiple Regimens and Implications in Clinical Trials. Neurol Med Chir (Tokyo). 53(11):741–754. Epub 2013 Oct 21.
16. Wang ZX, Cao JX, Liu ZP, Cui YX, Li CY, et al. (2014). Combination of chemotherapy and immunotherapy for colon cancer in China: a meta-analysis. World J Gastroenterol. 28;20(4):1095–1106. doi: 10.3748/wjg.v20.i4.1095.
17. Chang CN, Huang YC, Yang DM, Kikuta K, Wei KJ, et al. (2011) A phase I/II clinical trial investigating the adverse and therapeutic effects of a postoperative autologous dendritic cell tumor vaccine in patients with malignant glioma. J Clin Neurosci. 18(8):1048–1054. doi: 10.1016/j.jocn.2010.11.034. Epub 2011 Jun 28.
18. Yamanaka R, Homma J, Yajima N, Tsuchiya N, Sano M, et al. (2005) Clinical evaluation of dendritic cell vaccination for patients with recurrent glioma: results of a clinical phase I/II trial. Clin Cancer Res. 11(11):4160–4167.
19. Wheeler CJ, Das A, Liu G, Yu JS, Black KL. (2004) Clinical responsiveness of glioblastoma multiforme to chemotherapy after vaccination. Clin Cancer Res. 10(16):5316–5326.
20. Liau LM, Prins RM, Kiertscher SM, Odesa SK, Kremen TJ, et al. (2005) Dendritic cell vaccination in glioblastoma patients induces systemic and intracranial T-cell responses modulated by the local central nervous system tumor microenvironment. Clin Cancer Res. 11(15):5515–5525.
21. Kikuchi T, Akasaki Y, Irie M, Homma S, Abe T, et al. (2001) Results of a phase I clinical trial of vaccination of glioma patients with fusions of dendritic and glioma cells. Cancer Immunol Immunother. 50(7):337–344.
22. Yamanaka R, Abe T, Yajima N, Tsuchiya N, Homma J, et al. (2003) Vaccination of recurrent glioma patients with tumour lysate-pulsed dendritic cells elicits immune responses: results of a clinical phase I/II trial. Br J Cancer. 89(7):1172–1179.
23. Yu JS, Liu G, Ying H, Yong WH, Black KL, et al. (2004) Vaccination with tumor lysate-pulsed dendritic cells elicits antigen-specific, cytotoxic T-cells in patients with malignant glioma. Cancer Res. 64(14):4973–4979.
24. Jie X, Hua L, Jiang W, Feng F, Feng G, et al. (2012) Clinical application of a dendritic cell vaccine raised against heat-shocked glioblastoma. Cell Biochem Biophys. 62(1):91–99. doi: 10.1007/s12013-011-9265-6.
25. Cho DY, Yang WK, Lee HC, Hsu DM, Lin HL, et al. (2012) Adjuvant immunotherapy with whole-cell lysate dendritic cells vaccine for glioblastoma multiforme: a phase II clinical trial. World Neurosurg. 77(5-6):736–744. doi: 10.1016/j.wneu.2011.08.020. Epub 2011 Nov 7.
26. Van Gool S (2013) Immunotherapy for high-grade glioma: how to go beyond Phase I/II clinical trials. Immunotherapy. 5(10):1043–1046. doi: 10.2217/imt.13.86.

27. Shah AH, Bregy A, Heros DO, Komotar RJ, Goldberg J (2013) Dendritic cell vaccine for recurrent high-grade gliomas in pediatric and adult subjects: clinical trial protocol. Neurosurgery. 73(5):863–867. doi: 10.1227/NEU. 0000000000000107.

28. Izumoto S, Tsuboi A, Oka Y, Suzuki T, Hashiba T, et al. (2008) Phase II clinical trial of Wilms tumor 1 peptide vaccination for patients with recurrent glioblastoma multiforme. J Neurosurg. 108(5):963–971. doi: 10.3171/JNS/2008/108/5/0963.

29. Sampson JH, Heimberger AB, Archer GE, Aldape KD, Friedman AH, et al. (2010) Immunologic escape after prolonged progression-free survival with epidermal growth factor receptor variant III peptide vaccination in patients with newly diagnosed glioblastoma. J Clin Oncol. 28(31):4722–4729. doi: 10.1200/JCO.2010.28.6963. Epub 2010 Oct 4.

30. Schreiber RD, Old LJ, Smyth MJ (2011) Cancer immunoediting: integrating immunity's roles in cancer suppression and promotion. Science. 331(6024):1565–1570. doi: 10.1126/science.1203486.

31. Wheeler CJ, Black KL, Liu G, Mazer M, Zhang XX, et al. (2008) Vaccination elicits correlated immune and clinical responses in glioblastoma multiforme patients. Cancer Res. 68(14):5955–5964. doi: 10.1158/0008-5472.CAN-07-5973.

32. Hussain SF, Heimberger AB (2005) Immunotherapy for human glioma: innovative approaches and recent results. Expert Rev Anticancer Ther. 5(5):777–790.

33. Ogbomo H, Cinatl J Jr, Mody CH, Forsyth PA (2011) Immunotherapy in gliomas: limitations and potential of natural killer (NK) cell therapy. Trends Mol Med. 17(8):433–441. doi: 10.1016/j.molmed.2011.03.004. Epub 2011 Apr 19.

34. Grivennikov SI, Greten FR, Karin M (2010) Immunity, inflammation, and cancer. Cell. 140(6):883–899. doi: 10.1016/j.cell.2010.01.025.

35. Jackson C, Ruzevick J, Brem H, Lim M. (2013) Vaccine strategies for glioblastoma: progress and future directions. Immunotherapy. 5(2):155–167. doi: 10.2217/imt.12.155.

36. Reardon DA, Wucherpfennig KW, Freeman G, Wu CJ, Chiocca EA, et al. (2013) An update on vaccine therapy and other immunotherapeutic approaches for glioblastoma. Expert Rev Vaccines. 12(6):597–615. doi: 10.1586/erv.13.41.

37. Li Z, Lee JW, Mukherjee D, Ji J, Jeswani SP, et al. (2012) Immunotherapy targeting glioma stem cells-insights and perspectives. Expert Opin Biol Ther. 12(2):165–178. doi: 10.1517/14712598.2012.648180. Epub 2011 Dec 26.

38. Prins RM, Soto H, Konkankit V, Odesa SK, Eskin A, et al. (2011) Gene expression profile correlates with T-cell infiltration and relative survival in glioblastoma patients vaccinated with dendritic cell immunotherapy. Clin Cancer Res. 17(6):1603–1615. doi: 10.1158/1078-0432.CCR-10-2563. Epub 2010 Dec 6.

39. Jackson C, Ruzevick J, Phallen J, Belcaid Z, Lim M. (2011) Challenges in immunotherapy presented by the glioblastoma multiforme microenvironment. Clin Dev Immunol. 2011:732413. doi: 10.1155/2011/732413. Epub 2011 Dec 10.

18

Adoptive Immunotherapy of Cytokine-Induced Killer Cell Therapy in the Treatment of Non-Small Cell Lung Cancer

Min Wang[1][⦾][¶], Jun-Xia Cao[1][⦾][¶], Jian-Hong Pan[2], Yi-Shan Liu[1], Bei-Lei Xu[1], Duo Li[1], Xiao-Yan Zhang[1], Jun-Li Li[1], Jin-Long Liu[1], Hai-Bo Wang[1], Zheng-Xu Wang[1]*

1 Biotherapy Center, General Hospital of Beijing Military Command, Beijing, China, 2 Department of Biostatistics, Peking University Clinical Research Institute, Peking University Health Science Center, Beijing, China

Abstract

Aim: The aim of this study was to systemically evaluate the therapeutic efficacy of cytokine-induced killer (CIK) cells for the treatment of non-small cell lung cancer.

Materials and Methods: A computerized search of randomized controlled trials for CIK cell-based therapy was performed. The overall survival, clinical response rate, immunological assessment and side effects were evaluated.

Results: Overall, 17 randomized controlled trials of non-small cell lung cancer (NSCLC) with a total of 1172 patients were included in the present analysis. Our study showed that the CIK cell therapy significantly improved the objective response rate and overall survival compared to the non-CIK cell-treated group. After CIK combined therapy, we observed substantially increased percentages of $CD3^+$, $CD4^+$, $CD4^+CD8^+$, $CD3^+CD56^+$ and NK cells, whereas significant decreases were noted in the percentage of $CD8^+$ and regulatory T cell (Treg) subgroups. A significant increase in Ag-NORs was observed in the CIK-treated patient group ($p = 0.00001$), whereas carcinoembryonic antigen (CEA) was more likely to be reduced to a normal level after CIK treatment ($p = 0.0008$). Of the possible major side effects, only the incidence of fever in the CIK group was significantly higher compared to the group that received chemotherapy alone.

Conclusion: The CIK cell combined therapy demonstrated significant superiority in the overall survival, clinical response rate, and T lymphocytes responses and did not present any evidence of major adverse events in patients with NSCLC.

Editor: Nupur Gangopadhyay, University of Pittsburgh, United States of America

Funding: This research work was supported by the National Natural Science Foundation of China (No. 31171427 and 30971651 to Zheng-Xu Wang), Beijing Municipal Science & Technology Project; Clinical characteristics and Application Research of Capital (No. Z121107001012136 to Zheng-Xu Wang) and the Postdoctoral Foundation of China (No. 20060400775 to Jun-Xia Cao). Zheng-Xu Wang designed the research; Jun-Xia Cao is one of the people who performed the research and wrote the paper. The funders had no role in study design, data collection and analysis, decision to publish, or preparation of the manuscript.

Competing Interests: The authors have declared that no competing interests exist.

* Email: zhxwang18@hotmail.com

⦾ These authors contributed equally to this work.

¶ These authors are co-first authors on this work.

Introduction

Lung cancer is the leading cause of cancer-related mortality worldwide [1]. According to the 2012 Chinese cancer registration annual report, more than 3 million new cases of lung cancer will be diagnosed every year, and the approximately 2.7 million deaths from lung cancer will account for 13% of allmortalities. There is no doubt that the incidence and mortality of lung cancer are far too prevalent [2]. In patients with advanced lung disease, 1-year survival rates are typically 35%, and 2-year survival rates were shown to approach 15%-20% in recent studies [3]. At best, the 5-year overall survival rate of localized cancer is 15.9%, and only half of extended-stage patients have a 3.7% chance of surviving 5 years [4]. Most NSCLC patients have locally advanced or metastatic cancer at stage IIIB-IV at the time of diagnosis, leaving only palliative therapeutic options. Based on the existing clinical data, chemotherapy appears to have limited benefits and disappointed prognoses [5].

The novel approach of adoptive cell immunotherapy relies on an ex vivo expansion of the autologous tumor-specific effector cells before their reinfusion into the host [6]. Since the development of this immunotherapy, a number of immunological effector cells have been employed to treat cancer and eliminate residual tumor cells after surgery, such as CIK cells, lymphokine-activated killer cells (LAKs), tumor-infiltrating lymphocytes (TILs), natural killer cells (NKs), and cytotoxic T lymphocyte cells (CTLs) [7,8]. Among them, LAKs, which are a mixture of lymphokine-activated $CD3^+$ T lymphocytes and $CD3^-CD56^+CD16^+$ NK cells, were cultured with recombinant interleukin-2 (rIL-2) for 3 days, and CTLs were isolated from a patient's own tissues, including peripheral blood mononuclear cells (PBMCs), TILs, draining lymph nodes, or PBMCs after vaccination with irradiated autologous tumor cells (ATCs) [7,8]. After adoptive cell immunotherapy made great strides due to the efforts of several generations of researchers, CIK cells were found to possess greater proliferative and cytolytic capacities than NK or LAK cells. CIK cells are MHC-unrestricted cytotoxic lymphocytes that can be generated in vitro from PBMCs and cultured with the addition of IFN-γ, IL-2 and CD3 monoclonal antibody (CD3mAb). Anti-tumor cytotoxic activity is represented by surface markers for both T cells (TCR-α/β, CD3) and NKT cells (CD3$^+$CD56$^+$) [9].

The first clinical trial using CIK cell therapy for cancer patients was reported in 1999 [10]. Soon afterward, a growing number of clinical trials have suggested that CIK therapy yields highly compelling objective clinical responses in several solid carcinomas compared to other immunological effectors. A pooled analysis of 792 patients with solid carcinomas indicated that treatment with CIK cells is associated with a significant prolonging of the mean survival time and disease control rate [11]. Recently, both chinese clinical trials with 563 patients and international registered clinical trials with 426 cases of CIK cell therapy provided evidence for a broad clinical application based on a positive evaluation of the immunological and clinical responses [12,13]. Some systematic reviews have analyzed CIK cell therapy and shown it to be safe and efficient to treat renal cell carcinoma, hepatocellular carcinoma, and colon cancer [14–16]. Furthermore, CIK cell therapy has been perceived to have significant survival benefits in a few NSCLC clinical trials [17–22]. These studies showed that the immunotherapy of cancers with CIK cells may improve immunological and clinical responses, promote the quality of life (QoL) of cancer patients, and extend their life spans under certain conditions. However, there is no systematic review to assess the therapeutic efficacy of CIK cell therapies combined with chemotherapy in NSCLC; therefore, we performed a systematic meta-analysis of CIK cell therapy with randomized controlled trials on NSCLC. Our large-scale CIK cell immunotherapy clinical trials systematically analyzed the clinical efficiency and safety considering the overall survival, clinical response, immunological assessments and side effects.

Methods

Study design, search strategy and eligibility criteria

The relevant studies were identified by searching PubMed, the Cochrane Center Register of Controlled Trials, Science Direct, Embase, and China National Knowledge Infrastructure for randomized controlled trials (RCT) in the most recent decades. The search strategy included the keywords 'non-small-cell lung cancer,' 'adoptive immunotherapy,' and 'cytokine induced killer cells' adoptive immunotherapy arms with no adjuvant treatment in NSCLC patients except those who had undergone the same chemotherapy compared with control arms. In addition, we manually searched a website of clinical trials for ongoing trials. We searched keywords 'non-small-cell lung cancer' and 'cytokine induced killer cells' on the website http://www.clinicaltrials.gov/. The registered clinical trials with publication citations are displayed at the bottom of the Full Text View tab of a study record, under the More Information heading. Reference lists of previously published trials and relevant review articles were examined for other eligible trials. No language restriction was applied. Review papers and postgraduate theses were also examined for published results. Furthermore, we performed manual searches in reference lists and conference proceedings of the American Society of Clinical Oncology (ASCO) annual

meetings and the European Cancer Conference (ECCO). We excluded abstracts that were never subsequently published as full papers and studies on animals and cell lines.

Data selection criteria

Data extraction was independently conducted by two reviewers (Min Wang and Jun-Xia Cao) using a standardized approach. Disagreement was adjudicated by a third reviewer (Zheng-Xu Wang) after referring back to the original publications. The selection criteria were as follows: (1) English language studies on human clinical trials with patients at all stages of NSCLC were included; (2) RCT with CIK cell-based immunotherapy combined with chemotherapy versus chemotherapy alone for the treatment of NSCLC were included; (3) all trials approved by the local ethical committee and in which all patients signed a study-specific consent form prior to study entry were included; (4) case studies, review articles, and studies involving fewer than 10 patients were excluded; (5) uncontrolled metabolic disease, inadequate hepatic function, renal dysfunction, neurological disorders and other infectious diseases were excluded from the study; and (6) blood samples receiving any chemotherapy or radiotherapy within one month before treatment were excluded.

The overall quality of each included paper was evaluated by the Jadad scale [23]. A few of the major criteria were employed as a grading scheme: (1) randomization; (2) allocation concealment; (3) blinding; (4) lost to follow up; (5) ITT (intention to treat); and (6) baseline. We also used a funnel plot to evaluate the publication bias.

Definition of outcome measures

The primary clinical endpoints in RCT for cancer therapies employed the measures of median survival time (MST) and progression-free survival (PFS). The time to progression (TTP) may not consider those patients who die from other causes but is often used as equivalent to PFS. The secondary endpoints were the clinical response rate, including the objective response rate (ORR) and disease control rate (DCR). The ORR was defined as the sum of the partial rates (PRs) and complete response rates (CRs), and the DCR was defined as the sum of the stable disease (SD), PR and CR, according to the World Health Organization criteria. The side effects and toxicity were graded according to the National Cancer Institute Common Toxicity Criteria. The data were either obtained directly from the articles or calculated using the graphed data in articles using Photoshop and a software graph digitizer scout.

Statistical analysis

The analysis was performed using Review Manager Version 5.0 (Nordic Cochran Centre, Copenhagen, Denmark). Heterogeneity was assessed to determine which model should be used. To assess the statistical heterogeneity between the studies, the Cochran Q-test was performed using a predefined significance threshold of 0.1. The treatment effects are reflected by odds ratios (ORs), which were obtained using a method reported by Mantel and Haenszel. To evaluate whether the results of the studies were homogeneous, Cochran's Q test was performed. We also calculated the quantity I^2, which describes the percentage of variation across studies that is due to heterogeneity rather than chance. The OR was obtained using a fixed-effect model with no statistically significant heterogeneity; otherwise, a random-effects model was employed. P-values <0.05 were considered statistically significant. All reported P-values were two-sided.

Results

Selection of the trials

The data searches yielded 167 references, 91 of which were considered ineligible for different reasons (44 non-CIK immunotherapy, 19 multiple cancer analyses, 18 reviews, and 10 animal models). The remaining 76 articles were further evaluated, and 59 trials were excluded due to language, lack of an RCT, and insufficient data. The final 17 articles were included in the meta-analysis with RCTs of CIK cell-based therapy for the treatment of NSCLC (Figure 1, also see the checklist S1).

The quality assessment of the 17 studies is summarized in Table 1. We also used a funnel plot to evaluate the publication bias. In our analysis, overall survival, clinical response rate, and side effects suffered low published bias. However, immunological assessment and T cell subgroups observed a high published bias (Figure 2), which demonstrated that the node of the vertical line does not meet the horizontal one at the midpoint by analysis with Review Manager Version 5.0.

Characteristics of CIK cell-based therapy

The characteristics of the 17 trials are listed in Table 2. Our selected 17 trials with a total of 1172 NSCLC patients in stage I-IV were included in the present analysis, and 90% of them included

metastatic or locally advanced NSCLC. The enrolled ages were between 28 and 82 years of age, with a median age greater than 50.

In all 17 trials, the control arm was chemotherapy or cyberknife alone, whereas the treatment arm was chemotherapy or cyberknife combined with CIK cell therapy. In each trial, all of the patients in the CIK group were treated identically to those in the chemotherapy group in terms of chemotherapy doses and cycles. In all 17 trials of the treatment arm, most of the patients were treated with CIK cells plus DC immunotherapy combined with chemotherapy, although patients in four of the trials were injected with CIK cells combined with chemotherapy [6,30,38,39]. Most of the CIK groups used DCs without pulse, i.e., the DCs were only induced to become mature before co-culture with CIK cells. In 4 out of 17 studies, the DCs were injected while being pulsed with lung cancer antigens or tumor lysate [17,22,33,37]. Some of the necessary cytokines were supplied in a culture of CIK, IL-2, IFN-γ, and CD3mAb in a variety of culture media. The patients received cell infusions of 1×10^9 to 2×10^{12} cells per course, mostly at a 10^9 order of magnitude. Most of the treatments with repeated CIK cell infusions were administered for at least 2 weeks, and some of them lasted over 1 month. The injected route for immunotherapy was mainly intravenous for CIK cells and via subcutaneous injection for DCs (File S1 and File S2).

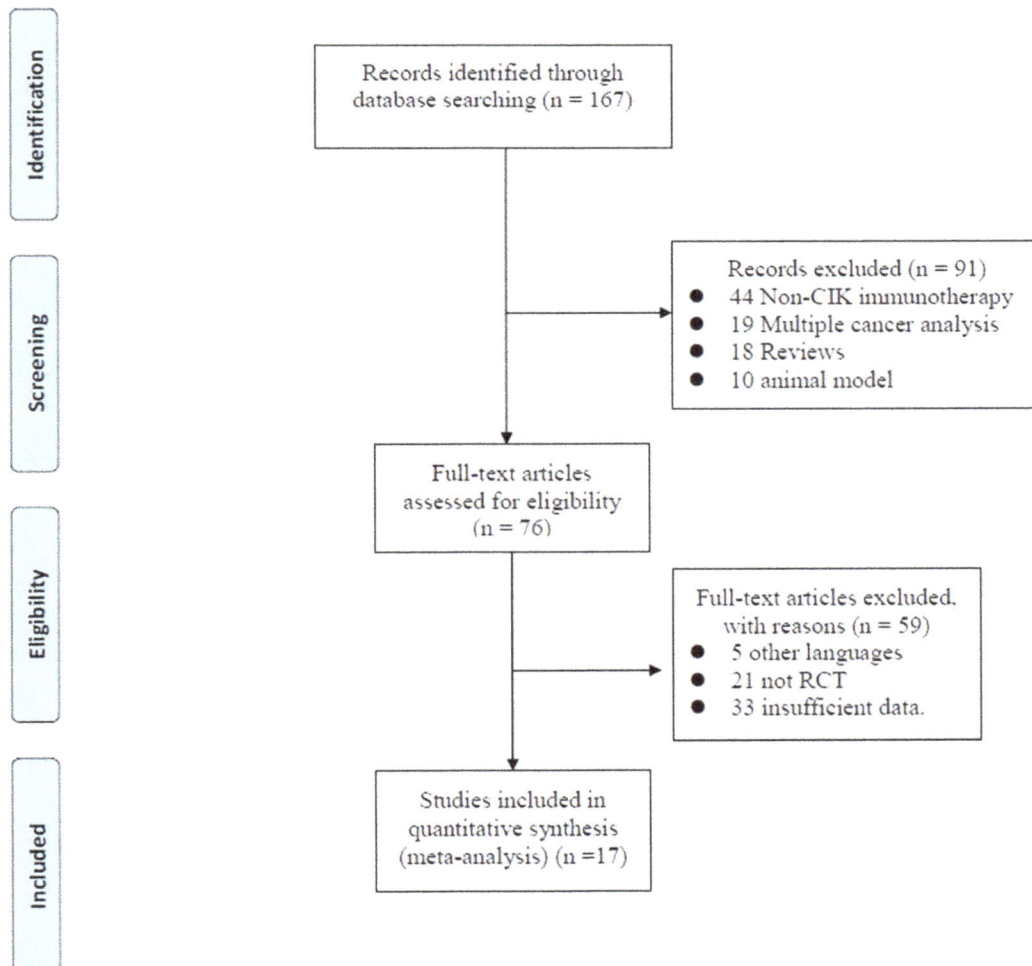

Figure 1. Flow diagram of the study selection process.

Table 1. Jadad Scale for the 17 randomized controlled studies.

Included studies	Randomization	Allocation concealment	Blinding	Lost to follow up ITT analysis	Baseline	Quality grading
Li 2009 [17]	Yes	Unclear	Unclear	No	Yes	Similar	B
Li 2012 [30]	Yes	Unclear	Unclear	No	Yes	Similar	B
Mo 2010 [18]	Yes	Unclear	Unclear	Yes	Unclear	Unclear	C
Peng 2012 [19]	Yes	Unclear	Unclear	No	Yes	Similar	B
Sheng 2011 [20]	Yes	Unclear	Unclear	No	Yes	Similar	B
Shi 2012 [21]	Yes	Unclear	Unclear	No	Yes	Similar	B
Wang 2013 [39]	Yes	Unclear	Unclear	Yes	Yes	Similar	B
Wu 2008 [6]	Yes	Unclear	Unclear	No	Yes	Similar	B
Xu 2010 [31]	Yes	Unclear	Unclear	No	Yes	Similar	B
Xu 2011 [32]	Yes	Unclear	Unclear	No	Yes	Similar	B
Yang 2013 [33]	Yes	Unclear	Unclear	No	Yes	Similar	B
You 2012 [34]	Yes	Unclear	Unclear	Yes	Yes	Unclear	B
Yuan 2011 [35]	Yes	Unclear	Unclear	Yes	Yes	Unclear	C
Zhang 2012 [36]	Yes	Unclear	Unclear	No	Yes	Similar	B
Zheng 2012 [38]	Yes	Unclear	Unclear	No	Yes	Similar	B
Zhong 2008 [37]	Yes	Unclear	Unclear	No	Yes	Similar	B
Zhong 2011 [22]	Yes	Unclear	No	No	Yes	Similar	B

ITT: intention-to-treat. A: adequate, with correct procedure; B: unclear, without a description of the methods; C: inadequate procedures, methods, or information.
Each criterion was graded as follows: Yes, adequate, with correct procedure; Unclear, without a description of the methods; No, inadequate procedures, methods, or information. Each involved study was graded as follows: A, studies with a low risk of bias and which were scored as grade of A for all items; B, studies with a moderate risk of bias, with one or more grades of B; and C, studies with a high risk of bias, with one or more grades of C.

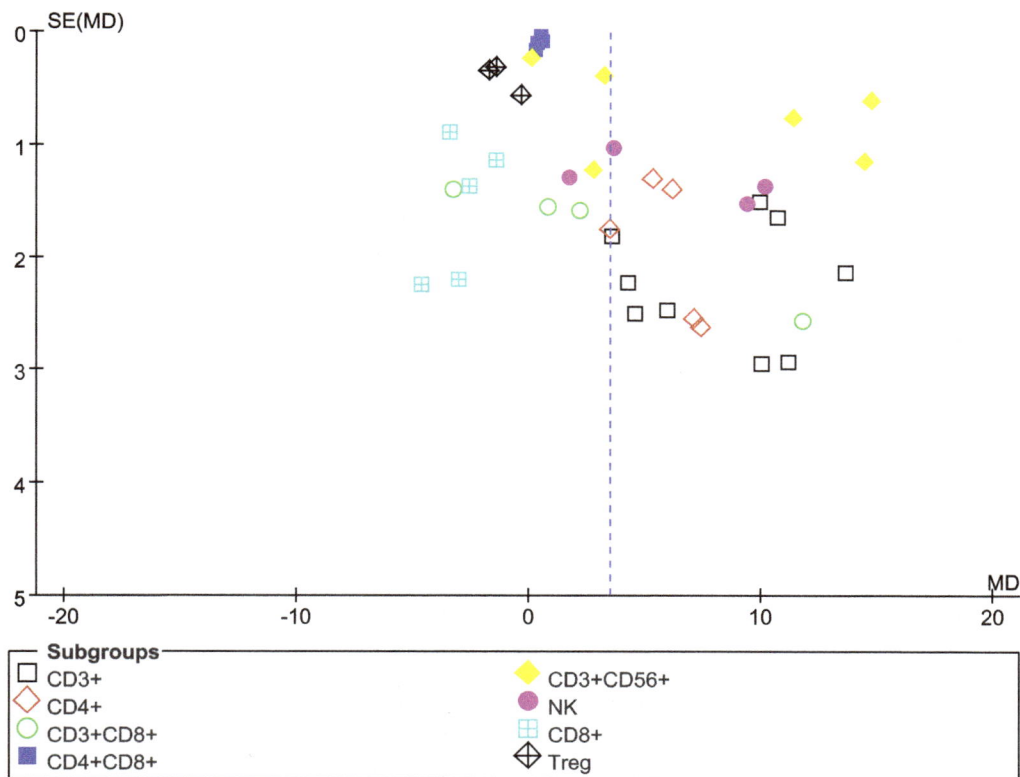

Figure 2. Funnel plot to evaluate the publication bias of T-cell subgroups. The analysis was performed using Review Manager Version 5.0.

Survival

The patients in the CIK group had significantly prolonged MST compared with those in the non-CIK group (95%CI -7.45 to -0.66, $p = 0.02$) (Table 3). The results of the pooled analysis showed that the CIK arm significantly extended overall survival at the end of follow-up, compared with the non-CIK group (Table 4). Three subgroups of patients of the CIK cell-based therapy group at 1-year survival, 2-year survival, and 3-year survival presented significant survival benefits compared to the patients in the non-CIK group (OR 0.64, 95%CI 0.46–0.91, $p = 0.01$; OR 0.36, 95%CI 0.22–0.59, $p < 0.0001$; OR 0.37, 95%CI 0.20–0.70, $p = 0.002$, respectively), which was consistent with the overall survival (OR 0.50, 95%CI 0.39–0.64, $p < 0.0001$). Based on the results of our analysis, the short-term survival subgroup showed a significant difference at the 1-year and 2-year survivals. The 1-year survival for the 282 patients in the CIK group was 56%, whereas a slightly lower 1-year survival rate was found for the non-CIK group (45% of 278 patients). A significant difference was also demonstrated in the 2-year survival group, which was 43.22% for 236 patients in the CIK group and 27.47% of 233 patients without the CIK cell treatment. The long-term survival rates in the CIK group showed a slight decrease compared with the short-term survival rate; however, a significant difference in the long-term survival rates was found compared to the non-CIK group ($p = 0.002$).

Concerning the median PFS, the CIK group did not produce any significant improvement compared with the corresponding control groups (95%CI -13.27 to 3.89, $p = 0.28$), whereas the median TTP clearly prolonged the median time to disease progression in the CIK group (95%CI -2.70 to -0.47, $p = 0.005$) (Table 3).

Response rate

The CIK cell-based therapy group showed favorable results when subjected to both analysis of the ORR (OR 0.58, 95%CI 0.44–0.78, $p = 0.00003$) and the DCR (OR 0.41, 95%CI 0.29–0.58, $p < 0.0001$), compared with the corresponding control arms. With no significant heterogeneity, a fixed-effect model was used in the ORR and DCR analyses (Table 4). Cochran's Q test resulted in a statistically significant P-value, and the corresponding quantity for I^2 was 0% for both groups, indicating that there was no evidence of heterogeneity among the individual studies.

Immunological assessment of T-cell subgroups

When heterogeneity was observed in the T-cell subgroups, a random-effects model was applied for the overall and subgroup analysis of T-cell immunological assessments (Table 5). The results demonstrated a substantially increased ratio of CD3$^+$ (MD 8.21, 95%CI 5.79–10.64, $p < 0.00001$), CD4$^+$ (MD 5.59, 95%CI 4.10–7.07, $p < 0.00001$), CD4$^+$CD8$^+$ (MD 0.49, 95%CI 0.37–0.61, $p < 0.00001$), CD3$^+$CD56$^+$ (MD 7.80, 95%CI 2.61–12.98, $p = 0.003$) and NK cells (CD3$^-$CD16$^+$CD56$^+$) (MD 6.21, 95%CI 2.25–10.17, $p = 0.002$), whereas the ratio of CD3$^+$CD8$^+$ (MD 2.55, 95%CI -2.46 to 7.56, $p = 0.32$) generated no statistical improvement after CIK treatment. In addition, the pooled analysis showed a significant decrease in the percentage of CD8$^+$ (MD -2.75, 95%CI -3.88 to -1.63, $p < 0.00001$) and Treg (CD4$^+$CD25$^+$CD127$^-$) (MD -1.26, 95%CI -1.94 to -0.58,

Table 2. Clinical information from the eligible trials in the meta-analysis.

Trials	Age	No. of pts	Operative method	Tumor Stage	CIK regimens	CIK culture	DC modification
Li 2009 [17]	40–80; (M61)	42;42	Chemo; Chemo+DC-CIK	I-IIIA	1.3×10^9/course, 4 treatments at intervals of a month	X-Vivo 20, IL-1α, IL-2, IFN-γ, CD3	ATL (100 μg/ml)
Li 2012 [30]	UK	37; 37	Chemo; Chemo+ CIK	III-IV	13×10^9/course, twice in a cycle, at least 3 cycles	X-Vivo 20,IL-1α, IL-2, IFN-γ, CD3	NO DC
Mo 2010 [18]	39–77; (M60)	20;21	Chemo; Chemo+ DC-CIK	IV	$2–6\times10^6$/course, 6 times every second day	RPMI1640, IL-1α, IL-2,IFN-γ, CD3mAb	NI-DC
Peng 2012 [19]	65–79; (M71)	23; 24	Chemo; Chemo+ DC-CIK	III-IV	$1\times10^{10}–2\times10^{12}$/course, 2–3 times a week, 7 days intervals for 4 cycles	CM, IL-1α, IL-2, IFN-γ, CD3	NI-DC
Sheng 2011 [20]	35–65; (M54)	33; 32	Chemo; Chemo+ DC-CIK	III-IV	5×10^9/course, 4 treatments in a week for 2 weeks	RPMI1640, IL-1α, IL-2, IFN-γ, CD3	NI-DC
Shi 2012 [21]	UK	30; 30	Chemo; Chemo+ DC-CIK	III-IV	5 times every second day	RPMI1640, IL-1, IL-2, CD3	NI-DC
Wang 2013 [39]	UK	11; 11	CK; CK+ CIK	AS	2×10^{10}/course, 2 courses in 2 months	UK	No DC
Wu 2008 [6]	38–78; (M60)	30; 29	Chemo; Chemo+ CIK	III-IV	1×10^9/course, 5 times every second day	RPMI1640, IL-1α, IL-2, IFN-γ, CD3	No DC
Xu 2010 [31]	47–75; (M59.6)	40; 38	Chemo; Chemo+ DC-CIK	III-IV	1.6×10^9/course, 2 times a week in next following 4–5 weeks	RPMI1640, IL-2, IFN-γ, CD3	NI-DC
Xu 2011 [32]	45–73; (M59)	40; 45	Chemo; Chemo+ DC-CIK	III	1.3×10^9/course, 2 times a week in 5–6 weeks	RPMI1640, IL-2, IFN-γ, CD3	NI-DC
Yang 2012 [33]	28–82; (M63.5)	61; 61	Chemo; Chemo + DC-CIK	III-IV	1.2×10^9/course, 30day intervals for 4 cycles	X-vivo 20, IFN-γ,IL-1α,IL-2,CD3McAb	ATL (100 μg/ml)
You 2012 [34]	M 52	50; 55	Chemo; Chemo+ DC-CIK	III-IV	5×10^9/course, 4 times a cycle, 2–6 cycles	RPMI1640, IL-1α, IL-2, IFN-γ, CD3mAb	NI-DC
Yuan 2011 [35]	M 66	32; 32	Chemo; Chemo+ DC-CIK	AS	4 times a cycle	Unknown	NI-DC
Zhang 2012 [36]	35–72; (M57)	50; 50	Chemo; Chemo+ DC-CIK	III-IV	28day intervals for 2 cycles	GT-T551,IL-2, IFN-γ, CD3	NI-DC
Zheng 2012 [38]	M 59	36; 36	γK; γK +CIK	III	1×10^{10}/course, 1 month intervals for 2 cycles	RPMI1640, IL-1α, IL-2,IFN-γ, CD3mAb	No DC
Zhong 2008 [37]	M 53.6	44; 22	Chemo; Chemo+ DC-CIK	IB	2 times in 4 days	UK	CEA PI-DC
Zhong 2011 [22]	40–65	14; 14	Chemo; Chemo+ DC-CIK	IIIB- IV	$1–1.7\times10^9$/course,30day intervals for 4 cycles	CM, IFN-γ, IL-2,CD3McAb	CEA, PI-DC (10 μg/ml)

M: median; UK: unknown; AS: advanced stage; Chemo: chemotherapy; CK: cyberknife; γK: γ-knife; NI-DC: non-impulsed DC; ATL: Autologous tumor lysate; PI-DC: peptide impulse DC; Pts: Patients. The selective data include the authors' names, year of publication, trial period, sample size per arm, regimen used, median or mean age of patients, cell preparation, CIK-based therapy treatment and information pertaining to the study design.

Table 3. Comparison of MTTP, MST, and MPFS between the non-CIK and CIK groups.

Event	No. of Trials [Ref]	No. of pts Non-CIK	CIK	Mean Difference	95% CI	P value	Heterogeneity (I^2)
MTTP	4 [6,21,31,36]	97	100	−1.59	−2.70 to −0.47	0.005	0%
MST	4 [6,31,32,37]	154	134	−4.06	−7.45 to −0.66	0.02	0%
MPFS	3 [21,30,37]	161	139	−4.69	−13.27 to 3.89	0.28	56%

MTTP: median time to progression; MST: median survival time; MPFS: median progression-free survival; Pts: patients; 95%CI: 95% confidence interval; significant difference: P value <0.05.

Table 4. Comparison of OS, ORR and DCR between the non-CIK and CIK groups.

Event	No. of Trials [Ref]	No. pts of Non-CIK	CIK	Odds Ratio (OR)|95% CI		P value	Heterogeneity (I^2)
1 yr OS	8 [6,18,19,22,31,32,33,36]	278	282	0.64	0.46 to 0.91	0.01	0%
2 yr OS	6 [6,17,18,31–33]	233	236	0.36	0.22 to 0.59	<0.0001	0%
3 yrOS	4 [17,20,31,37]	154	136	0.37	0.20 to 0.70	0.002	13%
ORR	11 [6,18–20,31–36,38]	401	410	0.58	0.44 to 0.78	0.0003	0%
DCR	10 [6,18–20,31–34,36,38]	369	378	0.41	0.29 to 0.58	<0.00001	0%

Forest plot comparing the 1-, 2- and 3-year OS between the non-CIK and CIK groups.OR, odds ratio; OS, overall survival. Due to the low heterogeneity detected, the fixed-effect model was used in this OS meta-analysis. Comparison of the ORR and the DCR between the non-CIK group and CIK group. OR, odds ratio; ORR, objective response rate; DCR, disease control rate. Due to the lack of heterogeneity, the fixed-effect model was used. OS: overall survival; ORR: objective response rate; DCR: disease control rate.

Table 5. Comparison of CD3[+], CD4[+], CD3[+]CD8[+], CD4[+]CD8[+], CD3[+]CD56[+], NK, CD8[+] and Treg before CIK treatment and after CIK therapy.

Event	No. of Trials [Ref]	No. of pts Before-CIK	CIK	Mean Difference	95% CI	P value	Heterogeneity (I²)
CD3[+]	9 [6,17,20,21,31–33,35,36]	359	359	8.21	5.79 to 10.64	<0.00001	67%
CD4[+]	5 [6,21,31,32,35]	174	174	5.59	4.10 to 7.07	<0.0001	0%
CD3[+]CD8[+]	4 [17,18,33,36]	174	174	2.55	−2.46 to 7.56	0.32	89%
CD4[+]CD8[+]	4 [6,31,32,35]	144	144	0.49	0.37 to 0.61	<0.00001	53%
CD3[+]CD56[+]	6 [6,18,19,30,36,38]	222	222	7.80	2.61 to 12.98	0.003	99%
NK	4 [6,21,32,36]	154	154	6.21	2.25 to 10.17	0.002	90%
CD8[+]	5 [6,21,31,32,35]	174	174	−2.75	−3.88 to −1.63	<0.00001	0%
Treg	3 [17,33,36]	153	153	−1.26	−1.94 to −0.58	0.0003	58%

Forest plot for the comparison of T-cell subgroups, before and after treatment with the CIK cell-based therapy. The random-effects meta-analysis model was used in this analysis.

$p = 0.0003$) subgroups after treatment with CIK cell-based therapy.

Immunological assessment of Ag-NORs and CEA expression

Due to the limited data presented in the published papers, only some of the immunological assessments, e.g., Ag-NORs (argyrophilic nucleolar organizer regions), and NSCLC tumor markers, e.g., CEA, were subjected to analysis. Heterogeneity was observed, and a random-effects model was therefore applied for the analysis of the subgroups and the overall analysis. The analysis showed that the CIK group significantly improved the patients' T lymphocyte immune activity, showing better Ag-NORs (MD −0.71, 95%CI −0.94 to −0.47, $p = 0.00001$) compared with the non-CIK therapy group (Table 6). The CEA expression level in the analysis was based on two trials [38,39]. The plasma CEA was markedly decreased in the CIK group compared to the non-CIK group (MD 3.96, 95%CI 1.64–6.28, $p = 0.0008$) (Table 6).

Toxicity and adverse reactions

The patients in the CIK group observed fewer severe side effects from chemotherapy, such as fewer cases of grade III and IV leucopenia, gastrointestinal adverse reactions, anemia and liver dysfunction (Figure 3). Without significant heterogeneity, a fixed-effect model (Mantel-Haenszel method) was used for the side effect analysis.

After CIK cell transfusion, most of the patients developed a slight fever, between 37.5 and 39 degrees, but the patients recovered within a few days without severe side effects. Four types of serious chemotherapy side effects could lead to toxic reactions in both groups of patients. The pooled analysis showed that the adverse effects of gastrointestinal adverse reactions (OR 1.77, 95%CI 1.20–2.59, $p = 0.004$) and anemia (OR 2.80, 95%CI 1.37–5.73, $p = 0.005$) generated a significant difference, with fewer episodes in the CIK group. Leucopenia and liver dysfunction were observed less frequently in the patients receiving the CIK treatment, but neither set of data displayed a significant difference compared with the non-CIK group (OR 1.59, 95% CI 0.93–2.72, $p = 0.09$; OR 1.11, 95%CI 0.60–2.06, $p = 0.73$).

Discussion

Immunotherapy has benefited from an increased understanding of tumor immunology and genetics. A number of studies have confirmed that immunotherapy is a safe and feasible treatment option for cancer patients [12–16]. Therefore, conventional therapy combined with adoptive cell immunotherapy is associated with a favorable prognosis compared to chemotherapy alone [18]. Our analysis was designed to elucidate the effects of CIK cell therapy on improving the therapeutic efficacy and safe treatment of NSCLC patients based on a variety of evaluation indexes, including clinical survival outcomes, clinical response rates, immunophenotypes and adverse effects.

In our study, 17 trials were selected for the analysis of the culture of CIK cells and treatment regimens. Most of the trials collected 50–100 ml of autologous peripheral blood and separated the mononuclear cells for further induction. Some of the necessary cytokines were supplied to the cultures of CIK cells, such as IL-2, IFN-γ, and CD3mAb, in 1640 or serum-free medium. Based on our study, most of the treatments with repetitive infusions of 1×10^9 to 2×10^{12} CIK cells were administered for at least 2 weeks on every second day for a minimum of two treatment cycles. However, the different doses and cycles of CIK cell transfusions may lead to different outcomes and immune responses.

Table 6. Comparison of the immunological assessment of Ag-NORs and CEA expression between the CIK and non-CIK group.

Event	No. of Trials [Ref]	No. of pts Non-CIK	CIK	Mean Difference	95% CI	P value	Heterogeneity (I^2)
Ag-NORs	2 [20,38]	69	68	−0.71	−0.94 to −0.47	0.00001	33%
CEA	2 [38,39]	47	47	3.96	1.64-6.28	0.0008	0%

Summary of the significant points in the Ag-NORs and CEA expression level between the CIK group and the non-CIK group with meta-analysis. The random-effects model was used for the calculations. Ag-NORs: argyrophilic nucleolar organizer regions; CEA: carcinoembryonic antigen; Pts: patients; 95%CI: 95% confidence interval; significant difference: P value <0.05.

In the present study, the CIK cell-based therapy group was associated with favorable results based on an evaluation of both the overall survival and clinical responses (Table 4). The 1-year survival (OR 0.64, 95%CI 0.46–0.91, $p = 0.01$), 2-year survival (OR 0.36, 95%CI 0.22–0.59, $p<0.0001$), and 3-year survival (OR 0.37, 95%CI 0.20–0.70, $p = 0.002$) showed significantly prolonged durations in the CIK cell therapy group. A favorable DCR and ORR were also observed in patients receiving CIK cell therapy ($p<0.0001$). The MTTP and MST also showed significant improvements in the CIK group ($p = 0.005$, $p = 0.02$). CIK cells, which are also known as NKT cells, exhibit both the cytotoxicity activities of T-lymphocytes and the restrictive tumor-killing activity by non-MHC of NK cells, among which the main effectors are CD3$^+$CD56$^+$ cells [7]. In total, 4 of 17 trials used DCs pulsed with lung cancer antigens or tumor lysate, whereas 9 trials used mature DCs co-cultured with CIK cells (Table 2). DCs possess antigen-presenting activities on the extracellular surface and are able to activate the proliferation of T cells and CIK cells. Therefore, considering the poor immunogenicity of NSCLC, CIK infusion with an immunoadjuvant or tumor-specific antigen pulsed DCs boosted the immune responses [24]. Therefore, CIK cell-based therapy even acting through completely different mechanisms for fighting cancer cells, can lead to an improvement in the clinical objective responses based on the assessment of traditional RECIST criteria [40].

The human immune response against cancer cells is mainly dependent on cellular immunity. Previous studies have found that the numerical ratios of T-lymphocyte subsets in the peripheral blood are disordered in tumor patients [17]. In the present study, we observed a substantially increased percentage of CD3$^+$ and CD4$^+$ ($p<0.001$), the ratio of CD4$^+$CD8$^+$ and CD3$^+$CD56$^+$ ($p< 0.001$) and NK cells ($p = 0.002$), but a significant decrease in the percentage of the CD8$^+$ ($p<0.001$) and Treg ($p = 0.0003$) subgroups after DC-CIK treatment by meta-analysis. Many studies have demonstrated that CIK cells possess strong cytotoxicity against a variety of T-lymphocyte populations, among which CD3$^+$CD56$^+$ is mainly responsible for the MHC unrestricted antitumor activity [8]. In addition, the number of CD4$^+$ and CD8$^+$ T-cells plays an important role in affecting clinical outcomes in NSCLC. The activation of CD4$^+$ T cells contributes to the secretion of immune regulatory cytokines, including IL-2, IL-12, and IFN-γ, which in turn facilitate an elevation in the cytolytic CD8$^+$ T cell responses, thereby inducing tumor cell death [25]. The activation of CD4$^+$ T cells also enhances the killing activity of NK cells and the phagocytic activity of macrophages, triggering a humoral immune response that leads to antibody production, thus CD4$^+$ and CD8$^+$ have a synergistic relationship in immune responses. Our meta-analysis demonstrated that CD3$^+$, CD4$^+$, CD4$^+$CD8$^+$, CD3$^+$CD56$^+$ and NK cells were increased after DC-CIK treatment, therefore suggesting the improvement of immune function after immunotherapy in the NSCLC patients.

In addition, we should note that CD8$^+$ T cells were not significantly increased after the immunotherapy, which also showed the varied immunophenotypes compared with the results of other T-cell assessments by the CIK treatment in different solid carcinomas [11–13]. Naïve CD4$^+$ T lymphocytes undergo cell differentiation in the presence of antigen, co-stimulatory molecules and cytokines, and these cells can be divided into several major groups: Th1, Th2 and Treg cells [26]. Th1 helper cells are the host immunity effectors against intracellular bacteria and protozoa. These are triggered by IL-12, IL-2 and the effector cytokine IFN-γ. The main effector cells of Th1 immunity are macrophages, CD8 T cells, IgG B cells, and CD4 T cells. Th2 helper cells are the host immunity effectors against multicellular helminthes [26]. The

Study or Subgroup	Non-CIK Events	Total	CIK Events	Total	Weight	Odds Ratio M-H, Fixed, 95% CI	Odds Ratio M-H, Fixed, 95% CI
4.1.1 Leucopenia							
Xu 2010	32	40	31	38	5.5%	0.90 [0.29, 2.79]	
Xu 2011	33	40	36	45	5.2%	1.18 [0.39, 3.52]	
Zheng 2012	28	36	20	36	3.9%	2.80 [1.01, 7.80]	
Zhong 2008	10	44	4	22	3.6%	1.32 [0.36, 4.82]	
Zhong 2011	13	14	10	14	0.6%	5.20 [0.50, 54.05]	
Subtotal (95% CI)		174		155	18.8%	1.59 [0.93, 2.72]	
Total events	116		101				
Heterogeneity: Chi² = 3.49, df = 4 (P = 0.48); I² = 0%							
Test for overall effect: Z = 1.70 (P = 0.09)							
4.1.2 Gastrointestinal adverse reaction							
Peng 2012	5	23	2	24	1.3%	3.06 [0.53, 17.66]	
Xu 2010	30	40	29	38	6.5%	0.93 [0.33, 2.62]	
Xu 2011	32	40	37	45	6.1%	0.86 [0.29, 2.57]	
You 2012	15	50	13	55	7.5%	1.38 [0.58, 3.30]	
Zhang 2012	27	50	16	50	6.4%	2.49 [1.11, 5.63]	
Zheng 2012	19	36	10	36	4.1%	2.91 [1.09, 7.74]	
Zhong 2008	6	44	2	22	2.0%	1.58 [0.29, 8.55]	
Zhong 2011	13	14	9	14	0.6%	7.22 [0.72, 72.70]	
Subtotal (95% CI)		297		284	34.5%	1.77 [1.20, 2.59]	
Total events	147		118				
Heterogeneity: Chi² = 6.93, df = 7 (P = 0.44); I² = 0%							
Test for overall effect: Z = 2.90 (P = 0.004)							
4.1.3 Anemia							
Zhang 2012	36	50	22	50	5.4%	3.27 [1.42, 7.52]	
Zhong 2008	1	44	0	22	0.6%	1.55 [0.06, 39.65]	
Zhong 2011	6	14	4	14	2.0%	1.88 [0.39, 9.01]	
Subtotal (95% CI)		108		86	7.9%	2.80 [1.37, 5.73]	
Total events	43		26				
Heterogeneity: Chi² = 0.51, df = 2 (P = 0.77); I² = 0%							
Test for overall effect: Z = 2.81 (P = 0.005)							
4.1.4 Liver dysfunction							
You 2012	26	50	20	55	8.0%	1.90 [0.87, 4.14]	
Zhang 2012	4	50	3	50	2.4%	1.36 [0.29, 6.43]	
Zhong 2011	1	14	8	14	6.5%	0.06 [0.01, 0.57]	
Subtotal (95% CI)		114		119	16.8%	1.11 [0.60, 2.06]	
Total events	31		31				
Heterogeneity: Chi² = 8.25, df = 2 (P = 0.02); I² = 76%							
Test for overall effect: Z = 0.34 (P = 0.73)							
4.1.5 No-infection fever							
Peng 2012	0	23	7	24	6.3%	0.05 [0.00, 0.93]	
Shi 2012	0	30	4	30	3.9%	0.10 [0.00, 1.88]	
Zhong 2008	0	44	4	22	5.1%	0.05 [0.00, 0.90]	
Zhong 2011	3	14	10	14	6.8%	0.11 [0.02, 0.61]	
Subtotal (95% CI)		111		90	22.1%	0.08 [0.02, 0.26]	
Total events	3		25				
Heterogeneity: Chi² = 0.39, df = 3 (P = 0.94); I² = 0%							
Test for overall effect: Z = 4.15 (P < 0.0001)							
Total (95% CI)		804		734	100.0%	1.33 [1.05, 1.70]	
Total events	340		301				
Heterogeneity: Chi² = 46.08, df = 22 (P = 0.002); I² = 52%							
Test for overall effect: Z = 2.33 (P = 0.02)							
Test for subgroup differences: Not applicable							

0.02 0.1 1 10 50
Favours CIK Favours Non-CIK

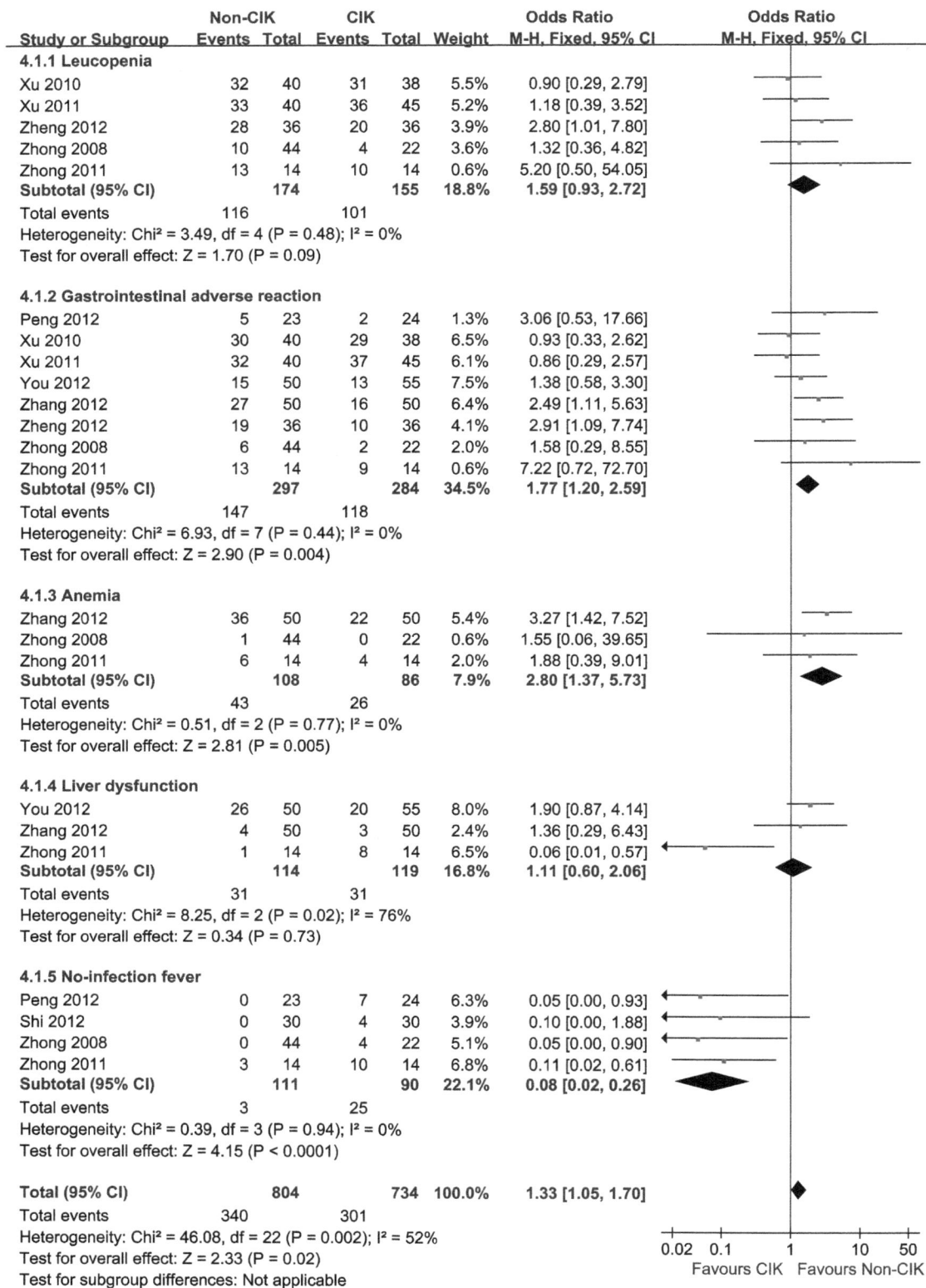

Figure 3. Forest plot comparing the toxicity and no treatment-related side effects between the CIK group and the non-CIK group.
Some serious adverse effects were observed significantly less frequently in the CIK group. Due to the lack of heterogeneity, the fixed-effect model was used.

main effector cells are eosinophils, basophils, and mast cells, as well as IgE B cells and IL-4/IL-5 CD4 T cells [27]. T regulatory cells express FoxP3 and produce TGF-β and CD4$^+$CD25$^+$CD127$^-$ T subgroups to suppress immune responses against Th1 and Th2. In addition, tumor cells also express high levels of CD4$^+$CD25$^+$ Treg cells, which help direct immunosuppressive cytokines to the tumor microenvironment [28], so the decrease of the Treg cell may be helpful to remove the immunosuppressive effect for NSCLC patients, and our results also demonstrated a lower number of Treg cells. Higher proportions of Treg and proliferating CD8$^+$ T cells were both associated with poor survival in malignancies lung cancer [41], suggesting that DC-CIK immunotherapy may play a role in enhancing the immune function of NSCLC patients.

Immunotherapy exerts its effect on the cellular immune response and requires time for immune cytokines to change the tumor burden or survival time. In our present study, we also evaluated T lymphocyte immune activity by Ag-NORs *in vivo* and the NSCLC tumor marker CEA. The significant increase in Ag-NORs ($p = 0.00001$) and the reduction in the CEA content ($p = 0.0008$) observed in the CIK group contributed to the prevention of short-term recurrence and improvement of clinical responses. We also analyzed clinical survival outcomes, clinical response rates, immunophenotypes and tumor markers, and we hypothesized that the CIK cells fight with tumor cells in several different ways, including direct cellular interactions (Fas/FasL pathway, granzyme B), the secretion of cytokines (IFN-γ, TNF-α, IL-2) and antibodies, and immune response regulations (T-lymphocyte variations) [29]. In all, our meta-analysis evaluated a variety of T-cell subgroups, and the differences in the cytokines used for immunotherapy, and we found that the results were consistent with the clinical therapeutic outcomes, such as the overall survival and clinical response.

In our analysis, CIK cell-based therapy yielded a disappointing result in non-infective fever (P<0.0001), and no other major side effect was observed. The pooled analysis showed that the adverse effects of gastrointestinal adverse reactions ($p = 0.004$) and anemia ($p = 0.005$) generated significant differences with fewer episodes in the CIK group. Thus, CIK cell immunotherapy with chemotherapy has proven to be a feasible and effective method for the treatment of NSCLC without severe side effects.

Limitation of the study

The 17 trials included in this meta-analysis were selected with an RCT to improve statistical reliability. To avoid bias in the identification and selection of trials, we minimized the possibility of overlooking published papers to the greatest extent. Although we selected using RCT as much as possible, there are some major criteria that did not receive a good grade under the Jadad scale, such as allocation concealment and intention-to-treat, meaning our study may have a moderate risk of bias. We also used a funnel plot to evaluate the publication bias. In our analysis, overall survival, clinical response rate, and side effects suffered low published bias; however, immunological assessment and T cell subgroups observed a high published bias. Therefore, there are some limitations to our study. First, CIK cell-based therapy is a greater concern for Chinese scholars; therefore, all 17 selected trials were from Asia, because there is a global lack of any multinational large-sample multicenter clinic research regarding CIK cell therapy for NSCLC. Second, some of the papers had to be excluded due to the lack of a control arm during the experimental design; however, some of the papers produced even

better prognosis after the CIK treatment. Third, our analyzed data were selected from published papers rather than drawn first-hand from patient records, potentially causing an overestimation of the analytical results. Therefore, only the enrollment of a larger sample could minimize this bias. However, various crucial issues for CIK cell-based immunotherapy need to be conquered before it can be approved as a standard treatment for NSCLC tumors due to several obstacles. First, the different dosage and treatment regimens of CIK cell transfusions may lead to different outcomes and immune responses. Second, although most of our selected papers focused on therapeutic outcomes based on chemotherapy RECIST criteria, due to the different tumor killing mechanisms, a novel immune-related response criterion (irRC) should also be used for the assessment of immunotherapy clinical activities [40]. Third, due to the poor immunogenicity of NSCLC, optimizing DC modifications combined with CIK cell infusion may contribute to more favorable clinical outcomes in NSCLC patients.

Taken together, the CIK-combined therapy for NSCLC presented a significantly prolonged overall survival, an improved clinical response rate, a strengthened immune system, and low rates of adverse side effects. The CIK therapy is more concerned with reducing the tumor burden stage than curing cancer. The CIK adoptive immune therapy showed potential regarding improved clinical outcomes, and there is increasing evidence that the CIK therapy treatment of NSCLC evokes specific humoral and cellular antitumor immune responses. However, the timing of the immunotherapy, dosage, regimens and efficient tumor antigens still require further research.

Conclusion

In total, 17 randomized controlled trials of NSCLC with 1172 patients were included in the present analysis. Combined CIK cell therapy for the treatment of NSCLC demonstrated significant superiority in terms of overall survival and objective response compared with the non-CIK group. The T-lymphocyte subgroups also seemed to favorably affect the immune system after chemotherapy. The data also indicated that CIK therapy relieves the side effects of chemotherapy without causing any additional major side effects aside from non-infective fever. This analysis supports a further larger-scale meta-analysis for the evaluation of the efficacy of CIK adoptive cell therapy for the treatment of NSCLC in the future.

Acknowledgments

This research work was supported by the National Natural Science Foundation of China (No. 31171427 and 30971651 to Zheng-Xu Wang), Beijing Municipal Science and Technology Project for Clinical Characteristics and Application Research of Capital (No. Z121107001012136 to Zheng-Xu Wang); the National Natural Science Foundation of China (No. 30700974 to Jun-Xia Cao) and the Postdoctoral Foundation of China (No. 20060400775 to Jun-Xia Cao).

Author Contributions

Conceived and designed the experiments: ZXW. Performed the experiments: MW JXC. Analyzed the data: MW JXC BLX XYZ J. Li J. Liu HBW. Contributed reagents/materials/analysis tools: JHP YSL DL. Wrote the paper: MW JXC.

References

1. Parkin DM, Bray F, Ferlay J, Pisani P (2005) Global cancer statistics. CA Cancer J Clin 55: 74–108.

2. Chen WQ, Zheng RS, Zhang SW, Zhao P, Li GG, et al. (2013) Chinese cancer registration annual report: National cancer registration center of lung cancer. Chin J Cancer Res 25(1): 10–21.

3. Arango BA, Castrellon AB, Santos ES, Raez LE (2009) Second-line therapy for non-small-cell lung cancer. Clin Lung Cancer 10(2): 91–98.

4. National Institutes of Health (2012) Cancer of the Lung and Bronchus-SEER Stat Facts Sheet. http://seer.cancer.gov/statfacts/htm/lungb.html.

5. Jiang J, Liang X, Zhou X, Huang R, Chu Z, et al. (2013) Non-platinum doublets were as effective as platinum-based doublets for chemotherapy-naïve advanced non-small-cell lung cancer in the era of third-generation agents. J Cancer Res Clin Oncol 139(1): 25–38.

6. Wu C, Jiang J, Shi L, Xu N (2008) Prospective study of chemotherapy in combination with cytokine-induced killer cells in patients suffering from advanced non-small cell lung cancer. Anticancer Res 28(6B): 3997–4002.

7. Choi D, Kim TG, Sung YC (2012) The past, present, and future of adoptive T cell therapy. Immune Netw 12(4): 139–147.

8. Sangiolo D (2011) Cytokine induced killer cells as promising immunotherapy for solid tumors. J Cancer 2: 363–368.

9. Rutella S, Iudicone P, Bonanno G, Fioravanti D, Procoli A, et al. (2012) Adoptive immunotherapy with cytokine-induced killer cells generated with a new good manufacturing practice-grade protocol. Cytotherapy 14(7): 841–850.

10. Schmidt-Wolf IG, Finke S, Trojaneck B, Denkena A, Lefterova P, et al. (1999) Phase I clinical study applying autologous immunological effector cells transfected with the interleukin-2 gene in patients with metastatic renal cancer, colorectal cancer and lymphoma. Br J Cancer 81: 1009–1016.

11. Ma Y, Zhang Z, Tang L, Xu YC, Xie ZM, et al. (2012) Cytokine-induced killer cells in the treatment of patients with solid carcinomas: a systematic review and pooled analysis. Cytotherapy 14(4): 483–493.

12. Hontscha C, Borck Y, Zhou H, Messmer D, Schmidt-Wolf IG (2011) Clinical trials on CIK cells: first report of the international registry on CIK cells (IRCC). J Cancer Res Clin Oncol 137(2): 305–310.

13. Li XD, Xu B, Wu J, Ji M, Xu BH, et al. (2012) Review of Chinese clinical trials on CIK cell treatment for malignancies. Clin Transl Oncol 14(2): 102–108.

14. Jäkel CE, Hauser S, Rogenhofer S, Müller SC, Brossart P, et al. (2012) Clinical studies applying cytokine induced killer cells for the treatment of renal cell carcinoma. Clin Dev Immunol 2012: 473245.

15. Ma Y, Xu YC, Tang L, Zhang Z, Wang J, et al. (2011) Cytokine-induced killer (CIK) cell therapy for patients with hepatocellular carcinoma: efficacy and safety. Exp Hematol Oncol 1(1): 11.

16. Wang ZX, Cao JX, Liu ZP, Cui YX, Li CY, et al. (2014) Combination of chemotherapy and immunotherapy for colon cancer in China: A meta-analysis. World J Gastroenterol 20(4): 1095–1106.

17. Li H, Wang C, Yu J, Cao S, Wei F, et al. (2009) Dendritic cell-activated cytokine-induced killer cells enhance the anti-tumor effect of chemotherapy on non-small cell lung cancer in patients after surgery. Cytotherapy 11(8): 1076–1083.

18. Mo C, Gao J, Wang J, Huang Y, Wu X, et al. (2005) Clinical efficacy of DC-activated and cytokine-induced killer cells combined with chemotherapy in treatment of advanced lung cancer. Chinese J Cancer Biotherapy 17(4): 419–423. doi: 10. 3872/j. issn. 1007-385X. 2010. 04. 011.

19. Peng D, Li J, Yuan J, Liu Y, Yu W, et al. (2012) Efficacy and safety of autologous DC and CIK cells cominedPemetrexed in the treatment of elderly patients with non-small cell lung cancer. Chinese J Immunol 28(7): 648–652. doi: 10.3969/ j.issn.1000-484X.2012. 07.017.

20. Sheng CH, Bao F, Xu S, Chang CY (2011) Clinical research on chemotherapy combined with dendritic cell-cytokine induced killer cells for non-small cell lung cancer. Journal of Practical Oncology 26(5): 503–506.

21. Shi SB, Ma TH, Li CH, Tang XY (2011) Effect of maintenance therapy with dendritic cells: cytokine-induced killer cells in patients with advanced non-small cell lung cancer. Tumori 98(3): 314–319.

22. Zhong R, Teng J, Han B, Zhong H (2011) Dendritic cells combining with cytokine-induced killer cells synergize chemotherapy in patients with late-stage non-small cell lung cancer. Cancer Immunol Immunother 60(10): 1497–1502.

23. Jadad AR, Moore RA, Carroll D, Jenkinson C, Reynolds DJ, et al. (1996) Assessing the quality of reports of randomized clinical trials: Is blinding necessary? Control Clin Trials 17: 1–12.

24. Shepherd FA, Douillard JY, Blumenschein GR Jr (2011) Immunotherapy for non-small cell lung cancer: novel approaches to improve patient outcome. J Thorac Oncol 6(10): 1763–1773.

25. Arens R, Schoenberger SP (2010) Plasticity in programming of effector and memory CD8 T-cell formation. Immunological Reviews 235: 190–205.

26. Mucida D, Cheroutre H (2010) The many face-lifts of CD4 T helper cells. Advances in Immunology 107: 139–152.

27. Neurath MF, Finotto S, Glimcher LH (2002) The role of Th1/Th2 polarization in mucosal immunity. Nature Medicine 8: 567–573.

28. Gallimore A, Godkin A (2008) Regulatory T cells and tumor immunity observations in mice and men. Immunology 123: 157–163.

29. Yu J, Zhang W, Jiang H, Li H, Cao S, et al. (2008) CD4+T cells in CIKs (CD4+ CIKs) reversed resistance to fas-mediated apoptosis through CD40/CD40L ligation rather than IFN-gamma stimulation. Cancer Biother Radio pharm 23(3): 342–354.

30. Li R, Wang C, Liu L, Du C, Cao S, et al. (2012) Autologous cytokine-induced killer cell immunotherapy in lung cancer: a phase II clinical study. Cancer Immunol Immunother 61(11): 2125–2133.

31. Xu Y, Xu D, Zhang N, Chen F, Liu J (2011) Observation of Chemotherapy Combined with Cytokine-induced Killer Cells and Dendritic Cells in Patients with the Advanced Non-Small Cell Lung Cancer. Prac J Cancer 25(2): 163–166.

32. Xu Y, Xu D, Zhang N, Chen F, Zhang G, et al. (2011) Effection of NP concurrent chemotherapy radiotherapy and sequential adoptive immunity cell for locally advanced non-small cell lung cancer. Chinese J Cancer Prev Treat 18(13): 1032–1035.

33. Yang L, Ren B, Li H, Yu J, Cao S, et al. (2013) Enhanced antitumor effects of DC-activated CIKs to chemotherapy treatment in a single cohort of advanced non-small-cell lung cancer patients. Cancer Immunol Immunother 62(1): 65–73.

34. You Z, Su X, Liu Y (2012) Observation on Clinical Efficacy of DC-CIK Biotherapy Auxiliary Interventional Chemotherapy on Central Non-Small-Cell Lung Carcinoma. Anti-tumor Phar 2(3): 193–196. doi: 10.3969/j.issn.2095-1264.2012.03.010.

35. Yuan J, Peng D, Li J (2011) Clinical effects of administering dendritic cells and cytokine induced killer cells combined with chemotherapy in the treatment of advanced non-small cell lung cancer. J Clin Pulmonary Med 16(12): 1910–1911.

36. Zhang J, Mao G, Han Y, Yang X, Feng H, et al. (2012) The clinical effects of DC-CIK cells combined with chemotherapy in the treatment of advanced NSCLC. Chin Ger J Clin Oncol 11(2): 67–71.

37. Zhong R, Han B, Zhong H, Gong L, Sha H, et al. (2008) Dendritic cells immunotherapy combined with chemotherapy inhibits postoperative recurrence and metastasis in stage IB of NSCLC after radical surgery. China Oncol 18(10): 760–764.

38. Zheng FC, Zhang XY, Feng HZ, Chen J, Sun Y, et al. (2012) Clinical Study of Stereotactic Conformal Body γ-knife Combined with Adoptive Immunotherapy (Dendritic Cell and Cytokine-induced Killer Cell) in the Treatment for Advanced Non-small Cell Lung Cancer. Journal of Chinese Oncology 18(11): 815–818.

39. Wang YY, Wang YS, Liu T, Yang K, Yang GQ, et al. (2013) Efficacy study of Cyber Knife stereotactic radio surgery combined with CIK cell immunotherapy for advanced refractory lung cancer. Exp Ther Med 5(2): 453–456.

40. Wolchok JD, Hoos A, O'Day S, Weber JS, Hamid O, et al. (2009) Guidelines for the evaluation of immune therapy activity in solid tumors: immune-related response criteria. Clin Cancer Res 15: 7412–7420.

41. McCoy MJ, Nowak AK, van der Most RG, Dick IM, Lake RA (2013) Peripheral CD8(+) T cell proliferation is prognostic for patients with advanced thoracic malignancies. Cancer Immunol Immunother 62(3): 529–539.

19

Copy Number Loss of the Interferon Gene Cluster in Melanomas is Linked to Reduced T Cell Infiltrate and Poor Patient Prognosis

Peter S. Linsley*, Cate Speake, Elizabeth Whalen, Damien Chaussabel

Department of Systems Immunology, Benaroya Research Institute, Seattle, WA, United States of America

Abstract

While immunotherapies are rapidly becoming mainstays of cancer treatment, significant gaps remain in our understanding of how to optimally target them, alone or in combination. Here we describe a novel method to monitor levels of immune cells and pathways in expression data from solid tumors using pre-defined groups or modules of co-regulated immune genes. We show that expression of an interconnected sub-network of type I interferon-stimulated genes (ISGs) in melanomas at the time of diagnosis significantly predicted patient survival, as did, to a lesser extent, sub-networks of T helper/T regulatory and NK/T Cytotoxic cell genes. As a group, poor prognosis tumors with reduced ISG and immune gene levels exhibited significant copy number loss of the interferon gene cluster located at chromosome 9p21.3. Our studies demonstrate a link between type I interferon action and immune cell levels in melanomas, and suggest that therapeutic approaches augmenting both activities may be most beneficial.

Editor: Maria G. Castro, University of Michigan School of Medicine, United States of America

Funding: The authors have no support or funding to report.

Competing Interests: This work comprises a portion of a patent application.

* Email: plinsley@benaroyaresearch.org

Introduction

Immunotherapy of cancer is assuming a growing importance [1], and has led to durable clinical responses to several immunotherapeutic agents in a broad range of human cancers [2]. Despite this encouraging activity, cancer immunotherapy is not always effective and may be associated with significant safety issues due to mechanism-based, immune-related adverse events [3,4]. Maximizing benefits and minimizing risks of immunotherapy will require new approaches for monitoring responses and toxicities, stratifying patients, and guiding combination therapies. Increasingly, high-throughput methods are being used to generate prognostic, predictive, and mechanistic signatures to guide treatment (reviewed in [5,6]). Genome-scale studies have an inherent problem with false positives because of the inequality between numbers of genes and samples [7]. One solution is to focus on pre-defined groups (modules) of coordinately expressed and annotated genes [8,9]. Here we describe a novel method to assess immune function and predict patient survival from solid tumor expression data using transcript modules identified in immune cells.

Materials and Methods

The Cancer Genome Atlas (TCGA) Data

TCGA data designated as available without restrictions were obtained from public repositories. TCGA data and sample annotation for SKCM set were obtained from the Broad Institute GDAC Firehose (https://confluence.broadinstitute.org/display/GDAC/Home). For the studies reported here, we used stddata and analyses Runs, 09/23/13. The sample annotation data were downloaded as: SKCM.clin.merged.picked.txt. The expression profiles were downloaded as: SKCM.rnaseqv2__illuminahiseq_rnaseqv2__unc_edu__Level_3__RSEM_genes_normalized__data.data. We obtained a curated set of 291 annotated RNAseq profiles, each comprising approximately 20 million reads normalized by the RSEM procedure [10]. Expression values for RNAseq data are reported as log2(Reads) or log2(Reads+1) for low expression values. The CNV data were downloaded as: all_data_by_genes_GISTIC2_level_4_052313.txt. The mutation data were downloaded as: SKCM-TM.cosmic_mutations.txt. RPPA measurements were downloaded as: SKCM.protein_exp__mda_rppa_Level_3__protein_norm.txt.

Transcript modules

Immune molecule modules were constructed de novo as simple co-expression matrices between levels of marker genes (cell surface and transcription factor genes) and all other genes across a dataset of RNAseq profiles. The dataset comprised profiles from 134 samples of whole blood and/or purified cells (CD4+ T cells, CD8+ T cells, NK cells, B cells, neutrophils, and macrophages) from healthy controls and individuals with autoimmune or infectious diseases. Notably, this dataset contained samples from multiple sclerosis patients before and 24 hr after treatment with AVONEX. Experiments to be described elsewhere show a strong type I interferon signature in patient samples taken after treatment when

compared with pre- treatment samples (C. Speake et al, manuscript in preparation). Here, we calculated Pearson correlation
coefficients between marker gene transcript levels and levels of all
50,484 ENSEMBL gene models, across all samples. The top 100
most positively correlated transcripts (Pearson correlation coefficients, 0.491–0.994, median = 0.863) were designated as immune
molecule modules and are presented in Table S1. These 111
modules comprised 5,149 named genes.

Analysis procedures

Tools from GenePattern (http://genepattern.broadinstitute.
org/gp/pages/index.jsf) were used to process data set
GSE39088 from GEO (http://www.ncbi.nlm.nih.gov/geo/). Data were downloaded using GEOImporter and probe-level data
collapsed into gene-level data using CollapseDataset. Normalized
data set GSE22153 was downloaded from GEO and probe-level
data were collapsed into gene-level data using the WGCNA
package in R. For network viewing, gene lists were projected on to
the STRING 9.1 [11] Network of Known and Predicted Protein-
Protein Interactions (http://string-db.org/). Nodes having ≥2
edges were then exported into Cytoscape [12] (http://www.
cytoscape.org/) for manipulation and visualization.

Other analyses were performed using the R language and core
packages [13], and additional packages: *ggplot2* [14]; *reshape2*
[15]; *party* [16]; and *survival* [17,18]. The *ggkm* function in R was
used for plotting enhanced KM plots [19].

Type I error correction and statistical significance

For *survdiff* p-values, we used permutation testing to correct for
type I error and to estimate statistical significance directly from the
data. From 10,000 random partitions of SKCM samples into two
equally sized groups, we observed 105 (~1%) that gave *survdiff* p-
values <0.01. We therefore used 1% of the total numbers of
module tested as the expected value for the null distribution of
survdiff having p-values <0.01. For all other tests used, we
considered p-values <0.05 as significant.

Accession codes

On publication, RNAseq profiles used for creating immune
molecular modules will be deposited into GEO, Accession
GSE60424.

Results

Three groups of immune molecular module genes predict patient survival

We hypothesized that transcript modules [8,20] would elucidate
how immune processes impact tumor prognosis and response to
therapy. Melanoma is the tumor type where immunotherapy is
most often effective [2], and one which may regress spontaneously
[21] or in response to therapy [22], concomitant with autoimmune
symptoms. We therefore focused on melanoma, where we
reasoned that immune processes might be active. We utilized
the SKCM (SKin Cutaneous Melanoma) dataset (Methods) from
The Cancer Genome Atlas (TCGA), a large-scale collaborative
effort to characterize genomic changes that occur in cancer.
Clinical characteristics of this data set are summarized in Table 1.
Tumor biopsy samples were taken at or near the time of diagnosis.

In preliminary analyses (not shown), we found that transcript
modules [9,20] suggesting immune surveillance (i.e., T cells,
Cytotoxic cells and ISGs) were expressed in SKCM melanomas
and could predict patient survival. To confirm and extend these
findings, we performed a systematic analysis with de novo
constructed immune molecular modules (Methods). These mod-

ules (Table S1) comprised genes most positively correlated with
levels of cell marker genes and transcription factors [23]).

We used the strategy shown in Figure 1A to test modules for
their ability to predict patient survival. We divided melanomas
into two groups for each module, one having higher than median
expression of module genes (module high), and the other, lower
than median expression (module low). We then compared survival
of the two sets of patients using log-rank test p-values and Kaplan-
Meier (KM) plots [18]. We tested all immune molecule modules
for their ability to predict melanoma patient survival and ranked
them by p-value (Table S2). We noted that many of the top
modules comprised highly overlapping sets of genes. To examine
this overlap more rigorously, we calculated the fraction of gene
overlap in pairwise comparisons between top modules and
subjected the resulting data matrix to hierarchical clustering
(Figure 1B). As expected, all modules showed strongest gene
overlap with themselves (on-diagonal), but many also showed
strong overlaps with other modules (off-diagonal). These off-
diagonal modules formed three major groups.

The first group included several modules giving very significant
p-values, including IRF7.mod, STAT2.mod, STAT1.mod, and
AFF1.mod, which gave a weaker p-value (Table S2). The markers
for these modules are well-known participants in interferon
pathways, and an average of eighty six percent of the genes in
them were found in the Interferome database (http://interferome.
its.monash.edu.au/interferome/home.jspx). Since genes in these,
but not other top modules, were up-regulated after in vitro
treatment of whole blood with type I interferon (Figure S1), we
refer to them as ISGs. Network analysis of the best-scoring module
in this group (IRF7.mod) revealed a highly interconnected sub-
network (Figure S2A) of ISGs (DDX58, ISG15, ISG20, IFIT2,
OAS3, etc.).

The second group of overlapping modules also comprised some
with very significant p-values (MAF.mod and CD28.mod), but
others that were less significant (RBL2.mod, IL2RA.mod, and
TCF.mod). The best-scoring module in this group (MAF.mod)
contained a sub-network of T cell activation and costimulatory
genes (Figure S2B). Many molecules in this module clearly indicate
T cells (CD2, CD5, CD6, CD28, ICOS, LCK, etc.), but gave
inconclusive evidence as to the type of T cell subset(s) they
represented. This module may therefore represent a mixture of
cells, or single cells with unique properties ('Th/Treg' cell genes).

The third group of overlapping modules gave only weakly
significant p-values (EOMES.mod, KLRD1.mod, and
NKG7.mod). The best-scoring module in this group
(KLRD1.mod) yielded a sub-network of genes characteristic of
cytotoxic cells ('Cytotoxic cell' genes), including CD160, NCAM1,
GZMA, GZMB, NKG7 and TBX21 (Figure S2C). Taken
together, these results give evidence for three sub-networks of
immune cell types/processes within tumors having significant
effects on melanoma patient survival: ISGs; Th/Treg cells; and
Cytotoxic cells.

To examine interconnections between the three sub-networks,
we combined them into a single, larger scale network graph
(Figure 2A). On this larger scale, Th/Treg and Cytotoxic cell sub-
networks collapsed into a single sub-network, which remained
separate but linked to the sub-network of ISGs. We also compared
expression of top module genes in the three sub-networks across all
tumor samples (Figure 2, B–D). Median levels of genes in each
module were strongly correlated across samples, and tended
towards higher expression in samples with longer survival. Thus,
better prognosis tumors with high levels of any of these three
molecular modules have a strong tendency also to have
correspondingly high levels of the other modules, and vice versa.

Table 1. Patient characteristics of the SKCM Melanoma data set.

Variable	Median
Age (years)	56
Survival (days)	3,136
Breslow thickness (mm)	2.5
Gender	**Number**
M	170
F	107
Primary site	
primary tumor	37
regional cutaneous or subcutaneous tissue	50
regional lymph node	157
distant metastasis	31
Clark stage	
Stage 0	3
Stage 1	53
*Stage 2	78
Stage 3	99
Stage 4	12
Radiation therapy	
yes	274
no	3
Ulceration	
yes	90
no	98

Shown are data summarized from TCGA clinical data. * includes 6 samples that were ambiguously classified as stage I or II.

To provide direct evidence for the functional relevance of our findings, we analyzed immune cell protein expression data determined by Reverse Phase Protein Array (RPPA) data for the SKCM study. Proteins measured in this analysis included the kinase, LCK, an integral component of T Cell Receptor signaling, a T cell marker and a node in the sub-network shown in Figure S2B. As shown in Figure 2E, ISG hi tumors expressed significantly higher levels of LCK protein (p-value = 1.6e-10), supporting the notion they contain higher levels of T cell infiltrate.

KM plots confirmed the effectiveness of the best-scoring module in each group at predicting patient survival (Figure 3A–C). However, since partitioning into two equally sized groups was arbitrary, we determined the optimal grouping for ISG expression in SKCM melanomas by subjecting them to hierarchical clustering according to expression of IRF7.mod. The resulting clustering dendrogram (not shown) revealed three groups of samples, termed ISG hi (N = 55), ISG med (N = 184) and ISG lo (N = 46), listed in Table S3. When we compared patient survival in these three sample groups (Figure 3D), we observed a graded increase in survival according to ISG expression (median survival of 5,106, 2,184 and 813 days for ISG hi, ISG med and ISG lo, respectively). The overall difference between the curves was significant (p-value = 5.7e-3), as were differences between the ISG hi and ISG lo groups (p-value = 1.7e-3), and the ISG hi and ISG med groups (p-value = 2.2e-2). The difference between the ISG med and ISG lo groups was not significant (p-value = 8.5e-2). Thus, ISG expression levels are dose-dependent in their ability to predict patient survival.

Association of immune molecule profiles in tumors with other clinical covariates

To better judge the clinical significance of ISG levels, we examined how they associated with other clinical covariates. We created contingency tables comparing six clinical covariates against samples split on ISG levels (Table S4). Measures of gender, stage, ulceration and age were not significantly different between the two groups. However, ISG lo tumors were more likely to originate from distant metastases and have greater Breslow scores, consistent with these tumors being more aggressive.

We also compared the predictive ability of ISG module expression signatures with other clinical parameters, alone and in combination using a Cox proportional hazards model. Several variables gave significant p-values in univariate predictive analysis (stage, Breslow thickness, ulceration and age), but only ISG set and stage reached significance in the multivariable analysis (Table S5). The combined model was highly effective at predicting survival (Wald test p-value = 3.4e-5). A conditional inference tree from the multivariable model showed that ISG set was the input variable giving strongest association with survival (Figure S3). Tumor stage and patient age then most significantly split the ISG lo and ISG hi sets, respectively. Patients with ISG hi tumors, but less than median age had the longest survival, whereas patients with ISG lo, Stage III-IV tumors had the shortest (Figure S3). These results show that ISG levels are not a trivial covariate of other clinical variables, but a significant indicator of patient survival.

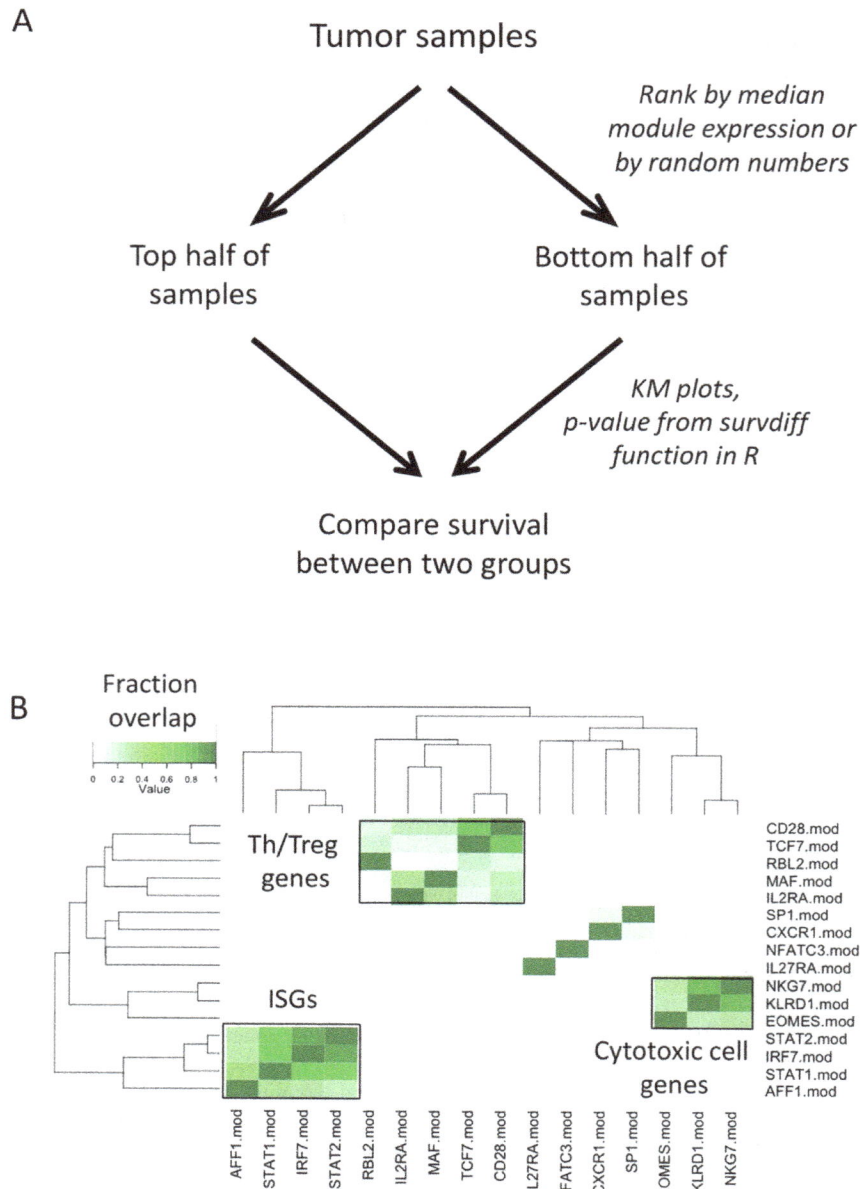

Figure 1. Using immune molecular modules to predict melanoma patient survival. A) Strategy to identify transcript modules most effective at predicting tumor prognosis. B) Overlapping gene sets comprise immune molecular modules best for stratifying melanoma patients. We identified immune molecular modules showing significant ability to stratify melanomas according to patient survival and determined the fraction of overlap between genes comprising the modules giving p-values <0.01 (Table S2). Shown here is a heatmap representation of the degree of overlaps between genes comprising the top modules. Molecular modules were clustered in both the X and Y dimensions according to the degree of gene overlap, as indicated by the color intensity scale. Although all modules showed strongest gene overlap with themselves (darkest green color on the diagonal), many modules also showed strong gene overlaps with other modules (lighter green off-diagonal color). Groups of modules comprising ISGs, Th/Treg and Cytotoxic cell genes are indicated.

Genetic characteristics of ISG hi and ISG lo tumors

It was also important to determine whether ISG hi and ISG lo tumor biopsies had distinctive genetic characteristics. We therefore searched for copy number variations that distinguish tumors with different ISG levels. We excluded ISG med samples from this analysis as the ISG hi and ISG lo samples were likely to show the greatest differences. We compared copy numbers for each gene in ISG hi and ISG lo samples using Wilcoxon p-values (Table S6). The top five most significantly different genes were from chromosome 9p21.3, including tumor suppressors CDKN2A and CDKN2B (Table S6). Genes from this region showed a large absolute difference between the groups, suggesting that a sizable fraction of tumors differed in copy number. Many genes from13q14.11 also showed significant differences, but these were of lower magnitude. Among the most significant genes at 13q14.11 was TNFSF11 (RANKL). These results show that at the group level, ISG hi and ISG lo tumors have distinct genetic differences.

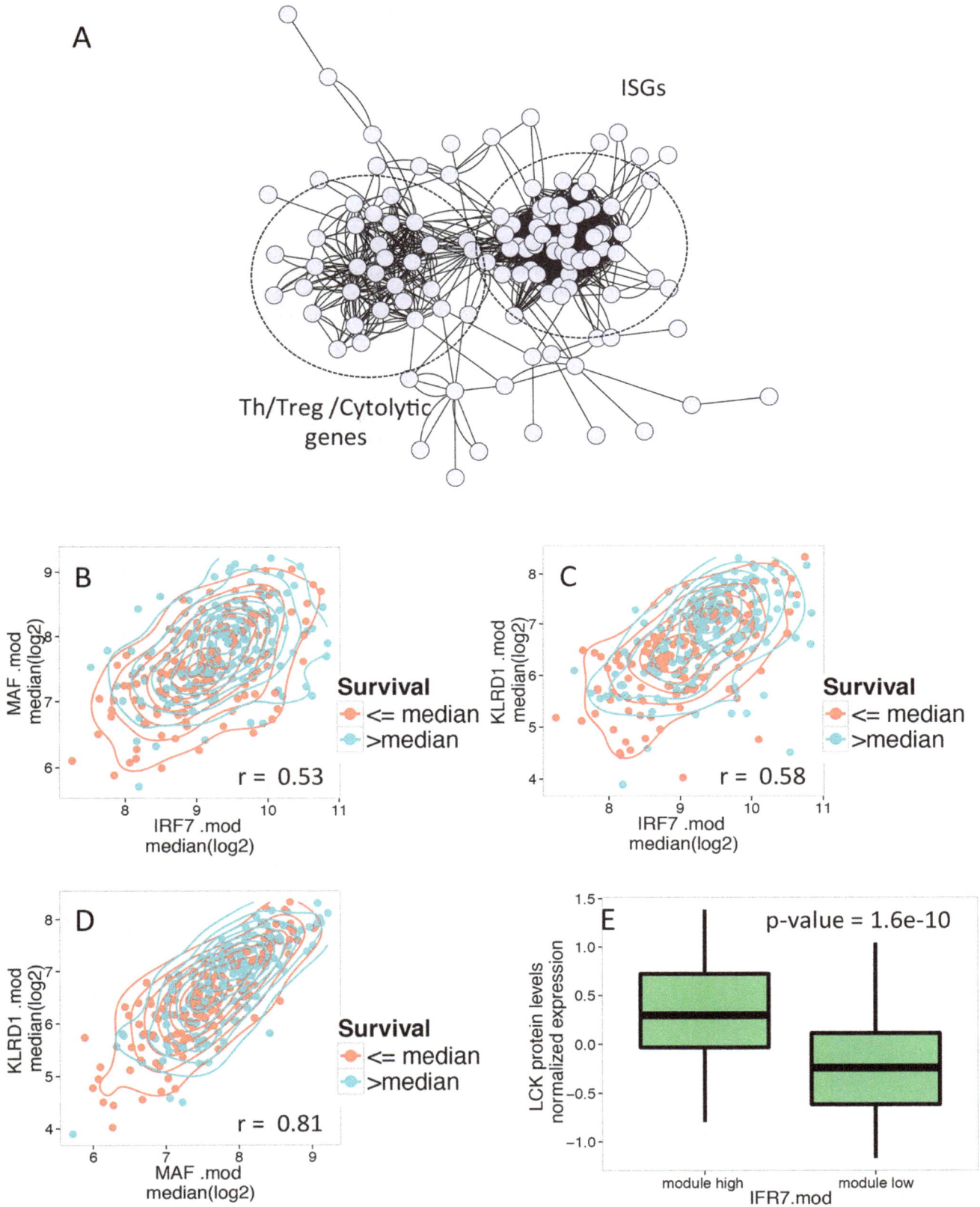

Figure 2. Relationship between genes in three modules effective at predicting patient survival. A) ISGs and T and Cytolytic cell genes comprise two interconnected sub-networks. Genes comprising combined IRF7.mod, MAF.mod and KLRD1.mod immune molecular modules were combined. Larger-scale sub-networks comprising T/NK genes and ISGs are labeled. Gene names of nodes have been omitted for clarity. B–D) Strong correlation between expression of genes in IRF7.mod, MAF.mod and KLRD1.mod. Shown are combination scatter/2D density plots of pairwise

comparisons of median expression of genes in IRF7.mod, MAF.mod and KLRD1.mod across SKCM samples. Magenta, samples with>median survival; teal, samples with≤median survival. Pearson correlation coefficients are indicated. B) median log2 expression of MAF.mod genes (Y axis) versus IRF7.mod genes (X axis). C) median log2 expression of KLRD1.mod genes versus IRF7.mod genes. D) median log2 expression of KLRD1.mod genes versus MAF.mod genes.

Because of the significance and magnitude of copy number differences at 9p21.3, we extended our analysis to determine how many genes from this locus were affected. As shown in Figure 4A, all genes from 9p21.3 showed significant copy number differences in comparisons between the ISG hi and ISG lo groups. The most significant copy number differences were at the CDKN2A and CDKN2B loci, extending in both directions and including the interferon gene cluster towards the top of the chromosome. This cluster encodes 17 type I interferons, the vast majority of this gene family in the human genome. Median copy numbers for all genes in the 9p21.3 region were consistent with the p-value determinations (Figure 4B). ISG lo samples showed copy number loss at 9p21.3, greatest in the region of the CDKN2A and CDKN2B genes, but extending in both directions and including the interferon gene cluster. Thus, poor-prognosis ISG lo samples were associated with significant copy number loss of 9p21.3 genes, which frequently includes the interferon gene cluster.

Validation of results on an independent cohort

It was important to validate our findings with an independent cohort. Jönsson et al [24] previously described studies using microarray profiles to classify melanomas into molecular subtypes. The samples from this study were from patients with similar demographic characteristics as in the SKCM study, and were well annotated with clinical information, and some genotyping data. Although these authors did not note ISGs in their profiles, our re-analysis of their data showed that IRF7.mod and MAF.mod gene sets were effective a stratifying patients according to survival, just as they were in the SKCM study (Figure S4). Moreover, although the Jönsson et al [24] studies were not adequately powered to definitively determine the effects of deletion of the CDKN2A locus on immune status, we noted that 5/6 samples with homozygous deletions of CDKN2A in their study were in both the IRF7.mod hi and MAF.mod hi subsets (p = 0.23). Finally, we examined the extent of tumor-infiltrating lymphocytes in the IRF7.mod hi and

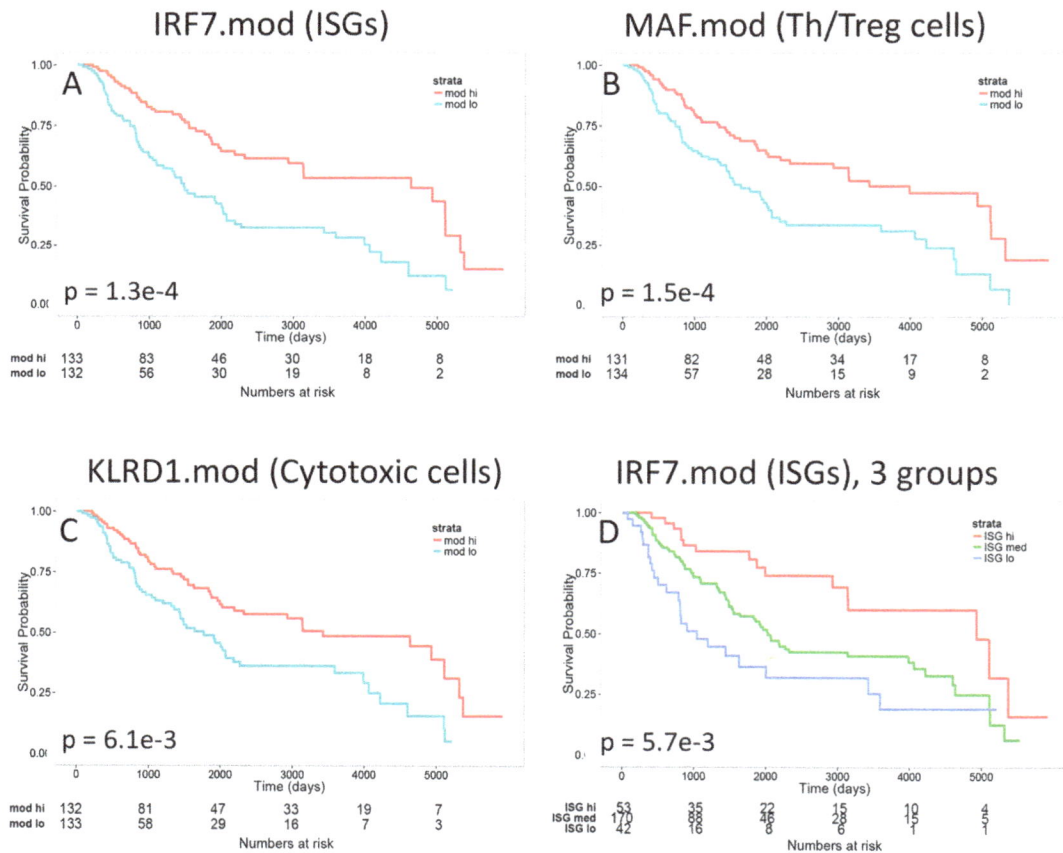

Figure 3. Expression of immune molecular module genes in melanomas predicts patient survival. We compared top-scoring immune molecular modules from the three effective groups for their ability to predict survival of melanoma patients. Shown are KM plots and p-values for the indicated modules. Magenta curves, patients having higher than median expression of module genes; teal curves, patients having lower than median expression of module genes. A) IRF7.mod; B) MAF.mod; and C) KLRD1.mod. D) Dose-dependent effect of ISG levels at predicting patient survival. Melanoma patients were stratified into three groups (ISG hi, ISG med and ISG lo) according to their expression of IRF7 marker modules genes (Table S3). E) LCK protein expression data supports higher levels of T cell immune filtrate in ISG hi samples. RPPA measurements for LCK from TCGA were compared for samples in ISG hi and ISG lo groups (N = 90 and N = 84 samples, respectively).

A

Chromosome 9p21.3

B

Chromosome 9p21.3

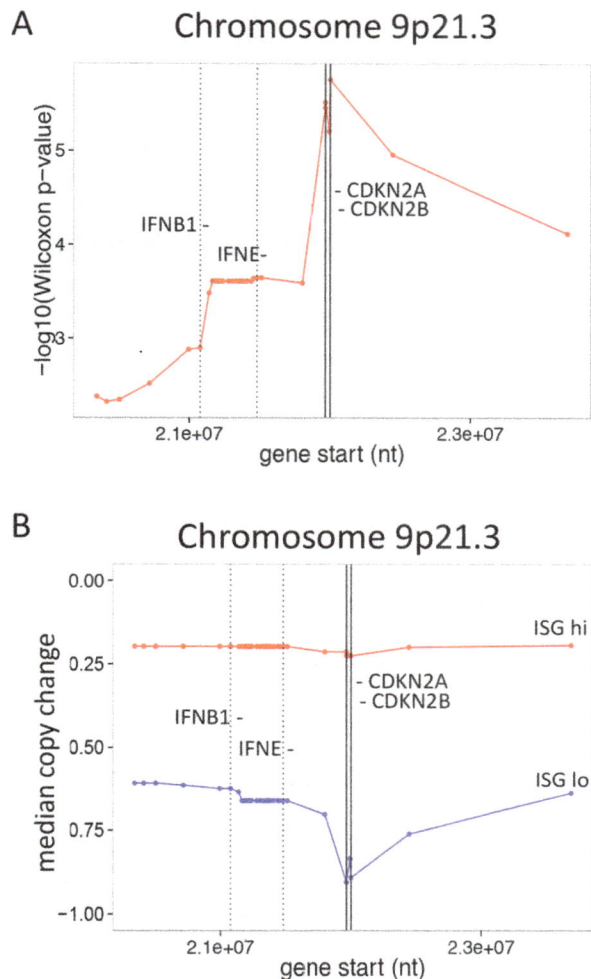

Figure 4. ISG hi melanomas show copy number loss chromosome 9p21.3. A) ISG lo samples have significant copy number differences at chr 9p21.3. We calculated Wilcoxon p-values and median copy numbers for all genes in ISG hi and ISG lo samples, and sorted genes by p-value (Table S6). Shown are -log10 p-values for differences in all genes chromosome 9p21.3 between ISG hi and ISG lo samples. Vertical lines indicate positions of the IFN gene cluster (17 IFN genes mapping between IFNB1 and IFNE) and CDKN2A and CDKN2B loci. B) Copy number loss encompassing the IFN gene cluster on chromosome 9 in ISG lo donors. Shown are median copy number changes for all genes at chromosome 9p21.3 in ISG hi and ISG lo samples.

MAF.mod hi subsets of the Jönsson et al [24] data, as determined by immunohistochemical staining of the T cell marker, CD3. As shown in Figure S4, both IRF7.mod hi and MAF.mod hi subsets were significantly enriched for samples scored by Jönsson et al as "CD3 brisk" (p-values 2.1e-2 and 1.8e-3, respectively), supporting tumor infiltration by T lymphocytes. Together, these studies with an independent data set support our observations with the SKCM study.

Discussion

Using a transcript module approach, we have demonstrated that expression levels of three distinct networks of immune genes in melanomas at time of diagnosis can predict patient survival. Two of these networks (Th/Treg and Cytotoxic cell genes) are likely derived from infiltrating immune cells. The third network (ISGs) is reduced in tumors having deletions at 9p21.3 and is likely derived, at least in part, from the tumors themselves. Expression of the ISG network is elevated in other tumors, but at present we do not know whether this elevation is due to the tumor itself, immune cell infiltrate or both.

Although themes of Cytotoxic and T cells have been noted in other signatures [5], there is very little gene overlap (not shown) between our modules and other published signatures [25–27]. Another novelty of our results is in the extent of type I interferon response we observe. While other profiling studies have implicated IFNG pathway (type II interferon) in immune cells [5], previous melanoma signatures [25–27] lack the prominent ISG response we describe. While the reason for this difference is unclear, possible explanations include differences in patient populations, and/or greater sensitivity of the module analysis approach, especially with highly co-regulated gene sets like ISGs. Type I interferons produced by immune cells [28] are important for immune surveillance and function in a way that does not completely overlap with IFNG [29]. Our results suggest a type I interferon response originating, at least partially, within tumors themselves, and link this response with levels of immune cell markers in tumors.

Chromosome 9p21.23 contains genes important in melanoma susceptibility [30–32], patient survival and success of interferon therapy [33]. This region encodes the CDKN2A and CDKN2B tumor suppressor genes, and may be deleted in several tumor types [34]. Deletion of this region occurs in early and late stages of melanoma, and may affect a large part of the chromosome [35]. Early studies of this locus ruled out the interferon gene cluster as a tumor suppressor [36], but suggested additional roles [37]. To our knowledge, our study is the first to link loss of this locus with reduced immune cell genes within tumors. Thus, loss of 9p21.3 may lead, or contribute to reduced immune surveillance and/or tumor destruction by the immune system. Recently, chromosomal instability was demonstrated to be a mechanism of modulating local cytokine expression in colorectal tumors [38]. Emerging evidence, therefore, suggests that genomic rearrangements within tumors may represent a broader mechanism for modulating anti-tumor immunity.

Interferon alpha, an approved therapy for late stage melanoma patients, is ineffective in some patients, but very effective in others, especially when treatment is accompanied by autoimmune symptoms [22]. Newer T cell directed therapies also are effective only in a subset of patients [2]. Significantly, our results show that best prognosis occurs when tumors show both ISG and T/NK cell responses. Furthermore, our results suggest that patients with tumors showing copy number loss at 9p21.3 will begin therapy with lower basal levels of ISGs and/or T/NK cells and may therefore require different treatment regimens. Combinations of interferon alpha with T cell-directed therapies could be more effective in these patients. Conversely, since individuals with tumors having high ISG responses already show evidence of an interferon response and T/NK cells, they may be more responsive to therapies augmenting one or both of these activities.

Supporting Information

Figure S1 Induction of ISG module transcripts following in vitro treatment of whole blood with interferon alpha. Shown are density plots of gene expression of genes in the indicated molecular modules in healthy control whole blood samples without (N = 46) or with (N = 18) in vitro treatment with alpha-interferon for 4 hrs. Genome scale microarray data were as described [39] and were obtained from GEO (GSE39088). Data were subsetted to show expression of genes from the indicated molecular modules in Untreated (pink) and IFNA-treated samples (teal). Rug plots along the x axes show distributions of the individual samples.

Figure S2 Immune molecular modules effective at stratifying patients contain distinctive sub-networks of genes. Genes in molecular modules (Table S1) were projected onto the STRING 9.1 Network (Methods). A) IRF7.mod sub-network, ISGs; B) MAF.mod sub-network, Th/Treg genes; and C) KLRD1.mod network, Cytotoxic cell genes.

Figure S3 Conditional inference tree from Cox proportional hazard model. We constructed a Cox proportional hazards model [17,18] using the clinical variables listed in Table S5 and created a conditional inference tree using the *ctree* function in R [40].

Figure S4 Validation in an independent cohort. We analyzed the data set published by Jönsson et al [24] (GSE22153) for validation of our findings with the SKMC set. A) Stratification of Jönsson et al samples by IRF7.mod; B) Stratification of Jönsson et al samples by MAF.mod; C) Contingency table showing distribution of samples classified as ISG hi and ISG lo by IRF7.mod expression, compared with those classified as "CD3 brisk" versus others ("non-brisk" and absent) by Jönsson et al; D) Contingency table showing distribution of samples classified as MAF hi and MAF lo by MAF.mod expression, compared with those classified as "CD3 brisk" versus others by Jönsson et al.

Table S1 Genes in immune molecular modules. Shown are the top 100 genes best correlated in expression levels with marker genes across row 1 (Methods).

Table S2 Groups of immune molecular modules best at predicting melanoma prognosis. Immune molecular modules were scored for their ability to predict survival of melanoma patients as described in Figure 1A. Shown are the results for the modules having unadjusted *survdiff* p-value <0.01. Permutation testing predicted ~1/111 of immune molecular modules to give *survdiff* p-values <0.01 by chance, as compared with the 16/111 we observed and show in this table (FDR~6%). Survdiff p-value, p-value calculated using *survdiff* function; group, identity of genes in the module (Figure 1B).

Table S3 Designation of melanoma samples according to immune molecular module expression. Shown are

results of melanoma sample stratification by immune molecular modules, IRF7.mod, MAF.mod and KLRD1.mod. For columns labeled as two variable mods, melanoma samples were identified as IRF7.mod, MAF.mod or KLRD1.mod hi or lo as described in Figure 1. For the column labeled three variable IRF7.mod, samples were divided into three groups, ISG hi, ISG med and ISG lo, as described Figure 2D.

Table S4 Clinical characteristics of ISG hi and ISG lo sets. Shown are the numbers of ISG hi and ISG lo samples with six clinical characteristic variables, and chi-square p-values for differences between ISG hi and ISG lo sets. Asterisks indicate degree of significance: *, p<0.05; **, p<0.01, ***, p<0.001.

Table S5 Univariate and multivariable models of survival. ISG expression and other clinical parameters were used to construct univariate and multivariable survival models. While we obtained similar results using patient age and Breslow thickness as discrete and continuous values, we show here only results obtained with the former. For univariate models, we show numbers of records and events for each variable, together with median survival, 95% confidence intervals and *survdiff* p-values. For the multivariable model, we show the Cox proportional hazard p-value. Asterisks indicate degree of significance: *, p< 0.05; **, p<0.01, ***, p<0.001.

Table S6 Copy number differences between ISG hi and ISG lo samples. Shown are median copy numbers for each gene in ISG hi and ISG lo samples, Wilcoxon p-values and absolute differences between the groups. Since adjacent genes subject to copy number variation at the chromosomal scale were unlikely to vary independently, we did not use multiple testing corrections for this analysis.

Acknowledgments

We gratefully acknowledge the TCGA Network for creating TCGA datasets. We also thank M. Carleton, M. Cheever, K.E. Hellstrom, L. Israelsson, J. Linsley and G. Nepom for insightful discussions and helpful comments on the manuscript.

Author Contributions

Conceived and designed the experiments: PSL. Performed the experiments: PSL. Analyzed the data: PSL EW. Contributed reagents/materials/ analysis tools: CS DC. Contributed to the writing of the manuscript: PSL CS EW DC. Provided statistical advice: EW. Provided the RNAseq data set used to construct immune molecular modules: CS DC. Conceived and executed the analysis: PSL.

References

1. Couzin-Frankel J (2013) Cancer Immunotherapy. Science 342: 1432–1433. doi:10.1126/science.342.6165.1432.
2. Chen DS, Mellman I (2013) Oncology meets immunology: the cancer-immunity cycle. Immunity 39: 1–10. doi:10.1016/j.immuni.2013.07.012.
3. Acharya UH, Jeter JM (2013) Use of ipilimumab in the treatment of melanoma. Clin Pharmacol Adv Appl 5: 21–27. doi:10.2147/CPAA.S45884.
4. Hamid O, Schmidt H, Nissan A, Ridolfi L, Aamdal S, et al. (2011) A prospective phase II trial exploring the association between tumor microenvironment biomarkers and clinical activity of ipilimumab in advanced melanoma. J Transl Med 9: 204. doi:10.1186/1479-5876-9-204.
5. Galon J, Angell HK, Bedognetti D, Marincola FM (2013) The continuum of cancer immunosurveillance: prognostic, predictive, and mechanistic signatures. Immunity 39: 11–26. doi:10.1016/j.immuni.2013.07.008.
6. Ascierto ML, De Giorgi V, Liu Q, Bedognetti D, Spivey TL, et al. (2011) An immunologic portrait of cancer. J Transl Med 9: 146. doi:10.1186/1479-5876-9-146.
7. Catchpoole DR, Kennedy P, Skillicorn DB, Simoff S (2010) The curse of dimensionality: a blessing to personalized medicine. J Clin Oncol Off J Am Soc Clin Oncol 28: e723–724; author reply e725. doi:10.1200/JCO.2010.30.1986.
8. Chaussabel D, Quinn C, Shen J, Patel P, Glaser C, et al. (2008) A modular analysis framework for blood genomics studies: application to systemic lupus erythematosus. Immunity 29: 150–164. doi:10.1016/j.immuni.2008.05.012.
9. Novershtern N, Subramanian A, Lawton LN, Mak RH, Haining WN, et al. (2011) Densely interconnected transcriptional circuits control cell states in human hematopoiesis. Cell 144: 296–309. doi:10.1016/j.cell.2011.01.004.

10. Li B, Dewey CN (2011) RSEM: accurate transcript quantification from RNA-Seq data with or without a reference genome. BMC Bioinformatics 12: 323. doi:10.1186/1471-2105-12-323.

11. Franceschini A, Szklarczyk D, Frankild S, Kuhn M, Simonovic M, et al. (2013) STRING v9.1: protein-protein interaction networks, with increased coverage and integration. Nucleic Acids Res 41: D808–815. doi:10.1093/nar/gks1094.

12. Shannon P, Markiel A, Ozier O, Baliga NS, Wang JT, et al. (2003) Cytoscape: a software environment for integrated models of biomolecular interaction networks. Genome Res 13: 2498–2504. doi:10.1101/gr.1239303.

13. R Core Team (2013) A language and environment for statistical computing. R Foundation for Statistical Computing. Vienna, Austria. Available: http://www.R-project.org/.

14. Wickham H (2009) ggplot2: elegant graphics for data analysis. Available: http://had.co.nz/ggplot2/book.

15. Wickham H (2007) Reshaping Data with the reshape Package. J Stat Softw 21: 1–20.

16. Hothorn T, Hornik K, Strobl C, Zeileis A (n.d.) party: A Laboratory for Recursive Partytioning. Available: http://cran.r-project.org/web/packages/party/index.html.

17. Therneau TM, Grambsch PM (2000) Modeling Survival Data: Extending the Cox Model. New York: Springer.

18. Therneau T (n.d.) A Package for Survival Analysis in S_. R package version 2.37-4. Available: http://CRAN.R-project.org/package=survival.

19. Abhijit GT, Cowley M (2011) An enhanced Kaplan-Meier plot. R. Available: http://www.r-bloggers.com/an-enhanced-kaplan-meier-plot/.

20. Banchereau R, Jordan-Villegas A, Ardura M, Mejias A, Baldwin N, et al. (2012) Host immune transcriptional profiles reflect the variability in clinical disease manifestations in patients with Staphylococcus aureus infections. PloS One 7: e34390. doi:10.1371/journal.pone.0034390.

21. Quaglino P, Marenco F, Osella-Abate S, Cappello N, Ortoncelli M, et al. (2010) Vitiligo is an independent favourable prognostic factor in stage III and IV metastatic melanoma patients: results from a single-institution hospital-based observational cohort study. Ann Oncol Off J Eur Soc Med Oncol ESMO 21: 409–414. doi:10.1093/annonc/mdp325.

22. Gogas H, Ioannovich J, Dafni U, Stavropoulou-Giokas C, Frangia K, et al. (2006) Prognostic significance of autoimmunity during treatment of melanoma with interferon. N Engl J Med 354: 709–718. doi:10.1056/NEJMoa053007.

23. Shay T, Jojic V, Zuk O, Rothamel K, Puyraimond-Zemmour D, et al. (2013) Conservation and divergence in the transcriptional programs of the human and mouse immune systems. Proc Natl Acad Sci U S A 110: 2946–2951. doi:10.1073/pnas.1222738110.

24. Jönsson G, Busch C, Knappskog S, Geisler J, Miletic H, et al. (2010) Gene expression profiling-based identification of molecular subtypes in stage IV melanomas with different clinical outcome. Clin Cancer Res Off J Am Assoc Cancer Res 16: 3356–3367. doi:10.1158/1078-0432.CCR-09-2509.

25. Ji R–R, Chasalow SD, Wang L, Hamid O, Schmidt H, et al. (2012) An immune-active tumor microenvironment favors clinical response to ipilimumab. Cancer Immunol Immunother CII 61: 1019–1031. doi:10.1007/s00262-011-1172-6.

26. Mann GJ, Pupo GM, Campain AE, Carter CD, Schramm S-J, et al. (2013) BRAF mutation, NRAS mutation, and the absence of an immune-related expressed gene profile predict poor outcome in patients with stage III melanoma. J Invest Dermatol 133: 509–517. doi:10.1038/jid.2012.283.

27. Ulloa-Montoya F, Louahed J, Dizier B, Gruselle O, Spiessens B, et al. (2013) Predictive gene signature in MAGE-A3 antigen-specific cancer immunotherapy. J Clin Oncol Off J Am Soc Clin Oncol 31: 2388–2395. doi:10.1200/JCO.2012.44.3762.

28. Fuertes MB, Woo S-R, Burnett B, Fu Y-X, Gajewski TF (2013) Type I interferon response and innate immune sensing of cancer. Trends Immunol 34: 67–73. doi:10.1016/j.it.2012.10.004.

29. Dunn GP, Bruce AT, Sheehan KCF, Shankaran V, Uppaluri R, et al. (2005) A critical function for type I interferons in cancer immunoediting. Nat Immunol 6: 722–729. doi:10.1038/ni1213.

30. Bishop DT, Demenais F, Iles MM, Harland M, Taylor JC, et al. (2009) Genome-wide association study identifies three loci associated with melanoma risk. Nat Genet 41: 920–925. doi:10.1038/ng.411.

31. Chatzinasiou F, Lill CM, Kypreou K, Stefanaki I, Nicolaou V, et al. (2011) Comprehensive field synopsis and systematic meta-analyses of genetic association studies in cutaneous melanoma. J Natl Cancer Inst 103: 1227–1235. doi:10.1093/jnci/djr219.

32. Falchi M, Bataille V, Hayward NK, Duffy DL, Bishop JAN, et al. (2009) Genome-wide association study identifies variants at 9p21 and 22q13 associated with development of cutaneous nevi. Nat Genet 41: 915–919. doi:10.1038/ng.410.

33. Lenci RE, Bevier M, Brandt A, Bermejo JL, Sucker A, et al. (2012) Influence of genetic variants in type I interferon genes on melanoma survival and therapy. PloS One 7: e50692. doi:10.1371/journal.pone.0050692.

34. Mitelman F, Mertens F, Johansson B (1997) A breakpoint map of recurrent chromosomal rearrangements in human neoplasia. Nat Genet 15: 417–474. doi:10.1038/ng0497supp-417.

35. Rákosy Z, Vízkeleti L, Ecsedi S, Bégány A, Emri G, et al. (2008) Characterization of 9p21 copy number alterations in human melanoma by fluorescence in situ hybridization. Cancer Genet Cytogenet 182: 116–121. doi:10.1016/j.cancergencyto.2008.01.008.

36. Fountain JW, Karayiorgou M, Ernstoff MS, Kirkwood JM, Vlock DR, et al. (1992) Homozygous deletions within human chromosome band 9p21 in melanoma. Proc Natl Acad Sci U S A 89: 10557–10561.

37. Olopade OI, Jenkins RB, Ransom DT, Malik K, Pomykala H, et al. (1992) Molecular analysis of deletions of the short arm of chromosome 9 in human gliomas. Cancer Res 52: 2523–2529.

38. Mlecnik B, Bindea G, Angell HK, Sasso MS, Obenauf AC, et al. (2014) Functional network pipeline reveals genetic determinants associated with in situ lymphocyte proliferation and survival of cancer patients. Sci Transl Med 6: 228ra37. doi:10.1126/scitranslmed.3007240.

39. Lauwerys BR, Hachulla E, Spertini F, Lazaro E, Jorgensen C, et al. (2013) Down-regulation of interferon signature in systemic lupus erythematosus patients by active immunization with interferon α-kinoid. Arthritis Rheum 65: 447–456. doi:10.1002/art.37785.

40. Hothorn T, Hornik K, Zeileis A (2006) Unbiased Recursive Partitioning: A Conditional Inference Framework. J Comput Graph Stat 15: 651–674.

20

Neuropilin-1 Expression is Induced on Tolerant Self-Reactive CD8+ T Cells but is Dispensable for the Tolerant Phenotype

Stephanie R. Jackson[1], Melissa Berrien-Elliott[1], Jinyun Yuan[1], Eddy C. Hsueh[2,3], Ryan M. Teague[1,3]*

1 Saint Louis University School of Medicine, Department of Molecular Microbiology and Immunology, St. Louis, Missouri, United States of America, **2** Saint Louis University School of Medicine, Department of Surgery, St. Louis, Missouri, United States of America, **3** Saint Louis University Cancer Center, St. Louis, Missouri, United States of America

Abstract

Establishing peripheral CD8+ T cell tolerance is vital to avoid immune mediated destruction of healthy self-tissues. However, it also poses a major impediment to tumor immunity since tumors are derived from self-tissue and often induce T cell tolerance and dysfunction. Thus, understanding the mechanisms that regulate T cell tolerance versus immunity has important implications for human health. Signals received from the tissue environment largely dictate whether responding T cells become activated or tolerant. For example, induced expression and subsequent ligation of negative regulatory receptors on the surface of self-reactive CD8+ T cells are integral in the induction of tolerance. We utilized a murine model of T cell tolerance to more completely define the molecules involved in this process. We discovered that, in addition to other known regulatory receptors, tolerant self-reactive CD8+ T cells distinctly expressed the surface receptor neuropilin-1 (Nrp1). Nrp1 was highly induced in response to self-antigen, but only modestly when the same antigen was encountered under immune conditions, suggesting a possible mechanistic link to T cell tolerance. We also observed a similar Nrp1 expression profile on human tumor infiltrating CD4+ and CD8+ T cells. Despite high expression on tolerant CD8+ T cells, our studies revealed that Nrp1 had no detectable role in the tolerant phenotype. Specifically, Nrp1-deficient T cells displayed the same functional defects as wild-type self-reactive T cells, lacking *in vivo* cytolytic potential, IFNγ production, and antitumor responses. While reporting mostly negative data, our findings have therapeutic implications, as Nrp1 is now being targeted for human cancer therapy in clinical trials, but the precise molecular pathways and immune cells being engaged during treatment remain incompletely defined.

Editor: Taishin Akiyama, University of Tokyo, Japan

Funding: Research reported in this publication was supported by the National Institute of Allergy and Infectious Disease/National Institutes of Health (R01AI087764) to RMT, by a Cancer Research Institute Investigator Award to RMT, and by a National Cancer Institute/National Institutes of Health fellowship (F30CA180375) to SRJ. The funders had no role in study design, data collection and analysis, decision to publish, or preparation of the manuscript.

* Email: rteague@slu.edu

Introduction

Activated cytotoxic T cells represent a powerful branch of the adaptive immune system, capable of detecting cellular abnormality and protecting the human host from microbial threats and malignancy. These cells are armed with a plethora of effector mechanisms, including cytolytic molecules and proinflammatory cytokines. While critical for host defense, CD8+ T cell responses can be detrimental or even fatal when deregulated [1,2,3,4,5]. Thus, T cell activation following antigen engagement must be tightly controlled. One mechanism of control is peripheral T cell tolerance, which is critical in preventing immunopathology mediated by excessive CD8+ T cell activity, and is especially important to limit the activation of self-reactive T cells harbored in the periphery of healthy individuals [6]. However, tolerance also presents a formidable barrier to eliciting anti-tumor immune responses since many cancer antigens are also expressed in healthy self-tissue [7]. In an effort to improve treatment options for patients with cancer, extensive work has gone into characterizing the factors that lead to T cell tolerance and the development of strategies that break tolerance toward tumor/self-antigens to augment immunotherapy [8].

We and others have reported that CD8+ T cell tolerance is regulated in part by the coinhibitory surface receptors PD-1, LAG-3 and CTLA-4 [9,10,11]. In our studies, these proteins were upregulated after antigen priming, particularly under tolerant conditions where these molecules proved fundamental for the dysfunctional phenotype [9]. Although not characterized as a coinhibitory receptor, a similar pattern of expression was also observed for the surface molecule, neuropilin-1 (Nrp1), implying a possible link between Nrp1 and the induction or maintenance of CD8+ T cell tolerance.

Nrp1 is a type-I transmembrane glycoprotein originally discovered for its role in neuron axon guidance and embryonic vessel formation [12,13,14,15]. Its expression has subsequently been reported on malignant cells and several immune cell subsets including dendritic cells (DC), conventional T cells, and regulatory T cells (Treg) [16,17,18]. Nrp1 has three extracellular domains important for ligand binding and receptor dimerization, and a short cytoplasmic tail that lacks a kinase domain. To support downstream signaling, Nrp1 dimerizes with other surface proteins such as plexin molecules, VEGFR2, TGFB-R, EGFR, HGFR, and PDGFR-α, allowing strong interactions with the multiple ligands. These varied binding partners permit Nrp1 ligation to modulate a variety of signaling pathways, contributing to the remarkable diversity in the physiological activities attributed to Nrp1 [16].

The first description of a possible role for Nrp1 in the immune system showed homotypic interactions between Nrp1 on mature DC and human T cells in the initiation of the primary T cell immune response [18]. Subsequent studies focused primarily on Nrp1 in murine Treg, as antigen engagement selectively supports Nrp1 expression on Treg versus conventional CD4$^+$ T cells [17]. In Treg, Nrp1 promotes synapse formation with DC and longer, more stable interactions leading to enhanced suppression [19]. The first in vivo reports found that Nrp1 helped suppress autoreactive CD4$^+$ T cells in a murine experimental autoimmune encephalomyelitis model [20]. More recently, Nrp1 was identified as a marker of natural versus induced Treg and shown to play a role in contact-independent suppression mediated by these cells [21,22]. Mechanistic studies by Delgoffe and colleagues demonstrated a role for Nrp1 in the stability and suppressive activity of Treg, involving phosphatase PTEN recruitment to the immunological synapse via association with the PDZ- protein interaction domain encoded in the cytoplasmic tail of Nrp1 expression [23]. Thus, there is a building consensus that Nrp1 is important for activation, synapse formation, and suppressive activity of CD4$^+$ Treg.

Few reports have explored the biology of Nrp1 on CD8$^+$ T cells. In a thorough analysis of the genes involved in CD8$^+$ T cells memory formation, Kaech et al. reported modest Nrp1 upregulation (2-fold higher) on effector and memory CD8$^+$ T cells relative to naive cells [24]. In 2012, Hansen et al comment briefly that a minor population of CD8$^+$ T cells in the spleen expressed Nrp1 (1%), which contrasted with 80% of Foxp3$^+$ Treg and 23% of CD4$^+$ T cells [25]. Nrp1 has been suggested as a potential marker for liver-sinusoidal endothelium-primed CD8$^+$ T cells that escape deletional tolerance [26]. These Nrp1$^+$ T cells formed a distinct memory cell population that lacked cytokine responsiveness, representing the first correlation between Nrp1 expression and CD8$^+$ T cells with a dysfunctional phenotype. However, these reports were correlative, and the functional relevance of Nrp1 in regard to CD8$^+$ T cell immunity and tolerance has not yet been determined.

In this study, we investigated the expression profile and functional role of Nrp1 on CD8$^+$ T cells under naive steady state conditions, and within distinct in vivo environments where antigen was encountered within immune, inflammatory, or tolerant contexts. We report that Nrp1 was selectively induced and highly expressed on CD8$^+$ T cells engaging self-antigen, both in mice and in human melanoma infiltrating T cells. Despite this unique expression pattern, Nrp1 appeared to play no part in the dysfunctional phenotype of murine self-reactive T cells. This was confirmed in Nrp1-deficient T cells, which performed similarly to wild-type T cells within both immune and tolerant environments, and when used in adoptive immunotherapy for cancer. These results support Nrp1 as a potential biomarker for dysfunctional

self-reactive CD8$^+$ T cells, which is dispensable for the induction and maintenance of T cell tolerance.

Results

Nrp1 is highly expressed on tolerant CD8$^+$ T cells primed by self-antigen in healthy hepatocytes

To define the intrinsic pathways regulating CD8$^+$ T cell tolerance versus immunity, the gene expression profiles of Gag-specific CD8$^+$ T cells (TCR^{Gag}) were defined after transfer into normal B6 mice (naive), B6 mice with an immunogenic Gag-positive FBL tumor (immune), or Alb:Gag mice that express the same Gag antigen under control of the Albumin promoter in healthy hepatocytes (tolerant) [27]. We previously reported that recognition of Gag in the immune context leads to CD8$^+$ T cell expansion, acquisition of effector function, and memory formation. However, in the tolerant context of an Alb:Gag host, these same T cells proliferate briefly but fail to acquire effector function and are largely deleted 8 days after transfer [9,28]. These tolerant T cells were characterized by high expression of multiple inhibitory receptors (e.g. CTLA-4, PD-1, LAG-3) vital for their dysfunctional phenotype [9]. Subsequent gene array analysis revealed that expression of the gene that encodes Nrp1 mirrored that of these co-inhibitory receptors on tolerant T cells. Specifically, like PD-1 (encoded by pdcd1), nrp1 gene expression was elevated upon engagement of antigen, but significantly upregulated in T cells engaging antigen under tolerant conditions (Fig. 1A). This expression profile was reflected on the surface of tolerant T cells relative to immunized T cells (Fig. 1B), which was evident as early as 2 days after T cell transfer into the tolerant environment (Fig. 1C). Collectively, these data demonstrate that Nrp1 marks tolerant T cells primed by a self-antigen in vivo, and compel further analysis of its possible role in the biology of tolerant CD8$^+$ T cells.

Nrp1 expression promotes optimal CD8$^+$ T cell proliferation in response to self-antigen

One of the earliest reported roles for Nrp1 in the immune system is the regulation of T cell proliferation. In these first reports, Nrp1 expression on human dendritic cells and CD4$^+$ T cells promoted prolonged T cell:DC interactions and more extensive proliferation of resting T cells [18]. However, these and other studies were limited only to in vitro analysis [19]. In the murine EAE model of multiple sclerosis, the exact opposite trend was observed, with Nrp1-deficient CD4$^+$ T cells proliferating more than Nrp1$^+$ cells [20]. Thus, there is still uncertainty surrounding the role of Nrp1 in T cell proliferation. More importantly, the impact of Nrp1 expression on CD8$^+$ T cell proliferation has not been analyzed. In our model, tolerance induction following engagement of antigen in the liver commences with extensive proliferation of responding CD8$^+$ T cells [28]. To examine the contribution of Nrp1 here, we evaluated the proliferation of transgenic Gag-specific T cells deficient for the gene that encodes Nrp1 via Lck-cre mediated gene deletion (Nrp1$^{f/f}$ Lck-cre TCR^{Gag}), referred to hereafter as nrp1$^{f/f}$.

WT Gag-specific CD8$^+$ T cells (CD90.1$^+$) were co-transferred with nrp1$^{f/f}$ Gag-specific CD8$^+$ T cells (CD90.1$^+$/90.2$^+$) into normal B6 recipients or Alb:Gag recipients. After 4 days in Alb:Gag hosts, surface expression of Nrp1 was evident on WT cells, but expression on nrp1$^{f/f}$ T cells was similar to naive T cells (Fig. 2A). This same nrp1 expression pattern was reflected at the gene expression level in identically treated cells (Fig. S1). While it is unlikely that Nrp1 expression was completely absent in all nrp1$^{f/f}$ T cells, we consistently observed a 5-10 fold reduction in surface

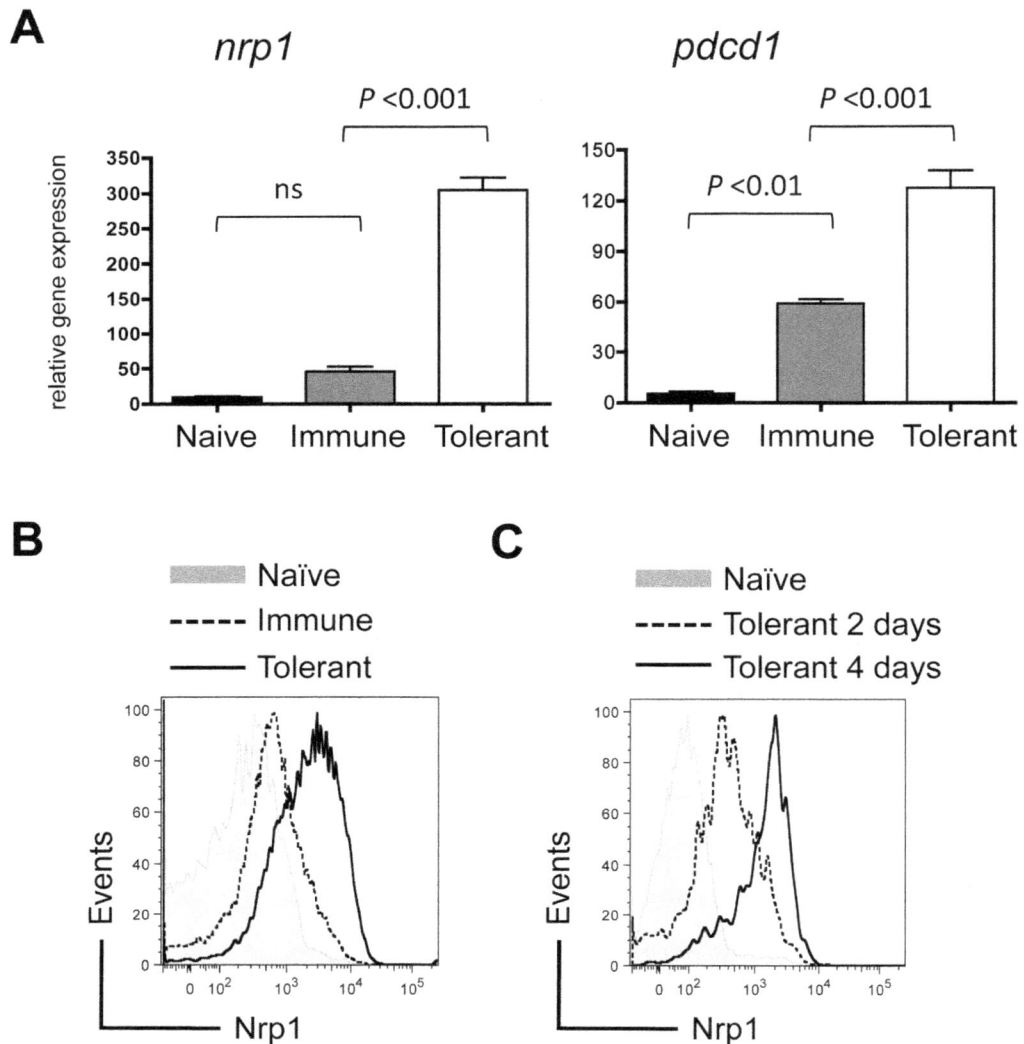

Figure 1. Nrp1 is highly expressed on tolerant CD8+ T cells primed by a self-antigen in healthy liver. Naive Gag-specific CD8+ T cells (CD90.1+) were transferred into B6 mice (naive), B6 mice bearing an immunogenic FBL tumor (immune), Alb:Gag mice (tolerant). (A) Two days after transfer, T cells were purified by cell sorting and RNA isolated for gene expression by microarray. Graphs displays *nrp1* and *pdcd1* relative gene expression pooled from biological triplicate samples, and error bars represent SD. (B) Nrp1 protein expression on T cells 3 days after adoptive transfer into the naive, immune or tolerant environment. Data are representative of 3 experiments, each with 3 recipient mice per group. (C) Nrp1 protein upregulation on T cells 2 and 4 days after transfer into Alb:Gag recipients. Data are representative of 2 time course experiments.

protein expression relative to WT T cells (Fig. S1). Both sets of transferred T cells underwent several rounds of cell division regardless of genotype but fewer *nrp1^{f/f}* T cells went into cell cycle and those that did underwent fewer rounds of division relative to WT T cells (Fig. 2B and 2C). These data demonstrate that Nrp1 is not essential for CD8+ T cell proliferation, but may be required for optimal responses, contributing modestly to the extent of CD8+ T cell activation during early induction of peripheral self-tolerance.

Nrp1 does not contribute to deficiencies in effector function by tolerant T cells

Negative regulatory receptor signaling has been shown to trigger dysfunction of tolerant CD8+ T cells [9]. If Nrp1 expression also contributes to poor effector activity, Nrp1-deficient T cells should have improved cytokine responses following self-antigen encounter. In support of this, studies by Bottcher *et al.* identified a distinct population of Nrp1+ CD8+ T cells lacking cytokine

responsiveness that correlated with high levels of Nrp1 expression [26]. To evaluate whether Nrp1 expression directly regulated effector function of tolerant CD8+ T cells, WT Gag-specific T cells (CD90.1+) were co-transferred with *nrp1^{f/f}* CD8+ T cells (CD90.1+/90.2+) into Alb:Gag hosts with or without acute *Listeria monocytogenes* infection. In agreement with our previous results [28], IFNγ production was not elicited in WT T cells within Alb:Gag recipients, but could be induced in these same hosts when accompanied by inflammation during an acute *Listeria* infection (Fig. 3). However, the same was true for Nrp1-deficient T cells, suggesting Nrp1 was not involved in the regulation of effector cytokine production by tolerant CD8+ T cells, nor was Nrp1 required for self-reactive CD8+ T cells to acquire effector functions during *Listeria* infection.

To further characterize the contribution of Nrp1 to the functional defects associated with tolerant self-reactive T cells, *in vivo* cytolytic activity was assessed. WT or *nrp1^{f/f}* T cells were

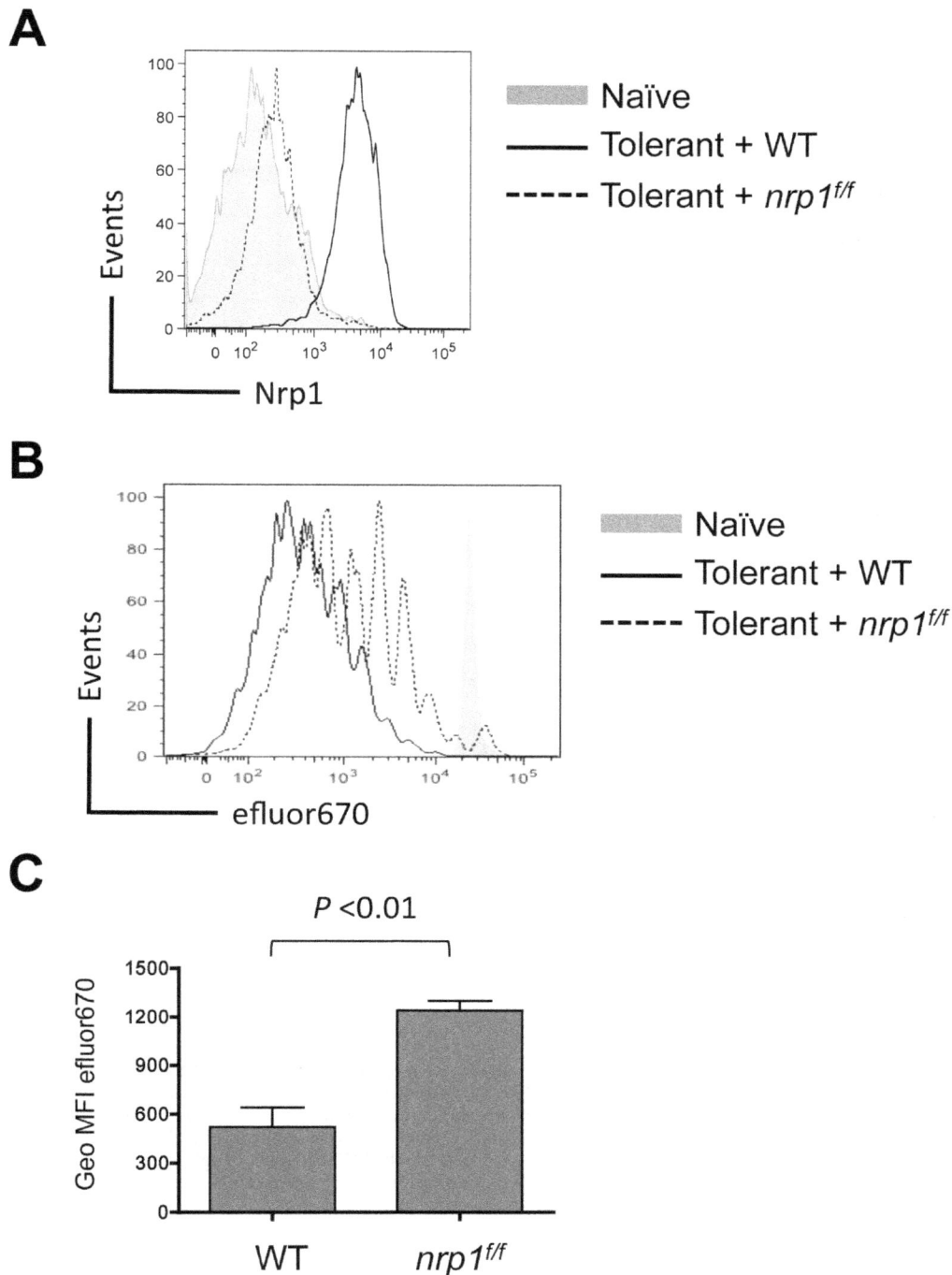

Figure 2. Nrp1 expression corresponds with a modest increase in CD8+ T cell proliferation in response to self-antigen. Naive WT or Nrp1-deficient CD8+ T cells were labeled with efluor670 cytoplasmic dye and co-transferred into B6 (naive) or Alb:Gag (tolerant) mice. (A) Nrp1 expression on WT and $nrp1^{f/f}$ T cells 3 days after transfer is compared in the overlaid histograms. (B) Dilution of efluor670 dye in transferred T cells was assessed 3 days after transfer and is displayed in overlayed histograms. (C) Geometric mean fluorescent intensity of efluor670 in T cells from either WT or Nrp1-deficient T cells (lower dye expression corresponds to more proliferation) is pooled from 4 separate experiments, each with 3 mice per group. Error bars are standard error of the mean (SEM) with P value indicated.

transferred separately into Alb:Gag recipient mice in the presence or absence of *Listeria*, followed 3 days later by an infusion of fluorescently labeled peptide-pulsed target cells. Consistent with our previous data [28], WT Gag-specific T cells failed to kill Gag-pulsed target cells within the tolerant environment, but specific

cytolytic activity was induced by self-antigen when encountered in conjunction with *Listeria* (Fig. 4). Cytolytic activity by Nrp1-deficient T cells was essentially identical to WT T cells under these same conditions. Likewise, blockade of Nrp1 by *in vivo* administration of anti-Nrp1 antibodies had no impact on WT T

A

B

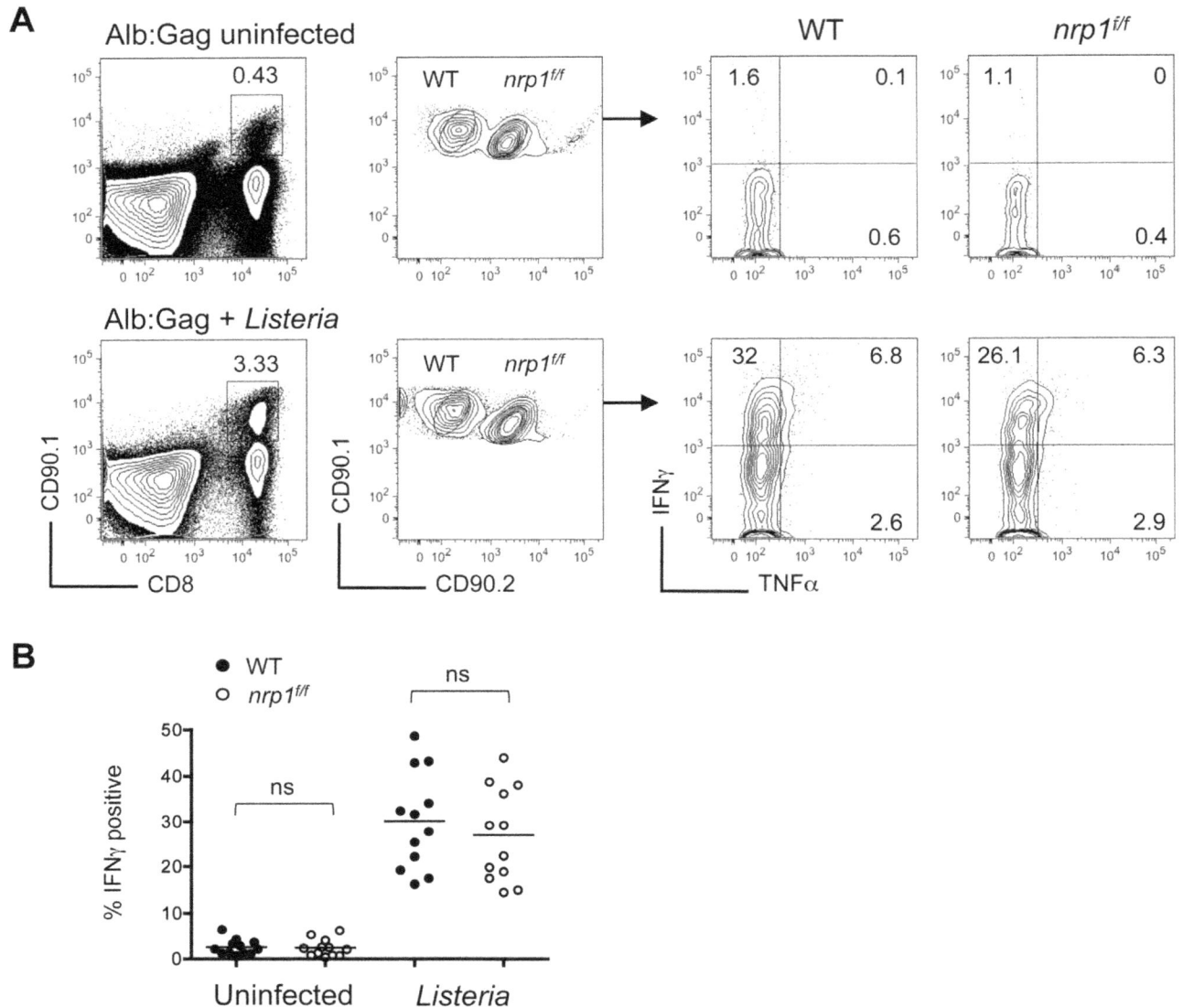

Figure 3. Nrp1 expression does not contribute to the lack of effector function in tolerant CD8+ T cells. Naive WT (CD90.1+) and Nrp1-deficient (CD90.1+/90.2+) Gag-specific CD8+ T cells were transferred into Alb:Gag recipients with (lower) or without (upper) a *Listeria* infection. Three days later, production of IFNγ and TNFα by transferred T cells was measured after overnight restimulation with Gag peptide. (A) Plots display T cell frequency (left) and IFNγ and TNFα production (right). Inset numbers are the percent of total splenocytes within the inscribed square region (left). Numbers in each quadrant represent the percent of gated CD8+ CD90.1+ T cells (right). (B) The percent of gated CD8+ CD90.1+ or CD8+ CD90.1+/90.2+ T cells that express IFNγ in differentially treated Alb:Gag recipients was graphed, with each circle representing individual mice pooled from 4 separate experiments. Horizontal bars represent the average for each group (ns = not significant).

cell effector function (data not shown). These data further support that Nrp1 neither hinders nor facilitates the cytolytic potential of self-reactive CD8+ T cells.

Nrp1 does not influence peripheral deletion of self-reactive CD8+ T cells

In tumor cells, ligation of Nrp1 can either promote cell survival or induce apoptosis, depending on the specific co-receptor and ligand involved [15]. Nrp1 ligation is reported to protect Treg against apoptotic cell death and induce a transcriptional profile enriched in pathways promoting survival and stability [23]. In our model, Nrp1 expressing self-reactive T cells are deleted by Bim-mediated apoptosis approximately 8 days after infusion into Alb:Gag recipients [9]. To identify any potential role of elevated

Nrp1 expression in the elimination of these T cells, WT (CD90.1+) and *nrp1^f/f* (CD90.1+/90.2+) Gag-specific CD8+ T cells were co-transferred into normal B6 or Alb:Gag host mice. Eight days later, the persistence of these transferred T cells was assessed in spleen, lymph node, bone marrow and liver. Under naive steady-state conditions, *nrp1^f/f* CD8+ T cells persisted slightly better than WT T cells in many of these tissues, but both cell types were deleted within the tolerant environment regardless of genotype (Fig. 5). Similarly, *in vivo* blockade by administration of anti-Nrp1 antibodies was also ineffective at preventing WT T cell deletion (data not shown). It was also evident that Nrp1expression did not affect T cell trafficking, as the relative proportion of WT to *nrp1^f/f* CD8+ T cells remained equivalent in all tissues analyzed. These

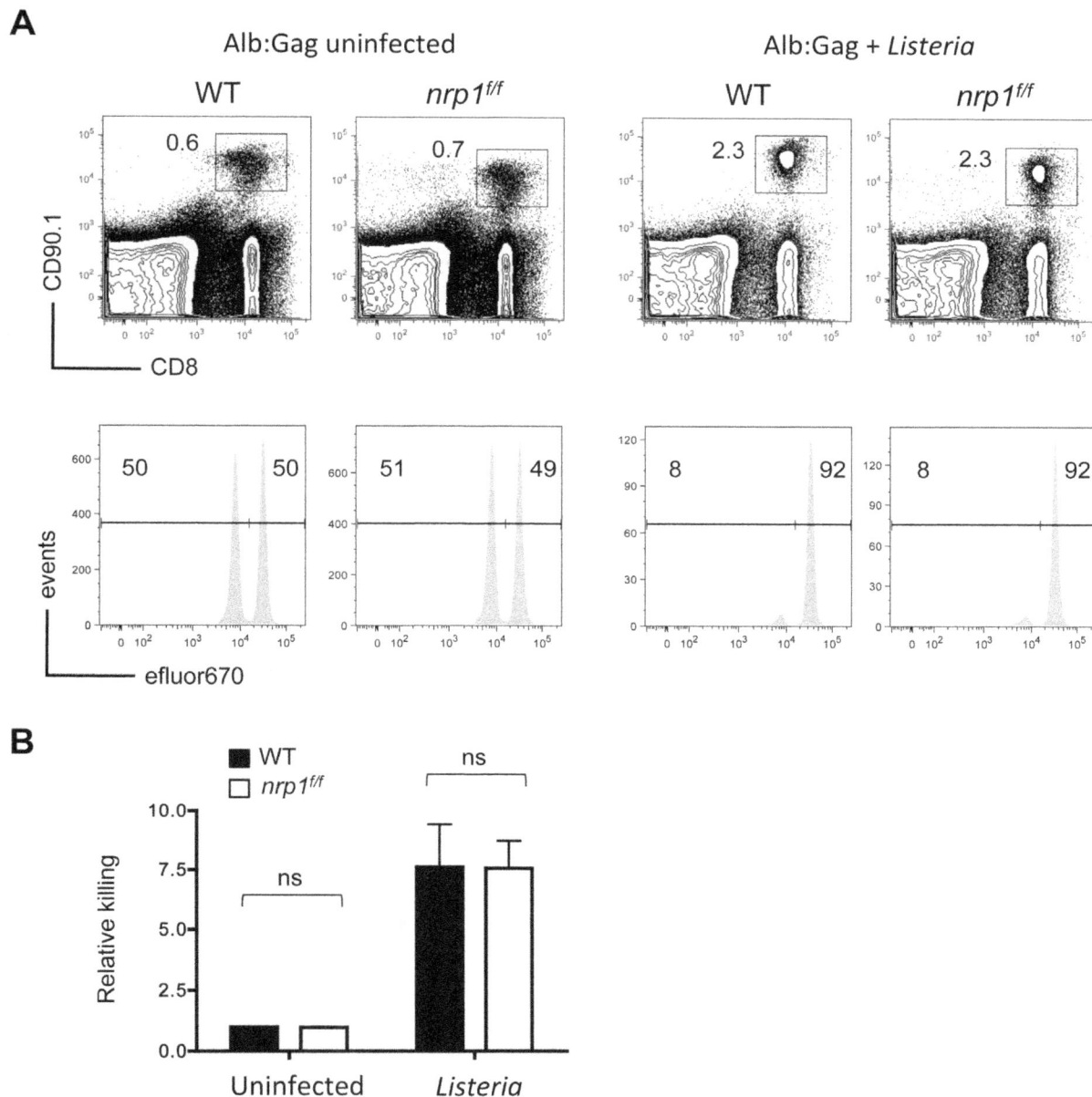

Figure 4. The cytotoxic potential of tolerant CD8$^+$ T cells is not regulated by Nrp1. WT or Nrp1-deficient CD90.1$^+$ Gag-specific CD8$^+$ T cells were transferred into Alb:Gag recipients with or without *Listeria* infection. Three days after transfer, recipients were infused with a 1:1 ratio of Gag (eFluor 670^{low}) and control (eFluor 670^{high}) peptide-pulsed target cells. Twenty hours later (day 4), recipient spleens were harvested and the frequency of transferred Gag-specific T cells was determined by flow cytometry (upper panels). Inset numbers are the percent of total splenocytes within the inscribed regions. Target cell frequency is displayed as histograms with the percentage of total eFluor 670-positive cells inset above the indicated regions (lower panels). (B) Graph displays relative target cell killing (% eFluor 670^{high}/% eFluor 670^{low}) pooled from 3 independent experiments. Error bars represent standard deviation (ns = not significant).

results suggest that Nrp1 had no role in peripheral deletion of self-reactive CD8$^+$ T cells following encounter with self-antigen.

Ablation of Nrp1 does not improve adoptive T cell immunotherapy for leukemia

Together, our data suggest that Nrp1 does not have an important role in the regulation of CD8$^+$ T cell function or survival, and has no real influence on the dysfunctional phenotype of tumor/self-reactive CD8$^+$ T cells. To definitively assess whether Nrp1 expression impacts CD8$^+$ T cell function over time, we

directly compared WT and *nrp1$^{f/f}$* T cells for efficacy in our model of adoptive T cell immunotherapy for cancer. A disseminated and progressive murine FBL leukemia was established in normal B6 or Alb:Gag host mice by i.v. injection, as previously described [28]. One week later, WT or *nrp$^{f/f}$* Gag-specific T cells were infused i.v. into the same recipients, which were monitored for health out to 40 days. Because WT T cells become tolerant in Alb:Gag recipients [9,28], adoptive immunotherapy is less effective and these recipients died of progressive tumor in less than 20 days (Fig. 6). Transfer of *nrp1$^{f/f}$* T cells provided a similarly low level of

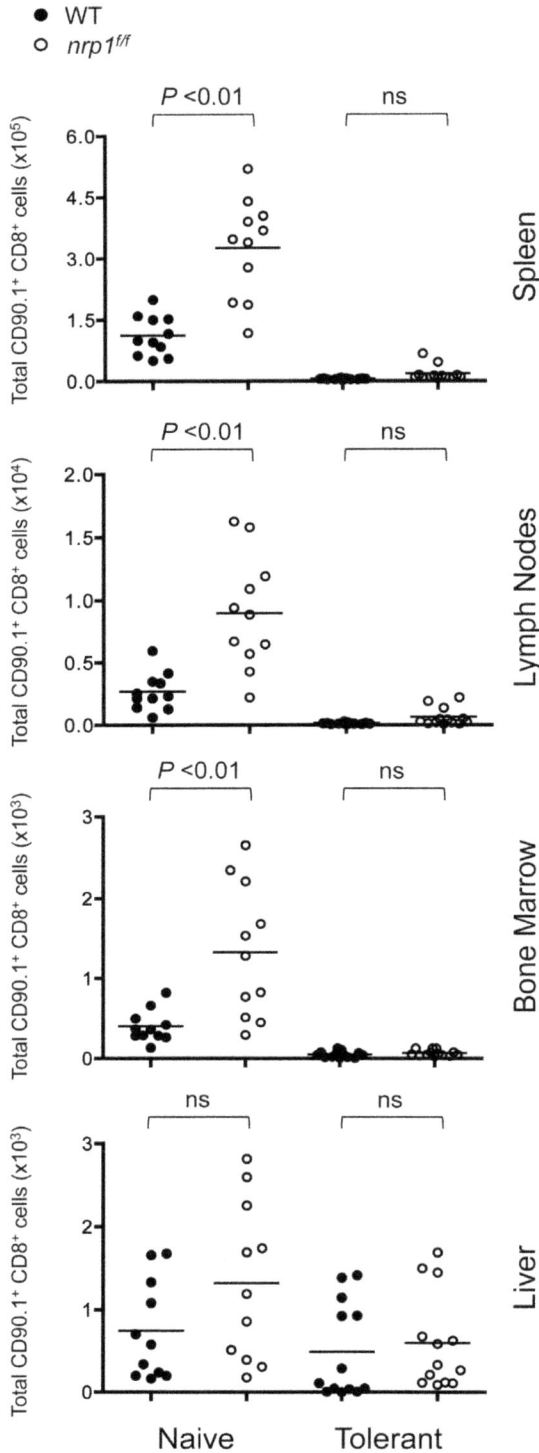

Figure 5. Deletion of self-reactive CD8⁺ T cells is not mediated by expression of Nrp1. Gag-specific CD8⁺ T cells from WT (CD90.1⁺) and Nrp1-deficient (CD90.1⁺/90.2⁺) donor mice were co-transferred into B6 or Alb:Gag recipients. The frequency of transferred T cells in recipient tissues was assessed after 8 days. The total number of WT or Nrp1-deficinet T cells in the indicated tissue is displayed graphically and shows pooled data from 4 independent experiments, with each circle representing data from one mouse. Horizontal bars represent the average for each group and P values are indicated (ns = not significant).

therapeutic benefit to tumor-bearing Alb:Gag recipients. Conversely, in tumor-bearing B6 recipients, transferred Gag-specific T cells are activated by the immunogenic FBL tumor [9]. Here, such T cells were capable of overcoming established leukemia in a majority (>75%) of recipient mice regardless of Nrp1 expression (Fig. 6). These results reinforce the notion that Nrp1 has no bearing on the *in vivo* persistence, trafficking, or function of CD8⁺ T cells despite high expression on tolerant versus immunized cells (Fig. 1).

Neuropilin-1 is expressed on human tumor infiltrating T cells

Expression of Nrp1 has been described on a variety of human tumor cells [16], tumor infiltrating Tregs [29,30,31], and peripheral blood lymphocytes [16,18]. However Nrp1 expression on human tumor-infiltrating CD8⁺ T cells has not been reported. Results from our mouse studies suggest that Nrp1 is expressed on tumor/self-reactive T cells, particularly under conditions that favor T cell dysfunction or tolerance. Despite a lack of involvement in the tolerant phenotype, Nrp1 may represent a valuable biomarker for such T cells in cancer patients. We evaluated tumor-infiltrating lymphocytes (TIL) derived from patients undergoing resection of metastatic melanoma. Nrp1 was not detected on the surface of either CD4⁺ or CD8⁺ T cells from the peripheral blood of patients or healthy donors (Fig. 7A). In contrast, Nrp1 was expressed on CD4⁺ and even more so on CD8⁺ TIL in a majority of patient tumor samples (Fig. 7A and 7B). Nrp1 expression on TIL corresponded with an antigen-experienced CD45RO⁺ phenotype (Fig. 7A), implying a possible connection with tumor/self-antigen reactive T cells. Although Nrp1 expression on tolerant mouse T cells did not contribute to the dysfunction, it did provide a unique marker of tumor/self-reactive T cells displaying a tolerant phenotype. To extend this observation to human T cells, *ex vivo* proliferation of CD8⁺ TIL and peripheral blood lymphocytes (PBL) derived from the same

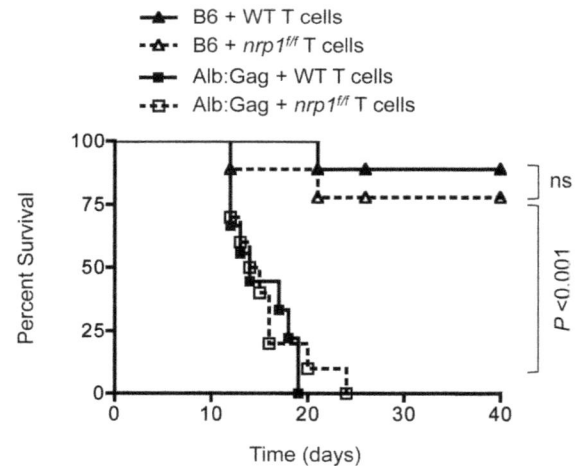

Figure 6. Nrp1 expression on adoptively transferred CD8⁺ T cells does not influence the efficacy of immunotherapy for leukemia. B6 or Alb:Gag recipient mice were inoculated with FBL leukemia. Seven days later, tumor-bearing recipients were infused with WT or Nrp1-deficient Gag-specific CD8⁺ T cells. Recipient survival was tracked for 40 days, and results pooled from 2 separate experiments are depicted in the graph showing percent survival (y-axis) over time in days (x-axis), with a total 10 mice in each treatment group. Data from B6 and Alb:Gag groups were compared and P values are indicated (ns = not significant).

patients was compared following stimulation with anti-CD3/CD28 beads. Data from 2 representative patients clearly demonstrates less proliferation from Nrp-1$^+$ tumor-infiltrating CD8$^+$ T cells relative to Nrp1-negative T cells isolated from PBL (Fig. 7C). Thus, while a case can be made that Nrp1 expression correlates with dysfunctional or tolerant T cells, the precise molecular mechanisms that lead to elevated Nrp1 under these conditions, and how Nrp1 contributes, if at all, in the process remains unknown.

Discussion

The receptor Nrp1 has been widely studied for its role in regulatory CD4$^+$ T cells [17,19,23,32]. However, the precise mechanism by which Nrp1 is involved in immunosuppression remains unclear. Nrp1 is also expressed on other cells of the immune system, but how Nrp1 contributes to the biology in these diverse populations is unknown. In our study of CD8$^+$ T cell tolerance, the negative regulatory receptors PD-1, CTLA-4, and LAG-3 were uniquely upregulated on CD8$^+$ T cells engaging self-antigen [9]. Similarly, Nrp1 was highly upregulated on the same T cells. Thus, we hypothesized that Nrp1, like these other molecules, might have an important role in the induction and/or maintenance of peripheral CD8$^+$ T cell tolerance.

Tolerant Nrp1$^+$ T cells have characteristic defects in the ability to produce effector cytokines, perform cytolytic functions, and are typically deleted from the periphery within 8 days of primary self-antigen encounter [9,28]. Therefore, we expected that a deficiency in Nrp1 might alter the induction of tolerance similar to what has been described when cells engage antigen in the absence of other negative regulatory receptors [33]. Instead, lack of Nrp1 expression had no impact on self-reactive T cells, which still failed to acquire effector capabilities and were deleted by apoptosis identically to WT self-reactive T cells. Additionally, Nrp1 deficiency did not affect the ability to boost self-reactive CD8$^+$ T cell activation under inflammatory conditions. Thus, in our model, Nrp1 held no perceivable influence over the phenotype and function of tolerant self-reactive CD8$^+$ T cells.

Coinhibitory molecules play an immunoregulatory role in controlling the balance between T cell activation and tolerance. Manipulation of these coinhibitory pathways provides a means to enhance immune responses to promote anti-tumor immunity [34]. Although antitumor immunity is often limited by self-tolerance, the outcome of antigen engagement within tumor versus healthy self-tissue can be quite different due to differences in costimulatory and coinhibitory signals received. The additional inflammatory and immunosuppressive mediators present in a tumor environment might alter the threshold for tumor/self-reactive T cell activation. Conversely, a role for Nrp1 expression on CD8$^+$ T cells that is distinct from tolerance might emerge under conditions in which tumor is present. To assess a potential role for Nrp1 in CD8$^+$ T cell function under these conditions, we evaluated the ability of Nrp1-deficient T cells to provide effective adoptive T cell immunotherapy for cancer. This is of special interest since anti-Nrp1 antibodies have recently completed phase I (NCT00747734) and phase Ib (NCT00954642) trials for patients with advanced solid tumors [35,36]. Thus, characterizing the immune subsets that anti-Nrp1 might target is important for evaluating potential mechanism of action and off-target toxicities. In our murine immunotherapy experiments, Nrp1 expression on adoptively transferred T cells had no influence on recipient survival outcomes, with treated mice uniformly succumbing to tumor under tolerant conditions but able to overcome the same tumors under immune conditions regardless of Nrp1 expression. Collec-

tively, these results support that expression of Nrp1 on CD8$^+$ T cells does not play a role in the tolerant phenotype that normally limits responses during adoptive T cell immunotherapy for cancer in mice.

In evaluations of Nrp1 on human CD8$^+$ T cells, we observed that some melanoma tumor-infiltrating T cells displayed significantly upregulated Nrp1 relative to T cells from normal adjacent skin tissue or peripheral blood. Thus, a correlation between Nrp1 expression and tumor/self-reactive could be made. However, the role Nrp1 plays in the biology of human CD4$^+$ and CD8$^+$ TIL remains unknown. Additionally, the tumor-derived factors that lead to elevated Nrp1 in some but not all patients with similar cancers have not been defined and warrant further investigation.

While we did not identify a role for Nrp1 in the regulation of CD8$^+$ T cell function or survival in a tolerant environment, our results should not be interpreted to imply a lack of utility for Nrp1 blockade in cancer therapy. Nrp1 function is complex, in part due to the multiplicity of co-receptors and ligands that Nrp1 can interact with, and its broad expression on a variety of cell types [17,18,37]. The impetus for using Nrp1 antibody blockade in cancer derives from its direct role in tumor cell survival and proliferation [38,39], its role in VEGF ligand-mediated angiogenesis [15,40,41,42], and also in the augmentation of Treg suppression [16,19,32]. Thus, Nrp1 may represent a direct tumor target and also a target for immunotherapy by modulation of Treg activity.

Our study evaluated the role of Nrp1 on tumor/self-reactive CD8$^+$ T cells, which has previously been underexplored. We conclude that the expression of Nrp1, although highly elevated on T cells engaging self-antigen in a tolerant context, does not regulate CD8$^+$ T cell tolerance. This has important clinical repercussions, as Nrp1 is being targeted therapeutically in cancer patients but the mechanism by which this strategy might enhance anti-tumor immunity is not completely understood. Additionally, while our results suggest Nrp1 may not represent a viable target for manipulation of self-reactive CD8$^+$ T cells during cancer immunotherapy, Nrp1 could represent a useful target in other scenarios, such as autoimmunity [20,43], or as a potential biomarker to help identify autoreactive T cells in patients.

Materials and Methods

Mice

$Rag1^{-/-}$ TCR^{Gag} transgenic mice have been previously described [9,28]. Alb:Gag mice express the H-2^b-restricted Friend murine leukemia virus-derived Gag glycoprotein in healthy hepatocytes under control of the Albumin promoter, as previously demonstrated [27]. C57BL/6 (B6) and Lck-cre mice were purchased from The Jackson Laboratory. Nrp1$^{f/f}$ mice were graciously provided by Dr. David Ginty and have previously been described [44]. Nrp1$^{f/f}$ and Lck-cre mice were crossed with $rag1^{-/-}$ TCR^{Gag} transgenic mice. To generate Gag-specific CD8$^+$ T cells deficient for neuropilin, Nrp1$^{f/f}$ x TCR^{Gag} mice were crossed with Lck-cre x TCR^{Gag} mice to generate Nrp1$^{f/f}$ x Lck-cre x TCR^{Gag} mice, which are $rag1$ sufficient. All animals were maintained under specific pathogen-free conditions and used in accordance with our animal protocol approved by the Animal Care Committee of the Department of Comparative Medicine, Saint Louis University School of Medicine (Saint Louis, MO).

Cell lines, peptides, and antibodies

FBL is a murine erythroleukemia cell line of B6 origin that expresses the H-2^b-restricted Friend murine leukemia virus-derived Gag glycoprotein as a tumor associated antigen [9,28].

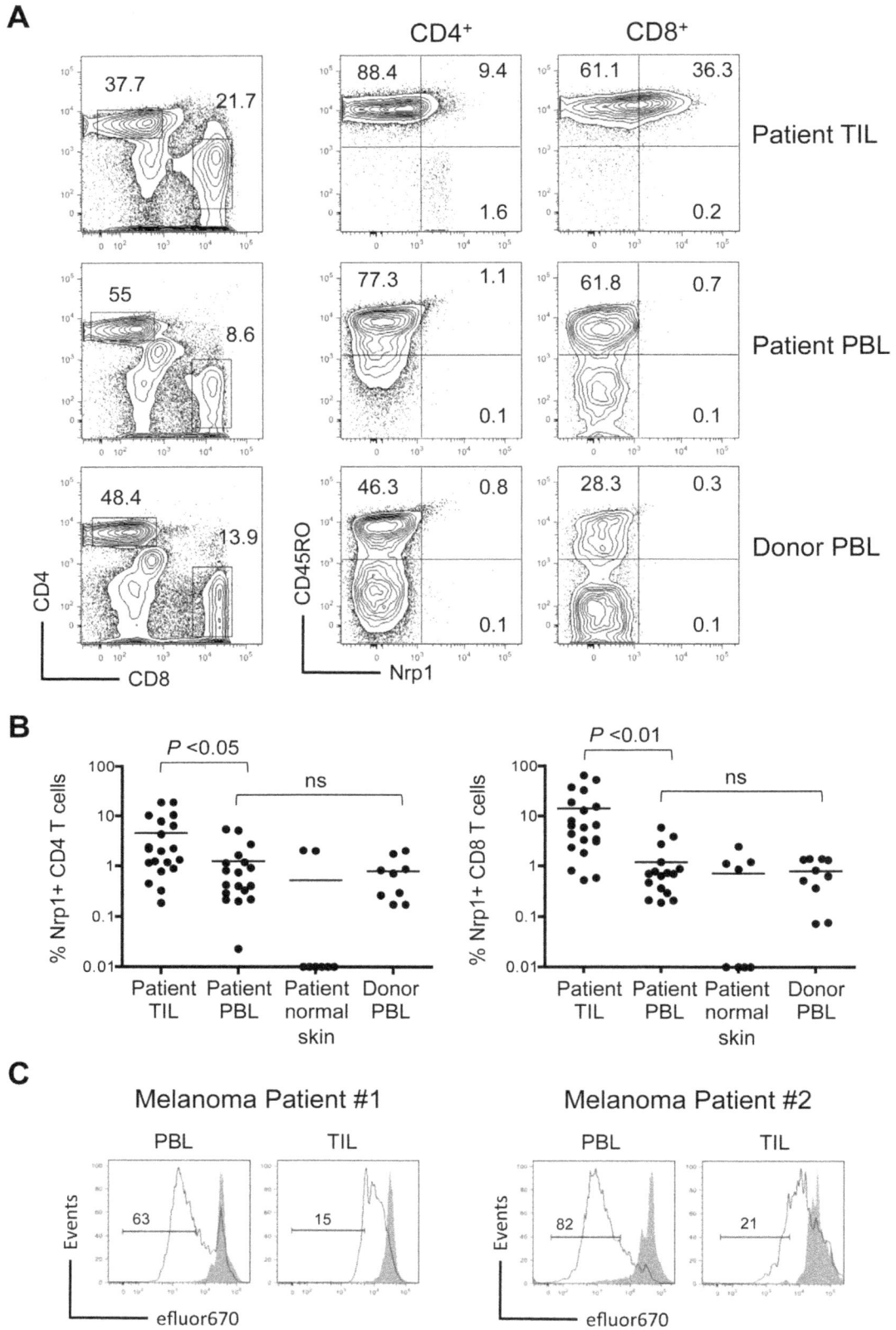

Figure 7. Nrp1 expression is increased on human tumor infiltrating T cells and corresponds with antigen experience. CD45$^+$ lymphocytes were analyzed from the blood (PBL) and tumor (TIL) of patients undergoing surgical resection of metastatic melanoma, and compared to lymphocytes from the blood of healthy donors. (A) The frequency of CD4$^+$ and CD8$^+$ T cells from the indicated tissues was compared (left) and co-expression of CD45R0 and Nrp1 assessed on these gated T cell populations (right). (B) The frequency of Nrp1$^+$ T cells among TIL, patient PBL, normal skin tissue adjacent to tumor, or healthy donor PBL is displayed graphically. Results are pooled from 8–20 independent samples, with each circle

representing data from one patient/donor. Horizontal bars represent the average for each group and P values are indicated (ns = not significant). (C) Proliferation of CD8$^+$ T cells from patient PBL or TIL was directly compared following 3 day *in vitro* stimulation with anti-CD3/CD28 beads. Histograms show relative dilution of efluor670 dye in stimulated (black line) versus non-stimulated (grey filled peaks) for 2 representative patients. Inset numbers are the percent of cells within the indicated region.

Gag peptide (CCLCLTVFL) and ovalbumin (SIINFEKL) control peptides were purchased from Pi Proteomics. Cell culture was conducted in complete RPMI-1640 with 10% FBS (Sigma). Fluorochrome-conjugated antibody to mouse CD8 (53–6.7) was purchased from eBiosciences. Fluorochrome-conjugated mouse antibodies to CD90.1 (OX-7), IFNγ (XMG1.2), TNFα (MP6-XT22), and human antibodies to CD4 (RPA-T4), CD8 (RPA-T8), and CD45RO (UCHL1) were purchased from BD Biosciences. Fluorochrome conjugated antibodies to mouse neuropilin-1 (761705) and human neuropilin-1 (446921) were purchased from R&D Systems. efluor-670 cell dye was purchased from Invitrogen. Anti-mouse Nrp-1A blocking antibody was provided by Genentech and administered intraperitoneally at 10 mg/kg every other day, similar to studies previously described [45].

T cell transfer, tumor inoculation, infection

Gag-specific T cells were isolated from spleens and lymph nodes of $rag1^{-/-}$ TCR^{Gag} or Nrp1$^{f/f}$ Lck-cre TCR^{Gag} donors. Whole-cell suspensions containing 2×10^6 Vα3-TCR$^+$ CD8$^+$ cells were intravenously injected into sex and age (6–8 week) matched recipients. In some experiments, transferred cells were labeled with efluor670 proliferation dye (eBioscience) before infusion according to the manufacturer's protocol. To provide an immunogenic environment, 5×10^6 FBL cells were established intraperitoneally in B6 recipients 3 days before T cell transfer. Infected recipients received 2×10^6 CFU attenuated (ΔActA) *Listeria monocytogenes* intravenously immediately prior to T cell transfer.

Gene array

Naive Gag-specific T cells were sorted or transferred into B6 mice with established FBL tumor (immune) and Alb:Gag mice (tolerant). Two days after T cell transfer, recipient spleen and lymph node were harvested and pooled. Transferred cells were sorted on a FACSAria (BD Biosciences). RNA was isolated using RNeasy Plus Mini Kit (Qiagen). Total RNA was used to generate aRNA (Affymetrix) and hybridized to the GeneChip Mouse Genome 430 2.0 Array (Affymetrix) and analyzed with a GeneChip scanner 3000 7G (Affymetrix). Data were obtained from 3 biological replicates per condition, and has been deposited in the Gene Expression Omnibus (GEO) with accession code GSE58722.

Flow cytometry

Recipient spleen and peripheral lymph nodes were harvested for analysis at indicated time points. Tissues were homogenized into single-cell suspensions before cell culture or staining for flow cytometry. Cell suspensions were stained for extracellular markers at 4°C for 30 minutes. *Ex vivo* cytokine production was assessed following overnight stimulation with 4 μg/mL Gag or Ova peptide in the presence of GolgiPlug (BD Biosciences). For intracellular staining of IFNγ and TNFα, cells were fixed and permeabilized in Cytofix/Cytoperm buffer (BD Biosciences), and proteins stained in Perm/Wash buffer (BD Biosciences) for 30 minutes at 4°C according to the manufacturer's protocol. All flow cytometry was conducted using either an LSR II or FACSCanto II (BD Biosciences), and resulting data analyzed using FlowJo software (Tree Star).

In vivo killing assay

Recipient mice received adoptive T-cell transfers and infections as described above. Three days after T cell transfer, B6 splenocytes (targets) were pulsed with 10 μg/ml Gag or control Ova peptide, and differentially labeled with 1 μM or 5 μM eFluor 670, respectively. Targets were then washed twice in phosphate buffered saline, combined at a 1:1 ratio, and injected into recipient mice intravenously. Twenty hours later, the frequency of eFluor^{high} versus eFluor^{low} targets from recipient spleens was assessed by flow cytometry.

Immunotherapy assay

One week prior to treatment, FBL leukemia was established in B6 or Alb:Gag mice by intravenous injection of 0.9×10^5 viable FBL tumor cells. Seven days after tumor inoculation, tumor-bearing mice received adoptive transfer of 2×10^6 Gag-reactive CD8$^+$ T cells by intravenous injection. Recipient survival was tracked for a minimum of 40 days with daily health monitoring, and recipients were euthanized upon moribund appearance.

Quantitative RT-PCR

Transferred T cells were sorted to better than 95% purity using a FACSAria III (BD Biosciences). Total RNA was isolated from sorted cells using RNeasy Mini Kit (Qiagen) and cDNA was synthesized using Transcriptor First Strand cDNA synthesis kit (Roche). Real-time PCR was performed with SYBR Select Master Mix (Life Technology) on a 7500 Real-Time PCR System (Applied Biosystems). Relative amplification values were calculated by normalizing to amplification of beta actin. The following primers were used: Nrp1 sense primer: 5′-CACCAACCCCACA-GATGTTGT-3′, Nrp1 antisense primer: 5′-CCAACATTCCA-GAGCAAGGAT-3′.

Statistical analysis

The Kruskal–Wallis test was used for statistical comparison (GraphPad Prism 4) of total cell numbers between different treatment groups. A one-way ANOVA was used for statistical comparison of cell frequencies between multiple treatment groups. Survival data were analyzed with a Mantel-Cox log-rank test. P values less than 0.05 were considered significant.

Patients and normal donors

Following a research protocol approved by the Saint Louis University School of Medicine Institutional Review Board (IRB), peripheral blood, tumor, and normal tumor-adjacent tissue were obtained from patients undergoing resections for metastatic melanoma. Blood samples were also obtained from normal healthy volunteers as separate controls. All subjects provided informed written consent by completion of an IRB approved consent form prior to participation in the study.

Isolation of human TIL and PBMC

Heparinized blood was diluted 1:1 (v/v) with PBS before Ficoll density centrifugation. The buffy coat containing PBMC was harvested, and washed twice in cold PBS and subjected to cell surface staining and flow cytometry analysis. Fresh pieces of tumor and normal adjacent tissue were minced into 1-mm-size pieces and tissue subjected to mechanical dissociation over 40 μm cell strainer. The resulting cellular suspension was diluted 1:1 (v/v) with PBS before Ficoll density centrifugation. The buffy coat containing TIL was harvested, washed twice in cold PBS, stained for expression of cell surface markers, and subjected to flow cytometry analysis.

Supporting Information

Figure S1 Nrp1 expression is significantly compromised in *nrp1^{f/f}* T cells. Naive WT or Nrp1-deficient CD8^+ T cells were transferred into B6 (naive) or Alb:Gag (tolerant) mice. (A) After 3 days, WT and *nrp1^{f/f}* T cells were sorted to better than 95% purity and mRNA isolated for quantitative RT-PCR analysis. Relative *nrp1* gene expression in WT and *nrp1^{f/f}* T cells from the indicated environments is shown. Samples were performed in triplicate and error bars represent standard deviation (B) Naive WT or *nrp1^{f/f}* CD8^+ T cells were transferred into B6 (naive) or Alb:Gag (tolerant) mice. The geometric mean fluorescent intensity

of anti-Nrp1-FITC (closed circles) and isotype-Ig (open circles) surface staining is shown for each of 3 separate mice per group. Horizontal bars represent the average for each group and *P* values are indicated (ns = not significant).

Acknowledgments

The authors would like to thank Sherri Koehm and Joy Eslick for technical assistance with flow cytometry and cell sorting. Collin Chen and Maureen Donlin provided assistance with the gene array studies identifying differences in Nrp1 gene expression. The authors thank Dr. David Ginty for providing the conditional *nrp1^{f/f}* mouse.

Author Contributions

Conceived and designed the experiments: SRJ RMT. Performed the experiments: SR JY MBE RMT. Analyzed the data: SRJ RMT. Contributed reagents/materials/analysis tools: ECH. Wrote the paper: SRJ RMT.

References

1. Nishimura H, Nose M, Hiai H, Minato N, Honjo T (1999) Development of lupus-like autoimmune diseases by disruption of the PD-1 gene encoding an ITIM motif-carrying immunoreceptor. Immunity 11: 141–151.
2. Tivol EA, Borriello F, Schweitzer AN, Lynch WP, Bluestone JA, et al. (1995) Loss of CTLA-4 leads to massive lymphoproliferation and fatal multiorgan tissue destruction, revealing a critical negative regulatory role of CTLA-4. Immunity 3: 541–547.
3. Waterhouse P, Penninger JM, Timms E, Wakeham A, Shahinian A, et al. (1995) Lymphoproliferative disorders with early lethality in mice deficient in Ctla-4. Science 270: 985–988.
4. Bennett CL, Christie J, Ramsdell F, Brunkow ME, Ferguson PJ, et al. (2001) The immune dysregulation, polyendocrinopathy, enteropathy, X-linked syndrome (IPEX) is caused by mutations of FOXP3. Nature genetics 27: 20–21.
5. Brunkow ME, Jeffery EW, Hjerrild KA, Paeper B, Clark LB, et al. (2001) Disruption of a new forkhead/winged-helix protein, scurfin, results in the fatal lymphoproliferative disorder of the scurfy mouse. Nature genetics 27: 68–73.
6. Bouneaud C, Kourilsky P, Bousso P (2000) Impact of negative selection on the T cell repertoire reactive to a self-peptide: a large fraction of T cell clones escapes clonal deletion. Immunity 13: 829–840.
7. Rosenberg SA (1999) A new era for cancer immunotherapy based on the genes that encode cancer antigens. Immunity 10: 281–287.
8. Jackson SR, Yuan J, Teague RM (2014 (in press)) Targeting CD8+ T cell tolerance for cancer immunotherapy. Immunotherapy.
9. Berrien-Elliott MM, Jackson SR, Meyer JM, Rouskey CJ, Nguyen TL, et al. (2013) Durable adoptive immunotherapy for leukemia produced by manipulation of multiple regulatory pathways of CD8+ T-cell tolerance. Cancer Res 73: 605–616.
10. Curran MA, Montalvo W, Yagita H, Allison JP (2010) PD-1 and CTLA-4 combination blockade expands infiltrating T cells and reduces regulatory T and myeloid cells within B16 melanoma tumors. Proc Natl Acad Sci U S A 107: 4275–4280.
11. Grosso JF, Goldberg MV, Getnet D, Bruno TC, Yen HR, et al. (2009) Functionally distinct LAG-3 and PD-1 subsets on activated and chronically stimulated CD8 T cells. J Immunol 182: 6659–6669.
12. Fujisawa H, Takagi S, Hirata T (1995) Growth-associated expression of a membrane protein, neuropilin, in Xenopus optic nerve fibers. Dev Neurosci 17: 343–349.
13. Kawakami A, Kitsukawa T, Takagi S, Fujisawa H (1996) Developmentally regulated expression of a cell surface protein, neuropilin, in the mouse nervous system. J Neurobiol 29: 1–17.
14. Kitsukawa T, Shimono A, Kawakami A, Kondoh H, Fujisawa H (1995) Overexpression of a membrane protein, neuropilin, in chimeric mice causes anomalies in the cardiovascular system, nervous system and limbs. Development 121: 4309–4318.
15. Soker S, Takashima S, Miao HQ, Neufeld G, Klagsbrun M (1998) Neuropilin-1 is expressed by endothelial and tumor cells as an isoform-specific receptor for vascular endothelial growth factor. Cell 92: 735–745.
16. Chaudhary B, Khaled YS, Ammori BJ, Elkord E (2014) Neuropilin 1: function and therapeutic potential in cancer. Cancer Immunol Immunother 63: 81–99.
17. Bruder D, Probst-Kepper M, Westendorf AM, Geffers R, Beissert S, et al. (2004) Neuropilin-1: a surface marker of regulatory T cells. Eur J Immunol 34: 623–630.
18. Tordjman R, Lepelletier Y, Lemarchandel V, Cambot M, Gaulard P, et al. (2002) A neuronal receptor, neuropilin-1, is essential for the initiation of the primary immune response. Nat Immunol 3: 477–482.
19. Sarris M, Andersen KG, Randow F, Mayr L, Betz AG (2008) Neuropilin-1 expression on regulatory T cells enhances their interactions with dendritic cells during antigen recognition. Immunity 28: 402–413.
20. Solomon BD, Mueller C, Chae WJ, Alabanza LM, Bynoe MS (2011) Neuropilin-1 attenuates autoreactivity in experimental autoimmune encephalomyelitis. Proc Natl Acad Sci U S A 108: 2040–2045.
21. Yadav M, Louvet C, Davini D, Gardner JM, Martinez-Llordella M, et al. (2012) Neuropilin-1 distinguishes natural and inducible regulatory T cells among regulatory T cell subsets in vivo. J Exp Med 209: 1713–1722, S1711–1719.
22. Weiss JM, Bilate AM, Gobert M, Ding Y, Curotto de Lafaille MA, et al. (2012) Neuropilin 1 is expressed on thymus-derived natural regulatory T cells, but not mucosa-generated induced Foxp3+ T reg cells. J Exp Med 209: 1723–1742, S1721.
23. Delgoffe GM, Woo SR, Turnis ME, Gravano DM, Guy C, et al. (2013) Stability and function of regulatory T cells is maintained by a neuropilin-1-semaphorin-4a axis. Nature 501: 252–256.
24. Kaech SM, Hemby S, Kersh E, Ahmed R (2002) Molecular and functional profiling of memory CD8 T cell differentiation. Cell 111: 837–851.
25. Hansen W, Hutzler M, Abel S, Alter C, Stockmann C, et al. (2012) Neuropilin 1 deficiency on CD4+Foxp3+ regulatory T cells impairs mouse melanoma growth. J Exp Med 209: 2001–2016.
26. Bottcher JP, Schanz O, Wohlleber D, Abdullah Z, Debey-Pascher S, et al. (2013) Liver-primed memory T cells generated under noninflammatory conditions provide anti-infectious immunity. Cell Rep 3: 779–795.
27. Ohlen C, Kalos M, Hong DJ, Shur AC, Greenberg PD (2001) Expression of a tolerizing tumor antigen in peripheral tissue does not preclude recovery of high-affinity CD8+ T cells or CTL immunotherapy of tumors expressing the antigen. J Immunol 166: 2863–2870.
28. Jackson SR, Yuan J, Berrien-Elliott MM, Chen CL, Meyer JM, et al. (2014) Inflammation programs self-reactive CD8+ T cells to acquire T-box-mediated effector function but does not prevent deletional tolerance. J Leukoc Biol.
29. Battaglia A, Buzzonetti A, Baranello C, Ferrandina G, Martinelli E, et al. (2009) Metastatic tumour cells favour the generation of a tolerogenic milieu in tumour draining lymph node in patients with early cervical cancer. Cancer Immunol Immunother 58: 1363–1373.
30. Battaglia A, Buzzonetti A, Monego G, Peri L, Ferrandina G, et al. (2008) Neuropilin-1 expression identifies a subset of regulatory T cells in human lymph nodes that is modulated by preoperative chemoradiation therapy in cervical cancer. Immunology 123: 129–138.
31. Piechnik A, Dmoszynska A, Omiotek M, Mlak R, Kowal M, et al. (2013) The VEGF receptor, neuropilin-1, represents a promising novel target for chronic lymphocytic leukemia patients. Int J Cancer 133: 1489–1496.
32. Glinka Y, Prud'homme GJ (2008) Neuropilin-1 is a receptor for transforming growth factor beta-1, activates its latent form, and promotes regulatory T cell activity. J Leukoc Biol 84: 302–310.
33. Probst HC, McCoy K, Okazaki T, Honjo T, van den Broek M (2005) Resting dendritic cells induce peripheral CD8+ T cell tolerance through PD-1 and CTLA-4. Nat Immunol 6: 280–286.
34. Page DB, Postow MA, Callahan MK, Allison JP, Wolchok JD (2014) Immune modulation in cancer with antibodies. Annual review of medicine 65: 185–202.
35. Weekes CD, Beeram M, Tolcher AW, Papadopoulos KP, Gore L, et al. (2014) A phase I study of the human monoclonal anti-NRP1 antibody MNRP1685A in patients with advanced solid tumors. Invest New Drugs.
36. Patnaik A, LoRusso PM, Messersmith WA, Papadopoulos KP, Gore L, et al. (2014) A Phase Ib study evaluating MNRP1685A, a fully human anti-NRP1 monoclonal antibody, in combination with bevacizumab and paclitaxel in

patients with advanced solid tumors. Cancer Chemother Pharmacol 73: 951–960.

37. Carrer A, Moimas S, Zacchigna S, Pattarini L, Zentilin L, et al. (2012) Neuropilin-1 identifies a subset of bone marrow Gr1- monocytes that can induce tumor vessel normalization and inhibit tumor growth. Cancer Res 72: 6371–6381.

38. Bielenberg DR, Pettaway CA, Takashima S, Klagsbrun M (2006) Neuropilins in neoplasms: expression, regulation, and function. Exp Cell Res 312: 584–593.

39. Beck B, Driessens G, Goossens S, Youssef KK, Kuchnio A, et al. (2011) A vascular niche and a VEGF-Nrp1 loop regulate the initiation and stemness of skin tumours. Nature 478: 399–403.

40. Kawasaki T, Kitsukawa T, Bekku Y, Matsuda Y, Sanbo M, et al. (1999) A requirement for neuropilin-1 in embryonic vessel formation. Development 126: 4895–4902.

41. Mamluk R, Gechtman Z, Kutcher ME, Gasiunas N, Gallagher J, et al. (2002) Neuropilin-1 binds vascular endothelial growth factor 165, placenta growth factor-2, and heparin via its b1b2 domain. J Biol Chem 277: 24818–24825.

42. Fuh G, Garcia KC, de Vos AM (2000) The interaction of neuropilin-1 with vascular endothelial growth factor and its receptor flt-1. J Biol Chem 275: 26690–26695.

43. Catalano A (2010) The neuroimmune semaphorin-3A reduces inflammation and progression of experimental autoimmune arthritis. J Immunol 185: 6373–6383.

44. Gu C, Rodriguez ER, Reimert DV, Shu T, Fritzsch B, et al. (2003) Neuropilin-1 conveys semaphorin and VEGF signaling during neural and cardiovascular development. Dev Cell 5: 45–57.

45. Pan Q, Chanthery Y, Liang WC, Stawicki S, Mak J, et al. (2007) Blocking neuropilin-1 function has an additive effect with anti-VEGF to inhibit tumor growth. Cancer cell 11: 53–67.

21

Exogenous Addition of Arachidonic Acid to the Culture Media Enhances the Functionality of Dendritic Cells for their Possible use in Cancer Immunotherapy

Jeetendra Kumar, Rupali Gurav, Vaijayanti Kale, Lalita Limaye*

Stem Cell Lab., National Centre for Cell Science, Ganeshkhind, Pune, India

Abstract

The development of dendritic cell based vaccines is a promising approach in cancer immunotherapy. For their successful use in the clinics, the propagation and functionality of DCs is crucial. We earlier established a two-step method for the large scale generation of DCs from umbilical cord blood derived MNCs/CD34+ cells. This work aims at improving their functionality based on the following observations: in vitro generated DCs can be less efficient in migration and other functional activities due to lower eicosanoid levels. The production of eicosanoids from Arachidonic Acid (AA) can be hampered due to suppression of the enzyme phospholipase A2 by IL-4, an essential cytokine required for the differentiation of DCs. We hypothesized that exogenous addition of AA to the culture media during DC generation may result in DCs with improved functionality. DCs were generated with and without AA. The two DC sets were compared by phenotypic analysis, morphology and functional assays like antigen uptake, MLR, CTL assay and in vitro and in vivo migration. Though there were no differences between the two types of DCs in terms of morphology, phenotype and antigen uptake, AA$^+$ DCs exhibited an enhanced in vitro and in vivo migration, T cell stimulatory capacity, CTL activity and significantly higher transcript levels of COX-2. AA$^+$ DCs also show a favorable Th1 cytokine profile than AA$^-$ DCs. Thus addition of AA to the culture media is skewing the DCs towards the secretion of more IL-12 and less of IL-10 along with the restoration of eicosanoids levels in a COX-2 mediated pathway thereby enhancing the functionality of these cells to be used as a potent cellular vaccine. Taken together, these findings will be helpful in the better contriving of DC based vaccines for cancer immunotherapy.

Editor: Thorbald van Hall, Leiden University Medical Center, Netherlands

Funding: The project received funds from Department of Biotechnology (DBT), Government of India via grant no. BT/PR13565/MED/31/89/2010. JK received his fellowship from Council of Scientific and Industrial Research (CSIR) India and from DBT (PR- 4930/31). The funders had no role in study design, data collection and analysis, decision to publish, or preparation of the manuscript.

Competing Interests: The authors have declared that no competing interests exist.

* Email: lslimaye@nccs.res.in

Introduction

Dendritic cells (DCs) are most efficient antigen presenting cells (APCs) which recognize the universe of antigens and control various types of responses [1,2]. DCs are capable of capturing antigens, processing them, and presenting them with appropriate costimulation molecules and initiate immune response [3,4]. DCs are not only critical for the induction of both primary and secondary T and B cell mediated immune responses, but are also important for the induction of immunological tolerance. DCs are at center of the immune system and modulation of the immune response is important in therapeutic immunity against cancer [5]. The unique ability of DCs in antigen presentation and regulation of immune response has made them an attractive adjuvant in cancer immunotherapy [6]. Advances in the *in vitro* DC generation protocols and better understanding of DC biology have resulted in their use as DC vaccines in the clinics. Since its first report in 1995, large numbers of clinical trials have been carried out to evaluate DC-based vaccines against more than a dozen different types of tumours [7,8,9]. Clinical use of DCs requires repeated vaccination to induce relatively high frequencies of tumor antigen specific Cytotoxic T lymphocytes (CTLs) and a complete response. This in turn requires a large number of DCs, generated *ex vivo* [10].

DCs can be generated from CD34$^+$ cells using a one step or a two step culture systems. In the first type of culture system CD34$^+$ cells are grown with a combination of growth factors, where in they are directly differentiated as dendritic cells [11,12,13]. On the other hand, in the two steps culture system CD34$^+$ cells are first expanded on a large scale as DC precursors. These expanded cells are further differentiated as DCs [14,15,16,17]. Despite the full understanding of the complex DC-mediated regulation of host leukocyte responses, *in vitro* generated DCs may not represent the equivalent of migratory DC *in vivo*, thereby limiting their use as magic bullets to improve the precision and effectiveness in cancer immunotherapy. Recent experimental evidence demonstrate that human monocyte-derived DC (MoDC) may be hampered in their ability to migrate in response to inflammatory as well as homeostatic chemotaxins [18]. Previous reports show that IL-4, which is an important cytokine for *in vitro* DC generation, inhibits many of the downstream pathways of Arachidonic Acid (AA) metabolism resulting in the impaired production of eicosanoids and platelet activating factor (PAF). Prostaglandin E_2 (PGE_2) is a member of the eicosanoid family of oxygenated AA derivatives. The first step of PGE_2 biosynthesis is the release of AA from membrane phospholipids by phospholipases such as phospholipase A2 (PLA_2). Since eicosanoids and PAF are known to play an important role in processes such as leukocyte migration, natural killer cell activation, and type 2 T helper cell differentiations, the deficiency in biosynthesis of these factors may be responsible for the observed handicaps of MoDCs [19].

We earlier established a two-step plastic adherence method for the large scale generation of DCs derived from both umbilical cord blood CD34+ cells [17] and MNCs (Mononuclear cells) [20]. The DCs generated by our method have a mature phenotype and are functionally active. However one of the cytokines used to generate DCs by our method is IL-4 and as mentioned above IL-4 may affect release of arachidonic acid from the membrane.We hypothesized that exogenous addition of AA to our cultures during the differentiation step may help in further improving the functions of DCs. The rationale for adding exogenous AA was that it may get converted into prostaglandins in a Cyclooxygenases-1 (COX-1) and Cyclooxygenases-2 (COX-2) dependent manner. To check this hypothesis, in the present study we tested the effect of AA addition on *in vitro* DC generation. Our data demonstrated that indeed AA+ DCs are superior in functions such as enhanced *in vitro* and *in vivo* migration, T cell stimulatory capacity, antigen uptake, CTL activity, significantly higher transcript levels of COX-2 and a favorable Th1 cytokine than AA- DCs. Thus our findings take us one step closer towards generating the ameliorate form of DC based cancer vaccine.

Materials and Methods

Cytokines

The recombinant human cytokines used for the study were Fms like tyrosine kinase 3 ligand (Flt-3L), Thrombopoietin (TPO), Stem Cell Factor (SCF), Interleukin-4 (IL-4), Granulocyte monocyte -colony stimulating factor (GM-CSF), Tumor necrosis factor-α (TNF-α), CD40 Ligand and Chemokine ligand-19 (CCL-19). All recombinant human cytokines were purchased from Peprotech Asia, Revohot Israel.

Antibodies

The antibodies used for flow cytometry were mouse anti human mAbs: CD1a, CD34, CD11c, CD40, CD8 -APC tagged; CD14, CD20, CD33, CD58, CD80, CD83, CD86, HLA-A2, CD45RA -PE tagged; CD3, CD54, HLA-DR, HLA-ABC -FITC tagged, anti murine CD 45.1 -PB tagged and CCR-7 (purified antihuman rat mAb). All monoclonal antibodies and respective isotype controls used for the study were purchased from BD pharmingen (San Diego, CA).

Other reagents used

Arachidonic Acid- (Cat. No. is A3555) from Sigma Aldrich, a tissue culture tested product derived from porcine liver. The purity of the product was ≥99% as analyzed by capillary Gas Chromatography.

Ficoll Hypaque-Histopaque (density 1.007 g/ml); Fluorescein isothiocyanate (FITC)-labeled dextran (40 kDa); Wright Stain, Giemsa Stain, Lipopolysaccharide, DMEM (Dulbecco's Modified Eagle Medium) and IMDM (Iscove's Modified Dulbecco's Medium) all were from Sigma Aldrich; ELISA kit (BD OptEIA); Heparin from SRL Pvt. Limited, Mumbai; Hydroxy Ethyl Starch (HES), Rosette sep for T cell isolation (Stem Cell Technologies, Vancouver, Canada); [³H] thymidine (240 GBq/milli mole,

BRIT, Navi Mumbai, India); Dimethyl sulfoxide (MP biomedical, Ohio, USA); Dynal kit for mRNA isolation (Dynal ASA, Oslo Norway).

Collection and Processing of Cord Blood Samples

Cord blood (CB) samples were obtained from the local hospitals according to the institutional review board [Institutional Ethics Committee (IEC) and Institutional Committee for Stem Cell Research (IC-SCRT)] –approved ethical guidelines which are in accordance with the Declaration of Helsinki. A prior informed written consent of the mother was obtained. The consent procedure was approved by IC-SCRT. The hard copies of the signed consent forms are numbered and filed with us. The samples were collected in sterile containers containing preservative-free heparin (40 IU of heparin/ml of blood) in plain IMDM. The samples were brought to the laboratory on ice packs and were processed to isolate mononuclear cells (MNCs).

Isolation of MNC

Cord Blood MNCs were separated by Ficoll- hypaque gradient centrifugation. The cells at the interphase were collected and washed to remove the Ficoll-hypaque. Nucleated cell count (Crystal violet staining) was taken and the MNCs were used for DC generation.

Isolation of T-Cells from Peripheral Blood

Peripheral blood was collected from healthy donors according to institutional review board. [Institutional Ethics Committee (IEC) and Institutional Committee for Stem Cell Research (IC-SCRT)] –approved ethical guidelines which are in accordance with the Declaration of Helsinki. A prior informed written consent of the healthy donor was obtained. The consent procedure was approved by IC-SCRT. The hard copies of the signed consent forms are numbered and filed with us. T cells were isolated from blood by using negative selection kit (Rosette Sep) as per the manufacture's instruction (Stem Cell Technologies). After Ficoll-hypaque gradient centrifugation cells at the interphase of Ficoll and medium were collected, washed then used in the experiments.

In Vitro Generation and Culture of DCs

Expansion cultures and Plastic adherence. MNCs (fresh or frozen) were expanded for 3 weeks, then enriched for CD14+ cells by plastic adherence and subsequently differentiated as described earlier [17,20]. Briefly, after 21 days of expansion the cells were washed and seeded at the density of 3×10^5 cells/well in six-well plate containing 2 ml of IMDM supplemented with 1% autologous plasma. The cells were kept for 1.5 hour at 37°C in 5% CO_2 incubator and the non-adherent and the loosely adherent cells were removed by washing with IMDM. The adherent cells were used for DC generation.

Differentiation of DCs from precursors in presence of AA (AA+ DCs) and absence of AA (AA- DCs). The precursor cell populations were divided into two sets. Cells were induced to differentiate as DCs by culturing them in GM-CSF (50 ng/ml) and IL-4 (30 ng/ml) for 3 days, on day 3rd GM-CSF (50 ng/ml) plus TNF-α (30 ng/ml) were added to cultures and further maintained for 4 days in IMDM supplemented with 5% autologous plasma. In order to assess the effect of AA, one set of culture was maintained with 100 μM of AA in addition to the conditions mentioned above. On day 7, the cells were subjected to maturation with a combination of TNF-α, lipopolysaccharide, and CD40L, at the concentration of 100 ng/ml each, for 48 hours. The experimental design is depicted in the form of a flow chart

Fig. S1. In all the experiments DCs generated without AA was considered as control set and with AA was considered as test set.

Morphological Analysis: Wright's and Giemsa Staining. The adhered cells in culture plates were fixed in methanol for 10 minutes at room temperature and stained with Wright's and Giemsa Stain. Observations were made under inverted microscope and images were taken (Olympus IX70).

Phenotypic Analysis: Flow cytometry. Mature AA$^+$ and AA$^-$ DCs were washed and suspended at 2×10^5 cells in 100 μL of cold phosphate-buffered saline (PBS) and staining was carried out as per the described protocol [17,20]. For CCR-7 staining, cells were incubated with primary followed by secondary and tertiary antibodies for 25 minutes each. Cells were washed twice, after each antibody incubations and finally resuspended in 1% paraformaldehyde. Cells were analyzed on a flow cytometer (FACS Canto II from BD Pharmingen- San Jose, California). Cell debris was eliminated from the analysis using a gate on forward and side scatters, and the total cells were analyzed. Data were analyzed and histogram overlays were prepared using computer software FACS Diva and Cell Quest Pro (Beckon Dickinson San Jose California), respectively.

Functional Characterization

Endocytosis assay with FITC-dextran. Immature DCs harvested on day 5 were incubated with FITC-dextran (20 μg/mL), either at +4°C (internalization control) or at +37°C, for 30 and 60 minutes. The cells were then washed thrice with cold PBS containing 0.01% sodium azide and 1% BSA. Cells were re suspended in 1% paraformaldehyde and were acquired on a flow cytometer (Canto II, BD).

Chemotaxis. The chemotaxis of the *in vitro* generated DCs toward CCL-19 was assessed in 24-well cell culture plates with BD Falcon ™ Cell culture 0.8 μm inserts. 500 μL of IMDM with or without rhCCL-19 (final concentration, 500 ng/mL) was added to the lower chamber as per the described protocol [17,20]. To check the specificity of chemokine receptor (CCR) interaction, in some experiments DCs were pretreated with CCR-7 blocking antibody for 1 hr in 1× PBS and then their migration towards CCL -19 were studied as described above. The migrated cells were stained by trypan blue dye and the viable cells were counted using hemocytometer. The results are expressed as the mean number of migrating cells ± standard deviation (SD).

Mixed Leukocyte Reaction (MLR). Allogeneic T cells were distributed at 10^5 cells per well into round bottom 96-well micro plates (Greiner Bio-One) and were cocultured in the presence of graded numbers of irradiated DCs (2500 rad, Co source) in 200 μL of medium containing 10% pooled cord blood AB+ plasma. Thymidine incorporation was measured on Day 3 after an 18-hour pulse with [³H] thymidine (1 μCi/well) by using standard procedures [17,20].

Cytokine measurement. Supernatants from the *in vitro* generated DC cultures were collected at 48 hrs after the addition of maturation stimuli and were kept frozen at −20°C. The supernatants were subsequently assayed for cytokine content (IL-10 and IL-12 p70) by ELISA using an ELISA kit as per the manufacturer's instructions. Amount of interleukins present in the supernatants were calculated by standard curve method.

In vitro CTL (Cytotoxic T lymphocytes) assay

Preparation of cell lysate. MCF-7 is a HLA-A2 restricted cell line and was used as the target cell line in the CTL assay. Lysis of MCF-7 cells was done by repeated freeze thawing then followed by sonication. After filter sterilization protein estimation was done and the lysate was stored at -80°C for antigen pulsing to the DCs.

Generation of effector cells and the CTL assay. HLA-A2 positive cord blood MNCs were used to generate DCs. Immature DCs were incubated with lysate of MCF-7 at a final concentration of 100 μg/ml of protein along with KLH (Keyhole limpet hemocyanin) 25 μg/ml for 48 hr as maturation stimuli in the culture medium for cross presentation of tumor antigen to autologous naïve T cells. For the control set of DCs, the maturation stimuli comprised of 100 ng/ml each of LPS, CD40L and TNF-α. The autologous naïve T cells were obtained by sorting of CD3, CD8, and CD45RA positive cells on FACS ARIA (BD). The naïve T cells were co cultured with MCF-7 lysate pulsed DCs that were generated from the same UCB sample with or without AA. DC-T cell co culture was maintained for 3 weeks with the addition of cytokines IL-2 (0.1 μg/ml) and IL-7 (5 μg/ml) and weekly re stimulation with fresh antigen pulsed DCs to generate effector Cytotoxic Killer Cells. CTLs thus generated from LPS pulsed and lysate pulsed AA$^+$ DCs/AA$^-$ DCs were co cultured with the target cells MCF-7 for 18 hours. Cells were then washed with plain media and then pulsed with [3H] thymidine for 8 hours. Percent killing of MCF-7 was calculated by P-JAM assay [21,22] using the formula- % killing = CPM [Target alone − Target + Killer] X 100/CPM Target Alone.

RT PCR analysis

mRNA was isolated from the AA$^+$ DCs and AA$^-$ DCs using Dynabeads mRNA DIRECT kit as per the manufacturer's instructions. The eluted mRNA were reverse transcribed to cDNA by using reverse transcriptase (Sigma Aldrich) and oligo-dT primers (Invitrogen) as per the instructions and PCR was performed with specific primers. The thermal cycle used was (95°C for 2 min, 95°C for 45 sec, annealing (as per different genes) for 45 sec, extension 72°C for 2 min) for 35 cycles and a final extension at 72°C for 5 minutes. The primer sequences used are described in Fig. S2.

Homing of mature DCs in NOD-SCID mice

The NOD/LtSZ-scid/scid mice were obtained from the Jackson Laboratories and were bred in the animal facility of our institute. The study was conducted adhering to the institution's guidelines for animal husbandry and has been approved by IAEC-NCCS/CPCSEA (Institutional animal ethical committee-NCCS/ Committee for the Purpose of Control and Supervision of Experiments on Animals. Approval number: IACUC-Institutional Animal Care and Use Committee, EAF-Experimental Animal Facility/2004/B-71). Animal procedures involving intra-venous infusion were carried out under anesthesia. Mice at 4–6 weeks of age were exposed to sub lethal dose of 300 rads total body irradiation from a ^{60}Co source (Gamma Chamber 5000, BRIT, Navi Mumbai, India). 10^6 AA$^+$ DCs and AA$^-$ DCs were infused through the tail vein into the sub lethally irradiated mice (n = 43; infusion of AA$^+$ DCs – 20 mice, AA$^-$ DCs – 20 mice and PBS – 3 mice). Mice were sacrificed after 18 hours to assess homing of human DCs in bone marrow. Homed cells were identified as DC by staining with human CD11c mAb. Murine CD 45.1 mAb was used to negate the presence cells of murine origin.

Statistical analysis

Different variables of AA$^+$ DCs and AA$^-$ DCs were compared. Statistical analysis was done using Sigma Stat (Version-2.03) and graphs were prepared using Sigma Plot software (Version 10) (Jandel Scientific, San Rafael, CA, USA) and GraphPad Prism 5 Software (San Diego, California, USA). Statistical analyses of differences between the two groups were performed using a t test.

Probability value: P≤0.05(*), P≤0.01(**) & P≤0.001(***) were considered statistically significant.

Results

Morphological and Phenotypic Characterization of DCs

The AA⁺ DCs and AA⁻ DCs show similar morphology. The DC precursors generated after 21 days of expansion of MNCs were enriched by the plastic adherence method and further differentiated as DCs [20]. There was marginal difference in the absolute number of DCs generated by the two methods from same number of starting population (approximately 3×10^7 AA⁺ DCs and 2.5×10^7 AA⁻ DC per 10^7 input MNCs). The morphology of AA⁺ DC and AA⁻ DCs was comparable. It was found that the DCs from both the sets exhibited the characteristic veiled morphology and DC clusters; Fig. S3. Phase contrast images showed typical adherent immature DCs, in both the sets [S-3(A)]. After addition of maturation stimuli typical nonadherent DC clusters were observed in both the cultures [S-3(B)]. Wright-Giemsa staining of mature adherent cells shows the presence of DCs with dendrites in the two sets [S-3(C)].

The AA⁺ DCs and AA⁻ DCs show similar DC phenotype. *In vitro* generated DCs were stained for a panel of DC specific and DC associated markers and analyzed on the flow cytometer. Fig. 1A depicts the flow cytometric profile of one representative sample with percent positive cells and MFI values in brackets. AA⁺ DCs and AA⁻ DCs showed a high and an equivalent percentage of cells expressing different costimulatory molecules like CD40, CD80, CD86, DC-associated integrin CD11c, adhesion molecules like CD54 and CD58, MHC class II molecules like HLA ABC and HLA DR. Fig. 1B and 1C depicts the phenotypic profile in terms of the percent positivity and MFI respectively, of three samples (mean ± SD, n = 3). The expression of myeloid lineage specific marker CD 33 was found significantly higher on AA⁺ DCs (67.4%) as compared to AA⁻ DCs (38.7%) Fig. 1B. MFI values of adhesion molecule CD 58 was found significantly higher on AA⁺ DCs (1423) as compared to AA⁻ DCs (1048) Fig. 1C. Taken together, AA⁺ DCs and AA⁻ DCs show similar morphology and typical interstitial DC phenotype.

Functional Characterization of DCs

The capability of endocytosis of AA⁺ DCs was higher as compared to AA⁻ DCs. Immature DCs are characterized by the ability of antigen uptake using different mechanisms. We analyzed the ability of the *in vitro* generated DCs for their receptor-mediated antigen uptake by measuring the FITC tagged dextran uptake. AA⁺ DCs and AA⁻ DCs were equally efficient in receptor-mediated uptake at 30 min and 60 min time intervals tested. AA⁺ DCs exhibited high and comparable FITC-dextran uptake as compared to AA⁻ DCs Fig. 1D (mean ± SD, n = 3). *In vitro* generated DCs exhibited more uptake at 60 min interval compared to 30 min, showing that they are functionally active and exhibit an increased uptake with increase in time.

Improved *in vitro* chemotaxis of AA⁺ DCs towards CCL19. Migration of DCs toward a chemokine gradient is an important functional property because in the immunotherapy protocols they must be capable of migration from the site of injection toward the lymph nodes, where they interact with the T cells and initiate the immune response. Fig. 2A shows, the cells suspended in IMDM added to the upper chamber in well at 0 hrs. No spontaneous migration was observed in the wells after 3 hrs, where CCL-19 was not added (Fig. 2B). More number of AA⁺ DCs (Fig. 2D) migrated towards CCL-19 as compared to AA⁻ DCs (Fig. 2C) and the difference was statistically significant (*p≤0.05,

**p≤0.01; n = 3; Fig. 2E). Migration towards CCL19 is mainly because the DCs express CCR7 receptor. When we stained the DCs of the two sets for the CCR-7 receptor antibody, the AA⁺ DCs and AA⁻ DCs showed 93.25% and 91.89% positive cells respectively along with MFI values in brackets (Fig. 2F). Mean MFI values of 3 samples for AA⁻ DCs were 821±156 and AA⁺ DCs were 1089±392. Thus both sets exhibited high and comparable level of CCR7 expression. The specificity of CCR7-CCL19 receptor ligand reaction was further confirmed by blocking the receptor with CCR-7 blocking Ab and then testing the migratory ability. As seen in Fig. 2G there was a significant reduction in migration of cells pretreated with blocking antibody in the two cultures. The migration of the test cells was once again significantly higher than control cells. This data indicated that, the addition of AA during differentiation step of DCs significantly improves their migratory ability.

AA⁺ DCs exhibited superior T-Cell stimulatory function. DCs are characterized by their ability to stimulate allogeneic T cells. This ability was assessed by MLR. The MLR was carried out by mixing the AA⁺ DCs and AA⁻ DCs with allogeneic T cells from peripheral blood in different proportions. Triplicates were taken for each concentration tested. Proliferation of T cells was measured by the thymidine uptake assay as described in methods. Data from Fig. 3 (mean ± SD, n = 3) indicate that the AA⁺ DCs have higher allostimulatory capacity. The differences were statistically significant at four out of six DC: T-cell ratios tested. At 1:10 ratio, thymidine incorporation in AA⁺ was higher than AA⁻ set.

Cytokine Profile of AA+ DCs is more favorable for adoptive immunotherapy. IL-12 not only signals for development of effector functions in T cells, but also programs the cells to survive as functional memory cells [23]. *In vitro* generated DCs were capable of secreting a high level of IL-12 p70 and a low level of IL-10. The AA⁺ DCs showed a better IL-12 p70 secretion profile as compared to AA⁻ DCs (Fig. 4). AA⁻ DCs on other hand had a higher level of IL-10 secretion compared to that of AA⁺ DCs (n = 3). The ratio of IL12/IL10 was higher in AA⁺ DCs as shown in Fig. S4. These observations suggest that the AA⁺ DCs have a better Th1 favorable cytokine profile as compared to AA⁻ DCs, making them a better choice for clinical application.

AA⁺ DCs demonstrate higher *in vitro* CTL activity

Figure 5A depicts CTL data from one representative sample. It is clearly seen that AA⁺ DCs are more efficient in effector function of T cells i.e. bringing about killing of MCF-7 cells in the CTL assay as compared to AA⁻ DCs. The killing is significantly higher at four ratios of effector target cell concentrations. The other two samples also showed similar trend (Fig. S5). CTLs derived from AA⁺ DCs exhibited an improved effector function i.e. enhanced overall killing as compared to CTLs derived from AA⁻ DCs. For the negative control set, AA⁺ DCs and AA⁻ DCs sets were matured with LPS, TNF-α and CD40L [20]. The CTLs thus generated were not effective in killing the target MCF-7 cell line. No killing was seen in either of these sets (data not shown). As an additional negative control for target specificity, CTLs obtained from MCF-7 lysate primed DCs were used in CTL assay against H1299 cell line but no killing effect was seen in these sets as well (CPM values for thymidine incorporation in case of control was 12649.33±30.73 SD. For pulsed and unpulsed group at highest target to T cell ratios were 12405.66±36.35 SD and 12537.33±27.47 SD respectively).

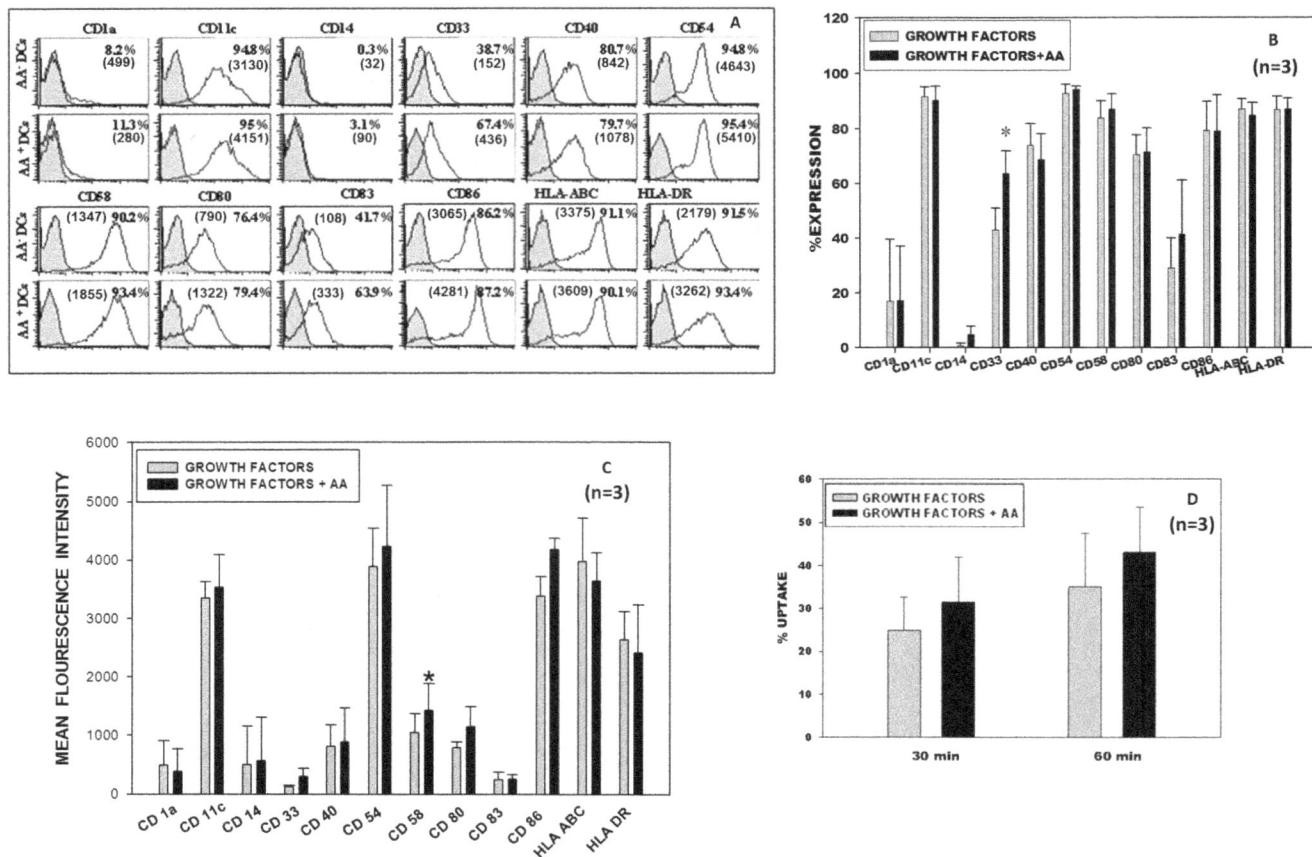

Figure 1. Phenotype and Antigen uptake of AA⁺ DCs and AA⁻ DCs: DCs were generated from the expanded DC precursor cells with and without AA. (A) FACS histogram profile of a representative experiment. Filled histograms show the isotype control and open ones show the specific phenotype with respective MFI values in the brackets. (B) It is seen that fully mature DCs were generated and there was not much difference in the expression levels of different surface markers, except CD33 (myeloid lineage) was higher in AA⁺ DC sets (mean ± SD, n = 3, P≤0.05 *). (C) Bar graph for DC specific and associated markers in terms of MFI, for CD 58 (adhesion molecule) the difference was found significantly higher (mean ± SD, n = 3, P≤0.05 *). (D) Receptor mediated antigen uptake of AA⁺ DCs and AA⁻ DCs: Dextran-FITC uptake by DCs (n = 3, mean ± SD). The control value (uptake at 4°C) is deducted from the respective test value (uptake at 37°C).

The mRNA levels of key enzymes involved in AA metabolism are higher in AA⁺ DCs

The transcript levels of three enzymes associated with arachidonic acid pathway, such as COX-1, COX-2, PLA$_2$, were detected by RT-PCR carried out as per standard methods. Gel images of RT-PCR are shown in Fig. 5B. There was a higher expression of COX-2 in the AA⁺ DCs set as compared to AA⁻ DCs set. Increased mRNA levels are indicative of active metabolism of the exogenously added AA in the test sets. However the differences in the expression of COX-1 and PLA2 between control and test sets were marginal. Taken together the *in vitro* data indicates that, AA⁺ DCs exhibited improved functional properties compared to AA⁻ DCs. Thus, though addition of AA does not alter the morphology and phenotype of DCs, the functions of these DCs are enhanced.

Enhanced homing of AA⁺ DCs to bone marrow in NOD SCID mice

To evaluate the *in vivo* homing ability of the *in vitro* generated DCs, we intravenously administered the cultured control and test DCs into sub lethally irradiated NOD/SCID mice as described in methods. 10⁶ AA⁺ DCs (test) and AA⁻ DCs (control) were used for

intravenous infusion. The animals were sacrificed after 18 hr and the ability of human DCs to home was assessed by staining the BM cells with anti hCD11c and anti murine CD45.1 mAb. Intravenous injected DCs have been reported to home to bone marrow [24]. The percent homing in each set was compared to the PBS infused irradiated recipient to detect the background staining if any. It was observed that, the animals, which received the AA⁺ DCs, showed a higher migration in BM than the animals that received the AA⁻ DCs generated with growth factors alone. This correlated well with the *in vitro* results. Fig. 6A shows that significantly higher number of AA⁺ DCs migrated to BM of individual animals as compared to AA⁻ DCs (P≤0.001). The representative dot and contour plots showing the gating strategy are exemplified in Fig. 6B. Expression of hCD11c in one representative mouse infused with PBS, AA⁻ DCs and AA⁺ DCs is shown in Fig. 6C 1, 2 and 3 respectively. Thus the presence of AA in the culture was found to be beneficial in generating the DCs with a higher migration capacity.

Discussion

DCs derived from UCB samples can serve as an allogeneic source of DCs for their potential use in cancer immunotherapy.

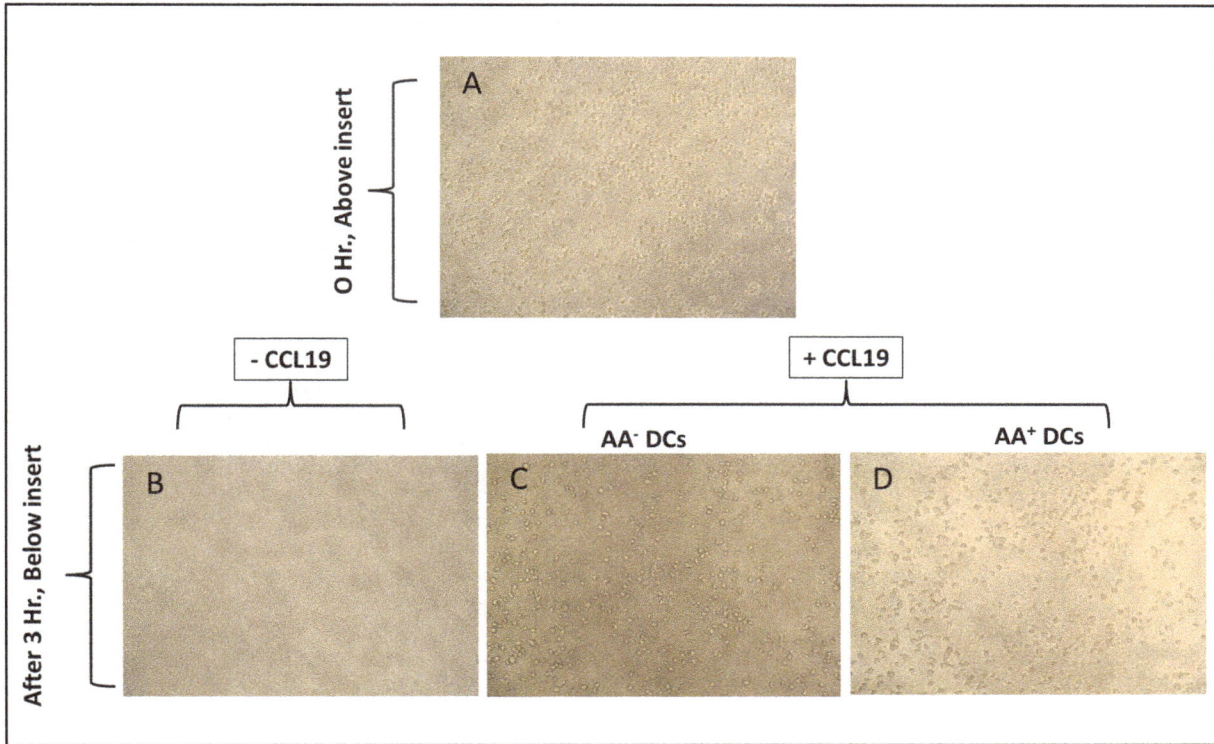

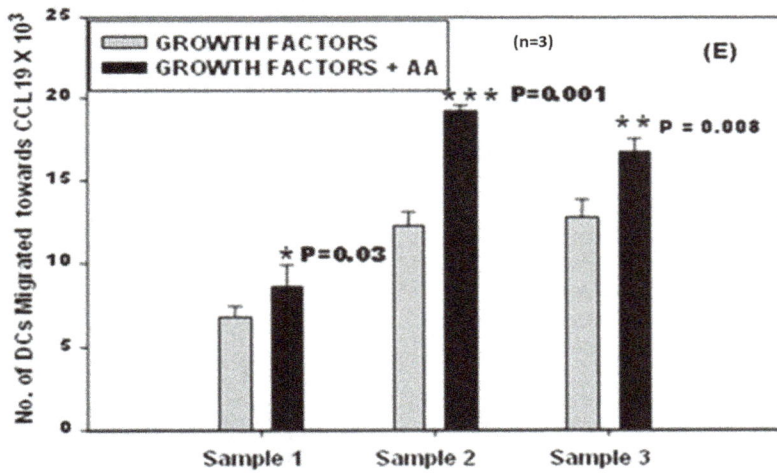

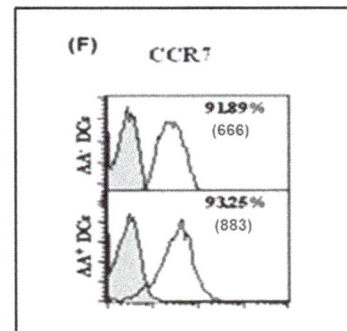

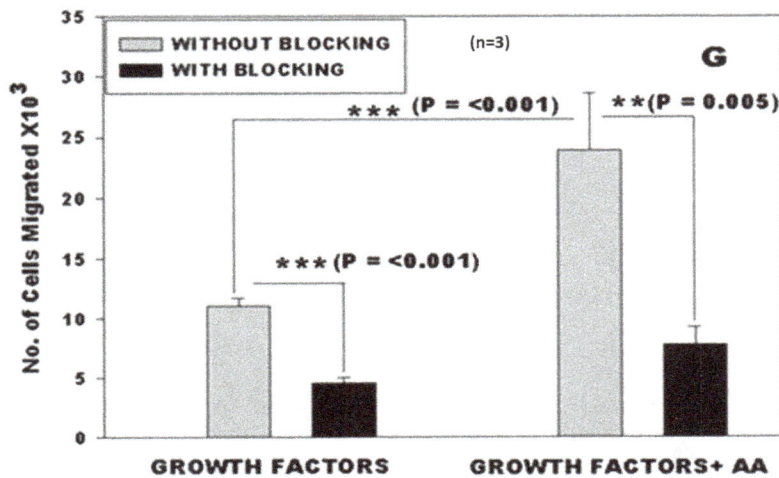

Figure 2. Chemotaxis and CCR7 expression: (A) DCs suspended in upper chamber of well before migration. After 3 hours (B) No spontaneous migration was observed in the wells, where CCL-19 was not added. Less no. of AA⁻ DCs (C) migrated towards CCL-19 than AA⁺ DCs (D). (E) AA⁺ DCs showed statistically efficient migration towards CCL-19 compared to AA⁻ DCs (n = 3, mean ± SD). (F) FACS histogram profile of a representative experiment showing expression of chemokine receptor CCR-7 along with MFI values in brackets. Filled histograms show the isotype control and open ones show the specific phenotype. (G) Blocking with CCR-7 Ab causes significant reduction in migration of both AA⁺ DCs and AA⁻ DCs (n = 3, mean ± SD). [P≤0.05(*), P≤0.01(**) & P≤0.001(***)].

Our published method leads to enrichment of a homogenous population i.e. myeloid interstitial DC subset [17,20]. Here we demonstrated for the first time that the addition of AA at the differentiation step of our culture method showed beneficial effects thus further improving the quality of DCs generated from cord blood. The maturation status plays a decisive role in antigen presentation, costimulation and ultimately adjudicates whether the outcome is immunogenic or tolerogenic. DCs used in cancer immunotherapy should have strong immunogenic response. DCs exhibit their anticancer effect by capturing the tumor antigens [7,8,9]. The AA⁺ DCs showed higher antigen uptake compared to AA⁻ DCs underscoring the beneficial effect of AA addition to the cultures. Another important feature of DCs is their capacity to stimulate the proliferation of T lymphocytes in an allogeneic MLR and to generate effector CTLs. The inflammatory nature of many cancers creates an immunosuppressive environment that leads to suppression of DC-instructed effector CD4+ and CD8+ T cell responses [6]. The enhanced MLR in the culture system with AA may be attributed to production of more mature DCs which may help to cope up with immunosuppressive environment of cancer seen in the *in vivo* situation.

The migratory properties of DCs are of fundamental importance for their function and have been extensively investigated [25,26]. DCs travel from bone marrow to the various tissues and from there to secondary lymphoid organs [1]. Our *in vitro* as well as *in vivo* data showed that DCs grown in presence of AA

exhibited enhanced migration to CCL19 (*in vitro*) and to BM (*in vivo*). Michael A. Morse *et al.* demonstrated that DCs injected I.V, initially localize in the lungs and then redistribute to the liver, spleen, and bone marrow, but apparently not to the lymph nodes or tumor masses [24]. We had not observed any differences in migration of AA⁻, AA+ DCs to the spleen. We had selected 18 hrs post infusion as the time point in homing experiment. Studying the homing at different time points probably may give a different picture. CCR-7 is selectively expressed on mature DCs. The CCR-7 receptor and CCL-19 ligand interaction facilitate migration of mature DCs [26,27]. Our data established the specificity of this interaction. Our results are in agreement with the findings of van Helden *et al.* where they report more efficient *in vitro* migration to CCL19 but no change in CCR7 expression on DCs after addition of PGE2 [28]. They attribute increase in migration to dissolution of podosomes by PGE2 as well as up regulation of MMP9 which is also essential for DC chemotaxis *in vitro* and *in vivo* migration. Whether the same mechanism operates in our system needs to be looked into.

DCs generated for immunotherapy purpose should have cytokine profile which supports the Th1 type of response. In other words, secretion of low levels of IL-10 and high levels of IL-12 is a desirable character for the DCs to be used for vaccination regimen. In our culture system AA addition results in improved IL12/IL10 ratio thus further improving their antitumor ability. Pawel Kalinski *et al.* [29] have shown that though PGE2 is

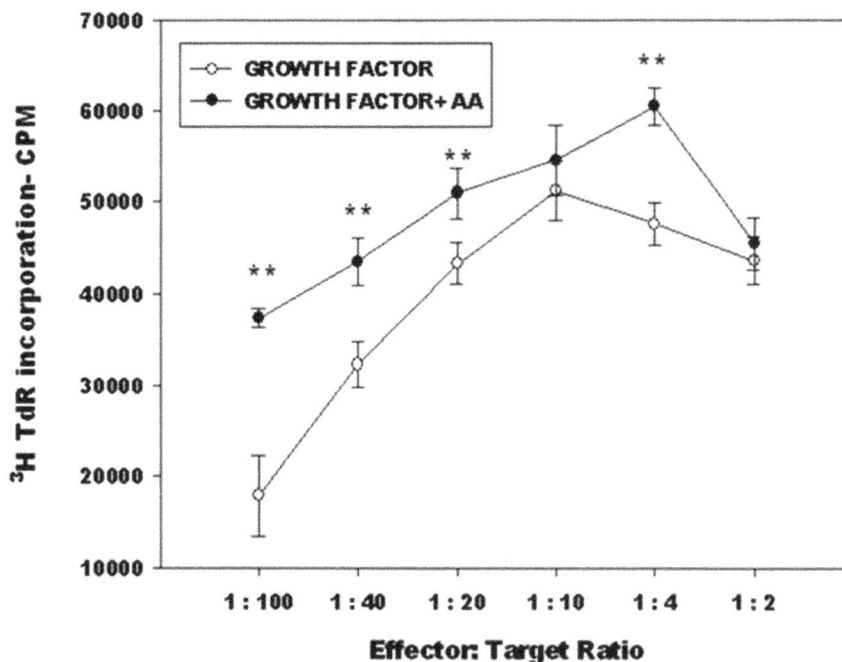

Figure 3. AA⁺ DCs exhibit better MLR than AA⁻ DCs: DCs generated were capable of efficient stimulation of allogeneic T cells. AA⁺ DCs showed better T-cell stimulation than the AA⁻ DC, differences were significant at four out of six DC:T-cell ratios tested (*P≤0.05,**P≤0.01). Representative data from three independent experiments is shown. TdR = thymidine.

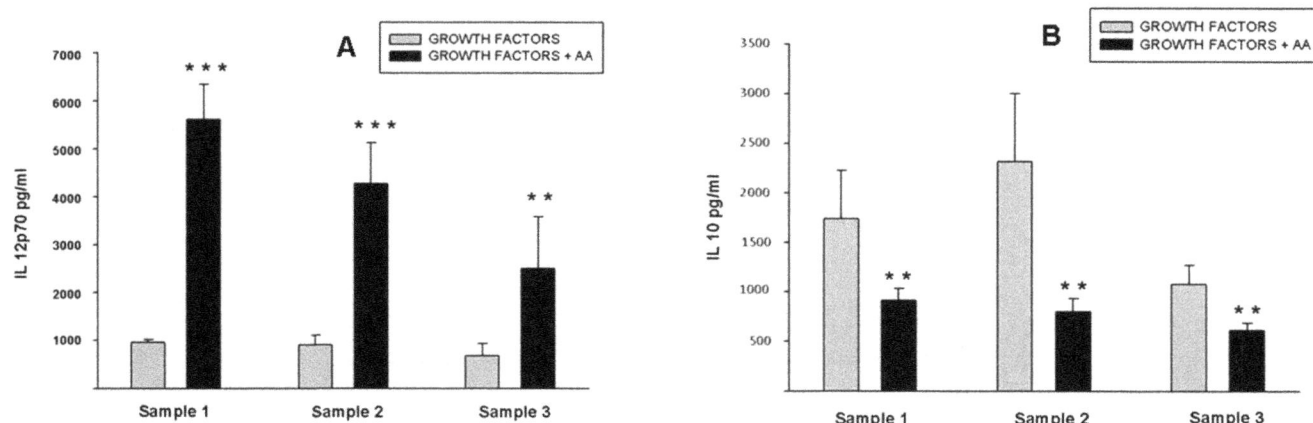

Figure 4. Detection of IL-10 and IL-12 p70 in the culture supernatants of AA$^+$ DCs and AA$^-$ DCs: *In vitro* **generated DCs were assessed for their ability to secrete IL-12 p70 and IL-10.** Results show that DCs generated by both culture conditions were capable of secretion of IL-12 p70 and IL-10. (A) AA$^+$ DCs showed a better IL-12 p70 secretion compared to AA$^-$ DCs. (B) Similarly, AA$^+$ DCs have low level of IL-10 secretion profile as compared to AA$^-$ DCs. The data of three independent samples are shown (n = 3, mean ± SD). [P≤0.05(*), P≤0.01(**) & P≤0.001(***)].

reported as a suppressive inflammatory factor, it also contributes to the initiation of primary immune responses by facilitating the cytokine-induced final maturation and the increase in immunostimulatory capacity of DC, confirming the role of PGE2 as a Th2-promoting factor, acting at the APC level. Enzymes Cyclooxygenases (COX-1 and COX-2) convert the AA released by cPLA2 to PG endoperoxide H2, which is the precursor of series 2 prostanoids such as PGD2 and PGE2. Unlike COX-1, COX-2 is an inducible enzyme involved in the sustained production of prostanoids by many cell types [30]. Notably, COX-2 activity is necessary for strong Ab response following vaccination; especially

when vaccines are poorly immunogenic or the target population is poorly responsive to immunization [31]. Thus the enhanced expression of COX-2 mRNA as seen in AA$^+$ DCs may be favorable for their use of as anticancer agents. However one wonders which of the following metabolites of AA downstream pathway like LTB4, cysteinyl leukotrienes, 12–15-hetes, PGE2, and PGD2 are actually responsible for the beneficial effect. In future we propose to address these issues of delineating the pathway by appropriate use of pharmacological inhibitors.

Many DC-based clinical trials for cancer treatment have shown its safety and feasibility [9,30]. The clinical efficacy of this therapy

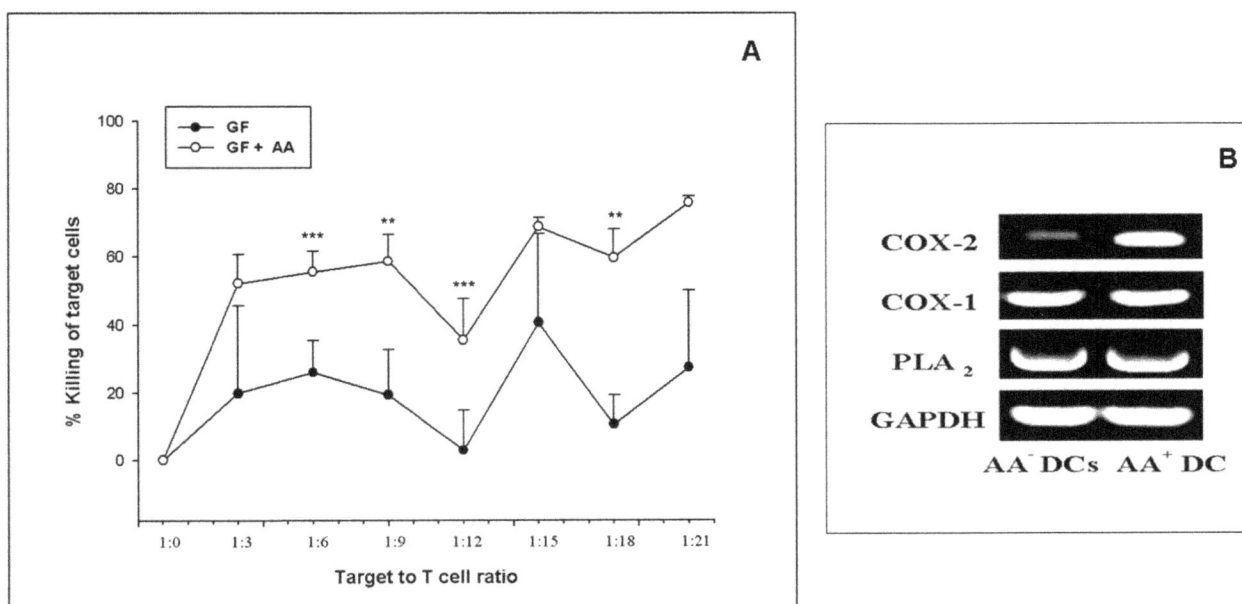

Figure 5. CTL and Transcript levels of key enzymes in AA$^+$ DCs and AA$^-$ DCs. (A) CTL data of one representative sample i.e. killing of the target (MCF-7) cells by CTLs generated by AA$^+$ DCs/AA$^-$ DCs pulsed with MCF-7 cell lysate. CTLs derived from AA$^+$ DCs exhibited an improved effector function i.e. enhanced overall killing as compared to CTLs derived from AA$^-$ DCs. The killing is significantly higher at four ratios of effector target cell concentrations. (*P≤0.05, **P≤0.01, ***P≤0.001). (B) Gene expression profile of three key enzymes associated with AA pathway along with the housekeeping gene GAPDH. There is a substantial up-regulation of transcript level of key enzyme COX-2 in the DCs cultured in presence of AA.

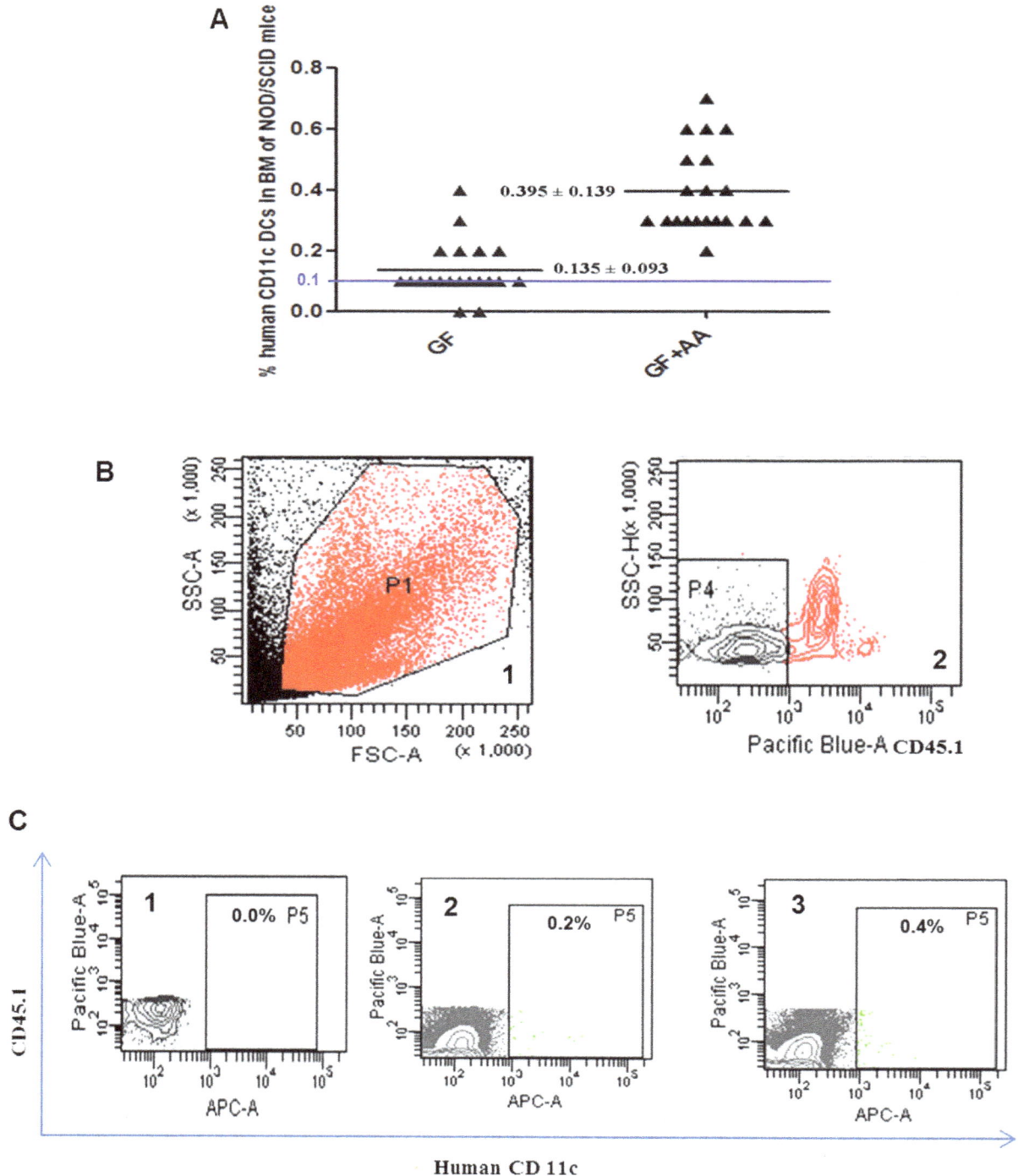

Figure 6. *In vivo* **homing of the human AA⁺ DCs and AA⁻ DCs in NOD/SCID mice.** (A) Scatter plot showing the percentage of DCs positive for human CD11c in bone marrow of individual mouse (n = 40), 18 hrs post-infusion. Significantly higher numbers of DCs were detected in BM of mice receiving AA⁺ DCs compared with mice receiving AA⁻ DCs (P≤0.001). Mice showing ≥0.1% human cells were considered positive for engraftment (Shown by a blue line). The bar indicates mean values with ± SD. (B) Representative Flow cytometry profile showing gating strategy 1) FSC/SSC, P1 gated cells were analyzes for mCD45.1 positive cells. 2) P4 represents gate for cells negative for mCD45.1, hCD11c were analyzed in P4 gate. (C) Representative Flow cytometry profile showing hCD11c positive cells in P5 gate of mice infused with 1) PBS, 2) AA⁻ DCs and 3) AA⁺ DCs.[Pacific blue-mCD45.1, APC- hCD11c].

still needs to be improvised. Advances in biology lead to frequent improvements in the vaccine production protocols and therapeutics [32,33,34,35,36,37]. Recent reports also illustrate that there is emerging evidence that PGE2 plays crucial roles in reciprocal crosstalk between dendritic cells and natural killer cell biology. Several NK cell functions (lysis, migration, proliferation, cytokine production) are influenced by PGE2, accentuating the role of PGE2 on DC– NK cell crosstalk and its subsequent impact on immune regulations in normal and immunopathological processes. [38] Some of the previous reports show that *in vitro* generated DCs are less efficient in migration and other functional activities [6,19,24] due to use of the cytokine IL-4 in the protocols [18]. IL-4 is known to adversely affect the AA metabolism. So we hypothesized that exogenous addition of AA in the culture medium may improve the functional activities of DCs. As per our expectation, AA^+ DCs exhibited a better *in vitro* chemotaxis, T cell stimulation, CTL activity, Th1 favorable cytokine profile, antigen uptake and *in vivo* migration. *In vitro* manipulation of cellular vaccines is crucial for their successful use in clinics and thus our methodology, though it shows an incremental increase in the output, may add a new dimension in improvising the production of a potent immunotherapeutic agent. In other words these findings will be helpful in the better contriving of DC based vaccines for cancer immunotherapy with enhanced functionality.

Supporting Information

Figure S1　Flow chart depicting the design of the experiment.

Figure S2　Sequence of four primers used in the study.

Figure S3　AA^+ DCs and AA^- DCs show similar morphology. Phase contrast images of (A) Immature adhered DCs. (B) Both cultures show the typical veiled clusters of mature DCs. (C) Wright-Giemsa images of adherent cells show typical DC morphology. Original magnification for A is 10X, for B and C is 20X. The phase contrast images were cropped and enlarged.

Figure S4　IL-12 p70/IL-10 ratio was higher in AA^+ DCs as compared to AA^- DCs. Concentrations of IL-12 p70 and IL-10 was in pg/ml.

Figure S5　CTL assay of other two samples showing improved killing in AA^+ DCs.

Acknowledgments

The authors thank Doctors Prakash Daithankar, Arvind Sangamnerkar, Girish Godbole and Ranjeet Bhosale for providing CB samples. We thank Ms. Nikhat Firdaus Q. Khan for technical help and the NCCS core facilities like flow cytometry and animal experimentation facility.

Author Contributions

Conceived and designed the experiments: LL. Performed the experiments: JK RG. Analyzed the data: JK VK LL. Contributed reagents/materials/analysis tools: LL VK. Wrote the paper: LL VK JK. P.I. in the project: LL. Co P.I. in the project: VK.

References

1. Banchereau J, Steinman RM (1998) Dendritic cells and the control of immunity. Nature, 392: 245–252.
2. Banchereau J, Briere F, Caux C, Davoust J, Palucka K, et al. (2000) Immunobiology of dendritic cells. Annu Rev Immunol 18: 767–811.
3. Cella M, Sallusto F, Lanzavecchia A (1997) Origin, maturation and antigen presenting function of dendritic cells. Curr Opin Immuno l 9: 10–16.
4. Bonasio R, von Andrian UH (2006) Generation, migration and function of circulating dendritic cells. Curr Opin Immunol 18: 503–511.
5. Palucka K, Banchereau J (2012) Cancer immunotherapy via dendritic cells. Nature Reviews Cancer 12: 265–277.
6. Melief CJ (2008) Cancer immunotherapy by dendritic cells. Immunity 29: 372–383.
7. Fong L, Engleman EG (2000) Dendritic cells in cancer immunotherapy. Annu Rev Immunol 18: 245–273.
8. Ridgway D (2003) The first 1000 dendritic cell vaccinees. Cancer Invest 21: 873–886.
9. Galluzzi L, Senovilla L, Vacchelli E, Alexander E, Wolf HF, et al. (2012) Trial watch: Dendritic cell-based interventions for cancer therapy. Oncoimmunology 7: 1111–1134.
10. Bontkes HJ, De Gruijl TD, Schuurhuis GJ, Scheper RJ, Meijer CJ, et al. (2002) Expansion of dendritic cell precursors from human CD34 (+) progenitor cells isolated from healthy donor blood; growth factor combination determines proliferation rate and functional outcome. J Leukoc Biol 72: 321–329.
11. Lee H, Kim M, Baek S (2008) In vivo efficacy of hematopoietic stem cell-derived allogeneic-DC vaccine in mouse melanoma metastasis model. Cancer Immunol Immunother 57: 1–53.
12. Santiago-Schwarz F, Rappa DA, Laky K, Carsons SE (1995) Stem cell factor augments tumor necrosis factor-granulocyte-macrophage colony-stimulating factor-mediated dendritic cell hematopoiesis. Stem Cells 13: 186–197.
13. Saraya K, Reid CD (1996) Stem cell factor and the regulation of dendritic cell production from CD34+ progenitors in bone marrow and cord blood. Br J Haematol 93: 258–264.
14. Arrighi JF, Hauser C, Chapuis B, Zubler RH, Kindler V (1999) Long-term culture of human CD34 (+) progenitors with FLT3-ligand, thrombopoietin, and stem cell factor induces extensive amplification of a CD34(-)CD14 (-) and a CD34(-)CD14(+) dendritic cell precursor. Blood 93: 2244–2252.
15. Encabo A, Solves P, Mateu E, Sepulveda P, Carbonell-Uberos F, et al. (2004) Selective generation of different dendritic cell precursors from CD34+ cells by interleukin-6 and interleukin-3. Stem Cells 22: 725–740.
16. Ryu KH, Cho SJ, Jung YJ, Seoh JY, Kie JH, et al. (2004) In vitro generation of functional dendritic cells from human umbilical cord blood CD34+ cells by a 2-step culture method. Int J Hematol 80: 281–286.
17. Balan S, Kale VP, Limaye LS (2009) A simple two-step culture system for the large-scale generation of mature and functional dendritic cells from umbilical cord blood CD34+ cells. Transfusion 49: 2109–2121.
18. Soruri A, Zwirner J (2005) Dendritic cells: limited potential in immunotherapy. Int J Biochem Cell Biol 37: 241–245.
19. Thurnher M, Zelle-Rieser C, Ramoner R, Bartsch G, Holtl L (2001) The disabled dendritic cell. FASEB J 15: 1054–1061.
20. Balan S, Kale VP, Limaye LS (2010) A large number of mature and functional dendritic cells can be efficiently generated from umbilical cord blood-derived mononuclear cells by a simple two-step culture method. Transfusion 50: 2413–2423.
21. Matzinger P (1991) The JAM test, A simple assay for DNA fragmentation and cell death. J lmm Meth 145: 185–192.
22. Usharauli D, Perez-Diez A, Matzinger P (2006) The JAM Test and its daughter P-JAM: simple tests of DNA fragmentation to measure cell death and stasis. Nat Protoc 1: 672–82.
23. Agarwal P, Raghavan A, Nandiwada SL, Curtsinger JM, Bohjanen PR, et al. (2009) Gene regulation and chromatin remodeling by IL-12 and type I IFN in programming for CD8 T cell effector function and memory. J Immunol. 183: 1695–1704.
24. Morse MA, Coleman RE, Akabani G, Niehaus N, Coleman D, et al. (1999) Migration of human dendritic cells after injection in patients with metastatic malignancies. Cancer Res 59: 56–58.
25. Verdijk P, Aarntzen EH, Lesterhuis WJ, Boullart AC, Kok E, et al. (2009) Limited amounts of dendritic cells migrate into the T-cell area of lymph nodes but have high immune activating potential in melanoma patients. Clin Cancer Res 15: 2531–2540.
26. Scandella E, Men Y, Gillessen S, Förster R, Groettrup M (2002) Prostaglandin E2 is a key factor for CCR7 surface expression and migration of monocyte-derived dendritic cells. Blood. 100: 1354–61.
27. Riol-Blanco L, Sanchez-Sanchez N, Torres A, Tejedor A, Narumiya S, et al. (2005) The chemokine receptor CCR7 activates in dendritic cells two signaling modules that independently regulate chemotaxis and migratory speed. J Immunol 174: 4070–4080.
28. van Helden SF, Krooshoop DJ, Broers KC, Raymakers RA, Figdor CG, et al. (2006) A critical role for prostaglandin E2 in podosome dissolution and induction of high-speed migration during dendritic cell maturation. J. Immunol. 177: 1567–1574.
29. Kaliński P, Schuitemaker JH, Hilkens CM, Kapsenberg ML (1998) Prostaglandin E2 induces the final maturation of IL-12-deficient CD1a+CD83+ dendritic cells: the levels of IL-12 are determined during the final dendritic cell maturation and are resistant to further modulation. J Immunol. 161: 2804–9.
30. Valera I, Fernandez N, Trinidad AG, Alonso S, Brown GD, et al. (2008) Costimulation of dectin-1 and DC-SIGN triggers the arachidonic acid cascade in human monocyte-derived dendritic cells. J Immunol 180: 5727–5736.
31. Ryan EP, Malboeuf CM, Bernard M, Rose RC, Phipps RP (2006) Cyclooxygenase-2 inhibition attenuates antibody responses against human papillomavirus-like particles. J Immunol 177: 7811–7819.

32. Steinman RM, Banchereau J (2007) Taking dendritic cells into medicine. Nature 449: 419–26.

33. Hsu AK, Kerr BM, Jones KL, Lock RB, Hart DN, et al. (2006) RNA loading of leukemic antigens into cord blood-derived dendritic cells for immunotherapy. Biol Blood Marrow Transplant 12: 855–867.

34. Thurner B, Roder C, Dieckmann D, Heuer M, Kruse M, et al. (1999) Generation of large numbers of fully mature and stable dendritic cells from leukapheresis products for clinical application. J Immunol Methods 223: 1–15.

35. Perroud MW Jr, Honma HN, Barbeiro AS, Gilli SC, Almeida MT, et al. (2011) Mature Autologous Dendritic Cell Vaccines in Advanced Non-Small Cell Lung Cancer: a Phase I Pilot Study. J Exp Clin Cancer Res 17: 30–65.

36. Kalinski P, Edington H, Zeh HJ, Okada H, Butterfield LH, et al. (2011) Dendritic cells in cancer immunotherapy: vaccines or autologous transplants? Immunol Res 50: 235–247.

37. Goessling W, Allen RS, Guan X, Jin P, Uchida N, et al. (2011) Prostaglandin E2 enhances human cord blood stem cell xenotransplants and shows long-term safety in preclinical nonhuman primate transplant models. Cell Stem Cell. 8: 445–458.

38. Harizi H (2013) Reciprocal crosstalk between dendritic cells and natural killer cells under the effects of PGE2 in immunity and immunopathology. Cellular & Molecular Immunology 10: 213–221.

Permissions

The contributors of this book come from diverse backgrounds, making this book a truly international effort. This book will bring forth new frontiers with its revolutionizing research information and detailed analysis of the nascent developments around the world.

We would like to thank all the contributing authors for lending their expertise to make the book truly unique. They have played a crucial role in the development of this book. Without their invaluable contributions this book wouldn't have been possible. They have made vital efforts to compile up to date information on the varied aspects of this subject to make this book a valuable addition to the collection of many professionals and students.

This book was conceptualized with the vision of imparting up-to-date information and advanced data in this field. To ensure the same, a matchless editorial board was set up. Every individual on the board went through rigorous rounds of assessment to prove their worth. After which they invested a large part of their time researching and compiling the most relevant data for our readers.

The editorial board has been involved in producing this book since its inception. They have spent rigorous hours researching and exploring the diverse topics which have resulted in the successful publishing of this book. They have passed on their knowledge of decades through this book. To expedite this challenging task, the publisher supported the team at every step. A small team of assistant editors was also appointed to further simplify the editing procedure and attain best results for the readers.

Apart from the editorial board, the designing team has also invested a significant amount of their time in understanding the subject and creating the most relevant covers. They scrutinized every image to scout for the most suitable representation of the subject and create an appropriate cover for the book.

The publishing team has been an ardent support to the editorial, designing and production team. Their endless efforts to recruit the best for this project, has resulted in the accomplishment of this book. They are a veteran in the field of academics and their pool of knowledge is as vast as their experience in printing. Their expertise and guidance has proved useful at every step. Their uncompromising quality standards have made this book an exceptional effort. Their encouragement from time to time has been an inspiration for everyone.

The publisher and the editorial board hope that this book will prove to be a valuable piece of knowledge for researchers, students, practitioners and scholars across the globe.

List of Contributors

Catherine Gérard, Nathalie Baudson, Thierry Ory and Jamila Louahed
GlaxoSmithKline Vaccines, Rixensart, Belgium

Hongsheng Miao, Carter M. Suryadevara, Luis Sanchez-Perez and Shicheng Yang
Duke Brain Tumor Immunotherapy Program, Division of Neurosurgery, Department of Surgery, Duke University Medical Center, Durham, North Carolina, United States of America

Bryan D. Choi and Elias J. Sayour
Duke Brain Tumor Immunotherapy Program, Division of Neurosurgery, Department of Surgery, Duke University Medical Center, Durham, North Carolina, United States of America
Department of Pathology, Duke University Medical Center, Durham, North Carolina, United States of America

Gabriel De Leon
Duke Brain Tumor Immunotherapy Program, Division of Neurosurgery, Department of Surgery, Duke University Medical Center, Durham, North Carolina, United States of America
Department of Molecular Cancer Biology, Duke University Medical Center, Durham, North Carolina, United States of America

Roger McLendon
Department of Pathology, Duke University Medical Center, Durham, North Carolina, United States of America
The Preston Robert Tisch Brain Tumor Center, Duke University Medical Center, Durham, North Carolina, United States of America

James E. Herndon II and Patrick Healy
Department of Biostatistics and Bioinformatics, Duke University Medical Center, Durham, North Carolina, United States of America

Gary E. Archer, Darell D. Bigner and John H. Sampson
Duke Brain Tumor Immunotherapy Program, Division of Neurosurgery, Department of Surgery, Duke University Medical Center, Durham, North Carolina, United States of America
Department of Pathology, Duke University Medical Center, Durham, North Carolina, United States of America

The Preston Robert Tisch Brain Tumor Center, Duke University Medical Center, Durham, North Carolina, United States of America

Laura A. Johnson
Duke Brain Tumor Immunotherapy Program, Division of Neurosurgery, Department of Surgery, Duke University Medical Center, Durham, North Carolina, United States of America
The Preston Robert Tisch Brain Tumor Center, Duke University Medical Center, Durham, North Carolina, United States of America

Mingjun Wang, Rong-Fu Wang and Helen Y. Wang
Center for Inflammation and Epigenetics, The Methodist Hospital Research Institute, Houston, Texas, United States of America
Center for Cell and Gene Therapy, Baylor College of Medicine, Houston, Texas, United States of America

Bingnan Yin, Lijuan Deng, Wei Zhao, Jia Zou, Qingtian Li and Christopher Loo
Center for Inflammation and Epigenetics, The Methodist Hospital Research Institute, Houston, Texas, United States of America

Satoko Matsueda and Ying Li
Center for Cell and Gene Therapy, Baylor College of Medicine, Houston, Texas, United States of America

Takeshi Ishikawa, Satoshi Kokura and Tetsuya Okayama
Department of Molecular Gastroenterology and Hepatology, Graduate School of Medical Science, Kyoto Prefectural University of Medicine, Kyoto, Japan
Department of Cancer ImmunoCell Regulation, Kyoto Prefectural University of Medicine, Kyoto, Japan

Tatsuji Enoki, Mitsuko Ideno and Junichi Mineno
Center for Cell and Gene Therapy, Takara Bio Inc, Otsu, Japan

Naoyuki Sakamoto, Naohisa Yoshida, Kazuhiro Kamada, Kazuhiro Katada, Kazuhiko Uchiyama, Osamu Handa, Tomohisa Takagi, Hideyuki Konishi, Nobuaki Yagi, Yuji Naito and Yoshito Itoh
Department of Molecular Gastroenterology and Hepatology, Graduate School of Medical Science, Kyoto Prefectural University of Medicine, Kyoto, Japan

Kazuko Uno
Division of Basic Research, Louis Pasteur Center for Medical Research, Kyoto, Japan

Toshikazu Yoshikawa
Department of Cancer ImmunoCell Regulation, Kyoto Prefectural University of Medicine, Kyoto, Japan

Tatsuya Moutai, Hideyuki Yamana, Takuya Nojima and Daisuke Kitamura
Division of Molecular Biology, Research Institute for Biomedical Sciences (RIBS), Tokyo University of Science, Noda, Chiba, Japan

Evripidis Lanitis and Denarda Dangaj
Ovarian Cancer Research Center, Department of Obstetrics and Gynecology, University of Pennsylvania, Philadelphia, Pennsylvania, United States of America
Department of Molecular Biology and Genetics, Democritus University of Thrace, Alexandroupolis, Greece

Ian S. Hagemann
Abramson Cancer Center, Department of Pathology and Laboratory Medicine, University of Pennsylvania, Philadelphia, Pennsylvania, United States of America

De-Gang Song, George Coukos and Andrew Best
Ovarian Cancer Research Center, Department of Obstetrics and Gynecology, University of Pennsylvania, Philadelphia, Pennsylvania, United States of America

Raphael Sandaltzopoulos
Department of Molecular Biology and Genetics, Democritus University of Thrace, Alexandroupolis, Greece

Daniel J. Powell, Jr.
Ovarian Cancer Research Center, Department of Obstetrics and Gynecology, University of Pennsylvania, Philadelphia, Pennsylvania, United States of America
Abramson Cancer Center, Department of Pathology and Laboratory Medicine, University of Pennsylvania, Philadelphia, Pennsylvania, United States of America

Kelcey G. Patterson, Jennifer L. Dixon Pittaro and Peter S. Bastedo
Department of Microbiology and Immunology, Western University, London, Ontario, Canada

David A. Hess
Department of Physiology and Pharmacology, Western University, London Ontario, Canada
Vascular Biology Research Group, Robarts Research Institute, London, Ontario, Canada

S. M. Mansour Haeryfar and John K. McCormick
Department of Microbiology and Immunology, Western University, London, Ontario, Canada
Centre for Human Immunology, Western University, London, Ontario, Canada
Lawson Health Research Institute, London, Ontario, Canada

Alexander M. Menzies, Lauren E. Haydu and Georgina V. Long
Melanoma Institute Australia, Sydney, Australia
The University of Sydney, Sydney, Australia

Matteo S. Carlino and Richard F. Kefford
Melanoma Institute Australia, Sydney, Australia
The University of Sydney, Sydney, Australia
Westmead Hospital, Crown Princess Mary Cancer Centre, Sydney, Australia
Westmead Institute for Cancer Research, Westmead, Australia

Mary W. F. Azer
Westmead Hospital, Crown Princess Mary Cancer Centre, Sydney, Australia

Peter J. A. Carr
The University of Sydney, Sydney, Australia
Westmead Hospital, Department of Radiology, Sydney, Australia

Arta M. Monjazeb
Department of Radiation Oncology School of Medicine, University of California Davis, Sacramento, California, United States of America

Julia K. Tietze, Steven K. Grossenbacher, Hui-Hua Hsiao, Anthony E. Zamora, Annie Mirsoian and Gail D. Sckisel
Department of Dermatology, School of Medicine, University of California Davis, Sacramento, California, United States of America

Brent Koehn and Bruce R. Blazar
Department of Pediatrics, Division of Blood and Marrow Transplantation and Masonic Cancer Center, University of Minnesota, Minneapolis, Massachusetts, United States of America

Jonathan M. Weiss and Robert H. Wiltrout
Cancer and Inflammation Program, National Cancer Institute, Frederick, Maryland, United States of America

William J. Murphy
Department of Dermatology, School of Medicine, University of California Davis, Sacramento, California, United States of America

Department of Internal Medicine, School of Medicine, University of California, Davis, Sacramento, California, United States of America

Huan Zhang, Xiaoming Cai, Junbao Yang, Yuewu Shen, Baofeng Chen and Suhua Liang
The Medical Biology Staff Room of North Sichuan Medical College, Sichuan Nanchong, the People's Republic of China

Bo Mu
The Medical Biology Staff Room of North Sichuan Medical College, Sichuan Nanchong, the People's Republic of China
Sichuan Key Laboratory of Medical Imaging, Affiliated Hospital of North Sichuan Medical College, North Sichuan Medical College, Nanchong, the People's Republic of China

Zineb Belcaid, Jillian A. Phallen, Alfred P. See, Dimitrios Mathios, Chelsea Gottschalk, Sarah Nicholas, Meghan Kellett, Jacob Ruzevick, Christopher Jackson, Xiaobu Ye, Betty Tyler and Michael Lim
Department of Neurosurgery, Johns Hopkins University School of Medicine, Baltimore, Maryland, United States of America

Jing Zeng, Phuoc T. Tran and John W. Wong
Department of Radiation Oncology and Molecular Radiation Sciences, Johns Hopkins University School of Medicine, Baltimore, Maryland, United States of America

Emilia Albesiano, Drew M. Pardoll, Charles G. Drake and Nicholas M. Durham
Department of Oncology and Medicine, Johns Hopkins University School of Medicine, Baltimore, Maryland, United States of America

Henry Brem
Department of Neurosurgery, Johns Hopkins University School of Medicine, Baltimore, Maryland, United States of America
Departments of Oncology, Ophthalmology, and Biomedical Engineering,
Johns Hopkins University School of Medicine, Baltimore, Maryland, United States of America

Sayeema Daudi and Shashikant Lele
Department of Gynecologic Oncology, Roswell Park Cancer Institute, Buffalo, New York, United States of America

Kevin H. Eng and Adrienne Groman
Department of Biostatisticsm, Roswell Park Cancer Institute, Buffalo, New York, United States of America

Paulette Mhawech-Fauceglia
Department of Pathology, University Southern California, Los Angeles, California, United States of America

Carl Morrison
Department of Pathology, Roswell Park Cancer Institute, Buffalo, New York, United States of America

Amy Beck
Center for Immunotherapy, Roswell Park Cancer Institute, Buffalo, New York, United States of America

Anthony Miliotto
Department of Gynecologic Oncology, Roswell Park Cancer Institute, Buffalo, New York, United States of America
Center for Immunotherapy, Roswell Park Cancer Institute, Buffalo, New York, United States of America

Junko Matsuzaki and Takemasa Tsuji
Center for Immunotherapy, Roswell Park Cancer Institute, Buffalo, New York, United States of America
Department of Immunology, Roswell Park Cancer Institute, Buffalo, New York, United States of America

Sacha Gnjatic
Department of Medicine, Mount Sinai Hospital, New York, New York, United States of America

Guillo Spagnoli
Department of Biomedicine, University Hospital Basel, Basel, Switzerland

Kunle Odunsi
Department of Gynecologic Oncology, Roswell Park Cancer Institute, Buffalo, New York, United States of America
Center for Immunotherapy, Roswell Park Cancer Institute, Buffalo, New York, United States of America
Department of Immunology, Roswell Park Cancer Institute, Buffalo, New York, United States of America

Kai-Lin Yang, Yu-Shan Wang, Chao-Chun Chang, Su-Chen Huang, Yi-Chun Huang and Mau-Shin Chi
Department of Radiation Therapy and Oncology, Shin Kong Wu Ho-Su Memorial Hospital, Taipei, Taiwan

Kwan-Hwa Chi
Department of Radiation Therapy and Oncology, Shin Kong Wu Ho-Su Memorial Hospital, Taipei, Taiwan
Institute of Radiation Science and School of Medicine, National Yang-Ming University, Taipei, Taiwan

Lawrence S. Lamb Jr
Department of Medicine, University of Alabama at Birmingham, Birmingham, Alabama, United States of America

Department of Surgery, University of Alabama at Birmingham, Birmingham, Alabama, United States of America

Joscelyn Bowersock, Yun Su and Austin Johnson
Department of Medicine, University of Alabama at Birmingham, Birmingham, Alabama, United States of America

Anindya Dasgupta and H. Trent Spencer
Emory University School of Medicine, Department of Pediatrics, Aflac Cancer Center and Blood Disorders Service, Atlanta, Georgia, United States of America

G. Yancey Gillespie
Department of Surgery, University of Alabama at Birmingham, Birmingham, Alabama, United States of America

Daiqing Gao, Changyou Li, Xihe Xie, Peng Zhao, Xiaofang Wei and Weihong Sun
Biotherapy Center, Qingdao Center Hospital, The Second Affiliated Hospital, Qingdao University Medical College, Qingdao, China

Hsin-Chen Liu, Jian Jian Li and Aris T. Alexandrou
Department of Radiation Oncology, NCI-Designated Comprehensive Cancer Center, University of California at Davis Sacramento, Sacramento, California, United States of America

Jennifer Jones and Ronghua Zhao
Department of Medicine, University of Saskatchewan, Saskatoon, Canada

Sébastien Anguille, Evelien L. Smits and Zwi N. Berneman
University of Antwerp, Faculty of Medicine and Health Sciences, Vaccine and Infectious Disease Institute (VAXINFECTIO), Laboratory of Experimental Hematology, Antwerp, Belgium
Antwerp University Hospital, Center for Cell Therapy and Regenerative Medicine, Antwerp, Belgium

Eva Lion, Karen Couderé and Viggo F. Van Tendeloo
University of Antwerp, Faculty of Medicine and Health Sciences, Vaccine and Infectious Disease Institute (VAXINFECTIO), Laboratory of Experimental Hematology, Antwerp, Belgium

Jurjen Tel and I. Jolanda M de Vries
Radboud University Nijmegen Medical Centre and Nijmegen Centre for Molecular Life Sciences, Department of Tumor Immunology, Nijmegen, The Netherlands

Phillip D. Fromm
ANZAC Research Institute, Dendritic Cell Biology and Therapeutics Group, Sydney, Australia

Xiao-Yan Zhang, Jin-Long Liu, Duo Li, Jun-Li Li, Yi-Shan Liu, Min Wang, Bei-Lei Xu, Hai-Bo Wang and Zheng-Xu Wang
Biotherapy Center, the General Hospital of Beijing Military Command, Beijing, People's Republic of China

Jun-Xia Cao
Biotherapy Center, the General Hospital of Beijing Military Command, Beijing, People's Republic of China
Tsinghua-Peking Center for Life Sciences, Laboratory of Dynamic Immunobiology, School of Medicine, School of Life Sciences, Tsinghua University, Beijing, People's Republic of China

Min Wang, Jun-Xia Cao, Yi-Shan Liu, Bei-Lei Xu, Duo Li, Xiao-Yan Zhang, Jun-Li Li, Jin-Long Liu, Hai-Bo Wang and Zheng-Xu Wang
Biotherapy Center, General Hospital of Beijing Military Command, Beijing, China

Jian-Hong Pan
Department of Biostatistics, Peking University Clinical Research Institute, Peking University Health Science Center, Beijing, China

Peter S. Linsley, Cate Speake, Elizabeth Whalen and Damien Chaussabe
Department of Systems Immunology, Benaroya Research Institute, Seattle, WA, United States of America

Stephanie R. Jackson, Melissa Berrien-Elliott and Jinyun Yuan
Saint Louis University School of Medicine, Department of Molecular Microbiology and Immunology, St. Louis, Missouri, United States of America

Ryan M. Teague
Saint Louis University School of Medicine, Department of Molecular Microbiology and Immunology, St. Louis, Missouri, United States of America
Saint Louis University Cancer Center, St. Louis, Missouri, United States of America

Eddy C. Hsueh
Saint Louis University School of Medicine, Department of Surgery, St. Louis, Missouri, United States of America
Saint Louis University Cancer Center, St. Louis, Missouri, United States of America

Jeetendra Kumar, Rupali Gurav, Vaijayanti Kale and Lalita Limaye
Stem Cell Lab., National Centre for Cell Science, Ganeshkhind, Pune, India

Index